Provided as an educational service by Genentech

The content of this text represents the independent opinion of the authors and not necessarily that of Genentech. Healthcare Professionals should consult full prescribing information before prescribing the product.

Genentech

10281000

PEDIATRIC PRACTICE

Endocrinology

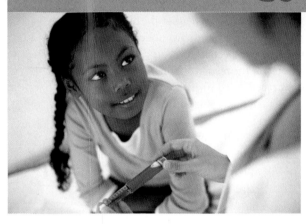

NOTICE

Medicine is an ever-changing science. As new research and clinical experience broaden our knowledge, changes in treatment and drug therapy are required. The authors and the publisher of this work have checked with sources believed to be reliable in their efforts to provide information that is complete and generally in accord with the standards accepted at the time of publication. However, in view of the possibility of human error or changes in medical sciences, neither the authors nor the publisher nor any other party who has been involved in the preparation or publication of this work warrants that the information contained herein is in every respect accurate or complete, and they disclaim all responsibility for any errors or omissions or for the results obtained from use of the information contained in this work. Readers are encouraged to confirm the information contained herein with other sources. For example and in particular, readers are advised to check the product information sheet included in the package of each drug they plan to administer to be certain that the information contained in this work is accurate and that changes have not been made in the recommended dose or in the contraindications for administration. This recommendation is of particular importance in connection with new or infrequently used drugs.

PEDIATRIC PRACTICE

Endocrinology

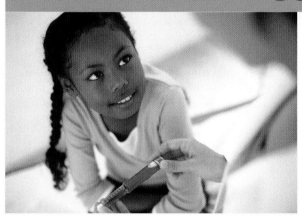

EDITORS

Michael S. Kappy, MD, PhD
Professor of Pediatrics
Section Head, Endocrinology
University of Colorado Health Sciences Center
Division of Endocrinology
The Children's Hospital
Denver, Colorado

David B. Allen, MD
Professor of Pediatrics
University of Wisconsin School of Medicine and Public Health
Head of Endocrinology
Director of Endocrinology and Diabetes Fellowship Training Program
UW American Family Children's Hospital
Madison, Wisconsin

Mitchell E. Geffner, MD
Professor of Pediatrics and Director of Fellowship Training
Division of Endocrinology, Diabetes, and Metabolism
Keck School of Medicine
University of Southern California
Division of Endocrinology and Metabolism
Children's Hospital Los Angeles
Los Angeles, California

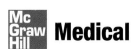
Medical

New York Chicago San Francisco Lisbon London Madrid Mexico City
Milan New Delhi San Juan Seoul Singapore Sydney Toronto

The McGraw·Hill Companies

Pediatric Practice: Endocrinology

1 2 3 4 5 6 7 8 9 0   CTP/CTP   12 11 10 9

ISBN 978-0-07-160591-5
MHID 0-07-160591-6

This book was set in Minion by International Typesetting and Composition.
The editors were Alyssa K. Fried and Robert Pancotti.
The production supervisor was Sherri Souffrance.
Project management was provided by Rajni Pisharody, International Typesetting and Composition.
The text designer was Janice Bielawa; the cover designer was David Dell'Accio.
China Translation & Printing Services, Ltd. was printer and binder.

This book is printed on acid-free paper.

Photo Credits:
Cover, main photograph and photograph of girl undergoing thyroid palpation: Credit: Tia Brayman, The Children's Hospital, Denver, Colorado.
Chapter 1 opener: Credit: GettyImages.
Chapter 2 opener: Credit: Michael S. Kappy, MD, PhD.
Chapter 3 opener: Credit: GettyImages.
Chapter 4 opener: Credit: Tia Brayman, The Children's Hospital, Denver, Colorado.
Chapter 5 opener: Credit: Photo Researchers, Inc.
Chapter 6 opener: Credit: GettyImages.
Chapter 7 opener: Credit: GettyImages.
Chapter 8 opener: Credit: GettyImages.
Chapter 9 opener: Credit: GettyImages.
Chapter 10 opener: Credit: Photo Researchers, Inc.
Chapter 11 opener: Credit: GettyImages.

Cataloging-in-Publication data for this title are on file at the Library of Congress.

McGraw-Hill books are available at special quantity discounts to use as premiums and sales promotions, or for use in corporate training programs. To contact a representative please e-mail us at bulksales@mcgraw-hill.com.

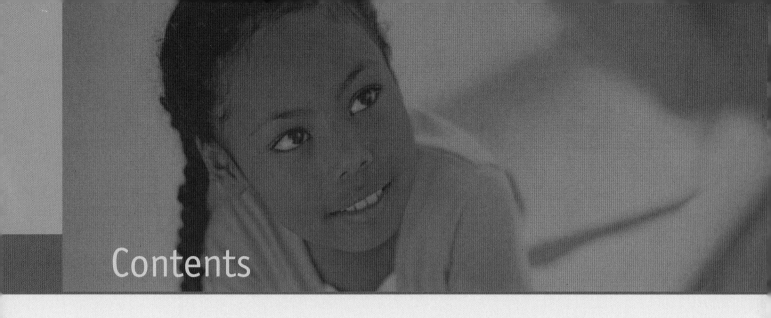

Contents

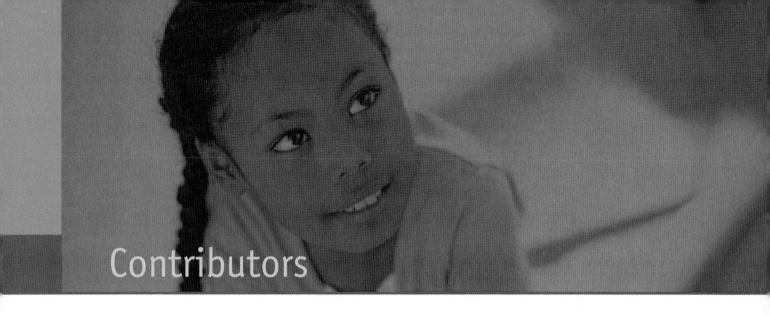

Contributors

David B. Allen, MD
Professor of Pediatrics
University of Wisconsin School of Medicine
  and Public Health
Head of Endocrinology
Director of Endocrinology and Diabetes Fellowship
  Training Program
UW American Family Children's Hospital
Madison, Wisconsin

Kathleen Bethin, MD, PhD
Division of Endocrinology and Diabetes
State University of New York at Buffalo
Women & Children's Hospital of Buffalo
Buffalo, New York

Bruce A. Boston, MD
Children's Diabetes Program
Doernbecher Children's Hospital
Oregon Health & Science University
Portland, Oregon

David W. Cooke, MD
Associate Professor of Pediatrics
Johns Hopkins University School of Medicine
Baltimore, Maryland

Paul Czernichow, MD
Head of Pediatric Endocrinology
Robert Debré Hospital
Paris, France

Dana Dabelea, MD, PhD
Associate Professor
Department of Epidemiology
University of Colorado Denver School of Medicine
Denver, Colorado

Patricia A. Donohoue, MD
Professor of Pediatrics
Chief, Section of Endocrinology and Diabetes
Medical College of Wisconsin
Milwaukee, Wisconsin

Robert J. Ferry, Jr., MD
Chief, Division of Pediatric Endocrinology
Department of Pediatrics
LeBonheur Children's Medical Center
University of Tennessee Health Science Center
St. Jude Children's Research Hospital
Memphis, Tennessee

Sherry L. Franklin, MD
Pediatric Endocrinology of San Diego Medical Group, Inc.
Rady Children's Hospital of San Diego
Assistant Clinical Professor
University of California
San Diego, California

John S. Fuqua, MD
Section of Pediatric Endocrinology and Diabetology
Indiana University School of Medicine
Indianapolis, Indiana

Lisa Gallo, MD
Fellow in Pediatric Endocrinology
University of Florida
Gainesville, Florida

Mitchell E. Geffner, MD
Professor of Pediatrics and Director of Fellowship
  Training
Division of Endocrinology, Diabetes, and Metabolism
Keck School of Medicine
University of Southern California
Division of Endocrinology and Metabolism
Children's Hospital Los Angeles
Los Angeles, California

Christopher P. Houk, MD
Division Chief of Pediatric Endocrinology
Associate Professor of Pediatrics
Medical College of Georgia
Augusta, Georgia

Stephen A. Huang, MD
Department of Endocrinology
Children's Hospital Boston
Boston, Massachusetts

Michael S. Kappy, MD, PhD
Professor of Pediatrics
Section Head, Endocrinology
University of Colorado Health Sciences Center
Division of Endocrinology
The Children's Hospital
Denver, Colorado

Andrea Kelly, MD
Attending Physician
Division of Endocrinology and Diabetes
Department of Pediatrics
The Children's Hospital of Philadelphia
University of Pennsylvania School of Medicine
Philadelphia, Pennsylvania

Georgeanna J. Klingensmith, MD
Professor
Department of Pediatrics
University of Colorado Denver School of Medicine
Director of Pediatric Clinics
Barbara Davis Center for Childhood Diabetes
The Children's Hospital
Denver, Colorado

Peter A. Lee, MD
Division of Pediatric Endocrinology
Pennsylvania State University College
  of Medicine
Milton S. Hershey Medical Center
Hershey, Pennsylvania

Michael A. Levine, MD
Division of Endocrinology and Diabetes
Department of Pediatrics
The Children's Hospital of Philadelphia
University of Pennsylvania School of Medicine
Philadelphia, Pennsylvania

Lisa D. Madison, MD
Department of Pediatrics
Doernbecher Children's Hospital
Oregon Health & Science University
Portland, Oregon

Joseph A. Majzoub, MD
Chief, Division of Endocrinology
Thomas Morgan Rotch Professor of Pediatrics
Harvard Medical School
Division of Endocrinology
Children's Hospital Boston
Boston, Massachusetts

Jon M. Nakamoto, MD, PhD
Managing Director
Quest Diagnostics Nichols Institute
San Juan Capistrano, California

Lindsey E. Nicol, MD
Fellow, Pediatric Endocrinology
Department of Pediatrics
University of Wisconsin School of Medicine
  and Public Health
Madison, Wisconsin

Leslie Plotnick, MD
Professor
Department of Pediatric Endocrinology
Johns Hopkins University School of Medicine
Baltimore, Maryland

Alan D. Rogol, MD, PhD
Professor
Division of Pediatric Endocrinology and Diabetes
Department of Pediatrics
University of Virginia Health System
Charlottesville, Virginia

Janet H. Silverstein, MD
Division of Endocrinology
Department of Pediatrics
University of Florida College of Medicine
Children's Medical Services Center
Gainesville, Florida

Abhinash Srivatsa, MD
Division of Endocrinology
Children's Hospital Boston
Instructor in Pediatrics
Harvard Medical School
Boston, Massachusetts

William Winter, MD
Professor
Departments of Pathology and Pediatrics
  (Division of Endocrinology)
University of Florida
Gainesville, Florida

Selma F. Witchel, MD
Division of Endocrinology
University of Pittsburgh Medical Center
Director, Pediatric Endocrinology
Fellowship Training Program
Children's Hospital of Pittsburgh
Pittsburgh, Pennsylvania

Philip Zeitler, MD, PhD
Division of Pediatric Endocrinology
University of Colorado Health Sciences Center
The Children's Hospital
Denver, Colorado

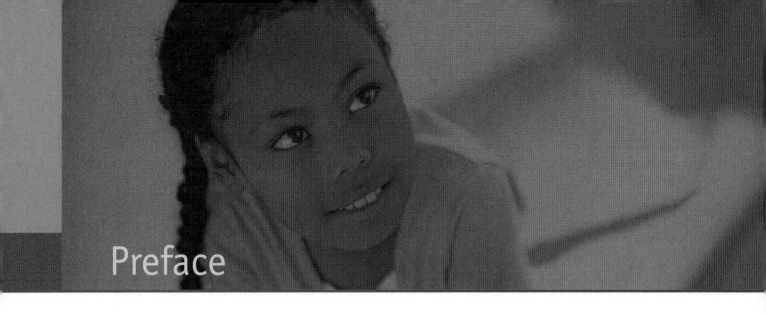

Preface

Of the many attractive qualities of pediatric endocrinology, two in particular—its diversity of disorders and its intrinsically pediatric focus on growth and physical development—amplify the importance of practical knowledge of this specialty for the primary care provider. In the past, apart from type 1 diabetes, endocrine problems in clinical practice were relatively rare; they required a pediatric health care expert to differentiate their distinguishing features from the breadth of normal variations in ruling such disorders *out* much more often than *in*. During the past 20 years, however, as the incidence of type 1 diabetes mellitus has increased, other diseases that were virtually unseen in children—obesity-associated insulin resistance, type 2 diabetes mellitus, and ovarian androgen excess—have emerged as common occurrences in pediatric primary care. Ethnic demographic changes, growth and puberty acceleration due to excess nutrition, and other factors have reduced the mean age of appearance of first puberty signs so that normal variations must now be distinguished more frequently from pathologic causes of precocious puberty. The expanded availability and variety of (often controversial) growth-promoting and puberty-altering treatments have created therapeutic options for a broadening spectrum of children, for whom critical evaluation of benefit, cost, and risk is required. Further, in most states of the United States, every new baby is now screened for congenital adrenal hyperplasia as well as for congenital hypothyroidism. Because of these changes among others, the primary child health care provider ponders possible endocrine diagnoses or therapeutics virtually every day.

With these thoughts in mind, the editors set out to create a pediatric endocrinology text that, first and foremost, would be an outstanding clinical analysis and decision-making resource. Since an understanding of the clinical manifestations and treatments of endocrine disorders begins with knowledge of concepts of hormone action and principles of feedback control, the first chapter, "General Concepts and Physiology," links genetics, cell biology, and physiology with pathophysiology to provide a clear and approachable overview of endocrine systems. Subsequent chapters are traditional in title—disorders of growth, water homeostasis, thyroid and adrenal glands, calcium and bone metabolism, puberty, sex differentiation, and carbohydrate metabolism—but innovative in organization and emphasis. Problem-oriented rather than diagnosis-oriented frameworks are emphasized so as to capture conceptual and practical approaches to clinical dilemmas of current general practice. Integration of pathophysiology with clinical management is emphasized, with extensive use of figures to illustrate principles of normal and abnormal physiology and treatment rationale and effects. Attention is paid to guiding readers in "how to think about" the evaluation of clinical problems and "when to refer" complex or worrisome patients. Through this approach, the editors' objective is to achieve a subspecialty text that, true to its inclusion in the "Pediatric Practice" series, is distinguished not only by its effective description of state-of-the-art science, but by its clinical utility as well.

It is our added hope that this text is an equally valuable education resource for pediatric endocrinology. Talented educators have a gift for making complex phenomena understandable, a gift that cannot be displaced by the unlimited and instant access to information now provided by web-based journals and databases. The task placed before our group of internationally recognized senior authors was daunting: concisely yet comprehensively review current knowledge, link these concepts with analysis of clinical situations suggesting endocrine system problems, and provide practical recommendations for rational and efficient evaluation and treatment of children with endocrine disorders. The skill with which they accomplished this synthesis is a testament to their far-reaching experience and thoughtful analysis and makes these chapters exceptional examples for young subspecialists developing their own conceptual approaches, and to all pediatric endocrinologists engaged in teaching others. It is the editors' hope that well-worn covers with many dog-eared pages will signify that this book has adeptly filled an important niche.

The editors wish to thank Alyssa Fried of McGraw-Hill for her expert assistance and firm yet always friendly prodding to remain on task and on time.

Michael S. Kappy, MD, PhD
David B. Allen, MD
Mitchell E. Geffner, MD

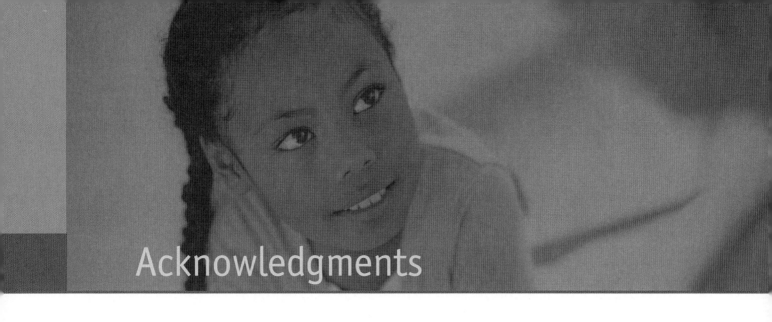

Acknowledgments

Once again, we get to acknowledge those family members, friends, and colleagues whose influence in our lives is inestimable. I would like to begin by expressing my gratitude for the support given to me over many years by my parents, Jack and Lil; my wife, Peggy; my sons, Doug and Greg; my granddaughters, Samantha and Summer; my brother, David; and my sister, Ellen. Other family members to thank are my brothers-in-law, Joe Suckiel and Jay Markson, and the entire Markson family. I am particularly saddened by the recent loss of my great-cousin, Ralph Kaplowitz, a member of the first NBA Championship team—the 1946-47 Philadelphia Warriors—and a good friend.

Of the many wonderful colleagues with whom I have worked for 50 years, I particularly thank the following for guidance and support at various times in my life: Lennie Licara, Saul Chavkin, Yvonne Brackbill, Kenneth Monty, Harry Harlow, Harry Waisman, Robert Metzenberg, Willam Middleton, Henry Kempe, Henry Silver, Vince Fulginiti, Grant Morrow, Claude Migeon, Bob Blizzard, Harold and Helen Harrison, and Elmer "Whitey" Lightner. A special thanks to Jules Amer, Irwin Redlener, Lew Barness, and Enid Gilbert-Barness for their guidance and friendship.

It goes without saying that this book and our previous one, "Principles and Practice of Pediatric Endocrinology," would not have been possible without the incredibly valuable collaboration and support given freely by Dave Allen and Mitch Geffner. There are many other colleagues and friends whom I would like to acknowledge, but space limitations do exist. To all of you, you know who you are, thank you.

Michael S. Kappy, MD, PhD

The work of this book has stimulated much positive personal and professional reflection—on the complexity, advancement, and expansion of our field of pediatric endocrinology, on the insights of countless brilliant contributors to this progress, on the joy and privilege of caring for children, and on the satisfaction of collaborating with such wonderful and talented colleagues: Michael Kappy, Mitch Geffner, and our contributing authors.

For inspiration, I am most indebted to my father, Rich Allen, a dedicated pediatrician in the truest and most profound sense of the word. In spite of my efforts to take a different path, the example he provided in caring for children brought me back to medicine, and then to pediatrics. For whatever perspective and humility I do have, I give thanks to my mother, Joyce, the most centered and loving individual I have ever known. And for everything else, I thank my wife, Sally, who has unselfishly and constantly supported and encouraged me for over 35 years; and my children, Brittany, Doug, and Nick, who provide immeasurable love and joy and the motivation always to do my best.

Professionally, I first acknowledge the generous spirit of Dr. Robert Blizzard for his invaluable advice and support early in my career. I also thank Ann Johanson, Ron Rosenfeld, Ed Reiter, Alan Rogol, Barbara Lippe, Margaret MacGillivray, and Ken Copeland, who have inspired and encouraged me to seek academic and leadership challenges. I am indebted to my University of Wisconsin mentors and colleagues Norm Fost and Aaron Friedman, who instilled in me a love for critical thinking and the importance of challenging conventional wisdom. And finally, a sincere thank you to my UW Endocrine Division co-workers—Michael MacDonald, Ellen Connor, Aaron Carrel, and Tracy Bekx—who make work in the real world so much fun, and without whose patience and support I could not have pursued so many opportunities.

Twenty-five years ago, the specialty of pediatric endocrinology captivated my interest because of its elegance, diversity, mystery, and intrinsically pediatric focus on the changes of childhood and adolescence. My hope for this book is that it both captures and conveys these qualities for the reader.

David B. Allen, MD

xii ■ *Acknowledgments*

I have once again had a professional thrill ride working with my close friends, Mike Kappy and Dave Allen, on our second endeavor into the world of textbook writing. Their endless knowledge, work ethic, and unyielding camaraderie are unmatched.

For the second time, I can see that editing and language are key essentials to the art of creating a textbook, talents for which my father (high school chemistry teacher and review book writer) and mother (high school French teacher) must be commended for providing the impetus (and genetics).

In my preface in our previous book, I acknowledged the many mentors, colleagues, and trainees who had inspired me to that point. That list is still true to this day, but I would like to expand it to make up for one inadvertent omission, Alan Morris, former fellow and longstanding friend, and to acknowledge my most recent fellow graduates: Josh May, Lily Chao, Christine Burt Solorzano, Avni Shah, and Nina Ma. I also can't say enough about Rob Rapaport, who is such a superb physician, scientist, and, most importantly, friend.

I must also pay special tribute to three people from my prior list who, tragically, met untimely deaths and who had major impacts in my professional life: Dave Golde, Joao Antunes, and Alan Herschenfeld.

But not to dwell on the obvious, I would never have had the opportunity to write this book or to have had any professional success were it not for the unwavering support of my family. My wife, Andrea, has been my rock and my children, Jenny and Eric, have always been there for me. I also want to acknowledge my soon-to-be daughter-in-law, Ashley King. I am so fortunate to have them all in my life.

Mitchell E. Geffner, MD

CHAPTER 1

General Concepts and Physiology

Kathleen Bethin and John S. Fuqua

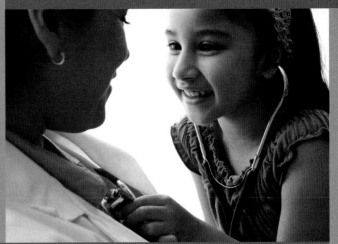

INTRODUCTION

There are broad principles and concepts in endocrinology that the reader must understand. Familiarity with concepts such as negative feedback loops, hormone-receptor function, and hormone replacement therapy allows the physician to generalize what is learned in one area and apply it to others. This gives the ability to predict the effects of an endocrine abnormality or perturbation on downstream hormones and its subsequent clinical effects. Conversely, it also allows the clinician to consider a set of symptoms, work backward to develop a differential diagnosis, and test this by looking for laboratory abnormalities that are diagnostic for an endocrine disease. This chapter will review many of these basic principles that are applicable across the field in order to provide groundwork for later chapters. Following a discussion of general hormone function and integration of endocrine systems, we will discuss the classification of hormones. Reviews of hormone synthesis, processing, and transport follow, and then we will outline the regulation of hormone secretion. Following this, we will examine the evolving field of hormone receptors and discuss nontraditional endocrine systems. The clinical relevance of the preceding material is apparent in the section covering principles of endocrine disease. Finally, we will summarize important principles in endocrine testing.

HORMONE FUNCTION

The endocrine system consists of a dizzying number of hormones, and newly discovered ones are added to the list on a regular basis. The word "hormone" comes from the Greek word "ormaein" meaning to set in motion or to spur on. This is an apt derivation, because hormones are chemicals secreted by one tissue that produce effects in distant tissues, leading to an array of physiological responses. In children, we can categorize hormones by the systems they affect, including growth, reproduction, homeostasis, and energy regulation. Many hormones play roles in multiple categories, emphasizing the complex network of interactions and the redundancy built into these processes. Table 1-1 shows how selected endocrine systems fit into this categorization, illustrating this redundancy

Growth

Growth is an exceedingly complex process that is unique to pediatric medicine. When considering the endocrine control of growth, many think first of growth hormone (GH), but growth involves many other hormones as well. For example, thyroid hormone and sex steroids are permissive for growth hormone secretion, and in the presence of hypothyroidism or hypogonadism, growth hormone is not secreted normally. Growth hormone itself is critical for the secretion of insulin-like growth factor-1 (IGF-1), a hormone that is responsible for many of the effects of GH on linear growth and other metabolic processes, both in fetal life and in childhood and beyond. Before birth, growth hormone's effects are less noticeable, and insulin serves an active role in promoting fetal growth. Insulin-like growth factor-2 (IGF-2), which is not under the regulation of GH, is also an important endocrine mediator of fetal growth. Each of the above hormones have their own sets of regulatory hormones and factors, such as growth-hormone-releasing hormone (GHRH) and somatostatin for GH and thyrotropin-releasing hormone (TRH) and thyroid-stimulating hormone (TSH) for thyroid hormone.

Table 1-1.

Classes of Hormone Function with Selected Examples of Endocrine Systems

Hormone Function	Regulatory Hormones	Effector Hormones
Growth	GHRH	GH
	Somatostatin	IGF-1
	TRH	T_4
	TSH	T_3
	LH	Estradiol
	FSH	Testosterone
		Insulin
Reproduction	GnRH	Estradiol
	LH	Testosterone
	FSH	MIS
		Prolactin
Homeostasis	TRH	T_4
	TSH	T_3
	CRH	
	ACTH	Cortisol
	GnRH	
	LH	Estradiol
	FSH	Testosterone
		ADH
		Renin
		Angiotensin
		Aldosterone
		PTH
		Vitamin D
		Insulin
		Epinephrine
		Leptin
Energy Balance	TRH	T_4
	TSH	T_3
	GHRH	GH
	Somatostatin	IGF-1
	CRH	Cortisol
	ACTH	
		Leptin
		Glucagon
		Insulin

ACTH, adrenocorticotrophic hormone; ADH, antidiuretic hormone; CRH, corticotrophin-releasing hormone; FSH, follicle-stimulating hormone; GH, growth hormone; GHRH, GH -releasing hormone; GnRH, gonadotropin-releasing hormone; IGF-1, insulin-like growth factor-1; LH, luteinizing hormone; MIS, Mullerian-inhibiting hormone; PTH, parathyroid hormone; T_3, triiodothyronine; T_4, L-thyroxine; TRH, thyrotropin-releasing hormone; TSH, thyroid -stimulating hormone

Deficiencies of the regulatory hormones have much the same effects on growth as deficiencies of the primary hormones. Some hormones also play less direct roles, primarily promoting processes important for homeostasis, but without which growth cannot proceed. Examples of these include the hormones required for normal calcium and bone mineralization such as parathyroid hormone (PTH), 25-hydroxy- and 1,25-dihydroxyvitamin D, and

fibroblast growth factor-23 (FGF-23). Hormones, particularly estrogens, also actively mediate the physiologic cessation of growth during adolescence, as indicated by the failure of growth plate fusion in an individual with an estrogen receptor mutation and in those patients carrying mutations in the gene for the aromatase enzyme, critical for the synthesis of estrogen.[1,2]

Reproduction

Reproduction is an essential function of every species, and the endocrine system plays critical roles in both the reproductive process itself and in the anatomic and physiological development essential for reproduction to occur in both males and females. Developmental defects of the internal and external genitalia and errors of puberty are also unique to pediatric endocrinology and comprise a significant percentage of patients seen in clinical practice. In the area of reproduction, as in other endocrine systems, there is a large degree of cross talk between different hormones and their receptors. Beginning with sexual differentiation, a coordinated network of genetic events results in the synthesis and secretion of testosterone and Müllerian inhibiting substance (MIS) that, interacting with their specific receptors, initiate the differentiation of nonspecific or bi-potential reproductive structures into either typical male or female features. Participating in this process are regulatory hormones such as chorionic gonadotropin, luteinizing hormone (LH), follicle-stimulating hormone (FSH), and inhibins.

The reproductive system is typically quiescent during the mid-childhood years, but at the time of puberty, gonadal activity restarts in both males and females under regulatory mechanisms involving the central nervous system as well as the gonadotropins LH and FSH. While MIS appears to be less critical for normal gonadal function in postnatal life, other gonadal factors such as the inhibins remain important. In the male, testosterone secretion during puberty causes various secondary sex characteristics such as muscularity, body hair, and voice deepening, and estrogen secretion in females causes breast development and the establishment of a female body habitus. In the case of the reproductive system then, across the life of a developing child a given hormone may have very different effects, depending on the physiological and developmental state of the individual, be it fetus or adolescent.

Although regulatory mechanisms are generally fixed, the reproductive system features one of the few feedback loops that changes. While gonadotropin secretion in sexually mature females causes ovarian estrogen secretion that leads to suppression of gonadotropin production by negative feedback, at the midpoint of the menstrual cycle this changes to a positive feedback system and results in the LH surge that causes ovulation.

Homeostasis

Homeostasis refers to the maintenance of the metabolic milieu of the individual at steady state, and this is arguably the most important function of endocrine systems in general. Homeostasis is not a single process; it consists of many very different aspects. Hormones tightly regulate diverse physiological features such as maintenance of normal serum osmolality, normal bone mineral content, normoglycemia, metabolic rate, and many others.

Osmoreceptors in the vasculature in part control the release of vasopressin (antidiuretic hormone [ADH]) from the posterior pituitary gland, which subsequently controls free water excretion and regulates water balance and serum osmolality. The renin-angiotensin-aldosterone system provides separate but overlapping regulation of sodium and potassium balance.

PTH and 1,25-dihydroxyvitamin D, the activated form of vitamin D, maintain bone mineral content, serum calcium, and phosphorus concentrations at a steady state. Other endocrine factors directly influencing this system include FGF-23, PTH-related protein (PTHrP), and calcitonin.

Glucose availability is critical for energy homeostasis, and a far-reaching system of apparently unconnected hormones (see the "Glucose Control" section later in the chapter) controls serum glucose levels. Basal metabolic rate, defined as the rate of oxygen consumption at rest, is partially under the influence of thyroid hormones, including the regulatory hormones TRH and TSH and the effector hormones L-thyroxine (T_4) and its activated or active form, triiodothyronine (T_3). It is T_3 that binds to the intracellular thyroid hormone receptor to alter the transcription of genes controlling metabolic rate.

Energy Production

Endocrine regulation is essential for handling of the body's energy needs, including the immediate use and storage of nutrients such as glucose, proteins, and lipids. Insulin permits the uptake of glucose into muscle cells where it is converted to energy in the form of adenosine triphosphate (ATP). At the same time, insulin suppresses the oxidation of fatty acids and promotes energy storage. Deficiency of insulin, as is seen in type 1 diabetes, leads to hyperglycemia, with lack of normal glucose utilization, as well as excessive lipolysis, fatty acid oxidation, and protein breakdown, resulting in the polyuria, polydipsia, weight loss, and ketoacidosis seen in untreated diabetes. Other hormones also influence energy storage and delivery, including cortisol and growth hormone. A complex neuroendocrine system controls food intake with remarkably fine regulation of body weight over years using leptin as the primary adipocyte-derived endocrine hormone leading to satiety.[3]

INTEGRATION OF HORMONE SYSTEMS

As seen from the above discussion, endocrine control of physiologic processes often features a rich interweaving of hormone systems, with a great deal of redundancy. Table 1-1 and Figure 1-1 illustrate this overlap, with several of the hormone systems, such as the growth and thyroid axes, being involved in more than one aspect of endocrine function. Such integration of multiple hormone systems in the regulation of a body process increases the robustness and stability of the system and

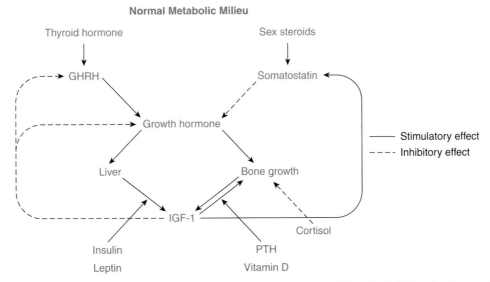

FIGURE 1-1 ■ There are many different endocrine influences in the process of growth, including the GH/IGF-1, thyroid, adrenal, insulin, and PTH/vitamin D axes, illustrating the integration of many systems in the regulation of complex physiologic processes.

allows for smoother and finer regulation. Two examples of this hormone integration are growth and the regulation of serum glucose levels.

Growth

Human growth involves not only the classic growth hormone axis, consisting of the hypothalamic regulatory hormones GHRH and somatostatin, GH itself, IGF-1, and various binding hormones, carrier proteins, and receptors, but also an array of other axes[4] (Figure 1-1). Thyroid hormone is essential for normal GH secretion and efficacy. During adolescence, the hypothalamic-pituitary-gonadal axis is also essential for normal growth. Delivery of adequate amounts of glucose, amino acids, and lipids to cells is clearly necessary for normal metabolism, and insulin, cortisol, and leptin are required for this to occur. Bone metabolism also needs to flourish for proper skeletal development, and this requires multiple steps of endocrine input, including PTH and vitamin D metabolites as well as input from GH and IGF-1. All of this must occur on a background of normal electrolyte balance and normal serum osmolality.

Glucose Control

Plasma glucose concentration is finely regulated within a relatively narrow range, and this also occurs through a complex interaction of numerous endocrine processes. Insulin provides the primary regulation within the normal physiologic range. If a large influx of glucose occurs, putting upward pressure on glucose concentration, insulin secretion also increases, promoting entry of glucose into muscle cells, glycogen synthesis, and lipogenesis. Serum glucose levels declining into the hypoglycemic range, however, suppress insulin secretion, leading to lipolysis and fatty acid oxidation which provide additional substrate for energy. Hypoglycemia also activates counter-regulatory hormone secretion. These counter-regulatory hormones consist of GH, epinephrine, glucagon, and cortisol, and cause increased hepatic glycogen breakdown and gluconeogenesis. Proteolysis releases amino acids for use in gluconeogenesis, again providing for system redundancy.

HORMONE TYPES

The signal transduction pathways of the endocrine system are very elaborate.[5] However, the processes are actually based on a simple concept. Hormone binding to its receptor causes a conformational change of the receptor, which transmits a signal that initiates the physiological response. The specificity of the receptor for its hormone, the specific cell type, and the specific signaling system in the cell all contribute to the specific response that is seen. There are three major classifications of hormones based

Table 1-2.

Classification of Some Known Hormones

Peptide Hormones	Steroid Hormones	Amine Hormones
GHRH	Cortisol	Epinephrine
Somatostatin	Estradiol	Norepinephrine
GH	Testosterone	Dopamine
IGF-1	25-hydroxyvitamin D	T_4
TRH	1,25-dihydroxyvitamin D	T_3
TSH		
GnRH		
LH		
FSH		
hCG		
MIS		
Prolactin		
Insulin		
ACTH		
CRH		
MSH		
PTH		
PTHrP		
ADH		

ACTH, adrenocorticotrophic hormone; ADH, antidiuretic hormone; CRH, corticotrophin releasing hormone; FSH, follicle stimulating hormone; GH, growth hormone; GHRH, G H-releasing hormone; hCG, human chorionic gonadotropin; IGF-1, insulin-like growth factor-1; LH, luteinizing hormone; MIS, Mullerian-inhibiting hormone; MSH, melanocyte-stimulating hormone; PTH, parathyroid hormone; PTHrP, PTH-related peptide ; T_3, triiodothyronine; T_4, L-thyroxine; TRH, thyrotropin-releasing hormone; TSH, thyroid-stimulating hormone

on chemical structure: proteins or peptides, steroids, and amines (Table 1-2). The structure of the hormone determines both the location of the hormone receptor (membrane or nuclear) and the half-life of the hormone in circulation. Since peptide hormones are water soluble, peptide hormones bind to membrane receptors. Most amine hormones also bind membrane receptors, except for thyroid hormone, which binds nuclear receptors. Steroid hormones also bind nuclear receptors. Thyroid hormones have the longest half-life, which is measured in days, but other amine hormones have the shortest half-life of only a few minutes. Peptide and steroid hormones fall in the middle, with half-lives ranging from a few minutes to several hours. Hormones that circulate in low concentrations rapidly associate and dissociate from the receptor, such that receptor occupancy is a function of both hormone concentration and receptor affinity.

Peptide

The majority of hormones are peptide hormones.[5] Peptide hormones vary greatly in size from as small as three peptides to large multi-subunit glycoproteins. Examples of peptide hormones are listed in Tables 1-2 and 1-3.

Table 1-3.

Membrane Receptor Families and Signaling Pathways

Receptors	Effectors	Signaling Pathways
G protein–coupled-seven transmembrane (GPCR)		
β-Adrenergic	$G_s\alpha$, adenylate cyclase	Stimulation of cyclic AMP
LH, FSH, TSH	Ca^{2+} channels	production, protein kinase A
Glucagon		
PTH, PTHrP		Calmodulin, Ca^{2+}-dependent kinases
ACTH, MSH		
GHRH, CRH		
α-Adrenergic	$G_i\alpha$	Inhibition of cyclic AMP production
Somatostatin		Activation of K^+, Ca^{2+} channels
TRH, GnRH	G_q, G_{11}	Phospholipase C, diacylglycerol-IP$_3$, protein kinase C, voltage-dependent Ca^{2+} channels
Receptor tyrosine kinase		
Insulin, JGF-1	Tyrosine kinases, IRS-1 to IRS-4	MAP kinases, PI 3-kinase, RSK
EGF, NGF	Tyrosine kinases, ras	Raf, MAP kinases, RSK
Cytokine receptor-linked kinase		
GH, PRL	JAK, tyrosine kinases	STAT, MAP kinase, PI 3-kinase, IRS-1, IRS-2
Serine kinase		
Activin, TGF-β, MIS	Serine kinase	Smads

IP$_3$, inostol triphosphate; IRS, insulin receptor substrates; MAP, mitogen-activated protein; MSH, metanocyte-stimulating hormone, NGF, nerve growth factor, PI, phosphatidylinostol, RSK, ribosconal S6 kinase; TGF-β, transforming growth factor β. For all other abbreviations, see text.
Reproduced from Jameson JL. Principles of endocrinology. In: Jameson JL, ed. Harrison's Endocrinology. New York, NY: McGraw-Hill; 2006:1-15.

Since peptide hormones are not fat soluble, they do not easily cross the cell membrane and thus bind membrane receptors. When protein hormones bind their receptors, there is an immediate induction of the intracellular signaling pathway associated with that particular receptor. Depending on the specific receptor, the signaling cascades may activate or inhibit cAMP production, activate calcium or potassium channels, or regulate other proteins by phosphorylation. The signaling pathways for many membrane receptors are depicted in Figure 1-2.

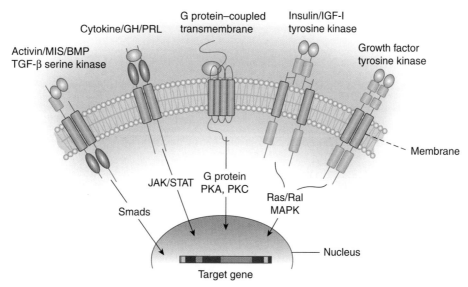

FIGURE 1-2 ■ Membrane receptor signaling. MAPK, mitogen-activated protein kinase; PKA, -C, protein kinase A, C; TGF, transforming growth factor. For other abbreviations, see text. (*From Jameson JL. Principles of endocrinology. In: Jameson JL, ed.* Harrison's Endocrinology. *New York, NY: McGraw-Hill; 2006:1-15.*)

The membrane receptor families and their associated signaling pathways are shown in Table 1-3.

The glycoproteins are structurally the most complex group of peptide hormones.[6] The carbohydrate moiety constitutes 15% to 35% of the hormone by weight. These hormones include: LH, FSH, TSH, and human chorionic gonadotropin (hCG). Glycoprotein hormones are composed of 2 subunits joined by noncovalent forces. They share a common α subunit and a hormone-specific β subunit. Although the β subunits are unique, they are homologous, with the β subunits of hCG and LH sharing the most homology. In order for hormones to affect the target organ, they must bind and activate their specific receptors. In the physiological state, hormones bind only their specific receptor. However, in the case of hormone excess, a hormone may bind to its receptor as well as closely related receptors. This is demonstrated by the use of synthetic hCG by endocrinologists to stimulate the LH receptor during testing of testicular function in prepubertal boys.[7] This also may be demonstrated in cases of severe hypothyroidism. At very high TSH levels may bind to the FSH receptor, activating the gonads, causing testicular enlargement in boys and ovarian stimulation in girls (van Wyk-Grumbach syndrome).[8] The receptors for the glycoprotein hormones are G protein–coupled receptors (GPCRs) that activate the adenylate cyclase and inositol triphosphate diacylglycerol pathways.[5,9]

Steroid

Steroid hormones are derived from cholesterol (Figure 1-3).[5] Steroid hormones include estrogen, testosterone, cortisol, vitamin D, and retinoids. Because of their lipophilic nature, steroid hormones readily cross the cell membrane and bind nuclear receptors. Once hormone is bound to its nuclear receptor, the receptor binds the DNA response element, usually as a dimer. Steroid hormone binding to its receptor results in activation or repression of gene transcription (Figure 1-4). Thus, the effects of steroid hormones are delayed compared to peptide hormones. However, since gene transcription is altered, the effect of steroid hormones is sustained.

Amines

Amine hormones are derived from the amino acid tyrosine.[9] This class includes dopamine, catecholamines, and thyroid hormone. Like the peptide hormones, the amine hormones usually bind membrane receptors. Thyroid hormone, however, binds nuclear receptors. Similar to steroid hormones, it takes longer to see the effects of increases in thyroid hormone, but the effects are sustained. Epinephrine, norepinephrine, and dopamine induce rapid- and short-lived changes, even more rapidly than seen with the peptide hormones.

HORMONE PRECURSORS AND PROCESSING

There are numerous steps involved in the production of the active hormone. Some hormones are directly synthesized in the active form and others require further processing to the active hormone, or more active form.

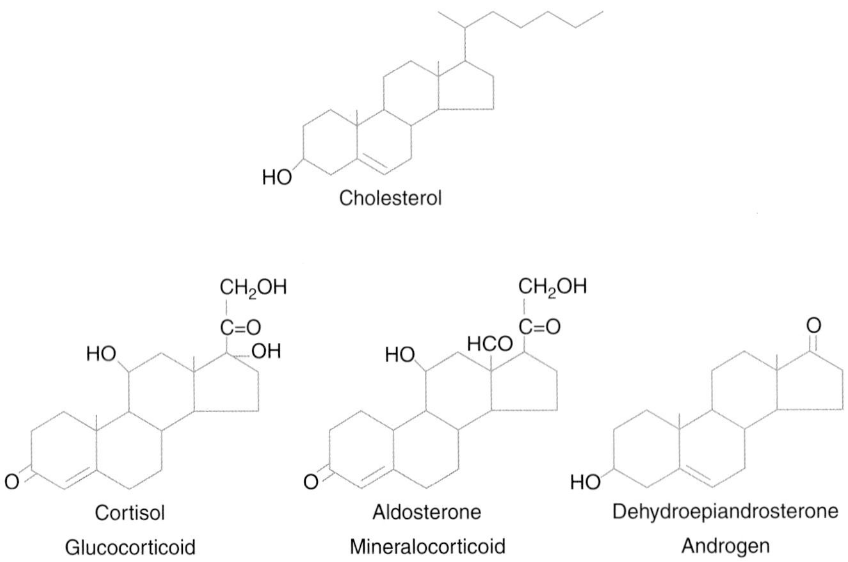

FIGURE 1-3 ■ Hormones of the adrenal cortex. The principal hormones synthesized and released by the adrenal cortex are the glucocorticoid (cortisol), the mineralocorticoid (aldosterone), and the androgen (dehydroepiandrosterone). These steroid hormones are derived from cholesterol. (*From Molina PE. Adrenal gland. In: Molina PE. Endocrine Physiology. 2nd ed. New York, NY: McGraw-Hill; 2006:123-156*)

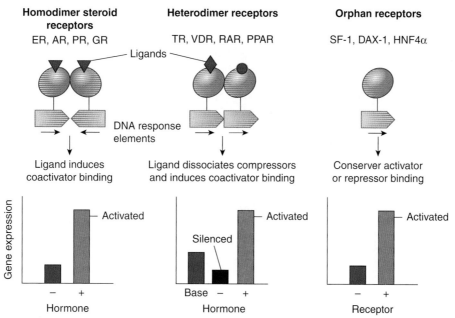

FIGURE 1-4 ■ Nuclear receptor signaling. ER, estrogen receptor; AR, androgen receptor; PR, progesterone receptor; GR, glucocorticoid receptor; TR, thyroid hormone receptor; VDR, vitamin D receptor; RAR, retinoic acid receptor; PPAR, peroxisome proliferator activated receptor; SF-1, steroidogenic factor-1; DAX, *dosage sensitive sex-reversal, adrenal hypoplasia congenita, X-chromosome;* HNF4α, hepatic nuclear factor 4α. *(From Jameson JL. Principles of endocrinology.* In: Jameson JL, ed. Harrison's Endocrinology. *New York, NY: McGraw-Hill; 2006:1-15.)*

Hormone Synthesis

No matter which class a hormone belongs to, the rate-limiting step in hormone activation is usually the synthesis of the hormone.

Protein/peptide hormones

The synthesis of peptide hormones is dependent on classical gene expression.[5] The gene for a peptide hormone is transcribed into mRNA which is then translated into a protein. The protein is further modified by posttranslational processing. Synthesis of peptide hormones is regulated by DNA regulatory elements found on many genes. However, the peptide hormone genes also contain specific hormone response elements, resulting in very precise control of synthesis. This is exemplified by direct repression of TSH synthesis by binding of thyroid hormone to a thyroid hormone response element on the TSH gene. Peptide hormones are synthesized in the endoplasmic reticulum and then transferred to the Golgi apparatus, where they are packaged into secretory granules (Figure 1-5). Mature secretory granules sit immediately beneath the plasma membrane. Typically, the signal for granule release causes a change in intracellular calcium, resulting in fusion of the granule to the plasma membrane and, finally, release of its contents.

Steroid hormones

Steroid hormones are derived from cholesterol.[10] The first and rate-limiting step in hormone synthesis is the cleavage of cholesterol to pregnenolone in the inner mitochondrial membrane by the enzyme CYP11A1 (cholesterol side-chain cleavage). The hormone precursors are shuttled back and forth between the endoplasmic reticulum and the mitochondria until the final product is produced. The basic steroid backbone is depicted in Figure 1-3. There is very little storage of steroid hormones, with the finished product usually diffusing into circulation after synthesis.

Amines

The amine hormones are derived from tyrosine.[9] Thyroid hormone synthesis is critically dependent on iodine ingestion.[11] Thyroglobulin is a large glycoprotein that contains multiple tyrosine residues. It is synthesized in thyroid follicular epithelial cells. Thyroglobulin is secreted into the follicular lumen where it undergoes posttranslational modification. TSH binding to its receptor on the basolateral membrane of thyroid follicular epithelial cells results in stimulation of the enzymatic steps involved in thyroid hormone synthesis, thyroid hormone release, and growth of the thyroid gland.[11] In hypothyroidism, the high levels of TSH stimulate thyroid growth, resulting in a goiter. In hyperthyroidism, stimulation of the TSH receptor by the thyroid antibodies results in thyroid growth and development of a goiter. The thyroid hormones, T_4 and T_3, are both secreted from the thyroid gland. However, T_4 is produced in far excess compared to T_3.

Catecholamines are synthesized from tyrosine in the adrenal medulla.[10] Tyrosine is actively transported into the cell, where the first and rate-limiting step is catalyzed by tyrosine hydroxylase. A total of four enzymatic

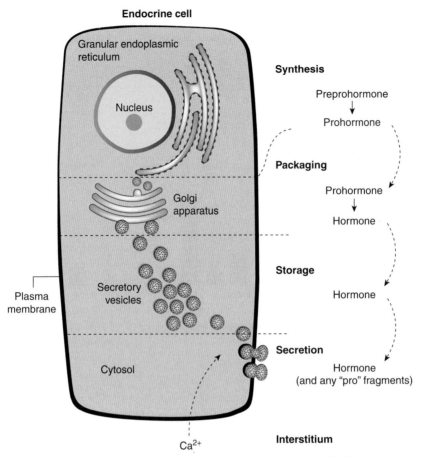

Endocrine cell

FIGURE 1-5 ■ Peptide hormone synthesis. Peptide hormones are synthesized as preprohormones in the ribosomes and processed to prohormones in the granular endoplasmic reticulum (ER). In the Golgi apparatus, the hormone or prohormone is packaged in secretory vesicles, which are released from the cell in response to an influx of Ca^{2+}. The rise in cytoplasmic Ca^{2+} is required for docking of the secretory vesicles in the plasma membrane and for exocytosis of the vesicular contents. The hormone and the products of the posttranslational processing that occurs inside the secretory vesicles are released into the extracellular space. Examples of peptide hormones are ACTH, insulin, growth hormone, and glucagon. (*From Molina PE. General principles of endocrine physiology. In: Molina PE.* Endocrine Physiology. 2nd ed. *New York, NY: McGraw-Hill; 2006:1-24*)

reactions produce the final product, epinephrine. Dopamine and norepinephrine are precursors to the final epinephrine product.

Prepro- and Prohormones

Many hormones are first synthesized as pro- or prepro-hormones and then posttranslationally modified to the active hormone. Typically, hormones that are to be secreted contain an N-terminal signal sequence that directs the prohormone to the endoplasmic reticulum, where this signal sequence is then cleaved.

In the follicular lumen of the thyroid cells, thyroglobulin undergoes iodination of multiple tyrosine residues followed by coupling of the iodotyrosines in a reaction catalyzed by thyroid peroxidase.[12] After coupling, thyroglobulin is processed in lysosomes to produce T_4 and T_3.

Parathyroid hormone (PTH) is also synthesized as a preprohormone.[9,13] The initial translational product of the PTH gene is preproPTH, which contains hydrophobic amino acids on the N terminus which are critical for

efficient transport of the hormone into the endoplasmic reticulum for further processing. In the endoplasmic reticulum, the preproPTH is quickly cleaved to proPTH which contains 6 amino acids at the N-terminal end in addition to the bioactive 84 amino acid PTH.

Other peptide hormones are made up of subunits that must be associated before the hormone is active. The initial insulin translational product, preproinsulin, consists of an α and β subunit connected by C-peptide.[14] During insertion into the endoplasmic reticulum the signal peptide is cleaved, producing proinsulin. Prohormone convertases cleave the C-peptide, generating the active insulin hormone. C-peptide and insulin are packaged together in secretory granules in the Golgi apparatus and released together. Thus in certain instances, both C-peptide and insulin are measured to distinguish endogenous causes of hypoglycemia from exogenously administered insulin.

Luteinizing hormone, follicle stimulating hormone, chorionic gonadotropin and thyroid stimulating hormone are comprised of a common α subunit and unique β subunits, encoded for by distinct genes.[5]

Some genes encode for a prohormone that can be cleaved to multiple hormones.[5] The prohormone proopiomelanocortin (POMC) is posttranslationally cleaved to several different hormones. POMC is cleaved to ACTH, β-endorphin, α-, β-, and γ-melanocyte–stimulating hormone (MSH). This is why patients with Addison disease who have supraphysiological levels of ACTH (and POMC) are hyperpigmented.

Glycosylation

Glycoproteins are the largest hormones and consist of a common α subunit and a unique β subunit.[5] The carbohydrate moiety which is cotranslationally attached to the glycoprotein hormone protects the nascent polypeptide from intracellular degradation. Carbohydrate attachment is also essential for correct folding and combination of the subunits. The carbohydrate attachment is also required for secretion of the mature hormone from the cell. After secretion of the hormone, the carbohydrate moiety is important in stabilizing the hormone in circulation and appears to be important for receptor signaling, but does not affect affinity for the hormone receptor. The glycoprotein hormones bind the G protein–coupled receptors (GPCRs).

Postsecretion Activation

Some hormones are modified after secretion into the circulation. Although testosterone is the major androgen in the circulation of men, dihydrotestosterone (DHT) is the more potent androgen.[15] In the peripheral tissues (primarily the skin and prostate) DHT is formed by the actions of two isoenzymes, 5α-reductase types 1 and 2. In males, the majority of circulating estradiol is produced by aromatization of testosterone by the aromatase enzyme, primarily found in adipocytes as well as Leydig cells and placenta. The increase in adipocyte-derived aromatase is largely responsible for gynecomastia seen in overweight men.

Vitamin D is either absorbed from the gut (vitamin D_2) or synthesized in the skin from 7-dehydrocholesterol and the actions of sunlight (vitamin D_3).[16] These two forms are converted to 25-hydroxyvitamin D_3 in the liver, which is the major circulating form of vitamin D. In the kidney, the 25-hydroxyvitamin D_3 form is hydroxylated to the active form, 1, 25-dihydroxyvitamin D_3.

Although both T_4 and T_3 are secreted from the thyroid, the majority of T_3 comes from postsecretion conversion of circulating T_4 to T_3.[11] This occurs primarily in the liver by deiodination of T_4 to form T_3.

Hormone Degradation

The half-life of a hormone in circulation is dependent on its synthesis rate, amount of binding to proteins and rate of degradation.[5] Some hormones such as somatostatin vanish quickly whereas other hormones such as TSH have a prolonged half-life. Since somatostatin has effects on almost every organ, its short half-life allows for more local control of its activity. Modification of the somatostatin structure to lengthen its half-life has allowed pharmaceutical companies to develop analogues of somatostatin for treatment of diseases such as acromegaly and hyperinsulinism.

Most peptide hormones have a relatively short half-life of 20 minutes or so. Hormones such as growth hormone, ACTH, LH, PTH, and prolactin have sharp peaks of secretion and decay. Therefore, to accurately measure these hormones they must be either measured frequently (every 10-20 minutes) over many hours (8-24 hours) or in response to a stimulatory event. The short half-life of PTH has proven to be advantageous in being able to detect intraoperatively whether or not a parathyroid adenoma has been removed. The long half-life of T_4 (7 days) allows replacement therapy to be dosed daily. However, this also requires 4 weeks for steady-state levels to be reached. T_3, on the other hand, has a half-life of only 1 day, requiring dosing two-three times per day.

Hormones may be degraded through enzymatic modifications in the liver.[9] These modifications include hydroxylation, oxidation, glucuronidation, sulfation, and reduction with glutathione. They may also be degraded at their target site by lysosomal degradation of the hormone with recycling of the receptor. The inactivated hormone is then excreted through the feces or the urine.

Many hormones circulate bound to proteins, protecting hormones from rapid degradation.

HORMONE TRANSPORT

Carrier Proteins

Many hormones exist in circulation in equilibrium between free hormone and hormone bound to a carrier protein.[9] Specifically, thyroid hormone (T_4 and T_3) circulates bound to thyroxine-binding globulin (TBG), albumin and prealbumin; cortisol binds to cortisol-binding globulin; testosterone and estrogen bind to sex hormone binding globulin (SHBG); insulin-like growth factors bind to the IGF-binding proteins; and growth hormone circulates bound to GH-binding protein. These carrier proteins protect the hormone from rapid degradation and prolong the hormones' half-lives. Most binding proteins are synthesized in the liver. Therefore, liver disease may increase the metabolic clearance of a hormone by decreasing the amount of bound hormone.

Binding proteins not only increase hormone half-life, but also provide a readily available pool of hormone. Protein binding of hormones also may modulate access of the hormone to its receptors.

Importance of Free Hormone

Free or unbound hormone is the form of the hormone that binds its receptor and is important in maintaining homeostasis.[5] It is also the free hormone that provides feedback to regulate synthesis of new hormone. The free hormone and its binding proteins are in dynamic equilibrium. Conditions that affect binding protein levels usually do not affect hormone balance, but do affect the assays we use. For example, TBG deficiency results in a low measured total T_4, but does not affect free T_4 levels. Patients with TBG deficiency are euthyroid and do not require any intervention. Other conditions that affect binding protein levels and thus may cause abnormal total hormone measurements include liver disease, which causes loss of binding protein, and the use of birth control pills, which raises levels of binding proteins. Alteration in binding proteins, as occurs in pregnancy, with the use of birth control pills, and in critical illness, results in a rapid adjustment of the free hormone level to normal. In cases where binding proteins are known to be affected, the free hormone must be measured to know the hormonal status of the patient.

When a young female has an elevated total T_4 but normal TSH, pregnancy or use of birth control pills should be the top considerations in your differential. In euthyroid sick syndrome total T_4 and TBG are decreased, but free T_4 is often normal. Similarly, patients in the ICU may be misdiagnosed with adrenal insufficiency because total cortisol is low when in fact free cortisol is normal.

HORMONE REGULATION

A variety of regulatory mechanisms finely controls circulating levels of hormones within narrow physiologic ranges. As with other aspects of endocrine physiology, there are many levels to this regulation, ranging from macroscopic control of plasma concentrations down to pinpoint control of local tissue and pericellular levels. Traditionally, regulatory mechanisms have been categorized as endocrine, paracrine, or autocrine (Figure 1-6). Endocrine regulation involves secretion of a hormone by a specific cell type, with the hormone passing into the circulation and acting on a distant cell in a separate organ. Paracrine regulation consists of secretion and subsequent diffusion of a hormone within the local environment to act on another cell, either one directly contacting the source of the hormone or within a small pericellular region. Autocrine control refers to secretion of a hormone into the cell's microenvironment, with the hormone then interacting with membrane-bound or nuclear receptors within the same cell. In every endocrine system, all of these control mechanisms are relevant. As our understanding of endocrinology improves, the importance of

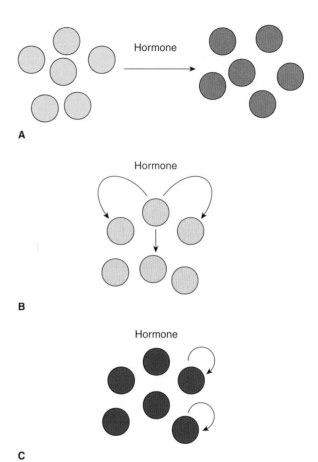

FIGURE 1-6 ■ Three different mechanisms of hormone function. **(A)** Endocrine action of hormones involves secretion of a hormone and its transport via the vasculature to interact with a distant target tissue. **(B)** Paracrine action involves secretion of a factor that diffuses within a tissue to affect adjacent cells. **(C)** Autocrine action involves secretion of a factor that acts on the secreting cells themselves.

paracrine and autocrine mechanisms has become increasingly apparent.[17]

Negative Feedback

Much of classical endocrinology involves negative feedback loops. In this setting, central trophic hormones often released from the hypothalamus and/or pituitary gland stimulate production of an effector hormone from hormone-secreting tissues. In addition to its end organ effects, the effector hormone limits its own secretion by suppressing production of its stimulating central trophic hormone. In the example of the thyroid axis, neurons in the supraoptic and paraventricular nuclei of the hypothalamus produce thyrotropin-releasing hormone (TRH) and transport it to the median eminence of the hypothalamus. From there, they secrete TRH into the hypothalamic-pituitary portal system, allowing it to reach the thyrotrope cells in the anterior lobe of the pituitary gland. Under TRH stimulation, TSH gene expression increases and the thyrotropes release stored

TSH that passes into the systemic circulation. In the thyroid gland, TSH causes increased activity of the biosynthetic enzymes necessary for thyroid hormone synthesis. TSH also leads to higher rates of absorption of the thyroglobulin-containing colloid within the thyroid follicles. The absorbed thyroglobulin is digested within the thyroid follicles, releasing T_4 and T_3, which exit the cells and enter the systemic circulation (Figure 1-7). Triiodothyronine (T_3) is the active form of thyroid hormone that binds to nuclear receptors in thyroid hormone-responsive cells. The thyroid gland directly secretes only between 10% and 40% of the circulating T_3, with the remainder arising from local tissue conversion of T_4 to T_3. T_3 resulting from this conversion in the pituitary thyrotropes blunts the stimulatory effect of TRH by suppressing synthesis of TSH. Thyroid hormone also exerts negative feedback on hypothalamic secretion of TRH. Additional factors, such as body temperature, physiologic stress, cortisol levels, and hypothalamic dopamine and somatostatin also control TRH and TSH secretion. These factors are discussed in more detail in Chapter 4.

This negative feedback system results in the control of circulating thyroid hormones within a narrow range that is constant within an individual and is smaller than published reference intervals for populations. What may appear to be trivial changes in thyroid hormone concentrations induced by small doses of

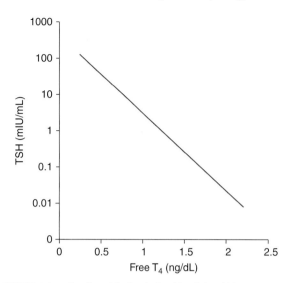

FIGURE 1-8 ■ Semilogarithmic relationship of thyroid hormone concentrations and TSH levels. Small increases and decreases in the free T_4 concentration lead to very large changes in TSH concentration.

levothyroxine or increased iodine supplementation lead to large changes in TSH levels according to a log-linear relationship (Figure 1-8) as the negative feedback effect is increased or decreased.[18] Additionally, the intensity of the negative feedback may vary with age across the pediatric population. Newborn infants and babies in the first few years of life maintain concentrations of thyroid hormones that are significantly higher than those seen in older children and adults, with the upper end of the reference range for T_4 typically being 16 to 17 mcg/dL in the newborn and 14 to 15 mcg/dL in infants up to 2 years of age. This compares to the reference range in older children and adults of 5 to 12 mcg/dL. At the same time, TSH levels are actually higher in the first year of life, indicating a relatively blunted degree of negative feedback. As the child gets older, the intensity of the negative feedback response increases, thus decreasing TSH levels and lowering T_4 and T_3 concentrations into the usual adult ranges.

This phenomenon of negative feedback variability also occurs in other hormone systems, including the hypothalamic-pituitary-gonadal axis. Hypothalamic gonadotropin-releasing hormone (GnRH) stimulates secretion of the pituitary gonadotropins luteinizing hormone (LH) and follicle-stimulating hormone (FSH). In the male, gonadotropins then stimulate testicular secretion of testosterone, with testosterone having a negative feedback effect on both gonadotropin and GnRH secretion. During infancy, the negative feedback response is relatively weak, and this leads to relatively high circulating levels of LH, FSH, and testosterone. Testosterone concentrations peak at about 6 to 8 weeks of age, reaching near pubertal levels. Over the next few months, negative feedback strengthens, and testosterone

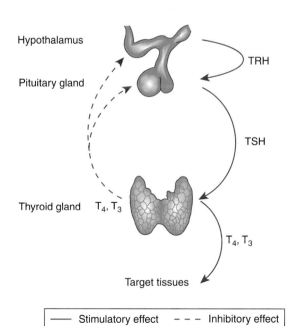

FIGURE 1-7 ■ Negative feedback regulation of thyroid hormone. Thyrotropin-releasing hormone (TRH) stimulates secretion of thyroid stimulating hormone (TSH), which in turn stimulates L-thyroxine (T_4) and triiodothyronine (T_3) secretion from the thyroid gland. T_3 suppresses TSH and TRH secretion by a negative feedback effect, regulating circulating levels of thyroid hormone.

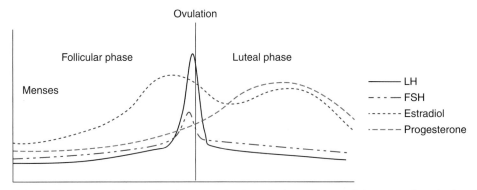

FIGURE 1-9 ■ Positive feedback occurs during the female menstrual cycle as the increasing estradiol concentration stimulates luteinizing hormone (LH) secretion, which in turn stimulates ovulation at mid-cycle.

levels decline to prepubertal values of less than 10 ng/dL by 6 to 8 months. At the time of puberty, negative feedback again relaxes, leading to a gradual increase of testosterone concentrations over the course of puberty, up to the adult levels of 300 to 1000 ng/dL.

Positive Feedback

In contrast to very prevalent negative feedback loops, positive endocrine feedback regulatory mechanisms are infrequent. The female hypothalamic-pituitary-ovarian axis during the menstrual cycle provides a good example of positive feedback (Figure 1-9). During the follicular phase of the menstrual cycle, the developing follicle produces gradually increasing amounts of estradiol under the influence of LH and FSH. Due to the positive feedback effect of estradiol on LH at mid-cycle, pituitary secretion of LH gradually increases and accelerates to form the mid-cycle LH surge that induces ovulation. Follicular secretion of progesterone enhances this positive feedback. The positive feedback occurs at both the pituitary gland and the hypothalamus, with estradiol increasing pituitary responsiveness to GnRH and promoting higher LH secretion and, along with progesterone, increasing GnRH secretion from the hypothalamus.

Paracrine/Autocrine Actions of Hormones

Besides the classical endocrine effects of hormones, in which a secreted molecule acts on a target cell at a distance, hormones also may cause physiological effects within the same tissue. If the target cell is adjacent to the secreting cell, these effects are termed paracrine. If the hormone acts on the same cell that secretes it, the effect is known as autocrine (Figure 1-6).

Paracrine actions

One of the best known paracrine actions of a hormone in pediatric endocrinology is the local effect of growth hormone on chondrocytes. As part of its endocrine action, GH causes hepatic secretion of IGF-1. However, in the growth plate, circulating GH binds to its receptors on chondrocytes, stimulating them to secrete locally derived IGF-1 into the extracellular matrix. This IGF-1 in turn stimulates proliferation of the growth plate chondrocytes, leading to increased thickness of the growth plate that ultimately translates into linear growth. In studies of tissue-specific knockout mice that have a deletion of the IGF-1 gene only in hepatocytes, growth is nearly normal, despite much lower circulating levels of hepatically derived IGF-1. However, knocking out the gene for acid labile substance (another IGF-1 binding protein) in liver reduces circulating IGF-1 to near zero, and these mice are growth restricted. This indicates that although locally derived IGF-1 is important, chondrocytes do require some plasma-derived IGF-1.[19] Paracrine actions of other hormones are frequently physiologically important in other endocrine systems as well.

Autocrine actions

Autocrine action refers to the effects of a secreted hormone on the same cell that secreted it. These actions lead to very fine control of hormone secretion at the tissue level. The intra-pituitary effects of activins and follistatins on FSH regulation demonstrate these autocrine effects (Figure 1-10). In the pituitary, hypothalamic GnRH arriving via the pituitary portal system leads to increased production of FSH. Activins are members of a group of hormones produced by the gonadotroph cells in the pituitary that stimulate FSH production by potentiating the effects of GnRH stimulation. Gonadotroph cells secrete activin that acts on the same cell to stimulate FSH production. An ultra-short loop negative feedback system regulates activin secretion, also involving autocrine action. Gonadotroph-derived activin stimulates production of follistatin from the gonadotroph. Follistatin then acts to inhibit activin production. This negative feedback loop acts by the same principle as the

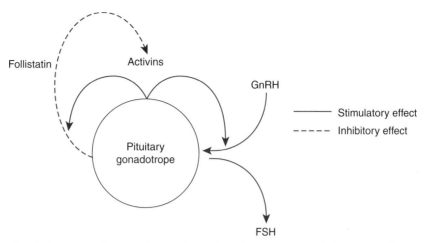

FIGURE 1-10 ■ Within the pituitary gland, the gonadotrope cells secrete activins, which have dual autocrine effects, acting both to increase responsiveness to gonadotropin-releasing hormone (GnRH) and to regulate their own secretion via the autocrine negative feedback production of follistatin.

classic endocrine negative feedback systems, but it occurs within and around a single cell by autocrine mechanisms. In this example, there are two interrelated autocrine processes: activin stimulation of FSH production and the negative feedback regulation of activin production. This example illustrates the exquisite local control of gonadotropin secretion superimposed upon the classic endocrine feedback loops. Similar local regulatory mechanisms exist in other endocrine systems.

Endocrine Cyclicity

Pulsatile secretion

Many hormones are secreted in a rhythmic or pulsatile fashion, with the frequency varying from as short as hourly up to daily or more. In prepubertal children, the hypothalamus secretes gonadotropin-releasing hormone (GnRH) in low amplitude pulses, and as puberty ensues both the amplitude and frequency increase, starting at night (Figure 1-11). This GnRH pulsatility leads to peripheral venous LH concentrations that clearly vary with time. Although the pituitary secretes FSH with a similar pulsatility, the longer half life of FSH blurs this in peripheral blood, and levels appear more constant over the short term. Pulsatile GnRH exposure is essential for normal gonadotropin secretion. In the treatment of central precocious puberty, long-acting GnRH analogs suppress LH and FSH secretion by eliminating exposure to pulsatile GnRH. The pituitary gland also secretes growth hormone in a pulsatile fashion, but instead of a regular rhythm, the pulses occur in a less predictable fashion, typically with the largest burst of secretion after the onset of sleep and with several irregularly spaced bursts of variable intensity during the rest of the night. Smaller bursts of secretion occur infrequently during the day.

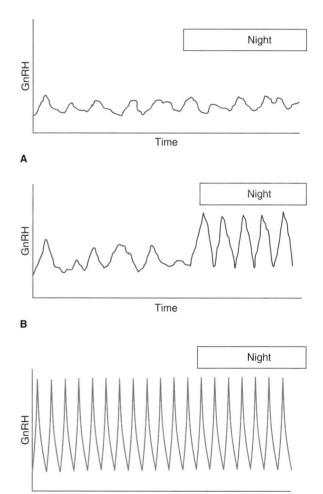

FIGURE 1-11 ■ Establishment of pulsatile secretion of gonadotropin releasing hormone (GnRH). **(A)** In childhood, GnRH secretion occurs in irregular, low amplitude pulses. **(B)** Early in puberty, pulsatility increases, particularly at night during sleep. **(C)** After puberty, GnRH release occurs in regular, high amplitude pulses every 60 minutes during the entire 24-hour cycle.

Circadian rhythms

Several hormones have diurnal variation, with their concentrations cycling over the course of approximately 24 hours. These include cortisol, testosterone, estradiol, TSH, and prolactin. Early in infancy, the diurnal variation is not present, and levels of these hormones remain relatively constant. By approximately 3 to 4 months of age, however, the mature secretory pattern is in place, being maintained by the light/dark cycle. Individuals with severe visual impairment have disordered diurnal variability of these hormones. Some pathologic conditions may alter diurnal patterns. For example, patients with endogenous Cushing syndrome lose this secretory pattern and consistently have elevated evening cortisol levels.[20]

Long-term cyclicity

The estrus cycle in animals and the menstrual cycle in humans are examples of long-term cyclicity. The length of the menstrual cycle is typically 28 days. The time required for follicular maturation contributes largely to the length of the cycle up to ovulation, and the lifespan of the corpus luteum contributes to the length of the cycle from ovulation to the onset of menses.

HORMONE RECEPTORS

Membrane Receptors

The membrane receptors are grouped into families based on their structural similarities.[5,9] The four membrane receptor families include: seven-transmembrane G protein-coupled receptors (GPCRs), tyrosine kinase receptors, cytokine receptor-linked kinase receptors, and serine kinase receptors (Table 1-3).

The GPCRs are composed of three subunits, α, β, and γ, and are classified by their alpha subunit. They are so named because they bind guanine nucleotides (GDP and GTP). With more than a 1000 members, the GPCRs are the largest family of proteins in the human body.[5,9] Activity of the signaling pathway is regulated by GTP hydrolysis and the interactions between the subunits. When hormone is not bound to the receptor, GDP binds to the alpha subunit. Hormone binding to the receptor induces a conformational change that leads to dissociation of GDP, facilitating GTP binding to the α subunit, resulting in a dissociation of the α subunit from the $\beta\gamma$ complex (Figure 1-12). This allows the α subunit to activate adenylate cyclase, phospholipase C or protein kinase A. These enzymes produce secondary messengers (ie, cAMP, diacyl glycerol, mobilization of calcium) that activate or inactivate target proteins in the cell. Hydrolysis of GTP to GDP by GTPase restores the inactive state by allowing the α subunit to reassociate with the $\beta\gamma$ complex.

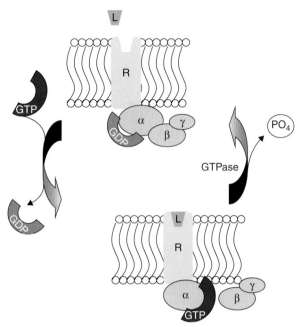

FIGURE 1-12 ■ Hormone binding to the G protein-coupled receptor (GPCR). Shown at the top of the figure is the unbound GPCR with GDP bound. The α subunit is associated with the $\beta\gamma$ complex. Hormone binding to the GPCR allows GTP to replace GDP. The $\beta\gamma$ complex then dissociates from the α subunit. GTPase activity of the α subunit forms GDP, allowing the $\beta\gamma$ complex to reassociate with the α subunit. R, receptor, L, ligand or hormone

There are more than a dozen isoforms of the α subunit.[5,9] $G\alpha_s$ stimulates and $G\alpha_i$ inhibits adenylate cylcase while $G\alpha_q$ stimulates phospholipase C. The β-adrenergic receptors are associated with the $G\alpha_s$ receptor, and binding to these receptors activates adenylate cyclase, increasing cyclic AMP levels. The α-adrenergic receptors are associated with the $G\alpha_i$ receptors, inhibiting adenylate cyclase and activating potassium and calcium channels. Both the α- and β-adrenergic receptors bind catecholamines. TRH (thyrotropin-releasing hormone) and GnRH (gonadotropin-releasing hormone) both act through the $G\alpha_q$ receptor and stimulate phospholipase C.

Other membrane receptors include the receptor-protein tyrosine kinase, cytokine receptor-linked kinase and serine kinase receptors.[5,9] The receptor-protein tyrosine kinases are single-transmembrane proteins. The intracellular portion of the receptor has intrinsic enzyme activity causing auto-phosphorylation of the receptor as well as phosphorylation of downstream proteins. Signaling pathways involved include the MAP kinases and Raf pathways. Insulin and growth factors are examples of hormones that bind the receptor-protein tyrosine kinases.

The cytokine receptor-linked kinases dimerize upon hormone binding and, similar to the tyrosine kinase receptors, activate their signaling pathway via phosphorylation and autophosphorylation. The cytokine receptor family also activates the MAP kinases as well as the JAK/STAT pathways. GH and prolactin bind to the cytokine receptors.

The serine kinase receptors signal through the Smads. Mullerian-inhibiting substance, activin, bone morphogenic proteins (BMPs), and TGF-β all bind to the serine kinase receptors.

Nuclear Receptors

The steroid receptors are located intracellularly.[5,9] Some steroid receptors are located in the cytoplasm and are translocated to the nucleus after ligand binding (glucocorticoid receptors) and others are located exclusively in the nucleus (thyroid hormone). There are at least 100 nuclear receptors identified. The receptors are classified by the ligands that they bind (Figure 1-4). Many of these receptors are still classified as orphan receptors, as their ligands have yet to be identified. Some of the orphan receptors are SF-1 and DAX-1, both of which play a role in adrenal and gonadal development, and HNF4$_\alpha$ which plays a role in the development of the pancreas.

The nuclear receptors have binding sites for their ligand and for DNA. Ligand binding results in either activation or repression of gene transcription. Most nuclear receptors bind the DNA as dimers. The estrogen, androgen, prolactin, and glucocorticoid receptors bind as homodimers (Figure 1-4). The thyroid, vitamin D, retinoid, and peroxisome proliferator-activated receptors bind DNA as heterodimers with the retinoid X receptors (Figure 1-4). Receptor specificity is determined by the DNA sequence, the orientation of the half-binding sites, and the spacing between the half-sites.

Receptors such as the thyroid hormone and retinoid receptors are bound by corepressor proteins in the absence of hormone binding. The corepressor proteins silence gene transcription. When hormone binds the receptor, the corepressor proteins dissociate allowing coactivator proteins that enhance transcription to bind. Mutations in the receptor binding sites for the corepressor and coactivator proteins may result in disease states. For example, mutations in the thyroid receptor resulting in defective dissociation of the corepressor may result in hormone resistance.

Coactivators may stimulate transcription by recruiting histone acetyl transferases (enzymes that open chromatin), interaction with other transcription factors, or direct interaction with transcription enzymes.

NONTRADITIONAL ENDOCRINE SYSTEMS

Although the focus in pediatric endocrinology is usually on the classic endocrine organs and systems, many endocrine systems exist that involve other organs, such as the heart, kidney, and bowel. These systems feature secretion of a circulating factor that acts on another organ at a distance and have a feedback system of regulation.

Heart

The heart (see Chapter 3) is the source of circulating natriuretic peptides. Several forms of natriuretic peptides exist, but the major ones involved in endocrine control of sodium balance and intravascular volume are atrial natriuretic peptide (ANP) and B-type natriuretic peptide (BMP). The right and left atria and ventricles are the major sources of both ANP and BNP. Cardiac tissue secretes these peptides after increases in atrial and ventricular pressure. ANP and BNP act in the kidney to promote renal sodium and volume loss by reducing sodium reabsorption, inhibiting the antidiuretic effect of vasopressin, and counteracting the sodium-retaining effect of aldosterone. In the adrenal gland, they inhibit aldosterone production. These actions have the net effect of lowering intravascular volume and decreasing the intracardiac pressures, providing negative feedback for ANP and BNP release.[21]

Kidney

In addition to its involvement in classic endocrine systems such as the control of calcium and phosphorous concentrations via PTH and vitamin D and the regulation of fluid and electrolyte balance via antidiuretic hormone and aldosterone, the kidney also serves as a primary endocrine organ in the regulation of red blood cell (RBC) mass and hematocrit. If the RBC mass drops, oxygen delivery also declines, leading to relative local hypoxia. The peritubular fibroblasts in the renal cortex sense this decline in oxygen tension and secrete erythropoietin into the circulation. In the bone marrow, erythropoietin stimulates the erythroid precursor cells to produce more RBCs, thus increasing the oxygen delivery to tissues, including the kidney, and regulating erythropoietin production.[22]

Gut

The gastrointestinal system secretes a large number of gastroenteropancreatic hormones that regulate aspects of function as diverse as carbohydrate metabolism, gastric acid secretion, intestinal motility, exocrine pancreatic function, and gallbladder motility. Additionally, gut hormones partially modulate appetite, acting in concert with adipose tissue-derived factors such as leptin and with complex CNS regulatory mechanisms. In this setting, ghrelin appears to act as an endocrine hunger signal. Although first discovered as a GH secretogogue, ghrelin's physiologic importance in the control of GH secretion is unclear. Secreted into the systemic circulation by cells predominantly in the gastric fundus, ghrelin crosses the blood–brain barrier to the hypothalamus and stimulates hunger and food intake. Feeding suppresses ghrelin secretion, providing short-term feedback regulation. Ghrelin may also be involved in long-term control of energy balance.[23]

ENDOCRINE DISEASE

Classification of diseases of the endocrine glands are typically based on the functional status of the hormone involved and include states of true hormone deficiency, resistance to the end organ effects of a hormone that mimic deficiency, true hormone excess, and activating mutations of hormone signaling pathways that mimic excess (Table 1-4).

Hormone Deficiency

Hypofunction of endocrine organs leading to hormone deficiency is the most common type of endocrinopathy. This hypofunction may be due to many different causes. Autoimmune destruction of a tissue leading to deficiency is quite common, and examples include chronic lymphocytic thyroiditis (Hashimoto thyroiditis) and type 1 diabetes mellitus, among others. In pediatric patients, developmental defects of the endocrine glands may occur, as in congenital hypothyroidism due to thyroid dysplasia. Additionally, specific gene defects may lead to enzymatic dysfunction also causing endocrine deficiency, such as the hypocortisolism seen in congenital adrenal hyperplasia. Injury to endocrine tissues may

occur from mechanisms such as trauma, infection, surgical removal, or irradiation. In many cases of endocrine hypofunction, the concentration of the secreted hormone may be low and that of the relevant trophic hormone may be abnormally high. A simple example of this is the low level of T_4 and the elevated level of TSH seen in cases of primary hypothyroidism. The exception to this is when the endocrine deficiency is due to lack of normal secretion of the trophic hormone itself. In that case, both the trophic and effector hormones will circulate at abnormally low concentrations. In the thyroid example above, central hormone deficiency would manifest as a low level of T_4 and either a low or inappropriately normal level of TSH (Table 1-5).

Hormone Resistance

Because hormone action occurs through specific cell membrane or nuclear receptors, mutation of the genes for any of these receptors may mimic deficiency of the hormone itself. Although each of these conditions is relatively uncommon, knowledge of the relevant endocrine physiology allows the clinician to predict the symptoms and signs that will be present and to predict the pattern of hormone levels seen on endocrine testing. One of the better known examples is complete androgen insensitivity syndrome (CAIS), in which the patient carries a mutation in the androgen receptor. Beginning in fetal life, affected patients are insensitive to the effects of androgens. Hence in the developing 46,XY fetus, normally androgen responsive tissues behave as if no androgen is

Table 1-4.

Mechanisms of Endocrine Disease

Class of Defect	Pathogenic Mechanisms	Representative Diseases
Hormone deficiency	Developmental defects	Thyroid dysplasia
	Enzymatic defects	Congenital adrenal hyperplasia
	Autoimmune disorders	Autoimmune thyroiditis
	Infection	Post meningococcal adrenal insufficiency
	Trauma	Post head injury hypopituitarism
	Irradiation	Radiation-induced hypopituitarism
	Surgical removal	Postsurgical hypothyroidism
Hormone resistance	Genetic mutation	AIS, pseudohypoparathyroidism, Laron syndrome, etc.
Hormone excess	Exogenous	Topical androgens
	Autoimmune stimulation	Graves disease
	Tumor	Cushing disease
	Dysregulation	Persistent hyperinsulinemic hypoglycemia of the neonate
Activating mutations of Hormone receptors	Genetic mutation	MAS, FMPP

AIS, androgen insensitivity syndrome; FMPP, familial male limited precocious puberty; MAS, McCune-Albright syndrome

Table 1-5.

Patterns of Effector and Trophic Hormones in Endocrine Disease

Category of Disease	Concentration of Effector Hormone	Concentration of Trophic Hormone	Example
Primary endocrine gland deficiency	Low	High	Autoimmune thyroiditis ($\downarrow$ T$_4$, $\uparrow$ TSH)
Central endocrine deficiency	Low	Low or normal	Growth hormone deficiency ($\downarrow$ IGF-1, $\downarrow$ GH)
Hormone resistance	High	High	Androgen insensitivity syndrome ($\uparrow$ testosterone, $\uparrow$ LH)
Primary endocrine gland hyperfunction	High	Low	Graves disease ($\uparrow$ T$_4$, $\downarrow$ TSH)
Central endocrine hyperfunction	High	Normal or high	Cushing disease ($\uparrow$cortisol, $\uparrow$ ACTH)
Activating receptor mutation	High	Low	FMPP ($\uparrow$ testosterone, $\downarrow$ LH)

ACTH, adrenocorticotrophic hormone; FMPP, familial male-limited precocious puberty; GH, growth hormone; IGF-1, insulin-like growth factor-1; LH, luteinizing hormone; T4, L-thyroxine; TSH, thyroid-stimulating hormone

present. Thus, instead of developing normal external male genitalia, the infant is a phenotypically normal female at birth. Testes are present and secrete testosterone normally, but the androgen resistance also prevents testosterone's normal negative feedback on gonadotropin secretion. Hence both testosterone and LH levels are high in the affected patient. Other well-known examples of hormone resistance include pseudohypoparathyroidism resulting from a mutation in the receptor for parathyroid hormone (PTH) and Laron syndrome owing to a mutation of the receptor for growth hormone. Many other similar conditions exist, and these are discussed in their respective chapters.

Insulin resistance is perhaps the most common syndrome of hormone resistance, but this does not usually result from defects of the receptor itself but from a variety of abnormalities of postreceptor signal transduction mechanisms. Syndromes of resistance to other hormones may also arise from similar defects.

Hormone Excess

Conditions of hormone excess feature high circulating levels of the hormone in question. This may arise either from hypersecretion of the hormone or from exogenous sources: ingestion or transdermal exposure to inappropriate amounts of the hormone or of hormonally active substances.

Exogenous

The surreptitious administration of insulin may cause hypoglycemia, while hyperthyroidism may be a result of self-administration of levothyroxine in an attempt to lose

weight. Although uncommon, cases of precocious puberty have arisen from transdermal absorption of topical androgens used by the patient's family members or other adults.[24] Similarly, while gynecomastia may be caused by high circulating levels of endogenous estradiol, reports of several cases show that it can arise from estrogenic actions of lavender and tea tree oils or other estrogens.[25]

Hypersecretion

Autoimmune stimulation. Other than Graves disease, hypersecretion of hormones is relatively uncommon in pediatric patients. Graves disease, however, has an incidence of approximately 1% in children and adolescents.[26] Graves disease results from stimulation of the TSH receptor by pathogenic autoantibodies.

Tumor. Other causes of hormone excess include tumoral secretion of either an effector hormone or a trophic hormone. Two examples of this include secretion of androgen by an adrenocortical adenoma leading to virilization in childhood and unregulated production of ACTH by a pituitary adenoma leading to excessive production of cortisol by the adrenals with resulting Cushing syndrome.

Altered regulatory mechanisms. Alteration of normal endocrine regulatory mechanisms may lead to disorders such as persistent hyperinsulinemic hypoglycemia of the newborn or central precocious puberty.

Diagnosis of hormone excess

In many cases of hormone excess, endocrine testing will reveal high levels of the effector hormones and low or suppressed concentrations of the respective trophic hormones. Hence in cases of hyperthyroidism due to both ingestion of excess thyroid hormone and Graves disease, the T_4 level will be high and the TSH level will be low. The exception to this occurs when the hormone excess is caused by hypersecretion of the trophic hormone itself, such as secretion of ACTH from a pituitary adenoma leading to hypercortisolism and resulting Cushing syndrome. In this case, cortisol levels will be high and the ACTH level will be inappropriately normal or elevated (Table 1-5).

Activating Mutations of Hormone Receptors

In addition to true hypersecretion, several conditions exist in which activating mutations of the hormone receptor mimic hypersecretion. Although rare, these conditions shed light on endocrine physiology. The two most commonly seen in pediatric patients are McCune-Albright syndrome (MAS) and familial male-limited precocious puberty (FMPP), also known as testotoxicosis. Patients with FMPP carry an activating mutation in the LH receptor. Hence, the Leydig cells of the testes act as if they are being stimulated by LH and constitutively secrete testosterone from infancy, leading to signs and symptoms of precocious puberty at an early age. Sexual precocity does not occur in females carrying the mutation, because the action of both the LH and FSH receptors are required for ovarian estrogen secretion. A variety of disorders may affect patients with MAS, including café au lait macules, fibrous dysplasia of bone, and forms of endocrine hyperfunction such as precocious puberty, hyperthyroidism, or acromegaly. At first, this array of disorders may seem confusing, but it can be explained by a somatic or postzygotic activating mutation in the $G\alpha_s$ subunit of the heterotrimeric G protein signal transduction mechanism (see "Membrane Receptors" section earlier in this chapter). Signal transduction occurs through G protein–coupled receptors for many hormones. However, because the mutation in affected individuals occurs on a somatic or postzygotic basis, not all endocrine tissues carry the mutated $G\alpha_s$ allele, and only tissues carrying this mutation will be affected. Hence, if skin melanocytes carry the mutation, the melanocyte-stimulating hormone receptor is activated, forming café au lait macules. If osteoclasts have the mutation, their PTH receptor is activated, forming fibrous dysplasia lesions. If ovarian tissue carries the mutation, gonadotropin receptors are chronically activated, and the cells secrete estradiol.

On a purely biochemical basis, one cannot distinguish the endocrine disorders of FMPP and MAS from disorders of exogenous hormone exposure or tumoral secretion of hormone (Table 1-5). Endocrine testing for MAS or FMPP will likely only provide supporting evidence.

Diagnosis of these conditions requires attention to the clinical picture, which may be pathognomonic, although confirmation by genetic testing is helpful in some cases.

PRINCIPLES OF ENDOCRINE TESTING

In clinical endocrine practice, the use of laboratory assays is ubiquitous. Practitioners use assays to investigate clinical findings, to confirm diagnoses, and to monitor and adjust treatment. The clinical laboratory is also essential for most clinical research. With the rapidly expanding armamentarium of tests available to the clinician and clinical researcher, the ability to assess a laboratory assay critically and to understand its application is an essential skill. Important analytic variables include aspects of the assay itself that may affect the outcome, such as the assay type, antibody specificity, and the effect of interferences in the assay. Preanalytic variables are conditions that exist before the sample is actually processed by the lab and which may affect the outcome; these may include patient variables or specimen handling conditions.

Assay Types

Immunoassays

Immunoassays have been a feature of endocrinology since the development of the radioimmunoassay (RIA) in the 1960s. The unifying features of immunoassays is the use of one or more antibodies directed against the particular hormone of interest and a reporter system that produces a quantifiable signal, such as a radioactive particle, light, or fluorescence. Immunoassays are broadly grouped into competitive and noncompetitive assays (Table 1-6).

Table 1-6.

Examples of Competitive and Noncompetitive Assays

Class of Assay	Assay	Label Type
Competitive	Polyclonal RIA	Radioisotope
	Monoclonal RIA	Radioisotope
	Radioreceptor assay	Radioisotope
Noncompetitive	ELISA	Enzyme-mediated color change
	IRMA	Radioisotope
	ICMA	Emission of light
	IFMA	Emission of fluorescent light

ELISA, enzyme-linked immunosorbent assay; ICMA, immunochemiluminescent assay; IFMA, immunofluorimetric assay; IRMA, immunoradiometric assay; RIA, radioimmunoassay

Competitive immunoassays. The RIA is the most well known of the competitive immunoassays. Competitive immunoassays are so named because the hormone being measured competes for antibody binding sites with a labeled version of the hormone that is added to the sample during the assay. After separation of the antibody-bound hormone from the reaction, the laboratory quantifies the signal arising from the antibody-hormone complexes. Newer modifications of the RIA replace the radioactive label with an enzyme-mediated colorimetric change, a fluorescent label, or a light-emitting chemical reaction (Table 1-6).

Noncompetitive assays. Noncompetitive immunoassays (often called immunometric assays) also use the concept of antibody specificity to measure an analyte. Unlike RIAs, the analyte does not compete with a labeled version for scarce antibody binding sites. Instead, immunometric assays use two antibodies directed against different epitopes on the hormone to deliver improved specificity. These antibodies form a "sandwich" with the hormone in the middle and are often called sandwich assays.

Noncompetitive assays differ from each other in the type of signal used to detect the sandwich formation (Table 1-6). Unlike RIAs, most immunometric assays do not use a radioisotopic label. This is less expensive, in terms of both reagents and disposal of radioactive waste and allows for increased sensitivity of these assays.

Nonimmunoassay measurement techniques

An alternative to antibody-based assays are assays that rely on the physicochemical properties of a molecule to separate it from other substances in solution. Chromatography is one such technique. Typically, this takes the form of high performance liquid chromatography (HPLC). Additionally, mass spectrometry is rapidly gaining popularity as the technique of choice for measuring concentrations of certain hormones. Mass spectrometry can detect an array of molecules based on the ratio of their atomic mass to electric charge, termed the m/z ratio. Clinical laboratories often place two sequential mass spectrometry units in tandem to improve accuracy.

Sensitivity and specificity considerations

Although increasing analytic specificity sounds as if it should always be a good thing, in some cases it may not be the best choice. Many hormones exist in multiple forms, such as multiple differentially glycosylated forms of LH, FSH, and TSH. Each of these glycosylated forms has different bioactivity. The more specificity an assay offers, the fewer of these potentially bioactive forms will be detected. Because there is not one single bioactive form of the hormone, it may be more clinically relevant to measure the entire mixture of glycosylated versions via a less specific assay.

Calibration Standards

All endocrine assays require comparison of the measured hormone to a designated standard preparation of the hormone at a known concentration. These typically are international standards used throughout the world to calibrate assays so that an assay performed in North America gives similar results to an assay done in Europe or Asia. Obviously, the use of different assay techniques and different calibration standards causes confusion at the least and jeopardizes patient care at worst. This has led to efforts to harmonize measurement of many hormones around the world.

Preanalytic Variables

Because of the complex interplay of endocrine systems and the negative and positive feedback loops that are integral to endocrinology, there are many subtleties and nuances that the clinician must take into account when requesting and interpreting hormone assays. Collectively, these are known as "preanalytic variables" because they are factors that exist prior to the analysis of the hormone. Table 1-7 summarizes many of these.

Clinical optimization of testing

Many endocrine diseases are relatively rare, and symptoms of many endocrine diseases may also exist in other nonendocrine conditions. Because of the low prevalence of some endocrine disorders (low pretest probability), laboratory tests often have high false positive rates and low positive predictive values. This may easily result in an

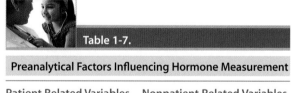

Table 1-7.

Preanalytical Factors Influencing Hormone Measurement

Patient Related Variables	Nonpatient Related Variables
Age	Plasma vs serum vs whole blood
Sex	Storage temperature
Pubertal status	Storage duration
Diurnal variation	Number of freeze/thaw cycles
Pulsatile secretion	Time before processing
Episodic secretion	EDTA vs heparin plasma
Nutritional status	Erroneous collection of timed
Posture	specimens
Exercise	
Pain/stress	
Medications	
Menstrual cycle	
Seasonal changes	
Body size	

EDTA, Ethylenediaminetetraacetic acid

erroneous diagnosis. The physician may increase the pretest probability by restricting testing to only those individuals with predetermined symptoms or physical findings or to those with clearly abnormal screening test results. An example of this would be restricting the use of growth hormone stimulation testing only to those patients who have a low height velocity or severe short stature. This group of patients is a population with a relatively high prevalence of growth hormone deficiency. If growth hormone stimulation testing is done on all children with heights at or below the fifth percentile, there will be many normal children who will have a low stimulated GH level (false positive test), because that population has a low prevalence of growth hormone deficiency.

Additionally, the physician should consider whether the results of a test would actually affect the management of the patient. It is not cost-effective to perform testing that will probably not be useful. One should avoid "shotgun testing," or ordering panels of tests without clear thought into the reasons for the tests. Not only might they be expensive, but the results may not be applicable to the patient and the chance of an erroneous result might be high. Many healthy individuals will have at least one lab value that falls outside of the reference interval if enough tests are performed. Labeling these people as having a disease may be inaccurate and harmful.

Reference Intervals

The term "reference interval" is preferred to "reference range" or "normal range," because it refers to the interval between the upper and lower limits of normal. However, values outside of the interval do not always indicate the presence of a disease. An example would be the value of 17-hydroxyprogesterone (17-OHP) in the diagnosis of

congenital adrenal hyperplasia (CAH). A full-term newborn may have a 17-OHP level of 300 ng/dL, which is above the reference interval. However, the diagnosis of CAH is unlikely, because infants with CAH typically have 17-OHP levels over 5000 ng/dL.

Additionally, just because a value falls within the reference interval does not mean that it is necessarily normal. Because of the dynamic relationship of hormones to other factors, including stimulating hormones and regulating substances, the clinician cannot interpret the concentration of many hormones without considering the levels of other compounds. For example, an insulin level within the reference interval is abnormal in the presence of hypoglycemia, when it should be low in a healthy person. As another example, the level of parathyroid hormone is often meaningless without a simultaneous calcium concentration (Figure 1-13). In a normal individual, calcium and PTH vary inversely, while in pathologic situations, they may vary directly. Although one would expect the level of PTH normally to be high in cases of hypocalcemia, individuals with hypoparathyroidism may have PTH concentrations that are either low or inappropriately normal. Hence, an isolated PTH level without knowledge of a simultaneous calcium level is not helpful. These examples illustrate that knowledge of a disease state and familiarity with the performance of a particular lab test in its diagnosis are critical.

In order to establish a reference interval, the clinical lab must assemble a large number of healthy individuals of ages, sexes, and stages of puberty that match the population that will have the test done clinically. This may be difficult to do, but failure to establish proper reference intervals makes the test less useful. Additionally, the assay used to establish the reference interval must be the same assay that is used clinically.

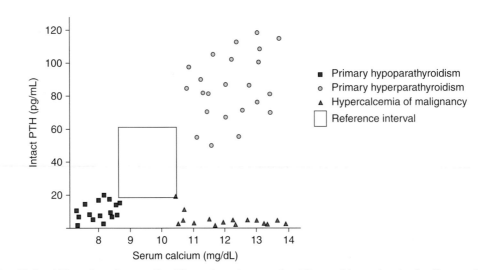

FIGURE 1-13 ■ Distinguishing primary hypoparathyroidism, primary hyperparathyroidism, and hypercalcemia of malignancy. The concentration of parathyroid hormone (PTH) may be normal in each of these conditions. They can only be distinguished from each other by comparing simultaneously obtained PTH and calcium concentrations.

If laboratory personnel subsequently refine the assay or replace it with a different assay, they must also replace the old reference interval or risk misclassifying patients due to false positive or false negative results. In some cases, the reference population may be difficult to define. For example, normal individuals who live in warm, sunny areas have higher levels of vitamin D precursors than normal individuals living in cold, rainy areas. Which population should be used to develop reference intervals? Laboratories must address questions such as this when developing these data.

REFERENCES

1. Woods KA, Camacho-Hubner C, Savage MO, Clark AJ. Intrauterine growth retardation and postnatal growth failure associated with deletion of the insulin-like growth factor I gene. *N Engl J Med.* 1996; 335:1363-1367.

2. Rochira V, Balestrieri A, Madeo B, Spaggiari A, Carani C. Congenital estrogen deficiency in men: a new syndrome with different phenotypes; clinical and therapeutic implications in men. *Mol Cell Endocrinol.* 2002; 193:19-28.

3. Farooqi S, O'Rahilly S. Genetics of obesity in humans. *Endocr Rev.* 2006; 27:710-718.

4. Rosenfeld R, Cohen P. Disorders of growth hormone/insulin-like growth factor secretion and action. In: Sperling M, ed. *Pediatric Endocrinology.* Philadelphia, PA: Saunders; 2002:211-288.

5. Jameson JL. Principles of endocrinology. In: Jameson JL, ed. *Harrison's Endocrinology.* New York, NY: McGraw-Hill; 2006:1-16.

6. Vassart G, Pardo L, Costagliola S. A molecular dissection of the glycoprotein hormone receptors. *Trends Biochem Sci.* 2004; 29:119-126.

7. Kauschansky A, Dickerman Z, Phillip M, Weintrob N, Strich D. Use of GnRH agonist and human chorionic gonadotrophin tests for differentiating constitutional delayed puberty from gonadotrophin deficiency in boys. *Clin Endocrinol (Oxf).* 2002; 56:603-607.

8. van Wyck JJ, Grumbach MM. Syndrome of precocious menstruation and galactorrhea in juvenile hypothyroidism: an example of hormonal overlap in pituitary feedback. *J Pediatr.* 1960; 57:416-435.

9. Molina PE. General principles of endocrine physiology. In: Molina PE, ed. *Endocrine Physiology.* New York, NY: McGraw-Hill; 2006.

10. Molina PE. Adrenal gland. In: Molina PE, ed. *Endocrine Physiology.* New York, NY: McGraw-Hill; 2006:123-156.

11. Molina PE. Thyroid gland. In: Molina PE, ed. *Endocrine Physiology.* New York, NY: McGraw-Hill; 2006:69-93.

12. Jameson JL, Weetman AP. Disorders of the thyroid gland. In: Jameson JL, ed. *Harrison's Endocrinology.* New York, NY: McGraw-Hill; 2006:71-111.

13. Murray TM, Rao LG, Divieti P, Bringhurst FR. Parathyroid hormone secretion and action: evidence for discrete receptors for the carboxyl-terminal region and related biological actions of carboxyl-terminal ligands. *Endocr Rev.* 2005; 26:78-113.

14. Molina PE. Endocrine pancreas. In: Molina PE, ed. *Endocrine Physiology.* New York, NY: McGraw-Hill; 2006:157-179.

15. Penning TM, Jin Y, Rizner TL, Bauman DR. Pre-receptor regulation of the androgen receptor. *Mol Cell Endocrinol.* 2008; 281:1-8.

16. Bringhurst FR, Demay MB, Krane SM, Kronenberg HM. Bone and mineral metabolism in health and disease. In: Jameson JL, ed. *Harrison's Endocrinology.* New York, NY: McGraw-Hill; 2006:411-430.

17. Denef C. Paracrinicity: the story of 30 years of cellular pituitary crosstalk. *J Neuroendocrinol.* 2008; 20:1-70.

18. Baloch Z, Carayon P, Conte-Devolx B, et al. Laboratory medicine practice guidelines. Laboratory support for the diagnosis and monitoring of thyroid disease. *Thyroid.* 2003;13:3-126.

19. LeRoith D. Clinical relevance of systemic and local IGF-I: lessons from animal models. *Pediatr Endocrinol Rev.* 2008; 5(2)(Suppl):739-743.

20. Elamin MB, Murad MH, Mullan R, et al. Accuracy of diagnostic tests for Cushing's syndrome: a systematic review and metaanalyses. *J Clin Endocrinol Metab.* 2008; 93:1553-1562.

21. Espiner EA, Richards AM, Yandle TG, Nicholls MG. Natriuretic hormones. *Endocrinol Metab Clin North Am.* 1995; 24:481-509.

22. Dunn A, Lo V, Donnelly S. The role of the kidney in blood volume regulation: the kidney as a regulator of the hematocrit. *Am J Med Sci.* 2007; 334:65-71.

23. Wren AM, Bloom SR. Gut hormones and appetite control. *Gastroenterology.* 2007; 132:2116-2130.

24. Franklin SL, Geffner ME. Precocious puberty secondary to topical testosterone exposure. *J Pediatr Endocrinol Metab.* 2003; 16:107-110.

25. Henley DV, Lipson N, Korach KS, Bloch CA. Prepubertal gynecomastia linked to lavender and tea tree oils. *N Engl J Med.* 2007; 356:479-485.

26. Hollowell JG, Staehling NW, Flanders WD, et al. Serum TSH, T(4), and thyroid antibodies in the United States population (1988 to 1994): National Health and Nutrition Examination Survey (NHANES III). *J Clin Endocrinol Metab.* 2002; 87:489-499.

CHAPTER 2

Normal Growth and Growth Disorders

Lindsey E. Nicol, David B. Allen, Paul Czernichow, and Philip Zeitler

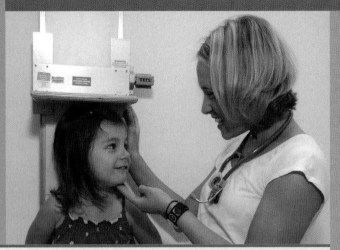

NORMAL GROWTH

Growth is a dynamic process influenced by many intrinsic and extrinsic factors that interplay to determine not only ultimate attained height but also the tempo and timing of height increase. Research continues to unravel hormonal and genetic complexities that account for variations in "normal" growth, and etiologies for disordered growth. Careful tracking of childhood growth is a sensitive indicator of health and well-being, and therefore an essential component of sound pediatric care. Detection of unexplained acceleration or deceleration in growth rate or tracking along a disparate percentile for family should prompt investigation. Endocrine disorders comprise an important, but only partial differential diagnosis of abnormal growth. This chapter discusses essential components of normal growth, the detection and evaluation of worrisome growth, and diagnosis and treatment of its multiple etiologies. The ultimate goal is to provide for those caring for children a conceptual framework for the assessment of and diagnostic approach to the child with abnormal growth.

Phases of Normal Growth

The rate of linear growth and the physiologic components regulating it vary with age. Conceptually, it is helpful to define growth as occurring in four discrete but congruent phases—prenatal, infancy, childhood, and adolescence (Figure 2-1). The range of growth velocities associated with these phases is depicted in Figure 2-2. Early detection of deviation from normal growth velocity is the key to prompt evaluation and diagnosis of a child with a growth abnormality.

Intrauterine growth occurs at a rate of approximately 1.2 to 1.5 cm per week, peaking at midstation (18 weeks) at 2.5 cm per week and slowing to 0.5 cm just before birth. There are both intrinsic and extrinsic factors contributing to prenatal growth and ultimate birth weight and length. Future growth patterns and genetic height tendencies, however, are not necessarily reflected at this stage. Hormonal control is largely caused by insulin and insulin-like growth factors 1 (IGF-1) and 2 (IGF-2). Maternal and uterine factors affecting fetal nutrition, insulin availability, and insulin sensitivity also have profound effects on intrauterine growth. By comparison, growth hormone (GH) and thyroid hormone have only modest effects on *in utero* somatic growth.

After birth the rate of growth is simultaneously the most rapid and rapidly slowing of a child's growth experience, peaking at approximately 25 cm per year then declining approximately 15 cm per year during the first 2 years of life. This rapid slowing in growth rate coincides with diminishing post-birth sex steroid production and influence of nutrition-responsive IGF effects to primary dependency on GH (Figure 2-1). Growth rate continues to steadily decelerate through 4 years of age when the child normally transitions to the childhood phase characterized by an average growth rate of 5 to 6 cm per year. Crossing of percentiles on the growth curve is not uncommon during the first 2 to 3 years of life. Genetic "channeling" (downward percentile crossing of a large baby born to short parents or upward crossing of small baby born to tall parents) is typically accomplished by 9 to 12 months of age. During 12 to 28 months, a tendency toward delayed growth is often manifest by growth rate deceleration that is more profound than average, resulting in down-channeling on the length-verses-age growth chart. After this time, growth should be expected to normally follow a consistent channel during the elementary school years. Depending upon the age of puberty onset, growth rate

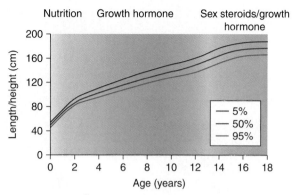

FIGURE 2-1 ■ Phases of childhood growth. (*Redrawn from Karlberg J. On the construction of the infancy-childhood-puberty growth standard.* Acta Paediatr Scand Supl. *1989;356:26.*)

may accelerate (early puberty) or decelerate (delayed puberty) compared to peers.

Adolescence is marked by a return of rapid growth with peak sustained growth rates of up to 15 cm per year. The timing and tempo of puberty and rate of skeletal maturation differs between boys and girls; ie, the pubertal growth spurt occurs earlier in girls than in boys, but boys will grow on average 13 cm taller prior to fusion of the epiphyseal growth plates. The greater average final height in boys is in part due to this extended time in the prepubertal phase allowing for a longer period of growth prior to plate fusion and partially due to the greater rate at which boys accrue height during their pubertal growth spurt.

The average onset of puberty not only differs between boys and girls but also amongst individuals of the same sex. The timing of sexual maturation plays a key role when assessing normalcy of growth rates and

formulating height prognoses, especially when comparing an individual to population averages. The relatively broad timing of the normal onset of puberty (boys ~9.5-14 years and girls ~7.5-13 years) can cause a "late bloomer" to move downward in growth percentiles relative to their peers who are entering into the accelerated growth phase of puberty. Most of the disparity in normal adult height is accounted for by differences in growth rate (and therefore height achieved) prior to puberty; thus, in most cases, age at onset of puberty (in contrast to height at the time of puberty onset) has relatively little effect on a child's final height.

Measurement

The most important tool in analysis of a child's growth is the plotting of accurate measurements on an appropriate growth chart. Although a seemingly simple process, correct positioning of a child during height or length assessment and accurate data recording is critical and should be done by a trained individual.

Children less than 2 years of age should be measured supine in full leg extension with the head in the "Frankfurt plane" (Figure 2-3). This is best done using a firm box with a head plate and a movable footboard. Once the child is over 2 years old and is physically able to stand on his/her own, a wall-mounted stadiometer is used for height measurement. The child, standing as erect as possible should have the back of his/her head; thoracic spine; buttocks; and heels, which are placed together, touching the vertical plane of the stadiometer (Figure 2-4). Both length and height should be measured three times

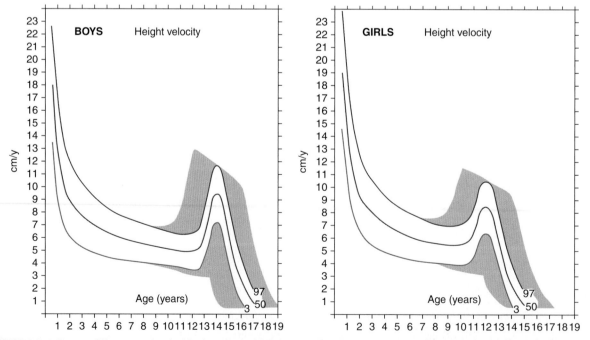

FIGURE 2-2 ■ Ranges of linear growth velocities in males and females. (*Modified from charts prepared by Tanner and Whitehouse, 1976, and reproduced with permission of Tanner JM and Castlemead Publications, Ward's Publishing Services, Herts, UK.*)

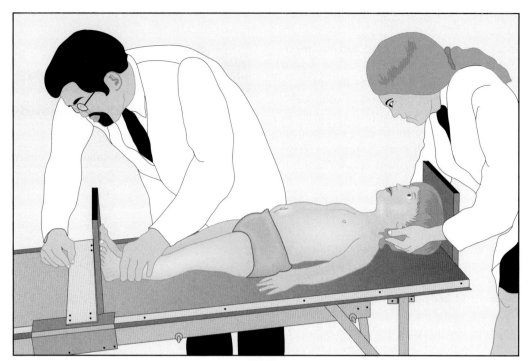

FIGURE 2-3 ■ Measurement of children less than 2 years of age should be obtained in the "Frankfurt plane" which places children in the supine position in full extension and other canthus of the eyes and the external auditory meatus perpendicular to the long axis of the trunk.

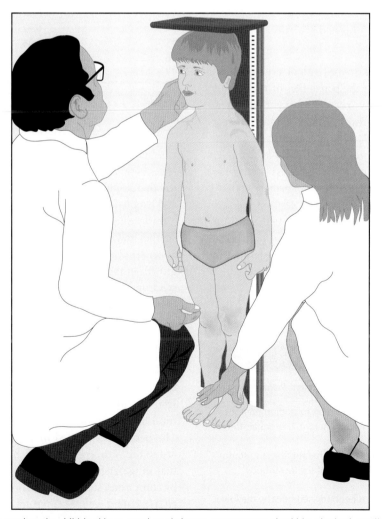

FIGURE 2-4 ■ After age 2 or when the child is able to stand on their own, measurement should be obtained standing erect against a wall-mounted stadiometer with the back of the head, thoracic spine, buttocks, and heels touching the vertical plane of the stadiometer.

with no more than 0.3 cm variation and the mean recorded. Serial measurements taken to assess growth velocity should be obtained by the same individual to eliminate variations between examiners or equipment. Recording of data over 9 to 12 months is preferable to minimize the effects of measurement error and seasonal variations. When 4 to 6 month intervals are used, extrapolation to an estimated "annual growth velocity" is necessary for comparison with growth velocity charts.

Body proportions, like growth velocity, also change with age; large-headed and short-limbed newborns gradually transition by late childhood to "adult" proportions, with arm spans roughly equivalent to height and upper-to-lower body segment ratios approximating one. Occipital-frontal head circumference, upper-to-lower (U/L) body segment ratio (Table 2-1), and arm span are useful in the assessment of short stature, tall stature, and markedly delayed or disproportionate growth. Detection of U/L ratio above expected is characteristic of short stature owing to some genetic conditions (eg, chondro-dysplasias, Turner syndrome), whereas a ratio below expected is observed in both short- (eg, spinal irradiation) and tall-statured (eg, Marfan syndrome) children.

Growth Charts

Measurement of the child (to the tenth of a centimeter) is plotted accurately against the percentiles of the population represented in the given chart. To construct a useful summation of a child's growth, at least annual measurement and plotting of height-for-age is recommended. Calculation and plotting of growth velocity for age on reference charts (www.cdc.gov/growthcharts) allows for comparison of short-term growth with normal standards.

Growth charts should always be selected based on gender, whether height or length will be plotted, and, if relevant, underlying syndrome. As noted above, both standing height- and length-for-age charts include data for

Table 2-1A.

Calculation of Upper-to-Lower Segment Ratio

1. Measure sitting height on block next to stadiometer. Subtract height of block from sitting height. This equals the height of the upper body segment.
2. Subtract the upper body segment height from the standing height. This equals the height of the lower body segment.
3. Divide the height of the upper body segment by the lower body segment.

Table 2-1B.

Upper to Lower Extremity Ratios in Boys and Girls

Age (Years)	Boys U/L Ratio	Girls U/L Ratio
Birth	1.70	1.70
1/2	1.62	1.60
1	1.54	1.52
1 1/2	1.50	1.46
2	1.42	1.41
2 1/2	1.37	1.34
3	1.35	1.30
3 1/2	1.30	1.27
4	1.24	1.22
4 1/2	1.22	1.19
5	1.19	1.15
6	1.12	1.10
7	1.07	1.06
8	1.03	1.02
9	1.02	1.01
10	0.99	1.00
11	0.95	0.90
12	0.98	0.99
13	0.97	1.00
14	0.97	1.01
15	0.95	1.01
16	0.99	1.01
17	0.99	1.01

Adapted from Wilkins L. The Diagnosis and Treatment of Endocrine Disorders in Childhood and Adolescence. IL: Springfield, Charles C. Thomas, Publisher; 1957.

children 2 to 3 years. Because of normal substantial differences between an individual's length and height, it is critical that height and length data only be plotted on height- and length-for-age growth charts, respectively. Otherwise, a misleading apparent discontinuity in the child's percentiles may prompt unnecessary concern and evaluation. Specialized growth charts are available for assessing growth in the context of genetic disorders such as Down syndrome (www.magicfoundation.org), Turner syndrome (www.magicfoundation.org), and achondroplasia.

In 2000 The National Center for Health Statistics (NCHS) (now part of the Centers for Disease Control and Prevention [CDC]) published charts based on cross-sectional data from physical exams across the entire country (via the National Health and Nutrition Examination Survey [NHANES]) better reflecting cultural and racial diversity (www.cdc.gov/growthcharts). The percentiles plotted in these charts range from the 3rd to the 97th. For children who are growing outside of that range, the degree of short stature can be described by computing standard deviation scores (SDS) from the NCHS data: *height SDS for age = (child's height − mean height for age and sex)/SD for height for age and sex.*

Although cross-sectional data is represented on standard height-for-age charts, and are useful in assessing growth during the infant and childhood phases, they neither take into account nor depict normal age variations in pubertal growth acceleration and growth termination. Height-for-age and growth velocity charts based on longitudinal data that also incorporate sexual development, such as those produced by Tanner and colleagues, are more useful when comparing late- or early-maturing adolescents to population standards (Figures 2-5 and 2-6). These charts help the examiner take into account the relatively broad timing of the pubertal onset and the acceleration of growth associated with the sexual development in an individual child.

Skeletal Maturation

Assessment of skeletal maturation provides information about the contribution of slowed or accelerated tempo of growth to a child's growth pattern, and is therefore

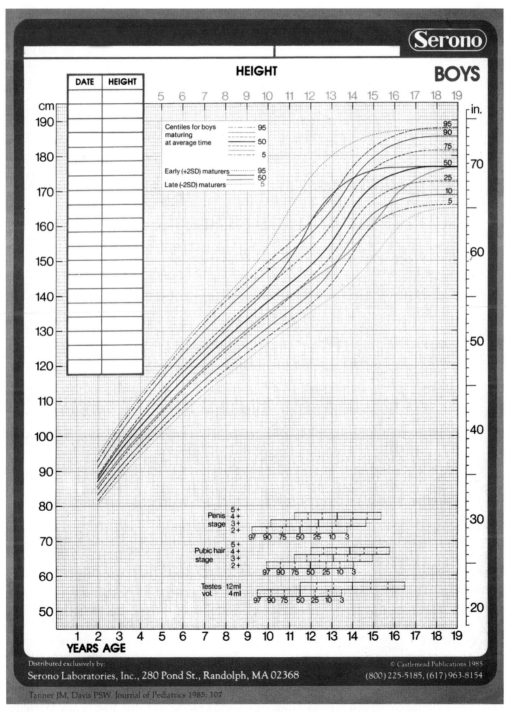

FIGURE 2-5 ■ Male height-for-age chart incorporating variations in timing of pubertal development.

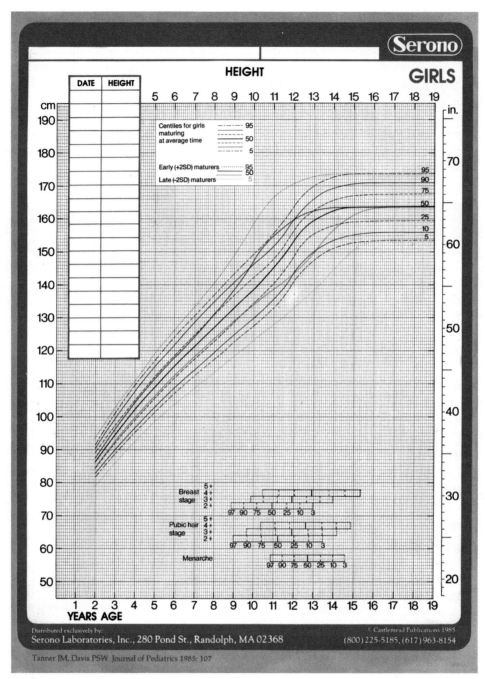

FIGURE 2-6 ■ Female height-for-age chart incorporating variations in timing of pubertal development.

another key component in the evaluation of an abnormally growing child. The multiple physiologic factors involved in growth plate elongation and maturation are still being unraveled, but it is currently well established that GH, IGF-1, thyroxine, and sex hormones play key roles in this process. While both androgens and estrogen are associated with acceleration in growth plate elongation and maturation, it is now known that estrogen has the predominating effect on this process. Estrogen (produced from androgens via the aromatase enzyme) controls the timing of the growth spurt, the conversion of proliferating into hypertrophic but senescent chondrocytes in the growth plate (and hence progress toward closure and bone mass accretion).[1] This phenomenon is an important pubertal process as 90% of skeletal mass is accrued by 18 years of age.

Skeletal maturation is assessed by examination of a "bone age"(BA) film, which is a radiograph of the left hand and wrist obtained after the neonatal period. Because the ossification of trabecular bone occurs in a predictable pattern, the evaluator can quantitatively assess the bone maturation of multiple ossification centers and compare it to standard male or female radiographs. The BA can then be compared to the patient's chronologic age as an indicator of growth tempo, remaining growth potential, and (with use of normative ± SD reference data) a judgment of statistically abnormal delay or advancement.

Although indispensable in the evaluation of growth, the use of a BA in practice also has its perils. The single film of the left hand is assumed to be representative of ossification centers in general and thus avoids radiation exposure required for radiographs of the entire skeleton. However, since the hand does not contribute to height, its accuracy in predicting growth potential can be limited. Most commonly, the radiograph is compared with the published standards of Greulich and Pyle (G-P),[2] a set of normal age-related standards that were collected from a small cohort of American white children between 1931 and 1942. Consequently, use of these dated standards has dwindling accuracy not only for the assessment of children in the twenty-first century but also in children from other ethnicities or children with intrinsic disease processes such as skeletal dysplasias. Nonetheless, G-P is still the most widely used skeletal development standard. An alternative method for assessing BA from radiographs of the left hand, involves a scoring system for developmentally identified stages of each of 20 individual bones, a technique that has been adapted for computerized assessment.[3] Further, assessment of BA can have substantial variability of intra-observer interpretation. It is thus optimal to have a consistent reviewer, especially in the context of serial BAs in the same patient.

Prediction of Adult Height and Parental Target Height

The extent of skeletal maturation can be employed to predict ultimate height potential. Several methods have been developed for the prediction of adult height (PAH) (Table 2-2). All are based on the premise that delay in BA relative to the chronologic age is proportionate to growth potential remaining. For each method, as BA advances the prediction of adult height becomes more accurate. The most commonly used is one developed by Bayley and Pinneau and is based on Greulich and Pyle's *Radiographic Atlas of Skeletal Development.* This calculation takes into account the BA, chronologic age, and current height and a semiquantitative allowance for chronological age (Table 2-3). Importantly, all methods of calculating PAH are based on data from normal children, and none has been documented to be accurate in children with growth abnormalities.

Assessment of the PAH is frequently used in conjunction with the mid-parental target height (MPH), which takes into account the familial genetic factors in growth and height potential. The MPH calculation is the average of the mother's and father's height adjusted by the average height difference of 13 cm between the sexes. Thus, if calculating the MPH of a female patient, 13 cm is subtracted from the father's height before it is averaged with the mother's. For the evaluation of a male, 13 cm is added to the mother's height before averaging the parents' heights. Like the PAH, this is a broad estimation (ie, two-SD range for this calculation is ±10 cm) but it can be useful in comparing a child's growth to that of their parents and siblings. The MPH is also useful for identifying whether a child's current and predicted growth trajectory differs from that expected; that is, significant disparity in the child's growth percentile (ie, ±10 cm) from the MPH percentile should prompt further investigation (most often revealing constitutional early or delayed growth and development) even if the child plots within the normal percentile range. Additionally, when there is a relatively large disparity between the parents' heights the calculated MPH

Table 2-2.

Methods for Prediction of Adult Height

Method	Parameters of Assessment	Reference
TW2	Height, BA, chronological age, pubertal height, pubertal bone age increments during previous year	Tanner J, et al. Assessment of skeletal maturity and prediction of adult height (TW2 Method). New York, Academic Press, 1983.
RWT	Height, BA, chronological age, MPH	Roche A, Wainer H, Thissen D. The RWT method for the prediction of adult height. *Pediatrics* (1975).
Khamis-Roche	Multiple regression analyses using height, weight, birth measurement, and MPH data	Khamis H, Roche A. Predicing adult stature without using skeletal age: The Khamis and Roche method. *Pediatrics* (1994).
Bayley and Pinneau	Height, BA, semiquantitative chronological age	Bayley N, Pinneau S. Tables for predicting adult height from skeletal age: Revised for use with the Greulich-Pyle hand standards. *J Pediatr* (1952).

Table 2-3.

Prediction of Adult Stature: Fraction of Adult Height Attained at Each Bone Age

Bone Age (year-month)	Girls			Boys		
	Delayed	Average*	Advanced	Delayed	Average*	Advanced
6-0	0.733	0.720		0.680		
6-3	0.742	0.729		0.690		
6-6	0.751	0.738		0.700		
6-9	0.763	0.751		0.709		
7-0	0.770	0.757	0.712	0.718	0.695	0.670
7-3	0.779	0.765	0.722	0.728	0.702	0.676
7-6	0.788	0.772	0.732	0.738	0.709	0.683
7-9	0.797	0.782	0.742	0.747	0.716	0.689
8-0	0.804	0.790	0.750	0.756	0.723	0.696
8-3	0.813	0.801	0.760	0.765	0.731	0.703
8-6	0.823	0.810	0.771	0.773	0.739	0.709
8-9	0.836	0.821	0.784	0.779	0.746	0.715
9-0	0.841	0.827	0.790	0.786	0.752	0.720
9-3	0.851	0.836	0.800	0.794	0.761	0.728
9-6	0.858	0.844	0.809	0.800	0.769	0.734
9-9	0.866	0.853	0.819	0.807	0.777	0.741
10-0	0.874	0.862	0.828	0.812	0.784	0.747
10-3	0.884	0.874	0.841	0.816	0.791	0.753
10-6	0.896	0.884	0.856	0.819	0.795	0.758
10-9	0.907	0.896	0.870	0.821	0.800	0.763
11-0	0.918	0.906	0.883	0.823	0.804	0.767
11-3	0.922	0.910	0.887	0.827	0.812	0.776
11-6	0.926	0.914	0.891	0.832	0.818	0.786
11-9	0.929	0.918	0.897	0.839	0.827	0.800
12-0	0.932	0.922	0.901	0.845	0.834	0.809
12-3	0.942	0.932	0.913	0.852	0.843	0.818
12-6	0.949	0.941	0.924	0.860	0.853	0.828
12-9	0.957	0.950	0.935	0.869	0.863	0.839
13-0	0.964	0.958	0.945	0.880	0.876	0.850
13-3	0.971	0.967	0.955		0.890	0.863
13-6	0.977	0.974	0.963		0.902	0.875
13-9	0.981	0.978	0.968		0.914	0.890
14-0	0.983	0.980	0.972		0.927	0.905
14-3	0.986	0.983	0.977		0.938	0.918
14-6	0.989	0.986	0.980		0.948	0.930
14-9	0.992	0.988	0.983		0.958	0.943
15-0	0.994	0.990	0.986		0.968	0.958
15-3	0.995	0.991	0.988		0.973	0.967
15-6	0.996	0.993	0.990		0.976	0.971
15-9	0.997	0.994	0.992		0.980	0.976
16-0	0.998	0.996	0.993		0.982	0.980
16-3	0.999	0.996	0.994		0.985	0.983
16-6	0.999	0.997	0.995		0.987	0.985
16-9	0.9995	0.998	0.997		0.989	0.988
17-0	1.00	0.999	0.998		0.991	0.990
17-3					0.993	
17-6		0.9995	0.9995		0.994	
17-9					0.995	
18-0		1.00			0.996	
18-3					0.998	
18-6					1.00	

Note that percentage of adult height attained at a given BA is influenced by whether BA is advanced or delayed; e.g. an 11 y.o, female with an "average" BA of 11 has attained 90.6% of adult height, a 12-year old female with a "delayed" BA of 11 has attained 91.8%, and a 10-year old female with an "advanced" BA of 11 has attained 88.3% of adult height, respectively. Thus, remaining growth potential at a given BA is slightly greater when the BA is achieved at a younger, rather than older age.
Table derived from Post EM Richman RA based on the data of Bayley and Pinneau (1952). These tables have been organized in an easy-to-use slide-rule format ("Adult Height Predictor," copyright 1987, Ron G Rosenfeld).
Copyright 2005 by Charles C Thomas, Publisher, LTD.

becomes less informative. While a child's growth can be disproportionately influenced by the pattern of one parent, statistical reassessment of population averages show that the final height of offspring tend to regress toward the mean. If this is not taken into account, the shorter calculated MPH may be used to inappropriately explain the short stature of a child.

Endocrine Regulation of Growth

Regulation of growth is provided by a complex interplay of stimulatory and inhibitory hormones influenced by afferent messages from the central nervous system (CNS) and periphery. The function of these systems reflects genetic programming, the nutritional and developmental state of the body, and the presence of interfering processes. Thus, evaluation for "endocrine" causes of abnormal growth includes, in addition to GH/IGF, gonadotropin/sex steroid, and thyroid function axes, an exploration for nutrition deficiencies, psychosocial stress, and occult organ dysfunction (eg, renal or gastrointestinal disease).

Regulation of somatic growth by endocrine systems varies significantly during a child's growing lifetime. During fetal life, GH is secreted readily, but seems relatively unimportant for fetal growth compared to the effects of nutrition, insulin, and non-GH dependent IGF influences on growth. Insulin's important role in fetal growth is highlighted by states of insulin excess (eg, maternal hyperglycemia stimulating fetal hyperinsulinemia) leading to overgrowth, while insulin deficiency (eg, pancreatic agenesis) or resistance (eg, leprechaunism) leads to growth restriction.

During the first few months of infancy, nutritional adequacy continues to exert strong influence on linear growth, so that infantile GH deficiency may not always be manifest by growth failure at this time. Thyroid hormone is a major contributor to postnatal growth but, like GH, it is of relatively little importance to growth of the fetus. On the other hand, postnatal hypothyroidism can cause profound growth failure and virtual arrest of skeletal maturation. In addition to having direct effects on epiphyseal cartilage, thyroid hormones appear necessary for normal GH secretion. Patients with hypothyroidism have decreased spontaneous GH secretion and blunted responses to GH stimulation tests.

Childhood growth is primarily regulated by nutrition, GH, and thyroid hormone. Gradually declining growth rates during childhood may be matched by declining laboratory evidence of GH secretion, particularly when pubertal onset is delayed. This phenomenon can create difficulty in distinguishing physiologic growth deceleration from true GH deficiency during the immediate prepubertal years. Growth during adolescence is regulated as much by estrogen and androgen as it is by nutrition, GH, and thyroid hormone. Gonadal steroids produce a growth spurt partially by enhancing GH secretion (via aromatization of testosterone to estrogen in the CNS), and also by stimulating IGF-1 production and chondrocyte proliferation in the growth plate directly. In addition, puberty-associated increases in serum insulin levels may independently contribute to the faster pubertal linear growth rate. Nevertheless, without GH an adolescent will not have a normal pubertal growth spurt.

During late adolescence and adulthood, GH continues to have important metabolic effects. These include: (1) stimulation of bone remodeling (by stimulating both osteoclast and osteoblast activity) with ultimate net increase in bone mass; (2) stimulation of lipolysis and fat utilization for energy expenditure; (3) growth and preservation of lean tissue mass and muscle function; and (4) facilitation of normal lipid metabolism. Sex-specific dimorphism in these metabolic effects, reflecting underlying sex steroid-mediated differences in GH sensitivity and secretion, become apparent during adolescence, leading to women having higher GH levels than men. Beyond linear growth, normal production of GH is needed for the adolescent to accomplish normal body composition maturation. Adults continue to secrete GH pulses, but the amplitude decreases with age, returning to a pattern more characteristic of the prepubertal child in early adulthood followed by a gradual but steady decline with aging.[4]

The GH and IGF axis

Growth hormone synthesis and secretion. While optimal growth and development occur only with the normal production and modulation of multiple hormones, the predominant common pathway for the endocrine regulation of childhood somatic growth is the GH/IGF-1 axis. GH synthesis and secretion occurs in/from the anterior pituitary (adenohypophysis). The gland itself originates from the floor of the primitive pharyngeal epithelium known as Rathke pouch. This in-folding occurs around the fifteenth to twentieth day of gestation and subsequently migrates caudally to meet a neural ectoderm extension from the floor of the midbrain that will develop into posterior pituitary. These two distinct embryological tissues form to create the pituitary gland, although the functions of the two halves remain distinct.

GH is produced in the somatotrophs of the anterior pituitary and is a single chain 191 amino acid, 22 kDa protein. GH synthesis and release starts with the stimulating affects of growth hormone-releasing hormone (GHRH). This neuropeptide is produced in neurons that have their bodies in the ventral arcuate nucleus of the hypothalamus and axons projecting into the median eminence, allowing the GHRH to be secreted into the portal system of the pituitary stalk. GHRH stimulates a cAMP–protein kinase A activation pathway causing an influx of calcium ions into the somatroph and subsequent synthesis and release of GH. Counter-regulation of GH release is directed by somatostatin SRIH (somatotropin release inhibitory hormone), produced in the periventricular nucleus of the hypothalamus and also released into the same portal system as GHRH. SRIH acts on the somatotroph K channels, preventing the outflow of K ions needed to accommodate the influx of positively charged calcium ions and subsequently blunts the release of GH.

It is the shifting balance between these two neuropeptides that determines the pulsatile release of GH. In general, GHRH stimulates release of GH while SRIH affects the timing and amplitude of the GH pulses. GHRH release during SRIH secretions allows for GH syntheses but not release from the somatotrophs. During times of decreased SRIH tone, stored GH is released in a pulse. Both GHRH and GH work in a negative feedback loop to stimulate SRIH release and GH itself, in a short feedback loop, will inhibit GHRH.

The production of SRIH and GHRH are influenced by multiple factors including other neuropeptides, downstream products of GH such as IGF-1, hormones such as cortisol and thyroxine, physical activity, sleep, fasting states, and dopamine agonists. During stage IV sleep, SRIH activity is low while GHRH activity persists, resulting in nocturnal pulses of GH that comprise the majority of growth-promoting stimulus during childhood. These pulses increase in both amplitude and frequency during puberty when the effect of estrogen in both males and females augments the release of GH. GHRH is also stimulated by triiodothyronine (T_3) and ghrelin, a synthetic hexapeptide secretagogue capable of binding a unique receptor and stimulating GH secretion at the hypothalamic and pituitary level. Ghrelin is secreted primarily from the stomach during fasting, implicating a role in the coordination of caloric balance. Persistent glucocorticoid excess negatively influences linear growth at the CNS level through inhibition of GHRH and augmentation of SRIH. This complex system of stimulatory and inhibitory feedback loops, which modulate GH production and secretion, is depicted in Figure 2-7.

Growth hormone action. In serum, GH is either free or bound to the GH-binding protein (GHBP), which is derived from cleavage of the extracellular portion of the GH receptor (GHR). GHBP in human plasma binds GH with high specificity and affinity but with relatively low capacity, as about 45% of circulating GH is bound. GHBP prolongs the half-life of GH, presumably by reducing its glomerular filtration, and modulates its binding to the GH receptor. Like GH, GHBP concentrations vary with age, estrogen levels, body mass index, and feeding states. At the target tissue cell membranes, steps in free GH action include: (1) binding of GH to the membrane-associated GH receptor; (2) sequential dimerization of the GH receptor through binding to each of two specific sites on GH; (3) interaction of the GH receptor with Janis

kinase 2 (JAK2); (4) tyrosine phosphorylation of both JAK2 and the GH receptor; (5) changes in cytoplasmic and nuclear protein phosphorylation and dephosphorylation; and (6) stimulation of target gene transcription. JAK2-dependent phosphorylation and activation have been demonstrated for many cytoplasmic signaling molecules which, after forming homodimers or heterodimers, translocate to the nucleus, bind DNA, and activate transcription of growth-promoting products, including IGF-1. Particularly in the liver, activation of GHRs also initiates the signaling pathway for the production of IGF-1 binding protein 3 (IGF BP3) and the acid-labile subunit (ALS). These components combine to form 150 kDa complex that transports IGF-1 in the blood and prolongs its half-life. Precisely how these varied pathways mediate the various anabolic and metabolic actions of GH remains to be elucidated.[5] (See Figure 2-8.)

Although, most measurable IGF-1 comes from the liver, GHRs are expressed in multiple tissues (including growth plates) providing a pathway for GH to have effects on growth independent of the hepatic production of IGF-1. GHRs are found in the epiphysis, the prechondrocytes of the cartilage precursor cells, and in the bone marrow. At these locations, autocrine and paracrine action of locally produced IGF-1 is the prime stimulator of somatic growth and elongation of bone. In other tissues, GH also has important body composition effects resulting in the promotion of lean mass accretion. GH provides counter-regulation to insulin, leading to an increase in lipolysis and inhibition of lipogenesis in adipose tissue as well as increase in amino acid transport and nitrogen retention in muscle.

Age-related issues in GH secretion. The connection between the hypothalamus and the pituitary portal system is developing by 9 weeks of fetal life and somatotrophs can be identified in the anterior pituitary. By 12 weeks of life the regulatory effects of SRIH and GHRH are in place. GH is secreted readily from this point in gestation on but, as mentioned earlier, plays only a small role in fetal linear and weight growth. A number of recently identified genetic mutations can result in GH deficiency, including HESX-1 (thought to be linked with septo-optic dysplasia), LHX-3 and 4 (pituitary hypoplasia), Pit-1 or PROP 1 (combined pituitary hormone deficiency), and GH1 (isolated GH deficiency). For a more extensive list see Table 2-4.

Immediately after birth GH levels are normally high through the first few days of life, with random values greater than 20 ng/mL being common. Since GH provides insulin counter-regulation (in conjunction with cortisol) during infancy, and its release is normally stimulated by hypoglycemia, a GH level below 20 ng/ml concurrent with hypoglycemia strongly suggests GH deficiency (GHD). In an infant with hypoglycemia, a simultaneous GH level below 20 ng/mL strongly suggests GH deficiency (GHD). GH is not the key regulator of linear growth velocity during

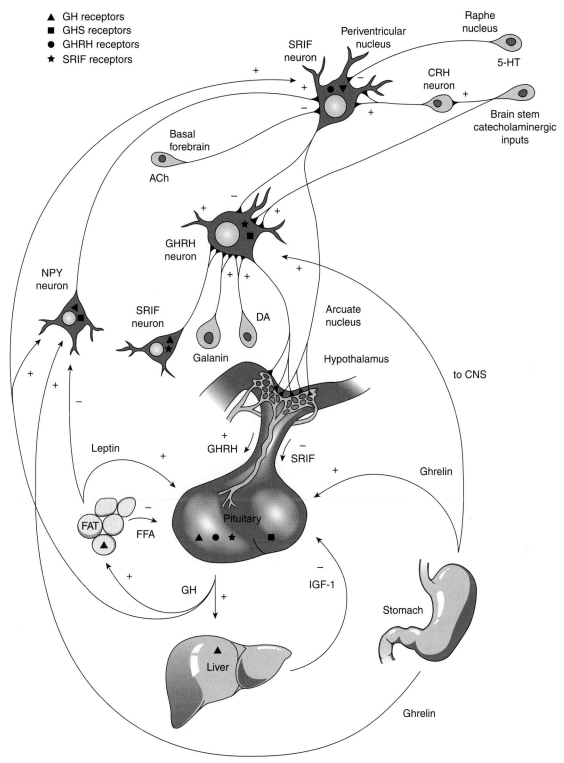

FIGURE 2-7 ■ Stimulatory and inhibitory feedback loops that modulate GH secretion. FFA, free fatty acids; NPY, neuropeptide Y; GABA, galanin, Á-aminobutyric acid; 5-HT, type 1D receptors; CRH, corticotropin-releasing hormone; Ach, acetylcholine; CNS, central nervous system; DA, dopamine. (*Redrawn with permission from Cone et al, 2003.*)

the primarily nutrition-dependent phase of very early infancy. Consequently, while neonates with hypopituitarism may show slowed linear growth resulting from GHD in the first few months of life, isolated GHD manifesting as growth failure may also not be detected clinically until 18 to 24 months of age.

During childhood, most GH secretion occurs in 2 to 5 discrete pulses during sleep. Because of this secretion pattern, GH is usually undetectable on random samples. A wide range of spontaneous GH secretion has been observed in both normal growing and short children, so testing this has not proven diagnostically useful. Since

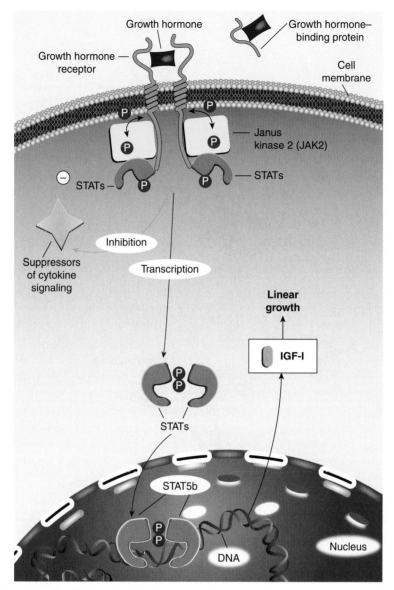

FIGURE 2-8 ■ GH Intracellular Signaling. (*Adapted from Eugster EA, Pescovitz OH. New revelations about the role of STATs in stature. N Engl J Med. 2003 Sep 18; 349(12):1110-1112.*)

the diagnosis of GHD usually does not connote a complete deficiency, affected children will often continue to grow, but at a sub-normal rate that results in a gradual downward crossing of percentile lines and slow decline in height SD.

During adolescence, a rise in estrogen leads to an increase in GH secretion and IGF-1 production (directly and indirectly). While this occurs in both sexes, higher levels of GH are typically observed in pubertal females, reflecting not only higher estrogen levels, but also the appearance of sex-specific differences in GH-induced hepatic IGF-1 production and feedback. GH pulses during the adolescent phase increase in frequency to occur both during the day and night and have higher amplitudes. GH bioavailability is also increased since production of its binding protein, GHBP, remains stable.

The IGF system. Two insulin-like-growth factors have been identified: IGF-1 and IGF-2. IGF-1 is a 70 amino acid peptide that is slightly alkaline and its sequence is encoded on the long arm of chromosome 12. IGF-2 has 67 amino acids, is slightly acidic, and encoded on the short arm of chromosome 11. Both peptides are composed of two amino chains connected by disulfide bonds. They share 45 amino acid positions and have approximately 50% homology to insulin. Depending on the tissue, there are multiple different messenger ribonucleic acid (mRNA) sequences as a result of variable splicing and regulation of transcription of the IGF-1 and 2 genes, adding another layer of sophistication to the affects of IGF expression and thus its growth effects.

The type 1 IGF receptor binds both IGF proteins with high affinity and both IGF-1 and 2 activate the tyrosine kinase stimulatory intracellular cascade

Table 2-4.

Genes Involved in Pituitary Hormone Deficiencies*

Gene	Protein Function	Human Phenotype	Inheritance
HESX1	Early developmental transcription factor (repressor)	Variable septo-optic dysplasia gene (SOD), combined pituitary hormone deficiency, idiopathic hormone deficiency (IGHD), ectopic posterior pituitary (EPP)	Dominant or recessive
SOX2	Early developmental transcription factor	Hypogonadotropic hypogonadism, anterior pituitary hypoplasia (APH), bilateral, abnormal corpus callosum, anophthalmia/microphthalmia, esophageal atresia, sensorineural hearing loss, learning difficulties	De novo
SOX3	Early developmental transcription factor	IGHD, mental retardation, APH, infundibular hypoplasia, EPP, midline abnormalities	X-linked recessive
GLI2	Early developmental transcription factor	Holoprosencephaly, hypopituitarism, craniofacial abnormalities, polydactyly, single nares, single central incisor, partial agenesis of the corpus callosum	Dominant
LHX3	Early developmental transcription factor	GH, TSH, gonadotropin deficiency, with pituitary hypoplasia, short, rigid cervical spine	Recessive
LHX4	Early developmental transcription factor	GH, TSH, cortisol deficiency, persistent craniopharyngeal canal and abnormal cerebellar tonsils	Dominant
PROP1	Terminal cell differentiation transcription factor	GH, TSH, prolactin, and gonadotropin deficiency, evolving adrenocorticotropic hormone deficiency, enlarged pituitary with later involution	Recessive
POU1F1	Terminal cell differentiation transcription factor	Variable APH with GH, TSH, and prolactin deficiencies	Recessive

*Adapted from Kelberman D, Dattani M. Hypopituitarism oddities: Congenital causes. Horm Res. 2007;68(5):138-144.

through the type 1 IGF receptor. It is through this receptor that the mitogenic and metabolic actions of IGF proteins are mediated. Like the GHR, the IGF receptor is expressed in a multitude of tissues. The type 1 receptor is made up of two transmembrane α subunits forming the IGF binding sites and two intracellular β subunits that make up the signal transduction component of the receptor. The type 2 IGF receptor only binds IGF-2 with high affinity and does not exert effects through the same tyrosine kinase activation pathway. The downstream effects of activating the type 2 receptor are more antimitogenic than growth stimulating. This receptor pathway may be involved in regulating the inhibitory effects of retinoids and modulation of growth inhibition of the IGF system.

In addition to the IGF receptors, the IGFBPs are also modulators of IGF action. Six IGFBPs are produced in response to GH stimulation and they bind 70% to 80% of IGF-1 and 2. They serve as carrier proteins for the IGF peptides, transport the IGFs to target cells, and modulate the interaction of the IGFs with their cell surface receptors. Highly conserved cysteine-rich regions of these carrier proteins are the sites of the disulfide bridges that play a key role in the structure and formation of the IGF binding site. When compared to IGF receptors, IGFBPs have a higher affinity for the IGF peptides. Bioavailability of free

IGFs appear dependent on the action of IGFBP proteases.[6] (See Figure 2-9.)

Developmental changes in IGFs. The IGF-1 levels vary substantially throughout life. At birth, the levels are relatively low (approximately 30%-50% of adult levels) and are influenced by gestational age and weight. Levels subsequently rise during childhood, reaching adult levels at the onset of puberty. Under the influence of gonadal steroids, both directly and indirectly via the increase in GH pulsations, IGF-1 levels will increase to 2 to 3 times the adult range. During this phase of growth the levels of IGF-1 more closely correlate with Tanner stage and BA rather than chronologic age. IGF-2 levels show less age variation and by 1 year of age, achieve adult levels with little subsequent decline.

The IGF system plays a central role in the regulation of fetal growth. IGF-1 levels in fetal and cord blood correlate with fetal size, and are reduced in SGA infants. Since deletion of the *IGF-1* gene leads to profound intrauterine growth retardation, normal local levels of IGF-1, largely independent of GH regulation, appear necessary for normal growth *in utero*. Animal studies suggest that IGF-2 is very important for gestational growth, but unlike IGF-1, does not appear to play a critical role in post-natal somatic growth. While IGFBPs are

The GH-IGF-IGFBP axis

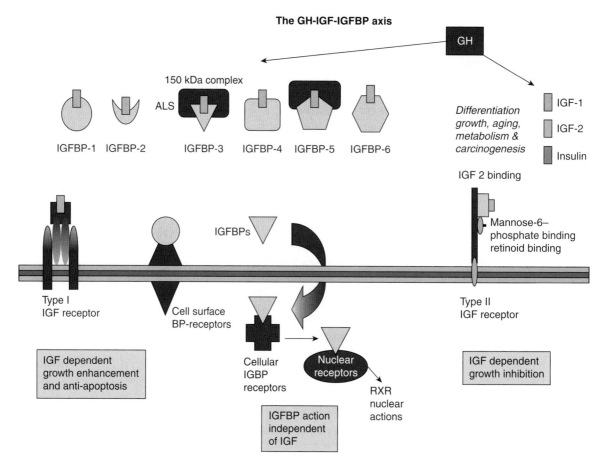

FIGURE 2-9 ■ The GH-IGF-IGFBP axis is shown with its ligands, binding proteins, receptors, and signaling pathways. (*Adapted from Cohen P. Overview of the IGF-1 system.* Horm Res. *2006; 65(1):3-8.*)

identifiable in the fetus and newborn, levels of IGFBP3 and ALS, the primary carriers of IGF-1 in postinfancy life, are low. Thus, it appears that fetal IGF-1 production is linked more tightly to nutrient supply and to insulin secretion than to GH regulation (Figure 2-10).

APPROACH TO THE CHILD WITH WORRISOME GROWTH

Normal growth rate is an important indicator of childhood. Therefore, proper growth assessment is a key component of pediatric care, requiring both careful measurement of length or height at discrete points and tracking of growth velocity over time. While accurate plotting of isolated linear growth measurements on growth charts will easily identify children who are abnormally short or tall in stature (ie, whose height falls outside + ~2 SD, <3rd or >97th percentile), early detection of a growth disorder frequently requires appreciation of both subtle changes in growth velocity or recognition that a growth pattern, while within the statistical normal range, is divergent from that expected for a particular child.

Evaluation of the child with worrisome growth begins by systematically answering the following questions:

(1) Is the growth rate normal or abnormally slow or fast? (2) What is the relationship between the linear growth rate and poor, normal, or excess weight gain? (3) What intrinsic, familial, or other genetic factors may be influencing this child's growth? (4) What is the family history for pubertal onset and age of adult height attainment, and is there BA evidence for delayed or accelerated growth? Since the normal range within the population is fairly wide, skillful and sensitive analysis that utilizes the answers to these questions can help in determining a more narrowly defined "expected" normal range for a specific child. Appreciation of the influences of superimposed factors in a single child usually provides either rationale for reassurance and observation, or reason to pursue diagnostic workup and possible treatment.

Is the growth rate normal or abnormally slow or fast? Growth rate is the change in height measured on separate occasions relative to the time elapsed. The normal range of growth velocities varies markedly with age, skeletal age, and pubertal stage. Growth rates estimated from measurements separated by months can be annualized to centimeters/year to allow comparison with normal growth rates charts for

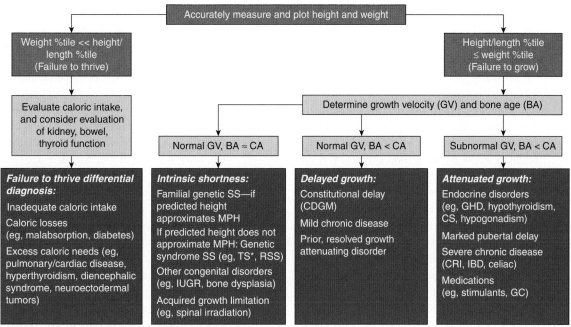

FIGURE 2-10A ■ Conceptual approach to the differential diagnosis of worrisome growth. Downward crossing of percentiles, height less than 3rd percentile, or height inappropriate for family, or abnormal body proportions. %tile, growth curve percentile; GV, growth velocity; BA, bone age; CA, chronological age; SS, short stature; TS, Turner syndrome; RSS, Russell Silver syndrome; IUGR, intrauterine growth restriction; CDGM, constitutional delay in growth and maturation; GHD, growth hormone deficiency; CS, Cushing syndrome; CRI, chronic renal insufficiency; IBD, inflammatory bowel disease.

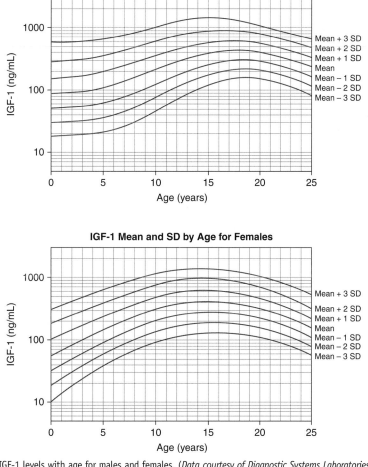

FIGURE 2-10B ■ Changes in IGF-1 levels with age for males and females. (*Data courtesy of Diagnostic Systems Laboratories, Inc., Webster, Texas.*).

age (Figure 2-2). To more precisely evaluate whether a growth rate is normal in children with delayed or accelerated growth patterns, determination of skeletal age and of "growth rate for BA" can also be helpful. Consistently diminished growth velocity becomes manifest as downward crossing of percentiles on the height or length for age growth chart, a situation that demands evaluation even when height remains within the normal range. Thus, careful attention to growth rate, and not only height, facilitates early detection of growth-slowing disorder in taller and shorter children alike.

What is the relationship between the linear growth rate and poor, normal, or excess weight gain? Both poor nutrition and excess caloric intake can influence linear growth. Particularly, early in life it is diagnostically helpful to distinguish between "failure to thrive" (ie, weight deficit > length deficit) (Figure 2-11) and "failure to grow" (length deficit > weight deficit), since the former should prompt initial evaluation of nutritional problems or undiagnosed illness, while the latter is more typical of growth-retarding endocrine disorders. On the other hand, overnutrition is a common cause of linear growth acceleration, with weight gain that precedes and exceeds in magnitude the increase in linear growth percentiles, usually accompanied by commensurate advancement in skeletal maturation and onset of puberty particularly in females (Figure 2-12). *Endocrine causes of obesity such as hypothyroidism and cortisol excess need not be considered when growth rate acceleration accompanies weight gain.*

What intrinsic, familial, or other genetic factors may be influencing this child's growth? Intrinsic and genetic influences on childhood growth rate and height attainment encompass a wide array of factors whose distinctive underlying physiologies are slowly yet steadily being unraveled. The parental contribution to a child's expected height percentile range is estimated using the MPH calculation described earlier. Important caveats include (1) diminishing accuracy of this calculation as parental height percentiles become more disparate and (2) the assumption that a parent's height represents his/her own genetic "potential" (ie, was not affected by an early life growth-restricting influence.) An extended family history is helpful in revealing sporadic growth disorders (eg, short-limb tendencies) that may not manifest in every generation. Determination of body proportions, in particular the upper-to-lower body segment ratio (corrected for age and BA, as this measurement normally varies throughout growth and development), may aid in the identification of some causes of short (eg, hypochondroplasia, Turner syndrome) or tall (eg, Klinefelter and Marfan syndromes) stature. Awareness of birth length and weight to determine whether the child was born small for gestational age (SGA) is critical to assess whether restriction of intrauterine growth may be persisting into childhood. Careful physical examination may detect stigmata of known chromosomal disorders associated with short (eg, Turner, Noonan, Down, Russell-Silver syndromes) or tall (eg, Marfan, Klinefelter, Soto [early in childhood] syndromes) stature.

What is the family history for pubertal onset and age of adult height attainment, and is there BA evidence for delayed or accelerated growth? The range of normal variations in "tempo" of childhood growth is not captured on most standard height-versus-age growth curves, but determination of this dimension is indispensable to evaluation of worrisome growth (variations in which determines the time required for an individual child to complete his/her growth). Differences in the time required to progress toward pubertal maturation and ultimate growth potential are influenced by biological variations in GH secretion and action, variations in suppression of the hypothalamic-pituitary-gonadal axis and its subsequent reawakening at pubertal onset during infancy and its subsequent reawakening at pubertal onset, and other factors (see Figures 2-5 and 2-6). Family history of early or late puberty or attainment of adult height is helpful in assessing the likelihood that a similar growth pattern in the child represents a normal variation. Helpful questions to elicit this history from parents include height at the beginning of high school, the maternal onset of menses, and continued paternal growth after high school. Objectively, the degree to which delay or acceleration in the growth process is contributing to a child's position on the growth curve is estimated by examination of BA.

The astute clinician assembles this information and then asks: "to what extent do the historical and physical examination findings explain the child's growth pattern and position on the growth curve?" Commonly, the process outlined above reveals historical and familial short or tall stature traits that, when combined with tendencies toward delayed or accelerated tempo of growth and pubertal development, provide a reasonable explanation. Further evaluation of the differential diagnosis outlined below, however, should be prompted by

2 to 20 years: Girls
Stature-for-age and Weight-for-age percentiles

NAME _____

RECORD # _____

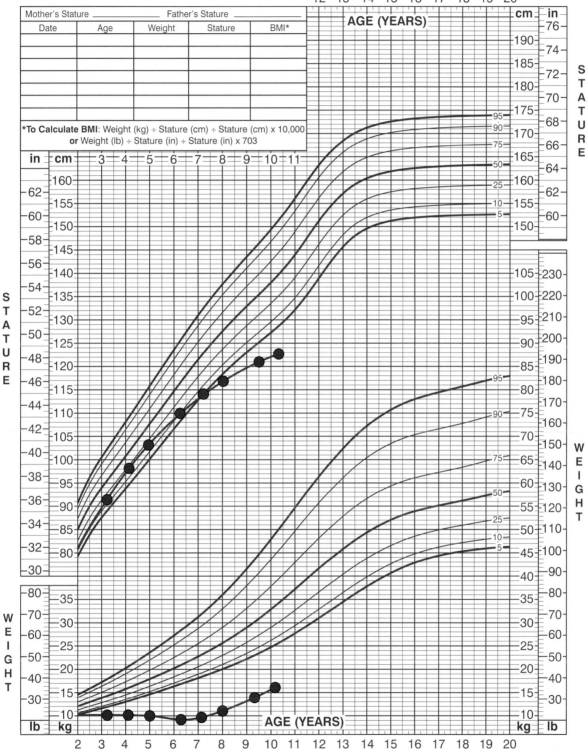

*To Calculate BMI: Weight (kg) ÷ Stature (cm) ÷ Stature (cm) x 10,000
or Weight (lb) ÷ Stature (in) ÷ Stature (in) x 703

Published May 30, 2000 (modified 11/21/00).
SOURCE: Developed by the National Center for Health Statistics in collaboration with
the National Center for Chronic Disease Prevention and Health Promotion (2000).
http://www.cdc.gov/growthcharts

CDC
SAFER·HEALTHIER·PEOPLE™

FIGURE 2-11 ■ In malnutrition, the weight deficit is greater than the length deficit.

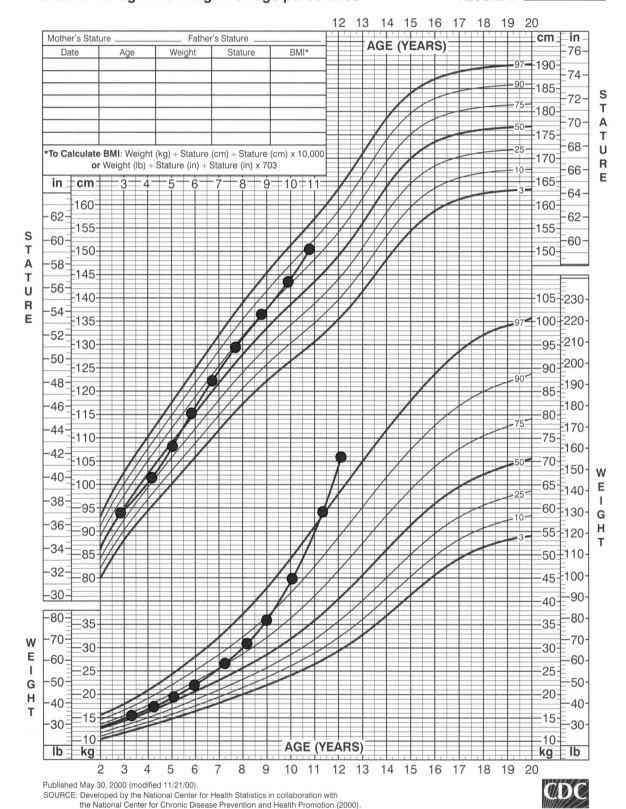

2 to 20 years: Boys
Stature-for-age and Weight-for-age percentiles

NAME _____

RECORD # _____

Published May 30, 2000 (modified 11/21/00).
SOURCE: Developed by the National Center for Health Statistics in collaboration with
the National Center for Chronic Disease Prevention and Health Promotion (2000).
http://www.cdc.gov/growthcharts

FIGURE 2-12 ■ In cases of excessive nutrition the weight gain exceeds the increase in linear growth acceleration.

(1) documented growth velocity less than 10th percentile or greater than 95th percentile for age (ie, any abnormally slow- or fast-growing child); (2) height-for-age less than 1st percentile (ie, any markedly short child); (3) height projection (current height percentile with correction for BA delay or advancement) that differs significantly from mid-parental height; and (4) detection of abnormal body proportion.

Diagnosis and Treatment of Worrisome Growth

Growth disorders in childhood generally display one or more of the following characteristics: (1) short stature with normal tempo of growth (ie, growth rate and skeletal maturation within the normal range, familial/genetic short stature); (2) short stature with normal growth rate but evidence for prior slowed tempo of growth (i.e. "constitutional growth delay" with delayed skeletal maturation); (3) abnormal growth rate with or without short stature (attenuated growth caused by systemic disease or hormonal deficiency); or (4) growth acceleration. Proper interpretation and diagnosis of growth disorders frequently requires appreciation of overlapping growth patterns in the same child. This is commonly observed in children with extreme "idiopathic (ie, nonpathological) short stature" resulting from combined influences of familial short stature and constitutional growth delay. Sound therapeutic decisions regarding growth problems must incorporate a clear understanding of both the complexity of multiple factors simultaneously influencing growth in an individual child and the natural history of these growth patterns. In many situations, careful watchful waiting is a critical first "intervention" that allows distinction of normal variations in growth from disorders for which treatment is needed. A conceptual approach to the differential diagnosis of a child with worrisome growth is depicted in Figure 2-10C. Box 2-1 lists the

circumstances in which a patient with growth disorders should be referred to a pediatric endocrinologist.

Growth hormone therapy overview

For many years, treatment of growth retarding disorders was confined to correction of underlying disease or hormonal disturbance. During the past 20 years, however, treatment of growth disorders has expanded beyond hormonal replacement therapy to include enhancement therapy to improve stature, body composition, and perhaps quality of life. One consequence of this expansion has been the evolution of complex ethical dilemmas in GH therapy regarding appropriate criteria for the initiation and discontinuation of therapy, responsible allocation of health care resources, and the growth of "cosmetic endocrinology".[7] While GH therapy has dominated as the growth-promoting therapy of choice, advances in the understanding of growth regulation and skeletal maturation by other factors (eg, estrogens and androgens, insulin, leptin) promise to lead to new innovations in manipulation of growth and stature.

In 1985, the first case of Creutzfeld-Jakob disease (CJD), a rare and fatal spongiform encephalopathy, was recognized in patients who had received GH derived from cadaveric pituitary glands; investigation disclosed that pituitary glands from which the GH was derived were contaminated with subviral particles. Fortunately, the FDA approved biosynthetic GH in the 1985, with production of GH by biological systems (*Escherichia coli* and, more recently, mammalian cells) transplanted with the *GH* gene now yielding a virtually unlimited supply of GH and eliminating risk of infection transmission. Virtually all GH prescribed currently is 191 amino-acid r-GH (recombinant GH).

Children with milder forms of inadequate GH secretion, previously excluded from GH, can now be considered for treatment. Increased availability of recombinant DNA-derived GH has also allowed investigation of its growth-promoting effects in poorly growing children who do not fit traditional definitions of growth hormone deficiency (GHD), many of whom were previously believed to be unresponsive to GH treatment. In addition, metabolic effects of GH apart from linear growth promotion are now being studied extensively, leading to new indications for and innovative dosing of GH therapy. The spectrum of disorders for which GH has been prescribed and the number of children receiving treatment continue to increase (Table 2-5).

Concern about social and psychological harm of short stature, and hope for effective therapy, has resulted in increased referrals for growth-promoting therapy. However, data confirming that stature per se is a primary determinant of psychological health is limited, although some have reported a higher frequency of underachievement, behavior problems, and reduced

---

Box 2-1.

When to consult or refer to a pediatric endocrinologist:

- Unexplained neonatal hypoglycemia, jaundice, microphallus
- Early signs of possible hypopituitarism, including GHD
- Unexplained abnormally slow or fast growth
- Persistent growth velocity less than 10th percentile or greater than 95th percentile for age
- Extreme short stature
- Height-for-age less than 1st percentile (< −2.25 SD)
- Growth pattern and prognosis at variance with family
- Height projection (current Ht-percentile corrected for BA) that differs significantly from MPH
- Detection of abnormal body proportion

Table 2-5.

FDA-Approved Indications for Growth Hormone Therapy

Indication	Dosage*
GHD	0.16-0.30 mg/kg/wk also dosed as 0.024-0.034 mg/kg/d
PWS	Up to 0.24 mg/kg/wk (or body surface area-based dosing at ~1 mg/m²BSA/day)
SGA/IUGR	Up to 0.48 mg/kg/wk
Turner syndrome	Up to 0.33-0.47 mg/kg/wk also dosed as up to 0.067 mg/kg/d)
Noonan syndrome	Up to 0.066 mg/kg/d
ISS	Up to 0.47 mg/kg/wk
Chronic renal insufficiency	Up to 0.35 mg/kg/wk (dose should be given 4 h after dialysis)
AIDS wasting	Consult adult text
Adult GHD	Starting 0.2 mg/d (range 0.15-0.30 mg/d) increase by increments of 0.1-0.2 mg/d every 1-2 m or starting 0.006 mg/kg/d up to 0.025 mg/kg/day depending on age
SHOX deficiency	Up to 0.35 mg/kg/wk

Depending on which brand of GH used the dosing may vary within the range listed.

social competency in short-statured children. Organic neuro-endocrine dysfunction (eg, classic GHD), rather than stature itself, may correlate most closely with psychological and scholastic impairment. While the physiologic benefits of GH supplementation to children with severe GH deficiency appear obvious, data confirming the efficacy of GH therapy in improving the quality of life of non-GH-deficient recipients are scarce.[8]

For many children, GH treatment will be appropriate therapy after the cause of the growth problem, the concerns of patients and parents, and likelihood of success have been assessed. For most short children, however, efforts to build self-esteem through parental support, judicious selection of activities, and counseling will be more effective than injected GH therapy. The decision to institute long-term GH therapy should include both careful physical and psychological evaluation, to determine whether the degree of disability and likelihood of therapeutic benefit justify investment of the required emotional and monetary resources. Although experience has shown that side effects appear minimal, the possibility of yet-unknown long-term adverse effects (or unexpected benefits) remains.[9]

Intrinsic Short Stature

Many children are born with intrinsic traits that predispose them to short stature despite normal endocrine systems. These factors affect either the absolute growth potential of stature-increasing growth centers (eg, children with short familial stature, born SGA, or with defined genetic syndromes or skeletal dysplasias) or the tempo at which such growth is accomplished (constitutional growth delay). The most severely affected children frequently demonstrate a combination of both traits. Standard laboratory evaluation usually reveals normal GH provocative testing and IGF-1 levels. However, recent discoveries (eg, mutation in the STAT5b component of GH signaling pathway) are beginning to provide physiological explanations for "normal" short stature. In addition, apparent normality of the GH/IGF-1 pathway does not preclude responsiveness to GH therapy, and several causes of intrinsic short stature are now included in approved indications for GH therapy.

Idiopathic short stature

Definition. Idiopathic short stature (ISS) is a diagnosis of exclusion applied to otherwise healthy short children with no identified etiology for poor growth; that is, no systemic illness, endocrine disorders, genetic syndromes, bone dysplasias, or low birth weight are identified. This group includes familial short stature (FSS) and constitutional delay of growth and maturation (CDGM) which together describe a fairly heterogeneous group of children (who often display evidence of both) and comprise nearly 80% of the short children who present to a pediatric clinic. By definition these children have heights less than 2 SD below the mean for a given age, sex, and, if available for comparison, specific population group.

Diagnosis, etiologies, and natural history. Familial short stature can be defined by a height below the 5th percentile, growth velocity that is parallel to but below the normal growth curve, and BA congruent with the child's chronologic age. When there is no concurrent constitutional delay, time of pubertal onset is normal with a projected final height near the current growth percentile. The height of both parents is often below the 10th percentile with the calculation of the MPH and PAH suggesting a final height that is reflective of the parents. As mentioned previously, marked difference between parental height percentiles can compromise the utility of the MPH calculation. While there is a tendency for a child's height to trend toward the MPH, some will clearly follow one parent's pattern closer than the other. Comparison with height percentiles of siblings is helpful in this situation.

Some cases of familial or genetic short stature are likely to represent heritable, subtle disruptions in the GH/IGF-1/growth plate axis. An example of such a defect may involve receptor and postreceptor signaling abnormalities that create reduce linear growth accomplished in response to normal GH secretion. For instance, heterozygous GHR mutations can be found in a minority of children with growth failure and poor response to GH, implicating receptor resistance to GH action. Given the complexity of possible genetic influences on the growth axis, the simple diagnosis of familial or genetic short stature will become increasingly inadequate to determine which children may warrant further evaluation and/or intervention.

CDGM refers to children with ISS who have delay in the tempo of growth and pubertal maturation. Children who are short due to CDGM usually show deviation from growth along normal percentiles between 12 and 28 months of age, and by 3 years of age begin to display normal growth velocity for age with height parallel to but below the 5th percentile. The slower tempo of growth and maturation leads to late onset of puberty, exaggerated slowing of prepubertal growth rate, and normal growth acceleration but slight attenuation of overall growth accomplished during puberty. Final height is usually within the normal range because of the longer period of growth prior to bone maturation but usually in the lower part of the MPH. By definition, children with pure CDGM should have BAs sufficiently delayed to result in normal predicted adult heights (> 163 cm in males and >150 cm in females). Marked delay in the pubertal growth can adversely affect spine mineralization, and osteopenia has been reported in men with a history of CDGM suggesting that bone mineral accretion may be an intrinsic defect in those with CDGM.[10]

During early- to mid-childhood, children with CDGM demonstrate normal GH secretion in response to provocative tests and have normal to slightly low serum IGF-1 and normal IGFBP-3 for skeletal age. However, in late childhood, children with severe CDGM may demonstrate low GH secretion in response to stimuli, suggesting transient GH deficiency corresponding to the delayed puberty and growth deceleration as a result of low gonadal steroid production. Thus, if this phenomenon is not appreciated (gonadal steroids are not administered before GH provocative testing), the diagnosis of GH deficiency is suggested and treatment often initiated. The fact that 30% to 70% of postpubertal adolescents diagnosed as GH deficient during childhood show restoration of normal GH secretion suggests that GH treatment in response to low prepubertal GH levels in CDGM patients is more common than generally recognized.

Treatment of ISS. Treatment of ISS with GH is vigorously debated for economic and ethical reasons, since it is still unresolved to what degree of shortness ISS should be considered a normal variant, and in what circumstances is treatment justified for a characteristic that is not caused definable disease or disorder. Thus, the decision to medically intervene for those who meet the criteria for ISS is individually based on the degree of current childhood shortness, likelihood for an acceptable adult height without intervention, psychological

stress associated with short stature, and evidence that treatment will have a positive effect on growth and quality of life. Currently the FDA approves GH for the treatment of ISS if the height is less than or equal to −2.25 SD (~1st percentile), the predicted adult height falls below the normal range (5 ft 3 in for males, 4 ft 11 in for females), epiphyses are open, and other causes of short stature are excluded.[11] The average height velocity in the first year of treatment typically increases to 8 to 9 cm per year compared to 4.5 cm per year before treatment. However, the effect on ultimate height gained is relatively modest, estimated to be approximately 1 cm per year of GH treatment.[12]

Long-term GH treatment of non-GH deficient short children with ISS at recommended doses (0.375 mg/kg/week) can lead to statistically significant increases in final height in some children. Since adult height is predominantly determined by the 85% of growth occurring before puberty, effective GH therapy requires substantial growth acceleration prior to puberty, and earlier treatment enhances outcome. Overall, girls appear to derive less height-increasing benefit, most likely related to later institution of treatment and earlier onset of puberty. Greater BA delay predicts greater response; otherwise there are presently no clinical (eg, pretreatment growth rate) or biochemical determinants that reliably predict long-term response to GH therapy. Future studies may discover in the ISS population-distinct genetic disturbances or subtle forms of GH deficiency that respond differently to treatment. In the meantime, whether meaningful improvements in final height are sufficient to justify cost and commitment to several years of GH therapy is still debatable.

Therapies that delay puberty and/or prevent bone maturation may be employed for use either on their own or in conjunction with GH therapy. Depot leuprolide, a long-acting GnRH analog (used to inhibit the endogenous pulsatile gonadotropin release) can be given in conjunction with GH in children with ISS to delay or stop puberty and slow growth plate maturation. The effectiveness of this combined approach is generally modest, with mean gains in height compared to predicted height approximately 4 cm.[13] These data, coupled with the expense of GnRH agonist therapy, concern about long-term bone mineralization effects, and the fact that pubertal delay is frequently and already a psychological concern for the short young adolescent, have caused enthusiasm for this approach to wane. Aromatase inhibitors (eg, letrozole and anastrazole), which markedly reduce conversion of androgens to estrogen and therefore limit estrogen-induced growth plate closure, have also been used. In adolescent males, reports of 3 to 5 cm gain in near final height have been reported when these drugs are used in conjunction with testosterone therapy in males with CDGM or with GH therapy in males with GHD.

Theoretically, aromatase inhibitors appear as attractive growth-extending alternatives for children with ISS, although use in ISS females is limited owing to the increase of peripheral androgen levels, and the potential for undiscovered adverse effects still merits attention.[14]

Intrauterine growth restriction or small for gestational age

Definition and etiology. Children born small for gestational age (SGA) are defined as having a birth weight and/or length less than two standard deviations below the mean given their gestational age and sex (below 3%). Although many of these children achieve a normal growth pattern, the 10% to 20% who fail to show linear catch-up growth by 2 to 3 years of age comprise a substantial population of children with small stature. The mean final adult height in SGA babies is reduced by a mean 3 to 4 cm compared to MPH, and severity of this effect is proportional to the extent of fetal impairment.

Diagnosis and natural history. Tests of the GH-IGF-1 axis are usually normal. Low levels of IGF-1 and IGFBP-3, suspected *in utero* secondary to fetal undernutrition, may persist and contribute to postnatal growth retardation, although levels of these proteins do not correlate with postnatal growth. Relative insensitivity to GH and IGF-1 is also possible, as elevations in GH levels before and IGF-1 levels after GH therapy are noted in some SGA infants.[15] Subsequent endocrine disorders associated with being born SGA include premature adrenarche, insulin resistance, ovarian hyperandrogenism, and reduced pubertal growth. A propensity for faster tempo in puberty and thus quicker rate of growth plate maturation and fusion can further jeopardize final height. Adults may also have difficulties with type 2 diabetes, hypertension, and cardiovascular disease.[16]

Treatment. Results of therapeutic trials of GH therapy for children born SGA with persistent growth retardation at 2 years of age have been sufficiently encouraging to justify FDA approval of GH therapy, with a dosing range up to (clearly supra-physiological) 0.48 mg/kg/week for this indication. Novel use of intermittent high-dose GH therapy has been successful for SGA patients, and could be potentially applied to other GH treatment indications; however, long-term studies suggest that additional height gained with either intermittent or high-dose GH treatment is modest (~0.5 SD or 1.25 inches) compared to sustained lower dose treatment. Whether children born SGA derive substantial psychological benefits from enhanced childhood stature (even without enhanced final stature) remains uncertain. However, there is some evidence that intelligence and psychosocial functioning may be enhanced for those SGA children on GH therapy.[16] Given the aforementioned propensity of insulin resistance in this population, concern of exacerbating this metabolic dysfunction has been a concern. Although, higher-dose GH therapy has increased insulin levels in some of these children, meaningful insulin resistance has not been identified. It is also reported that metformin treatment of female children born SGA not only reduces visceral fat, insulin resistance, and hyperandrogenism, but delayed menarche and appeared to improve height prognosis.[17]

Auxiliary height-enhancing treatment for short children born SGA may include administration of a GnRH analog (used to inhibit the endogenous pulsatile gonadotropin release) if accelerated pubertal tempo is observed. Similar to ISS, aromatase inhibition may prove useful in slowing growth plate maturation.

Turner syndrome

Definition and etiology. Turner syndrome (TS) is the result of a haplotype insufficiency of the X chromosome with approximately 50% of the diagnosis being the result of 45, X karyotype and the remainder resulting from the mosaicism and X chromosome structural abnormalities. While relatively common in live-born females (~1/2500), most affected fetuses are spontaneously aborted with those having a more mosaic pattern also having the greatest chances of survival.

Diagnosis and natural history. Clinical appearance is highly variable (Figure 2-13). At birth congenital lymphedema, low hairline, nuchal skin, and pterygium coli (webbed neck) may be present. Other features include small jaw, high palate, ptosis, downslanting palpebral fissures, epicanthal folds, midface hypoplasia, prominent ears, dysplastic nails, broad chest with hypoplastic nipples, cubitus valgus, multiple pigmented nevi, and short fourth metacarpals. Difficulties with recurrent otitis media may lead to conductive hearing loss, while sensorineural hearing loss of unknown etiology can also be present. Intelligence is within the normal range, although difficulties with visual-spatial organization and attention deficit are common. Autoimmune disorders, especially thyroiditis and (to a lesser extent) celiac disease, occur with sufficient frequency to warrant screening.

A high percentage of TS patients will have cardiac, renal, and urological abnormalities. The most common cardiac structural anomalies include bicuspid aortic valve, coarctation of the aorta, and aortic dilation. The urologic and renal defects include double collecting systems, horseshoe kidney, kidney rotational abnormalities, ureteropelvic and ureterovesical junction obstruction, and absence of kidney. All children with the diagnosis of TS should have both cardiac and renal imaging.

Approximately 95% to 100% of girls with TS experience short stature with an average growth velocity

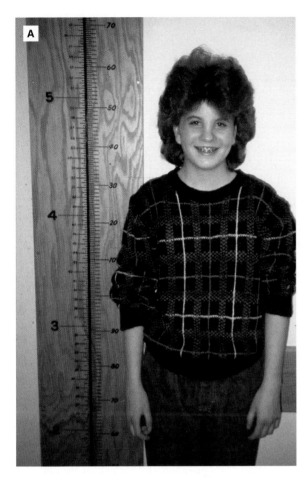

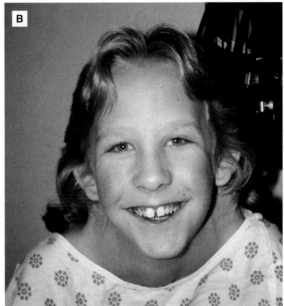

FIGURE 2-13 ■ Turner syndrome: Note the variation in clinical appearance between the adolescent female presenting for evaluation of primary amenorrhea (Figure 13A) compared with the patient demonstrating pronounced webbing of the neck, posterior rotation, and downward ear displacement, and down-slanting of the palpebral fissures (Figure 13B).

in childhood of 4.44 cm for each year of BA advancement. Specialized growth curves for girls with TS are available for download (www.magicfoundation.org). The cause of growth failure and short stature is likely related to the underlying mild bone dysplasia affecting limbs disproportionately, abnormal body segment ratios (U/L ratio significantly above normal for age), and estrogen deficiency with (if untreated) lack of increased GH secretion during adolescence. Haplo-insuffiency for the *SHOX* gene (short stature homeobox-containing gene) located on the long arm of the X chromosome is a key contributor to growth restriction. Evidence of growth failure may be present at birth but typically birth length is in the lower range of normal. Untreated mean final height, however, is approximately 20 cm below the female average (Figure 2-14).

Treatment. Although girls with TS have normal GH responses to provocative testing, abnormalities in growth plate cartilage rendering resistance to GH, and relatively low GH secretion after 8 years of age are reported as potential GH/IGF-1 axis contributors to poor growth. GH therapy can increase growth rate and height achieved in TS[18,19] and is an FDA-approved indication. Standard treatment utilizes a dose of approximately 0.35 mg/kg/week in daily subcutaneous injections as soon as

a girl with TS drops below the 5th percentile of the normal growth curve (as early as 2 years of age). In girls older than 8 years of age with marked short stature, concomitant administration of an anabolic steroid not aromatized to estrogen (eg, oxandrolone at 0.05 mg/kg/d) can be added for additional growth promoting effects. Possible side effects of oxandrolone that should be monitored include clitoral enlargement and glucose intolerance. Therapy is continued until a satisfactory height is achieved or until BA is more than 14 and annual growth rate is less than 2 cm. In a noncontrolled study, mean height of girls who completed an average of 7.6 years of GH therapy (n = 17) was 150.4 cm, a gain of 8.4 cm over the expected average height, while those treated with GH plus oxandrolone (n = 43) achieved a mean final height of 152.1 cm, an average gain of 10.3 cm over predicted height without treatment (Figure 2-15). Long-term follow-up of a Canadian controlled study showed that the treatment group achieved a mean height increase of 7.1 cm and height on average 5.1 cm. closer to MPH than the control group.[20] Thus, an adult height above the lower limit of normal for American women (150 cm) is now an attainable goal for many girls with TS.

Ovarian failure is another major issue for X haploinsufficiency, with either complete (~75%) or partial

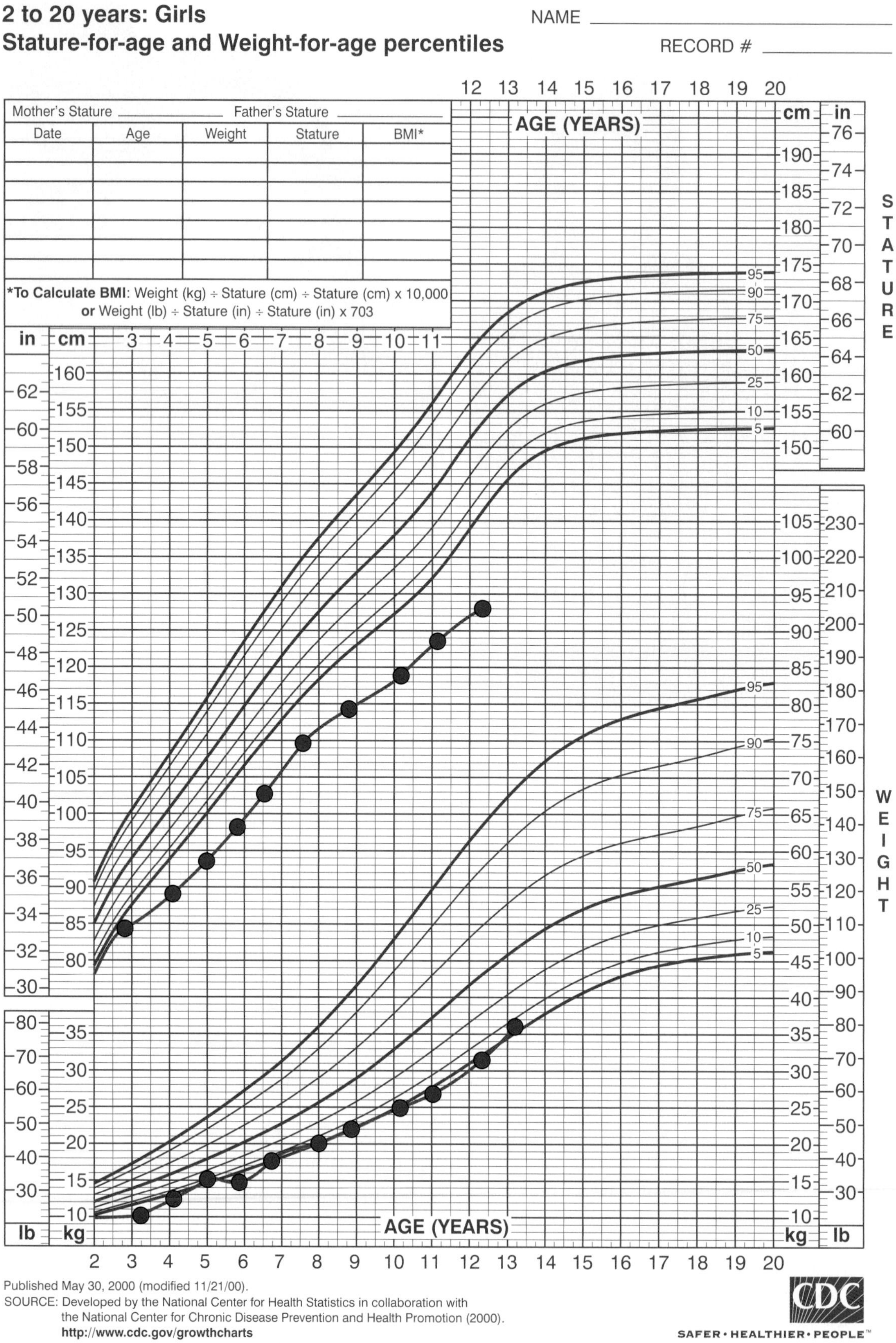
2 to 20 years: Girls
Stature-for-age and Weight-for-age percentiles
NAME
RECORD #
Mother's Stature
Father's Stature
Date
Age
Weight
Stature
BMI*
*To Calculate BMI: Weight (kg) ÷ Stature (cm) ÷ Stature (cm) x 10,000
or Weight (lb) ÷ Stature (in) ÷ Stature (in) x 703
AGE (YEARS)
STATURE
WEIGHT
cm
in
kg
lb
Published May 30, 2000 (modified 11/21/00).
SOURCE: Developed by the National Center for Health Statistics in collaboration with
the National Center for Chronic Disease Prevention and Health Promotion (2000).
http://www.cdc.gov/growthcharts
CDC
SAFER • HEALTHIER • PEOPLE™

FIGURE 2-14 ■ Example of a growth pattern chart seen in untreated Turner syndrome plotted on a standard growth curve. Note the abnormal growth velocity presenting in early childhood.

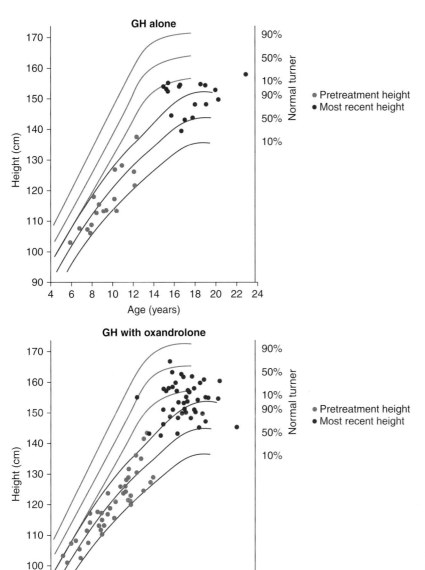

FIGURE 2-15 ■ Effect of GH therapy alone and with oxandrolone on last available height in girls with Turner syndrome. (*From Rosenfeld RG, Attie KM, Frane J, et al. Growth hormone therapy of Turner's syndrome: beneficial effect on adult height. J Pediatr. 1998 Feb; 132(2):319-324.*)

(~25%) absence of estrogen-induced sex characteristics (i.e. breast development, menses). Streak gonads can be seen in two-thirds of patients and one-third have below normal ovarian volumes. Ovarian function is related to underlying karyotype; those who achieve menarche or, very rarely, pregnancy are predominately those with mosaic karyotypes. Evidence of gonadal failure can be seen in the newborn period when gonadotropins are elevated until approximately 4 years of age when they decline to normal childhood level and then rise again to high levels at the usual age of pubertal onset. Estrogen replacement is necessary for those girls with complete ovarian failure or in those who demonstrate mid-pubertal arrest. Timing of estrogen treatment is individualized to maximize height attainment, psychological well-being, and bone mineralization. With oral estrogen therapy, there is a clear relationship between earlier treatment and reduced height achieved with GH therapy. However, awareness of likely GH response-inhibiting effects of orally administered estrogens (due to concentration-dependent inhibition of hepatic IGF-I production), and the advent of effective low-dose transdermal estrogen preparations may allow more age-appropriate sex hormone replacement without compromise of growth potential.[21]

Down syndrome

Definition diagnosis and natural history. Short stature is a prominent feature of Down syndrome (DS; trisomy 21). For reasons that remain obscure, children with DS are born approximately 500 gm and 2 to 3 cm smaller in length than normal and continue postnatal growth at subnormal rates. Although subnormal GH and IGF-1 levels have been identified in some children with DS, most show normal stimulated GH levels. Skeletal maturation is typically delayed and pubertal growth acceleration is blunted. A specialized growth chart is available for this population and provides a more realistic illustration of expected height-for-age and growth velocity (www.magicfoundation.org). Graphing a child with DS only on normal growth chart alone may lead to erroneously attributing declining growth percentiles solely to the syndrome rather than pursuing other etiologies such as hypothyroidism or celiac disease which occur with increased frequency.

Treatment. Periodic evaluation of thyroid status is indicated because of a strong association with autoimmune thyroid disease. GH treatment increases height SDS in children with DS but no significant increase in cognitive function. Concern regarding increased risk in DS of leukemia and diabetes mellitus, coupled with uncertainty about benefits of treatment, have limited enthusiasm for growth-promoting therapy, and GH therapy for DS is not a FDA-approved indication.

Noonan syndrome

Definition, diagnosis, and natural history. Noonan syndrome (NS) is an autosomal dominant disorder that shares many clinical features of Turner syndrome such as short stature (mean height 2 SD below population mean, usually in the absence of GH deficiency), webbing of the neck, low posterior hairline, ptosis, cubitus valgus, and ear malformations. However, it is clearly distinct from Turner in its genetic etiology, occurrence in both sexes, and mode of inheritance. Gonadal function is usually preserved, although small genitalia and cryptorchidism occur with increased frequency in males, and delays and incomplete progression in puberty can occur in both sexes. In contrast to left-sided heart defects typical for TS, heart defects in NS are primarily right-sided (pulmonic and peripheral pulmonic stenosis). Mental retardation of variable degrees is observed in 25% to 50% of children with NS. Multiple genes have been identified in populations sharing the Noonan characteristics with the PTPN11 (protein tyrosine phosphatase, nonreceptor type 11) mutation as the most well-defined and most common mutation found in this clinical syndrome.

Birth weights are typically normal but infancy and childhood growth diverge from normal percentiles, abnormal body proportions may be present, and there is an attenuated pubertal increase in growth rate. The precise etiology of poor growth remains unknown. GH secretion abnormalities do not explain the poor growth, although occasional reductions in GH production are reported.

Treatment. GH therapy recently received FDA approval for children with NS and short stature. In response to GH at doses up to 0.066 mg/kg/day, height SD scores improve, with the greatest effect on growth velocity occurring within the first 2 years of treatment. However, since height acceleration during the second or third years of treatment may not significantly increase compared to control subjects when pubertal subjects are excluded,[22] the long-term effect of GH on height achieved appears not as great as that observed in TS.

Osteochondrodyplasia (achondroplasia and hypochondroplasia)

Definition and diagnosis. Osteochondrodyplasias are a heterogeneous group of genetically transmitted bone and cartilage abnormalities that result in short stature with disproportionate size and/or shape of limbs, skull, and spine. There are over 100 osteochondrodysplasia conditions identified on the basis of the physical examination and radiologic findings. Abnormalities can predominantly involve epiphysial, metaphysial, or diaphysial bone growth. Further characterizations are made based on biochemical and genetic studies, but exact diagnosis is still often difficult. Body proportion measurement is critical, including arm span, sitting height, upper/lower body segment, and head circumference. Radiology studies clarify involvement of the long bones, skull, and vertebrae.

Etiologies, diagnosis, and treatment. Two of the more common osteochondrodyplasias are achondroplasia and hypochondroplasia. Both result from activating mutations in the fibroblast growth factor receptor 3 (FGR3) but in different domains. FGR3 is located on the short arm of chromosome 4 and normally functions to negatively regulate bone growth.[23] The spectrum of these disorders in is caused by different gain-of-function mutations in the *FGR3* gene that enhance growth-inhibiting effects through various downstream signaling pathways.

Achondroplasia occurs in approximately 1:26,000 live births. While inherited in an autosomal dominant pattern, most new cases are new, spontaneous mutations. Homozygous children usually die in infancy owing to restrictive lung disease. The classic clinical appearance of achondroplasia is almost ubiquitously caused by the same amino acid substitution in the transmembrane domain of the receptor and has 100% penetrance. This causes ligand-independent dimerization of the receptor, activation and up-regulation of cell-cycle inhibition, and likely down-regulation of expression of Indian hedgehog and parathyroid hormone–related peptide (PTHrP) receptor genes involved with bone formation.

Skeletal features include megalocephaly, low nasal bridge, lumbar lordosis, short trident hand, rhizomelia (shortness of the proximal legs and arms) with skin redundancy, and small iliac wings. The spinal abnormalities are small cuboid-shaped vertebral bodies with short pedicles and narrowing of the lumbar interpedicular distance. A small foramen magnum creates risk for hydrocephalus, while kyphosis and spinal stenosis may lead to spinal cord compression. Skeletal dysmorphology and abnormal growth velocity is present from infancy, although short stature may not be evident until after 2 years of age. Mean adult heights in males and females are 130 and 120 cm, respectively. Growth curves specifically for achondroplasia have been developed and are of value in following patients.[24]

Patients with achondroplasia demonstrate normal GH secretion, IGF-1 levels, and IGF-1 receptor activity. Reports of response to GH are variable both in terms of the improvement in linear growth and velocity but also in the degree of improved ratio of lower limb length. The largest published study in achondroplasia involved 40 children; during the first year of treatment, the height velocity increased from 3.8 to 6.6 cm per year and in the second year, the height velocity decreased to approximately 5 cm per year. A modest and variable improvement was seen in the ratio of lower limb length to height. Although GH was well tolerated, atlanto-axial dislocation during GH therapy was reported in one patient. In summary, most experts do not recommend GH therapy for achondroplasia.[24]

Hypochondroplasia is an autosomal dominant disorder, previously described as a "mild form" of achondroplasia but the two disorders do not occur in the same family. About 70% of affected individuals are heterozygous for a mutation in *FGFR3* gene, but locus heterogeneity exists as other unidentified mutations cause a very similar phenotype

The facial features of achondroplasia are absent, and both short stature and rhizomelia are less pronounced. In contrast to achondroplasia, poor growth may not be evident until after 2 years of age, but stature then deviates progressively from normal. Because of the more subtle changes compared to achondroplasia the diagnosis of hypochondroplasia can be exceedingly difficult to make in young children. Mild variants of the syndrome may be difficult to distinguish from normal without careful measurement of U/L ratios and consultative radiological opinions. Occasionally, severe short stature and body disproportion is not appreciated until near-adulthood when, following reduced growth achieved during the pubertal growth spurt, these features become more apparent. Adult heights typically are in the 120 to 150 cm range. Outward bowing of the legs may be accompanied by genu varum, lumbar interpedicular distances diminish between L1 and L5, and, there may be flaring of the pelvis and narrow sciatic notches.

Modest improvement in PAH for those receiving GH therapy are reported, but these estimates may be exaggerated by rapid growth during the first year of treatment. Proportionality of growth response (ie, spine versus extremity) to GH may be dependent on the genotype of *IGF-1* gene locus.[25] As in other conditions of intrinsic shortness, it is possible that higher GH dosage, concomitant GnRH analog treatment, and use of aromatase inhibitors could alter final height in these patients. It is likely that some mildly affected (and undiagnosed) children with hypochondroplasia are receiving GH treatment within the approved ISS indication. More severely affected patients would require leg-lengthening procedures to achieve a height in the normal range.

Prader-Willi syndrome

Definition, etiology, and natural history. Prader-Willi syndrome (PWS) results from deletion of the paternal allele or maternal disomy of a critical region of chromosome 15. Affected children are characterized by obesity, hypotonia, short stature, hypogonadism, and behavioral abnormalities. Many features of PWS reflect hypothalamic dysfunction; including hyperphagia, sleep disorders, deficient GH secretion, and hypogonadism. Interestingly, ghrelin levels in children with PWS are elevated compared with BMI-matched obese controls, a factor that may play a role as an orexigenic factor driving the insatiable appetite and obesity found in PWS. With an incidence of 1 in every 10,000 to 12,000 births, PWS is the most common syndrome associated with marked obesity.

Children with PWS display moderate intrauterine (average −1 SDS) and postnatal growth delay. Usually after age 2 or 3, when caloric intake increases and obesity begins to develop, growth rates increase, but normalization of length/height relationship is rare. Hands and feet tend to be particularly small. Childhood growth rates are close to normal, but lack of normal pubertal growth usually results in reduced adult stature (mean 152 cm for adult PWS male, 146 cm for adult PWS female). GH responses to provocative testing are low normal or blunted in PWS. Growth rates are borderline normal or diminished in the midst of excessive weight gain, in contrast to normal or accelerated growth typically seen in healthy non-PWS obese children. Levels of IGF-1 are relatively low (mean ~ −1.5 SDS) compared to normal-weight age-matched children, but not as low as in those with severe GHD. This likely reflects a stimulating influence of nutritional energy excess, which also sustains near-normal growth rates in children with PWS. Insulin levels are lower in children with PWS than in "healthy" obese children, and rise to the levels of obese children only with GH replacement therapy, suggesting relatively pretreatment heightened insulin sensitivity compatible with reduced GH secretion.

Treatment. Growth failure related to PWS is a recent approved indication for GH treatment in the United

States at a recommended dosage of approximately 1 mg/m²/day or 0.24 mg/kg/week, even in the absence of demonstrable GHD. (Approved indications in Europe include PWS-associated body composition abnormalities). GH treatment (1 mg/m²/day) leads to first-year growth rate of 10.1 ± 2.5 cm per year, a rate equal to that of other children with severe GHD, with a second year decrease in growth rate to 6.8 ± 2.3 cm, corresponding to a mean growth velocity SDS of 2.2 ± 2.2. Maintenance of catch-up growth rates in subsequent years often requires higher dosage of GH (eg, 1.5 mg/m²/day) leading to a cumulative change in height SDS during treatment of 1.8 ± 0.6. Mean increases in adult height of 10 cm and 6.5 cm in GH-treated males and female PWS patients, respectively, have also been reported.[26] (See Figure 2-16).

Patients with PWS also appear to benefit from the metabolic effects of GH therapy. Pretreatment body composition studies of children with PWS (utilizing DXA method) have revealed markedly increased percent of body fat (mean body fat 45%-49%) and low lean body mass; GH therapy leads to significant reductions in body fat (8%-10%) and increased lean body mass. With more prolonged treatment given at doses up to

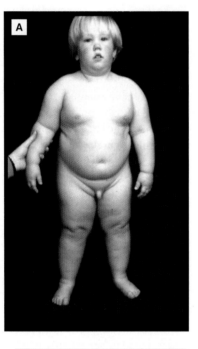
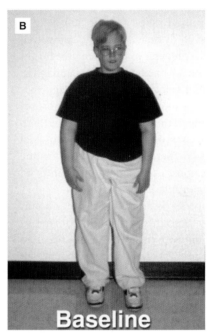
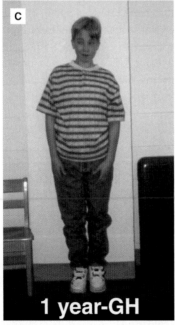
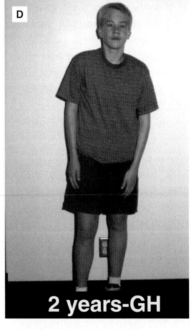

FIGURE 2-16 ■ Serial pictures of a child with Prader-Willi syndrome (PWS). Patient treated with human GH.

1.5 mg/m²/day, body composition, physical strength, activity, stamina, coordination ability, pulmonary function, and sleep quality continue to improve, but function in all parameters remains below normal. This likely reflects the influence of non-GH factors regulating body composition affected by the genetic mutation causing PWS and/or the relatively late institution of GH therapy. Studies currently underway of institution of GH therapy during infancy will address these possibilities.

Potential adverse effects of GH therapy of particular concern in PWS patients include changes in glucose tolerance, pseudotumor cerebri, scoliosis, and sleep-related death. However, fasting glucose, insulin, or HbA1c levels do not change during prolonged GH therapy in PWS patients. Rarely, symptoms consistent with pseudotumor cerebri occur, and resolve with temporary withdrawal and dose-graduated reintroduction of GH therapy. Baseline scoliosis screening and annual assessments during treatment have shown no differences between treated or observed PWS patients. Sleep-related death has been reported in a few morbidly obese PWS children receiving GH[27] prompting a labeling change (Genotropin) contraindicating GH therapy for treatment of children with PWS who have "severe obesity or severe respiratory impairment" and encouraging caution in those with "sleep apnea or other respiratory illnesses."

Endocrine Causes of Disordered Growth

Endocrine systems which control GH secretion and its downstream messenger IGF-1, pubertal development, thyroid activity, the adrenal cortex, calcium metabolism, and glucose homeostasis all have effects on childhood growth. Consequently, a wide variety of endocrine disorders, either congenital or acquired and resulting either in deficiency or excessive production of hormone effect, are associated with disordered growth.

Deficiency in the growth-promoting action of the GH/IGF-1 axis can result from any defect in the pathway from synthesis, release, or receptor binding of GH through the generation of its downstream messenger IGF-1, its association with IGF binding proteins and receptor binding, and subsequent cell signaling pathways. Genes regulating and physiologic pathways involved in this axis are continually being discovered, improving understanding and creating new diagnoses and treatment possibilities. The multitude of factors involved in just this one pathway illuminates why current diagnostic tests of the GH/IGF-1 axis are frequently inadequate to fully characterize the cause of a child's growth disorder.

IGF-1 deficiency

Definition. As IGF-1 is a major mediator of skeletal growth, its deficiency can result in severe growth failure. Causes of IGF-1 deficiency include: (1) central hypothalamic-pituitary dysfunction with failure of pituitary GH production, that is, hypopituitarism or GHD; and (2) primary or secondary GH insensitivity (GHI). IGF-1 deficiency syndrome describes the generic condition, whether caused by GH deficiency, dysfunction, or insensitivity, to illustrate this unifying concept. IGF-1 deficiency caused by hypothalamic dysfunction, with abnormalities of GHRH, endogenous growth hormone secretagogue (GHS) or SRIF synthesis or secretion, primary or secondary decreased pituitary GH production, or GHI share a common phenotype. If GH or IGF deficiency is acquired, clinical signs and symptoms will appear at a later age.

Natural history. Birth size is normal or within 10% of normal in most children with IGF-1 deficiency, but low in severe congenital GH deficiency or GHI. Many infants diagnosed before 2 years of age have birth lengths more than 2 SD below the mean (both in isolated GH and in multiple pituitary hormone deficiencies) and mean birth weight is around −1 SD, lending an appearance of relative adiposity, even in the neonatal period. Anatomic abnormalities include dysgenesis of the pituitary stalk, ectopic placement of the posterior pituitary inferior to the median eminence, and diminished volume of the anterior pituitary. Severe intrauterine growth restriction (IUGR) is *not* part of GHD-associated IGF deficiency, but can be seen in infants with profound IGF deficiency of other causes, confirming the critical role of IGF protiens in intrauterine growth. Breech deliveries and perinatal asphyxia are more common, and neonatal morbidity can include hypoglycemia and prolonged jaundice with direct hyperbilirubinemia caused by cholestasis and giant cell hepatitis. When GHD is combined with deficiency of ACTH and TSH, hypoglycemia may be severe. The combination of GHD with gonadotropin deficiency can cause microphallus, cryptorchidism, and hypoplasia of the scrotum. GHD (or GHI) should, therefore, be considered in the differential diagnosis of neonatal hypoglycemia and of microphallus/cryptorchidism.

Growth failure can, but does not always, occur during the first months of life, but by 6 to 12 months of age, the growth rate invariably deviates from the lower part of the normal growth curve. Skeletal proportions tend to be relatively normal but correlate better with BA than with chronological age. Skeletal age is delayed, and (in the absence of hypothyroidism) is similar to the height age. In acquired GHD, however, as from a CNS tumor, BA may approximate the chronological age. Weight/height ratios tend to be increased, and fat

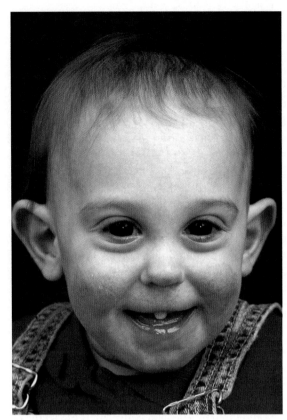

FIGURE 2-17 ■ Toddler with congenital GH and gonadotropin deficiency. Note the mid-facial hypoplasia and the single central incisor.

distribution is often "infantile" or "doll-like" in pattern. Musculature is poor, especially in infancy and can cause delay in gross motor development. Fontanelle closure is often delayed, the voice infantile because of hypoplasia of the larynx, hair growth is sparse and thin, and nail growth slow. Associated midline defects may be present including heart defects, cleft-palate and lip, and other mid-facial boney and soft-tissue abnormalities (Figure 2-17). Even with normal gonadotropin production, the penis is small, and puberty is usually delayed. Adult height data in patients with untreated GH deficiency are not plentiful, but a survey of reports indicates mean final height SDS between −3.1 and −4.7.[28]

Etiologies

1. Idiopathic, isolated GHD

Most children receiving GH are diagnosed as having either acquired, idiopathic, or isolated GHD (IGHD). This diagnosis should always be considered suspect, especially in the immediate prepubertal period owing to normal transient reduction in GH secretion at this time (Figure 2-18). Retesting of patients diagnosed with IGHD reveal normal GH secretion in 40% to 70%, the higher percentage occurring in those with "partial" GHD and normal MRI findings.[29] Additionally, IGHD

patients with normal MRI findings have mean adult heights equally to those with ISS treated with GH, supporting the likely biologic similarity of these two entities. In contrast, over 90% of patients with combined pituitary hormone deficiency, with or without structural abnormalities of the hypothalamic-pituitary area, demonstrate sustained GHD. Whether these results simply cast doubt upon the validity of the initial diagnosis or whether children with IGHD may truly normalize is not clear.

2. GHD following cancer treatment

Children who receive radiation to the hypothalamus/pituitary commonly develop IGF-1 deficiency caused by GHD. This effect is dose-dependent: above 18 Gy, the pubertal increase in spontaneous GH secretion is blunted, above 24 Gy all spontaneous GH secretion is diminished, and above 27 Gy GH response to provocative stimuli is reduced. The likelihood of GHD is increased by larger fraction size administered over shorter time intervals, younger age, and with increasing time following treatment. Growth failure is also observed commonly during the acute phase of chemotherapy, primarily because of poor nutrition, catabolic stress of illness, and growth suppressing effects of adjunct medications (eg, glucocorticoids). The addition of chemotherapy to radiation exacerbates growth failure. Thus, brain tumor survivors should be monitored every 3 to 6 months for reduction in growth rate and assessment of upper and lower segment lengths.

Other hormone deficiencies and direct effects on skeletal tissues can also adversely affect growth of children following radiation. Particularly at cumulative radiation doses exceeding 50 Gy, variable degrees of hypogonadism, thyrotropin deficiency, and ACTH deficiency is very likely to occur, with normal function in all pituitary hormone systems found in less than 10% of the subjects. Irradiation of skeletal tissues can arrest chondrogenesis at the epiphyseal growth plate, and spinal irradiation often results in loss of vertebral growth, scoliosis, development of abnormally low upper to lower body segment ratios, and, as a result, failure to show expected gains in height during puberty. These direct growth-inhibiting effects of radiation treatment are not corrected by GH therapy.

3. Insensitivity to GH action

There is increasing recognition of defects in the distal portion of the GH/IGF axis that extends from the binding of GH to its receptor and to the postreceptor actions of IGF-1. Aberrations in these

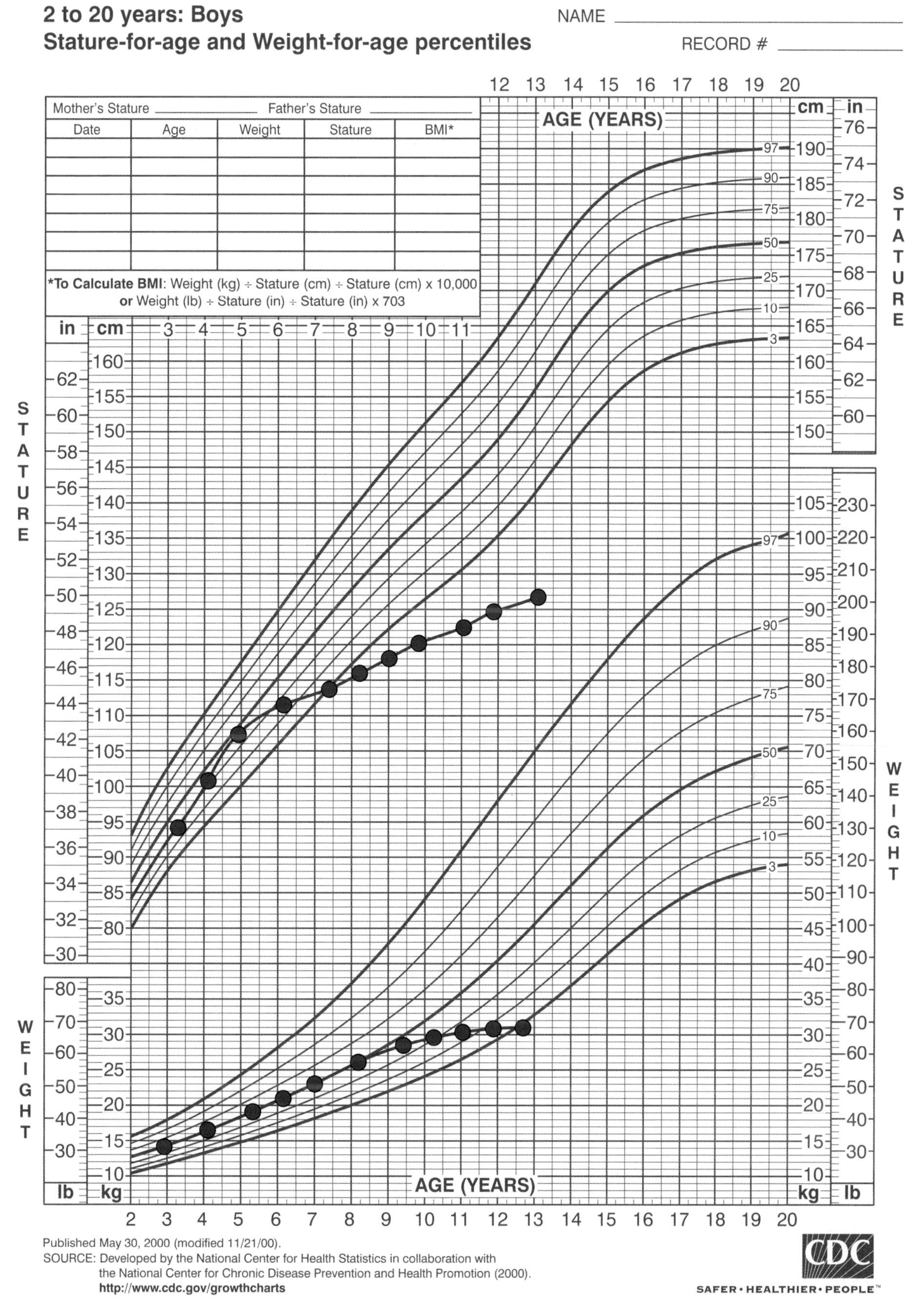
2 to 20 years: Boys
Stature-for-age and Weight-for-age percentiles
NAME
RECORD #
Mother's Stature
Father's Stature
Date
Age
Weight
Stature
BMI*
*To Calculate BMI: Weight (kg) ÷ Stature (cm) ÷ Stature (cm) x 10,000
or Weight (lb) ÷ Stature (in) ÷ Stature (in) x 703
AGE (YEARS)
STATURE
WEIGHT
cm
in
kg
lb
97
90
75
50
25
10
3
Published May 30, 2000 (modified 11/21/00).
SOURCE: Developed by the National Center for Health Statistics in collaboration with
the National Center for Chronic Disease Prevention and Health Promotion (2000).
http://www.cdc.gov/growthcharts
CDC
SAFER • HEALTHIER • PEOPLE™

FIGURE 2-18 ■ Growth chart of a child with acquired GHD. Note the more profound effect on height growth compared with the lesser effect on weight.

pathways create a physiology of GH insensitivity (GHI). The GHR is composed of three domains: an extracellular, hormone-binding domain, a single membrane-spanning domain, and a cytoplasmic domain. Some metabolic actions of GH, as well as its clearance, appear to be closely associated with GHBP concentrations. However, while GHBP levels generally reflect GH receptor levels and activity, levels of GHBP correlate only modestly with 24-hour GH production and growth rate. It is postulated that this reflects adjustments of GH secretion to accommodate GH receptor levels which may be genetically determined or modulated by environmental factors such as nutritional status. Levels of GHBP are low in early life, rise through childhood, and plateau during the pubertal years and adulthood. Impaired nutrition, diabetes mellitus, hypothyroidism, chronic liver disease, and a spectrum of inherited abnormalities of the GH receptor are associated with low levels of GHBP, while obesity, refeeding, early pregnancy, and estrogen treatment can cause elevated levels of GHBP.

Patients with GHI have the phenotype of GHD and diminished production of IGF-1 but with normal or elevated serum GH levels.[30] Measurement of abnormally low serum levels of GHBP is useful in identifying some subjects with GHI caused by genetic abnormalities of the GHR (Figure 2-19). However, patients with GH insensitivity caused by nonreceptor abnormalities, defects of the intracellular domain of the GHR, or inability of the receptor to dimerize may, however, have normal or even high serum levels of GHBP. Primary GHI can occur from: (1) abnormalities of the extracellular, dimerization, or intracellular domains of the GH receptor; (2) postreceptor abnormalities of GH signal transduction; (3) primary defects of IGF-1 biosynthesis; and (4) genetic insensitivity to IGF-1 action. Secondary GHI is an acquired and relatively common condition that can be caused by: (1) malnutrition; (2) hepatic, renal, and other chronic diseases; (3) circulating antibodies to GH; and (4) antibodies to the GH receptor.

Individuals with GHI show diminished response to exogenous GH, in terms of growth, metabolic changes, or of increases in serum levels of IGF-1 and IGFBP-3.[31] GHBP activity is undetectable in 75% to 80% of patients with this disorder. A wide variety of homozygous point mutations in this gene (missense, nonsense, and abnormal splicing) have been identified, with most existing in the extracellular or dimerization domain of the GH receptor. It is unclear whether substitutions identified in the intracellular GHR

domain in short children represent genuine mutations or innocent polymorphisms.

Heterozygosity for defects of the GH receptor may clinically suggest partial GHI, raising the question of whether some children labeled as "idiopathic short stature" may harbor such mutations. Given the requirement for dimerization of the GH receptor, an abnormal protein could exert varying degrees of dominant negative effect. However, inconsistencies in results studies relating identified GHR mutations with low GH/IGF-1 axis effect and vice versa justify maintaining healthy skepticism regarding the ability to precisely dissect out patients with varying degrees of GHI from the ISS group.

4. Post-GHR abnormalities leading to IGF-1 deficiency

At multiple sites, post-GHR defects in translation of GH message can result in growth impairment. Defects in JAK2 and MAPK leading to activate the STAT pathway have been described in children with profound short stature, failure to respond to GH, and normal GH binding and GHBP levels. Primary defects in IGF-1 biosynthesis caused by *IGF-1* gene deletions can lead to severe pre- and postnatal growth retardation, sensory-neural deafness, insulin resistance (caused by high GH levels), insensitivity to exogenous GH, but, reversal of growth and metabolic abnormalities with exogenous IGF-1 treatment.[32] Conditions of insensitivity to IGF-1 action also exist and include abnormalities of: (1) IGF transport and clearance which would alter presentation of IGF to its receptor; (2) the IGF receptor itself; and (3) postreceptor signaling activation. Such patients would be expected to be exceedingly small, both during pre- and postnatal life, have elevated GH and normal to high IGF-1 levels, and poor growth responses to GH and (presumably) IGF-1 administration. Primary defects of IGF transport and clearance, apparent deficient IGF-1 receptor production (eg, African Efe pygmies) or responsiveness (eg, leprechaunism) have also been reported as rare causes of growth failure.

Diagnosis

The foundation for the diagnosis of IGF deficiency is careful documentation of serial heights and determination of height velocity. Even in children below the 5th percentile in height, documentation of a consistently normal height velocity (above the 25th percentile) makes the diagnosis of IGF deficiency and GHD highly unlikely. Key history and physical examination findings indicating that GHD could be present are listed in Table 2-6.

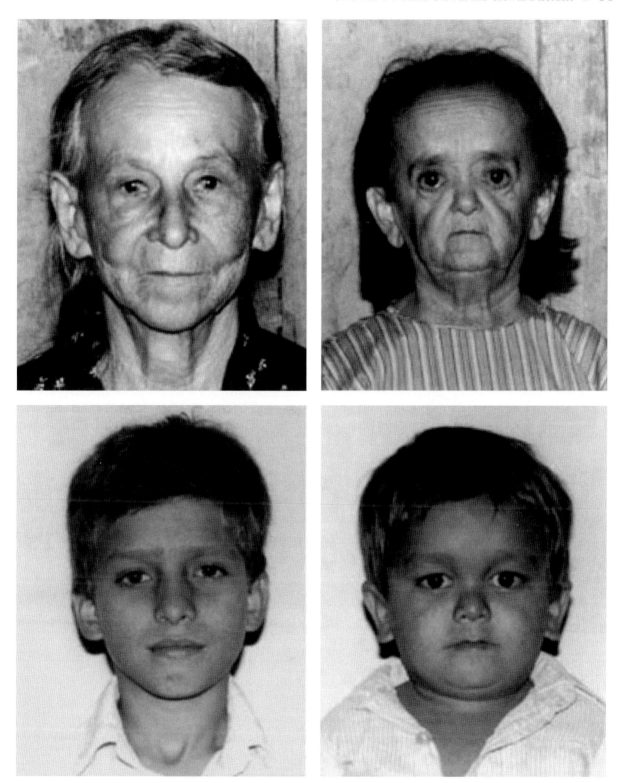

FIGURE 2-19 ■ Two patients (right panels) with GH resistance (Laron syndrome) caused a mutation in the *GHR* gene compared to nonaffected siblings (left panels). Note the "doll-like" features and mid-facial hypoplasia in Laron syndrome patients.

1. Assessment of GH secretion

The assessment of pituitary GH production is difficult because its secretion is pulsatile with the most consistent surges occurring at times of slow-wave EEG rhythms during phases 3 and 4 of sleep (see earlier in this chapter). Between normal pulses of GH secretion, serum GH levels are low (often < 0.1 µg/L), below the limits of sensitivity of most conventional assays (usually < 0.2 µg/L). Accordingly, measurement of a random serum GH

Table 2-6.

Key History and Physical Examination Findings Indicating that GHD Could Be Present

- In the neonate, hypoglycemia, prolonged jaundice, microphallus, or traumatic delivery
- Cranial irradiation
- Head trauma or central nervous system infection
- Consanguinity and/or an affected family member
- Craniofacial midline abnormalities
- Severe short stature (< −3 SD)
- Height < −2 SD and a height velocity over 1 y < −1 SD
- A decrease in height SD of more than 0.5 over 1 y in children over 2 y of age
- A height velocity below −2 SD over 1 y
- A height velocity more than 1.5 SD below the mean sustained over 2 y
- Signs indicative of an intracranial lesion
- Signs of multiple pituitary hormone deficiency (MPHD)
- Neonatal symptoms and signs of GHD

concentration is virtually useless in diagnosing GHD, but may be useful in the diagnosis of GHI and GH excess. Instead, physiologic and pharmacological stimuli are used to assess GH secretion ability. Physiologic stimuli include fasting, sleep, and exercise. Pharmacological stimuli include levodopa, clonidine, glucagon, propranolol, arginine, and insulin. Stimulation tests can be divided

into "screening tests" (exercise, fasting, levodopa, clonidine), characterized by ease of administration, low toxicity, low risk, and low specificity and "definitive tests" (arginine, insulin, glucagon). To improve specificity, provocative tests are performed in a fasting state, and sometimes sequentially. It is commonly required that a child "fail" two distinct provocative tests to be diagnosed with GHD. Standard provocative GH tests are summarized in Table 2-7.

Provocative GH testing, however, has a number of pitfalls. None of the standard pharmacological provocative tests satisfactorily mimic the normal secretory pattern of pituitary GH. Even when naturally occurring regulatory peptides are used for stimulation, their dosage, route of administration, and interactions with other regulatory factors are artificial. Second, the definition of "subnormal" response to provocative tests is arbitrarily defined, and has varied with time and by site. Before recombinant DNA GH was available, a cut-off level of 2.5 µg/L was often employed. In the era of plentiful therapeutic GH, this cutoff was increased to 7 µg/L and then to (the currently utilized) 10 µg/L, although there are no data for validating higher arbitrary cut-off values. Third, marked variability of GH assays (as much as threefold variability in the measurement of serum GH levels among established laboratories) limit their discriminatory power. Further,

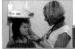

Table 2-7.

Tests to Provoke Growth Hormone Secretion

Stimulus	Dosage	Times Samples Are Taken (min)	Comments
Exercise	Step climbing; exercise cycle for 10 min	0, 10, 20	Observe child closely when on the steps
Levodopa	< 15 kg: 125 mg 10-30 kg: 250 mg > 30 kg: 500 mg,	10, 60, 90	Nausea, rarely emesis
Clonidine	0.15 mgs/m²	0, 30, 60, 90	Tiredness, postural hypotension
Arginine HCl (IV)	0.5 g/kg (mas 30 g) 10% arginine HCl in 0.9% NaCl over 30 min	0, 15, 30, 45, 60	
Insulin (IV)	0.05-0.1 unit/kg	0, 15, 30, 60, 75, 90, 120	Hypoglycemia, requires close supervision
Glucagon (M)	0.03 mg/kg (max 1 mg)	0, 30, 60, 90, 120, 150, 180	Nausea, occasional emesis
GHRH (IV)	1 (g/kg)	0, 15, 30, 45, 60, 90, 120	Flushing, metallic taste

Tests should be performed after an overnight fast. Many investigators suggest that prepubertal children should be "primed" with gonadal steroids, eg, 5 mg Premarin orally the night before and the morning of the test or with 50 to 100 µg/d ethinyl estradiol for 3 consecutive days before testing or 100 ng depot testosterone 3 days before testing. This, of course, alters patient's steady state and performs the provocative test in a steroid-rich environment. Patients must be euthyroid at the time of testing.

Documentation of appropriate lowering of blood glucose is recommended. If GHD is suspected, the lower dosage of insulin is usually administered, especially in infants. D10W and glucagon should be available.

newer GH assays measure GH immuno-potency at 30% to 50% of earlier assays, but "new normal" GH cut-off levels have been defined. Fourth, GH secretion normally varies with age, and prior to puberty and during the early phases of puberty, GH secretion may normally be so low as to blur the discrimination between GHD and constitutional delay of growth and maturation. Many children who "fail" provocative testing before the onset of puberty prove to have "normal" GH secretion after puberty or after administration of exogenous sex steroids. While it is well documented that such "priming" with sex steroids helps to identify the likely return of normal GH secretion with puberty, the role of such manipulations in guiding management of the poorly growing preadolescent remains obscure and vigorously debated. What is clear is that reliance on provocative testing alone without consideration of this peri-pubertal phenomenon can lead to erroneous and excessive diagnosis of GHD. Finally, provocative testing typically requires multiple timed blood samples and the parenteral administration of drugs. The resulting discomfort, occasional risk to the patient, and expense are self-evident.

Alternative approaches involve analysis of spontaneous GH secretion by multiple sampling (q 5-30 minutes) or by continuous blood withdrawal over 12 to 24 hours. The former method allows one to evaluate and characterize GH pulsatility, while the latter only permits determination of mean GH concentration. In spite of these apparent advantages, spontaneous GH secretion identifies only about half of the children with GHD as defined by provocative testing and approximately 25% of normally growing children show low overnight GH levels. These issues, combined with the obvious expense and discomfort of such testing, have precluded its widespread acceptance as a practical diagnostic alternative.

2. Measurement of the GH-dependent peptides (IGF and IGFBP determinations)

An important alternative means of diagnosing GHD is the assessment of IGFs and their binding proteins. IGF-1 levels are more GH-dependent than are IGF-2 levels and are more likely to reflect subtle differences in GH secretory patterns. However, serum IGF-1 levels are influenced by age, degree of sexual maturation, and nutritional status. IGF-1 levels in normal children less than 5 years of age are low with overlap between the normal range and values in GH deficient children. Assessment of serum IGF-2 levels is less age-dependent, especially after 1 year of age, but IGF-2 is less GH-dependent than is IGF-1. Serum levels of both peptides are relatively constant during the day so that provocative testing or multiple sampling is not necessary.

Limitations of reliance on IGF-1 measurement include: (1) interference in radioimmunoassays, radioreceptor assays and bioassays by IGFBPs, which must be removed or blocked; (2) age-dependency, being lowest in young children (< 5 years of age), a period during which one most wishes to have an accurate diagnostic test; (3) levels may be low in conditions other than GHD such as primary GH receptor dysfunction (Laron syndrome) and secondary GHI (malnutrition, liver disease, etc); (4) levels of IGF-1 (and IGFBP-3) are frequently normal in adult-onset GHD and in children with GHD resulting from brain tumors and/or cranial irradiation; and (5) imperfect correlation between serum IGF-1 levels and provocative or spontaneous GH measurements. In short-statured children less than 10 years of age, IGF-1 levels are below −2 SD in only approximately 50%. In fact, IGF-1 levels alone allow discrimination between GH deficiency and normal short children only in children with BAs more than 12 years. When serum levels of both IGF-1 and 2 are determined, the correlation with GH testing improves, because serum IGF-2 levels are low in GHD and normally do not increase with age after 1 year. The observation that "normal short" children may have low serum levels of IGF-1, IGF-2, or both calls into question the criteria by which the diagnosis of GH deficiency is made.

Given that provocative GH testing is both arbitrary and nonphysiologic and the inherent variability in GH assays, it is not surprising that the correlation between IGF-1 levels and provocative GH levels is imperfect. These points are further supported by recent observations with immunoassays for IGFBP-3. Measurement of IGFBP-3, normally the major serum carrier of IGF peptides, has clinical value because it is GH-dependent and its concentrations correlate with the sum of the levels of IGF-1 and 2. Serum IGFBP-3 levels vary with age to a lesser degree than is the case for IGF-1. Even in infants, serum IGFBP-3 levels are sufficiently high to allow discrimination of low values from the normal range. Serum IGFBP-3 levels are also less dependent on nutrition than IGF-1. Most important, IGFBP-3 levels are GH-dependent, with 97% of children diagnosed as GHD by conventional criteria (height < 3rd percentile, height velocity < 10th percentile, and peak serum GH < 10 µg/L) having

IGFBP-3 levels below the 5th percentile for age while 95% of non-GHD short children had normal IGFBP-3 levels.[33] However, it is likely that this study group included children with severe GHD, as such a clear correlation between provocative GH testing and serum IGFBP-3 levels is not observed in clinical practice. There is the additional concern that IGFBP-3 levels may be "falsely" normal in patients with GHD, resulting from acquired intracranial lesions.

3. Diagnosis of IGF deficiency caused by GHI

The combination of decreased serum levels of IGF-1, IGF-2, and IGFBP-3, plus increased or normal serum levels of GH suggests the diagnosis of GHI; namely, (1) basal serum GH more than 10 mU/L (~5 μg/L); (2) serum IGF-1 less than or equal to 50 μg/L; (3) height SDS less than −3; (4) serum GHBP less than 10% (based upon binding of [^{125}I]GH); and (5) a rise in serum IGF-1 levels after GH administration of less than twofold the intra-assay variation (~10%).[34] Unfortunately, in practice, there is striking discordance between serial studies in ISS patients for both IGF-1 and IGFBP-3 generation in response to GH, affirming the difficulty of assigning firm cutoff values of normal GH sensitivity. Decreased serum levels of GHBP also suggest the diagnosis of GHI. As mentioned above, though, individuals with GHI caused by mutations in the dimerization site or in the intracellular domain of the receptor or abnormalities of postreceptor signal transduction mechanisms have normal serum concentrations of GHBP. Consequently, definitive diagnosis of GHI requires: (1) the classical phenotype; (2) decreased serum levels of IGF-1 and IGFBP-3; and (3) identification of an abnormality of the GH receptor gene.

4. Possible partial GHI: idiopathic short stature and heterozygous defects of the GHR

Many children and early adolescents are short (< 3rd percentile), have slowed linear growth velocity (< 25th percentile), may have delayed skeletal maturation and an impaired or attenuated pubertal growth spurt, with or without a family history manifesting some or all of these clinical features, and have no chronic illnesses or apparent endocrinopathies. Such children usually have normal GH secretory dynamics, though provocative tests may be blunted under some circumstances; GH-dependent peptides are lower than expected on a chronological (though usually not skeletal age) basis; treatment with exogenous GH usually augments linear growth. Such children are usually considered variants of normal growth and achieve a final adult height within the range considered acceptable for the family. The etiology of the slowed childhood growth and frequently delayed pubertal spurt has not been established in most of these children. Eventually, causes of idiopathic short stature will likely be identified at each level of the hypothalamic-pituitary-GH-IGF axis.

Children with heterozygous mutations of the GH receptor have been considered as candidates to explain some cases of idiopathic short stature. Serum levels of GHBP in most children with ISS are lower than the normal mean; levels tend to be even lower in children with low IGF-1 and higher mean 12-hour levels of GH. These observations raise the possibility that an abnormality of GH receptor content or structure could impair GH action. In heterozygotes, protein from the mutant allele may disrupt the normal dimerization that occurs when GH interacts with its receptor, leading to diminished GH action and growth impairment. So far, however, analysis of GH-induced IGF-1/IGFBP-3 generation and genes in ISS children affirm that such heterozygotes explain only a small number of patients. Post-GH- and IGF-receptor dysfunction remains the potentially fertile area in which to uncover more causes of "idiopathic" growth failure.

Treatment. Treatment of IGF-1 deficiency begins with a trial of GH therapy. Subcutaneous daily GH administration is currently preferred, with most GHD children in the United States receiving daily treatment with 0.04 to 0.05 mg/kg/day, although many children show early satisfactory growth on smaller doses. Current GH preparations are essentially equivalent. Since growth before puberty is a major determinant of final adult height, early initiation of GH treatment allows more complete normalization of height. While there can be a temptation to defer injection therapy in young children in order to minimize discomfort and inconvenience, available evidence strongly supports early recognition, referral, diagnosis, and treatment of severely GH deficient patients as an important step toward optimizing growth potential.

Increasing the dose of GH improves growth rate; comparison of 0.025, 0.05, and 0.1 mg/kg daily in prepubertal severely GHD children showed significantly greater growth velocities and gains in cumulative height SDS in the 0.05 and 0.1 mg/kg/day groups compared with the 0.025 mg/kg/day group after 2 years of treatment. There were no significant differences between the 0.05 and 0.1 mg/kg/day groups.[35] Increased frequency of GH administration improves growth rate, suggesting the "pulsing" message of GH to its target cells, in addition to adequacy of GH levels, enhances linear growth. Nocturnal administration, which more closely mimics physiological GH secretion, may also add to efficacy, although this is not consistently observed.

The serum IGF-1 response to GH is dose-dependent, continuing to rise as GH is administered in doses above currently prescribed levels. Epidemiological studies that suggest an association between high serum IGF-1 levels and the incidence of malignancy have prompted a recommendation that IGF-1 and IGFBP3 levels be monitored on a regular basis. A younger age, greater delay in height age and BA, and greater severity of GH deficiency based upon provocative testing each correlate with improved *initial response* to GH therapy. Using multiple regression analysis, variables that have positive effects on *adult height* of GH-treated patients include taller parents, more frequent GH injections, longer duration of GH treatment, taller height at start of GH treatment, and greater severity of GH deficiency.

Regardless of the regimen chosen, the effect of GH wanes with time, and the first year of treatment usually produces the greatest growth increment. Following this early phase of rapid growth, short-term increased replacement doses of GH renews catch-up growth without adverse metabolic effects. Seasonal variation in growth rate during GH therapy, with peaks in the summer and nadirs in the winter (North American population) has also been described.

Children who have had removal of craniopharyngioma frequently experience growth acceleration in the absence of measurable GH. This phenomenon may be attributable to postoperative hypothalamic dysfunction resulting in nutritional excess and hyperinsulinemia, although other mechanisms (eg, GH variants, IGFs) are also postulated.[36] Polyphagia and significant weight gain are usually also observed. While supplementation with GH is not required to sustain linear growth, body composition analysis reveals increased fat mass and decreased lean mass typical for the GHD state. Unfortunately, post

surgical treatment with GH, while promoting linear growth, does not appear to slow the excessive weight gain commonly seen in this population. Avoidance of excessive cortisol replacement therapy is extremely important in these individuals. This growth pattern may persist, allowing attainment of normal adult stature without GH therapy, but GH may nevertheless be indicated to improve body composition and other metabolic consequences of GHD.

The issue of whether GH replacement doses should be increased substantially during puberty remains debated. While clearly insufficient dose and frequency of GH administration may reduce expected adult height, most studies show GH dose administered during puberty to be a relatively minor factor in determining total pubertal growth as compared to gender, chronologic age at pubertal onset, and prepubertal height relative to mid-parental height. On the other hand, an increase in dose to 0.7 mg/kg/week (in contrast to conventional dosage recommendations of 0.180.35-mg/kg/week) improves growth rates, near-adult height, and height SDS in GHD adolescents without evident adverse effects.[37] Since the cost of such treatment and the potential for inducing IGF-1 levels in the supra-physiologic range must be balanced with the possible added benefit achieved, the most effective frequency and dose of GH therapy during puberty is yet to be determined.

With early diagnosis, careful attention to accompanying hormonal deficiencies, and progressive dose adjustments, children with GH deficiency reach normal adult height (Figure 2-20). The BA will advance with GH treatment, but usually not more than height age. Linear growth often accelerates faster than BA following initiation of GH therapy, leading to increases in predicted final height. Even with successful long-term GH therapy, however, correction of disabling short stature does not consistently normalize the psychosocial outcome for adults with GH deficiency. Psychosocial counseling, which increases both therapeutic compliance during childhood

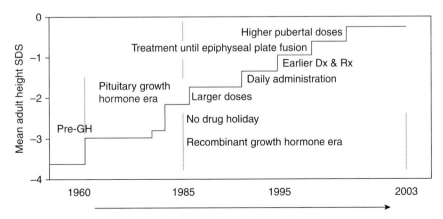

FIGURE 2-20 ■ Potential for attaining normal mean adult height in GHD treated with recombinant GH at contemporary dosing. (*Redrawn from Allen DB. Issues in the transition from childhood to adult growth hormone therapy. Pediatrics. 1999; 104:1004-1009.*)

and social outcomes during adulthood, should be a consistent adjunct to parenteral GH administration.

Failure to demonstrate an increase in growth rate and IGF-1 levels in response to GH therapy suggests the diagnosis of GH insensitivity and rationale for institution of IGF-1 treatment. An exception to the use of IGF-1 as a "second tier" therapy is known Laron syndrome, in which severe short stature and other characteristic features (Figure 2-15) are the result of GHI caused by GHR dysfunction. In these patients, doses of IGF-1 from 40 to 130 µg/kg given twice daily increase in first year growth rates by at least 2 cm and more commonly 4 to 6 cm per year. Unfortunately, longer term trial show waning of the growth-promoting effect, sometimes nearly to baseline levels. Reported side effects of IGF-1 therapy include hypoglycemia (IGF-1 has ~6% of hypoglycemia potency of insulin), headache, papilledema, and urolithiasis. Debate continues, however, regarding the use of IGF-1 to treat other short children showing either laboratory findings or a response to GH therapy suggesting GH resistance, including children with renal failure, liver failure, and children with ISS and low IGF-1 levels.[38]

The consequences of severe GHD in adult life and the beneficial effect of replacement therapy are increasingly well established. Accurate selection of appropriate candidates for adult GH treatment, and the transition of their care from pediatrics to adult medicine require careful consideration of several issues. Since the majority of children who are diagnosed as GHD and treated with GH do not have permanent GHD, anticipatory counseling regarding possible lifelong treatment should be focused on children with panhypopituitarism and those with severe isolated GHD associated with CNS abnormalities. Appropriate timing for termination of "growth-promoting" GH therapy should be guided by efforts to balance the high cost of late-adolescent treatment with the attainment of reasonable stature goals.

Confirmation of GHD following cessation of GH therapy for at least 1 month and provocation with appropriate stimuli (ie, insulin tolerance test, arginine or glucagon stimulation tests) and measurement of IGF-1 levels are appropriate for all candidates for adult GH therapy who do not have well-documented multiple pituitary hormone deficiencies. Testing of the GH axis can be performed within weeks of GH cessation, but confirmation of an emerging adult GHD state with body composition, blood lipid panel, bone densitometry testing, and quality of life assessments may require 1 or more years of pretreatment observation. While it remains unclear whether such a period of observation is necessary or advisable for late adolescents with suspected panhypopituitarism, such trials off GH do not appear to be detrimental. Those adolescents with a history of less severe GHD or those with "partial GHD" (ie, stimulated GH values of 5-10 µg/L on retesting as an adult) pose a

greater diagnostic and therapeutic challenge. If therapy is interrupted in this group, a minimum of close clinical, radiologic (if not previously performed), and laboratory monitoring for evidence of an evolving GHD state and/or other pituitary hormone deficiencies is required.

Hypothyroidism
Etiologies and effects on growth. Hypothyroidism (see Chapter 4) can be congenital or acquired. The congenital form (CH) is most commonly associated with aberrant embryologic glandular migration resulting in an absent or poorly functioning ectopic gland. Less commonly (~10% of cases), inherited enzyme deficiencies interfere with thyroid hormone synthesis. Untreated severe CH leads to jaundice, growth failure, anemia, and neurological damage. Fortunately, newborn screening programs have nearly eliminated the morbidity of severe undiagnosed CH in developed countries. Less commonly, CH results from deficient pituitary or hypothalamic function, usually more mild in severity and accompanied by other hormonal deficiencies. Acquired hypothyroidism is most commonly caused by chronic lymphocytic thyroiditis (Hashimoto thyroiditis); other causes include radiation exposure and iatrogenic surgery or medications (eg, lithium).

During early gestation, the developing child is dependent on maternal thyroid hormone *in utero* for normal neurological development, but less so for normal growth. After birth, in contrast, linear growth is heavily dependent on normal levels of thyroxine, and severe untreated CH leads to profound growth failure. In acquired states of thyroid deficiency, which usually evolve gradually, growth retardation may be subtle at first, but usually progresses in severity over ensuing years; that is, hypothyroidism should always be strongly considered in the child demonstrating near complete cessation of growth. Proportionally, linear height is more affected than weight acquisition, creating a growth stunted and often overweight for height child (Figure 2-21). Skeletal maturation is invariably delayed commensurate with the duration of thyroid hormone deficiency, and body proportion is immature with increased upper-to-lower segment ratios.

Diagnosis and treatment of hypothyroidism is described in Chapter 4. Treatment leads to prompt resumption of normal or supra-normal growth rates. Unfortunately, replacement therapy may not fully restore growth potential (especially if treatment is initiated near puberty) because of the associated rapid skeletal maturation once treatment is initiated. The deficit in final height correlates with the duration of hypothyroidism. In severe cases, pharmacological delay of puberty and growth plate fusion to improve height prognosis may be a consideration.

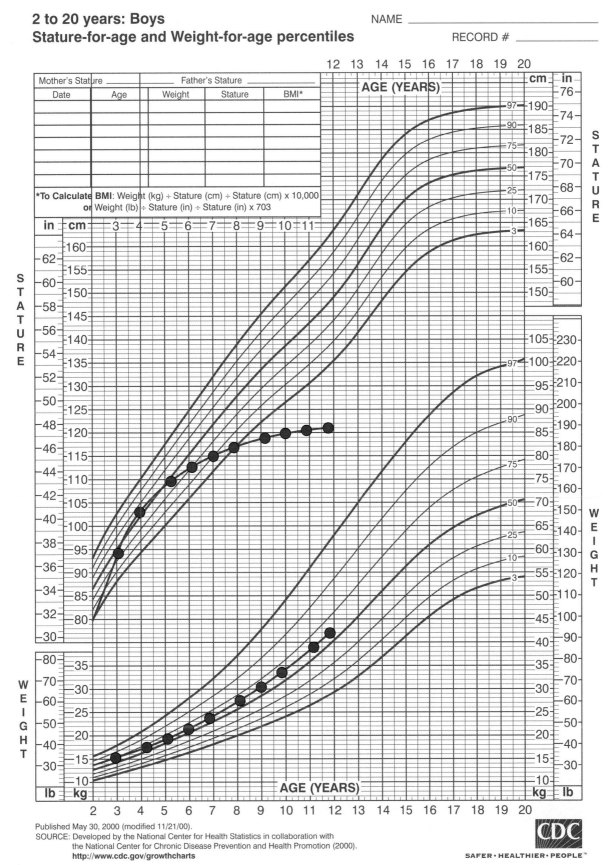

2 to 20 years: Boys
Stature-for-age and Weight-for-age percentiles

NAME _____

RECORD # _____

FIGURE 2-21 ■ Growth chart of a child with acquired hypothyroidism. Note the severe deceleration of growth velocity as weight acquisition remains relatively constant.

Glucocorticoid excess

Glucocorticoids interfere with normal bone growth and metabolism at multiple steps in the growth cascade: augmentation of somatostatin tone and suppression of GH secretion, impairment of IGF-1 bioactivity, suppression of new collagen synthesis and osteoblastic function, and enhancement of bone resorption and protein catabolism.[39]

Exposure to glucocorticoids in excess of normal physiologic production can occur (rarely) from endogenous production (eg, ACTH pituitary adenoma, adrenal tumor) or exogenous therapeutic preparations (eg, treatment of asthma, juvenile rheumatoid arthritis, renal transplantation, or inflammatory bowel disease—see chronic illness discussion below) (Figure 2-22).

Cushing syndrome in childhood (described in detail in Chapter 5), whether caused by an ACTH secreting tumor or an adrenal neoplasm, usually presents with growth failure accompanied by excessive weight gain (Figure 2-23). This effect on linear growth is a key finding differentiating glucocorticoid excess from the normal or accelerated linear growth resulting from exogenous obesity. Children with adrenal tumors may produce excess androgens as well as glucocorticoids, so that growth deceleration may be less apparent owing to the growth-promoting effects of androgens.

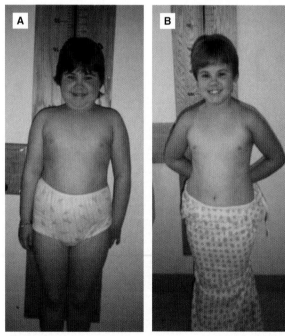

FIGURE 2-22 ■ Child showing growth failure and clinical features of glucocorticoid excess from prolonged excessive dose of inhaled corticosteroid treatment for asthma **(A)** and after reduction in dosage **(B)**. Note the resolution of the "moonfacies" and the truncal obesity.

Calcium, phosphate, and vitamin D abnormalities

The regulation of calcium, phosphate, and vitamin D levels and interactions is critical for formation and growth of normal bones. In a growing child, disruptions at any point in the parathyroid-vitamin D-kidney-bone system can result in skeletal abnormalities and short stature. Examples include dietary deficiencies or excessive losses of vitamin D, parathyroid hormone resistance syndromes, and disorders resulting in low levels of phosphate such as X-linked hypophosphatemia (XLH) (see Chapter 6 for details). Inherited disorders are often suggested by skeletal abnormalities and disproportional features in the parents.

Parathyroid resistance syndromes include a heterogeneous group of disorders that involve a state of hypocalcemia and hyperphosphatemia secondary to end-organ resistance to parathyroid hormone (PTH). The genetic defect is in the *GNAS1* gene encoding the α subunit of the stimulatory G protein leading to a diminished/absent response to PTH. Depending on the specific postzygotic mutation variable degrees of resistance may be present in various hormone axes utilizing the G-protein signaling pathway (TSH, ADH, gonadotropins, glucagon, ACTH, and GHRH) may also be affected. Children with PTH resistance usually have short stature owing to intrinsic bone abnormalities, but moderate degrees of accompanying hypothyroidism and/or GH deficiency should be excluded as potential contributors to growth failure. Distinctive shortening of metacarpals may be present, along with truncal obesity and mental retardation. Collectively these features are referred to as Albright hereditary osteodystrophy (AHO). Treatment of parathyroid resistance includes calcium and activated vitamin D such as calcitriol.

In vitamin D insufficient states there is a reduction in the intestinal reabsorption of calcium resulting in low serum ionized levels and a triggering of the release of PTH. Increases in PTH levels results in (1) increase in calcium absorption in the kidneys; (2) activation of 1-α-hydroxylase, which increases the conversion of the vitamin D to its active form of 1,25-dihydroxy vitamin D; and (3) the release of calcium from bone. Failure of calcification leads to rickets in growing bone and osteomalacia in mature bones. In spite of food supplementation, vitamin D insufficiency continues to be a cause of rickets and growth retardation, particularly in infants born premature or to vitamin D deficient mothers, especially if breast-fed exclusively for several months and exposed to low natural light. Characteristic findings include frontal bossing, craniotabes, rachitic rosary, bowing of the legs, and gross motor delays.

Phosphorous is also an important component in the physiologic processes involved in bone mineralization.

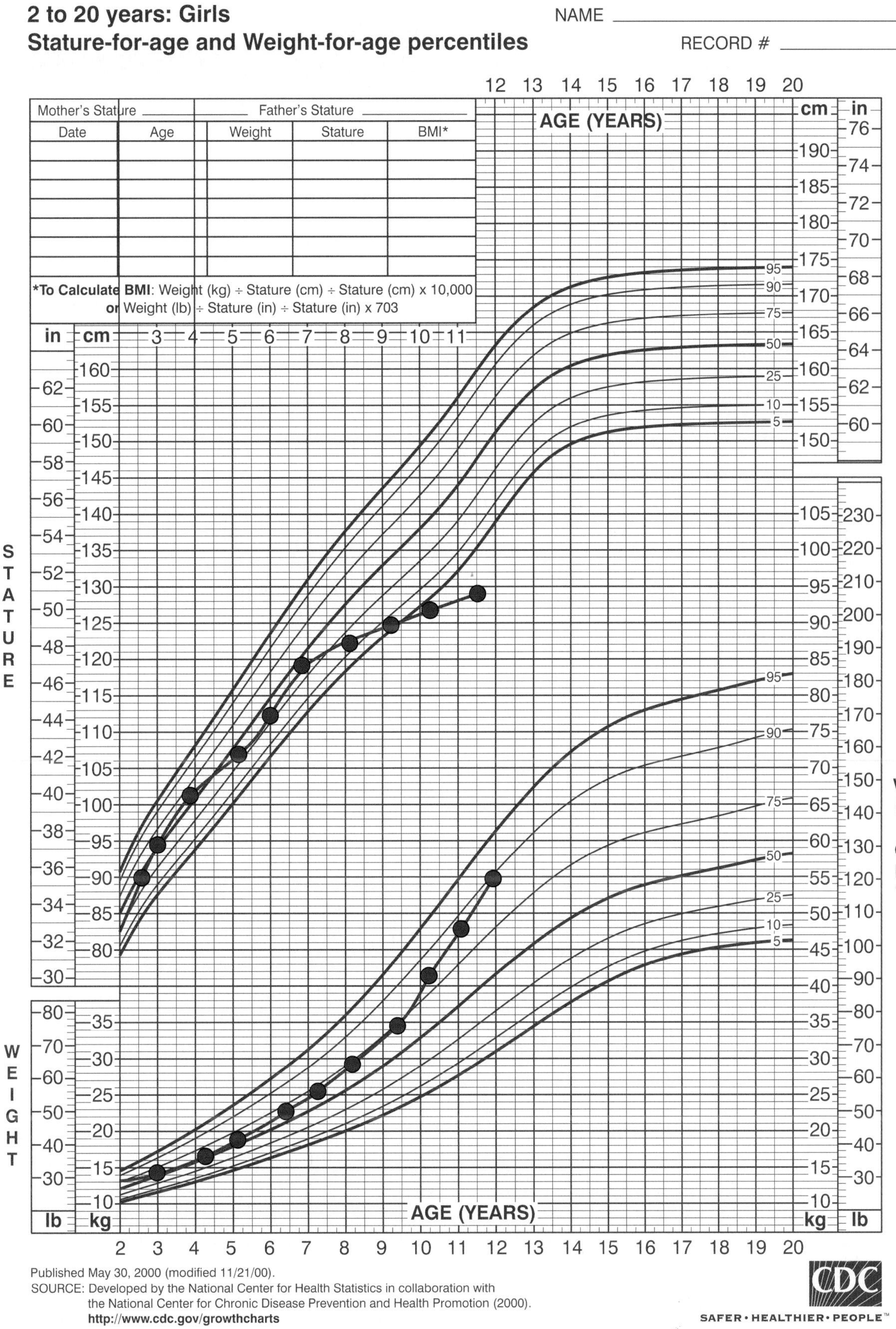

2 to 20 years: Girls
Stature-for-age and Weight-for-age percentiles

NAME _____

RECORD # _____

Published May 30, 2000 (modified 11/21/00).
SOURCE: Developed by the National Center for Health Statistics in collaboration with
the National Center for Chronic Disease Prevention and Health Promotion (2000).
http://www.cdc.gov/growthcharts

FIGURE 2-23 ■ Growth chart depicting declining growth velocity with acceleration of weight gain typical of cortisol excess.

A hypophosphatemic state leads to decreased mineralization and disorganization of the growth plates resulting in skeletal abnormalities. Various causes of low serum phosphorous include inherited disorders that result in the increased renal loss of phosphate. One such disease is X-linked hypophosphatemia (XLH) a disorder of phosphate homeostasis caused by a mutation in the *PHEX* gene encoding an endopeptidase expressed in bones and teeth. The pathophysiology of this mutation is still under investigation. Ultimately children with XLH have abnormal renal phosphate reabsorption and disruption of vitamin D metabolism resulting in disproportionately short-stature and radiologic evidence of rachitic disease. Serum phosphate levels are low but calcium levels are usually normal. Conventional treatment has included phosphate salts and vitamin D metabolites; however GH therapy has also been studied in this population because of its known effects on increasing renal phosphate retention. Consequently, GH has been administered to poorly growing children with X-linked hypophosphatemic rickets (XHR). Thus far, there is not enough conclusive evidence to show that GH treatment in this population is associated with changes in linear growth or improvements in bone mineralization or proportions.[40]

Abnormal Growth in Chronic Disease States

Growth impairment frequently accompanies chronic illness in children and adolescents (Table 2-8). In most circumstances, growth impairment is the result of multiple abnormalities. In the initial response to an acute illness, the anterior pituitary actively continues to secrete hormones into the circulation while in the periphery, anabolic target organ hormones are inactivated.[41] This response is thought to be beneficial and adaptive, causing reduced energy consumption, redirecting substrate utilization to make glucose, amino acids, and free fatty acid (FFA) preferentially available to critical organs, postponing catabolism, and inducing activation of immune response. However, when critical illness becomes prolonged, this initial positive adaptation becomes progressively more deleterious as mechanisms developed during evolution to allow survival during chronic stress become dominant. For example, during chronic illness pulsatile secretion of anterior pituitary hormones becomes uniformly reduced secondary to reduced hypothalamic stimulation, leading to decreased protein synthesis and increased protein degradation, reduced fat oxidation, insulin resistance resulting in impaired anabolism and reduced activity of target organs. In most cases, this chronic maladaption is combined with factors related directly to the primary illness itself. In rat models for inflammatory bowel

Table 2-8.

Chronic Disease, Systemic Disorders

Central nervous system
Cardiovascular system: Cyanotic heart disease, congestive heart disease
Lungs: Cystic fibrosis
Gastrointestinal system: Gluten enteropathy, Crohn disease, ulcerative colitis, chronic liver disorders
Urinary tract: Chronic renal failure, renal tubular acidosis
Connective tissue: Juvenile idiopathic arthritis, dermatomyositis
Chronic infections: HIV
Psychological disorders: Anorexia nervosa, psychosocial dwarfism

disease (IBD), for example, about 60% of the final growth impairment is attributable to undernutrition, while inflammation accounts for the remaining growth deficit. In humans, steroid treatment often further compromises growth.

Imbalance between energy supply and needs

Normal growth requires a balance between nutrient requirement and intake. Patients with cystic fibrosis (CF), for example, either lose weight or fail to grow normally if their absorbed energy intake is less than their total daily energy expenditure.

Reduced intake in chronic diseases. Reduced macro- and micronutrient intake and a disordered metabolic state result in both an insufficiency of substrate and abnormalities in enzyme function. A number of specific factors may contribute to reduced energy intake, including anorexia, mechanical problems, pain, malabsorption, and increased losses

Anorexia. The melanocortin system in the hypothalamus and brainstem is believed to have a central role in the regulation of feeding behavior. It is composed of two types of neurons situated in the arcuate nucleus of the hypothalamus: those that produce pro-opiomelanocortin (POMC) and induce an anorexic signal and those that produce the Agouti-related peptide (AgRP) and neuropeptide Y (NPY) and induce an orexic signal. POMC is cleaved into α melanocyte stimulating hormone (MSH), which acts on the melanocortin-3 receptor and/or the melanocortin-4 receptor. The AgRP/NPY neurons release AgRP, which is a natural antagonist of the melanocortin-3 and melanocortin-4 receptors and blocks the action of MSH-α. Together, then, the regulation of POMC and AgRP synthesis and secretion promote feeding stimulation or inhibition. It is currently believed that cytokines can influence the brain through modulating peripheral neurons that project to the brain through the vagus nerve, modulation of hormones such as leptin, and possibly acting directly in the brain, through the local production of cytokines and chemokines. The increased levels of cytokines stimulate the central melanocortin system and induce loss of appetite. Melanocortin inhibition has been shown to be a powerful tool in blocking the symptoms of cachexia.

Mechanical problems and pain. Children with genetic syndromes frequently have feeding problems and swallowing dysfunction as a result of a complex interaction of anatomic, physiologic, and behavioral factors. Oral dysfunction (cleft lip/palate), neuromotor impairments such as in hypotonia, and pain may lead to feeding difficulties.

Malabsorption. Growth retardation may reflect chronic malabsorption further complicated by increased catabolism. Failure of normal growth in a child with inflammatory bowel disease is an indicator of insufficient and unsuccessful therapy. Growth resumes after effective control of the disease and improvement in nutritional intake.

Increased loss. Chronic diarrhea, and vomiting such as in chronic regurgitation and gastro-esophageal reflux in infancy, cause poor weight gain and growth. In diabetes, urinary losses of glucose caused by poor control may also result in poor growth. Similarly chronic glucosuria may worsen growth in patients with CF-related diabetes (CFRD).

Increased energy needs in chronic diseases. Caloric expenditure is often increased in children with chronic disorders owing to increased cardiac or pulmonary work in congenital heart or lung disease, chronic infections in cystic fibrosis, chronic inflammation in Crohn disease (CD) or juvenile idiopathic arthritis (JIA), or increased protein catabolism owing to steroid therapy. Lung inflammation, in particular, has been associated with increases in resting metabolic rate (RMR); An HIV-associated hypermetabolic state has been described in adults and children

Growth-disrupting endocrine effects of malnutrition and chronic illness. Undernutrition leads to a fundamental shift in endocrine homeostasis, geared toward conserving energy and promoting diversion of substrate away from growth and reproduction toward critical body processes.

GH-IGF-1 axis. In patients suffering from chronic undernutrition, both relative GH resistance with low IGF-1 and IGFBP-3 and reduced GH secretion have been reported. In addition, energy deficiency can inhibit the hypothalamic-pituitary-reproductive axis, leading to delay in pubertal development or frank hypogonadotrophic hypogonadism.

GH resistance. Stunting of body growth is a significant complication of advanced chronic renal failure (CRF). However, circulating GH levels are normal to elevated in uremia, suggesting the presence of resistance to GH action. Indeed, this disease is the most well-studied example of GH resistance and serves as a good model for several other chronic disorders. Insensitivity to GH is the consequence of multiple defects in the GH/insulin-like growth factor-1 (IGF-1) system.[42]

Loss of GH pulsatility. In patients who are critically ill for a prolonged time, the pulsatile release of GH is suppressed, whereas the nonpulsatile fraction of GH release remains somewhat elevated.[41] This loss of GH pulsatility contributes to the low serum concentrations of IGF-1, IGFBP-3, and ALS. The origin of the loss of GH pulsatility resides within the hypothalamus and appears to be related to deficiency or inactivity of endogenous GHS, rather than to GHRH deficiency or resistance.

Changes in GH receptor expression. Serum growth hormone binding protein (GHBP), which is a cleaved product of the GH receptor, is a marker for GH receptor density in tissues. GHBP is low in children and adults with CRF and proportionate to the degree of renal dysfunction and to growth rate.

Janus kinase/signal transducer and activator of transcription signaling. The binding of GH to the growth hormone receptor (GHR) results in receptor dimerization, and autophosphorylation of the receptor tyrosine kinases and Janus kinase 2 (JAK2), which, in turn, stimulates phosphorylation of the STAT proteins (STAT1, STAT3, and STAT5).[42] Upon activation, these STAT proteins translocate to the nucleus and activate GH-regulated genes. In uremia, a defect in the postreceptor JAK2/STAT transduction has been documented. The JAK2/STAT pathway is regulated, among other factors, by suppressor of cytokine signaling (SOCS) proteins, which is induced by GH. These proteins bind to JAK2 and inhibit STAT phosphorylation. Up-regulation of SOCS has been described in inflammatory states and may play a similar role in CRF.

IGFs and IGFBPs. IGFs are transported in plasma bound to IGF binding proteins (IGFBPs), which are responsible for extending their half-life and controlling their bioavailability. Of the six

IGFBPs, IGFBP-1, IGFBP-2, and IGFBP-6, which are all inhibitors of IGF-dependant proliferation of chondrocytes, are elevated in CRF and correlate with the degree of renal dysfunction. Increased levels of IGFBP-1 and IGFBP-2 have been shown to correlate negatively with height. In addition to GH resistance, patients with CRF have poor growth during puberty as a result of delayed onset of pubertal growth, short duration of pubertal growth, and reduced gain of height during puberty. Reduced gain of height during puberty has been attributed to less frequent or absent LH pulses and reduced bioactivity. These abnormalities are partially restored after kidney transplantation.[43]

GH deficiency. Deficiencies in anterior pituitary hormone secretion, ranging from subtle to complete, occur following radiation damage to the hypothalamic-pituitary axis (HPA), correlated with the severity and frequency of total radiation dose delivered and the length of follow-up. The GH axis is the most vulnerable to radiation.

Leptin. Leptin is a circulating hormone derived from adipose tissue, regulates energy intake, energy expenditure, and energy partitioning. In malnourished children, circulating leptin concentrations are low and correlate with low IGF-1 concentration. In addition low leptin concentrations suppress gonadotropin secretion and may increase cortisol concentrations

KiSS-1 and GPR54. *KiSS-1* gene-derived kisspeptin, signaling through the G protein–coupled receptor 54 (GPR54) is a pivotal regulator of gonadotropin secretion and pubertal development. In prepubertal rats, food deprivation during a short-term fast induced a decrease in hypothalamic KiSS-1 and increase in GPR54 mRNA expression. Thus the hypothalamic KiSS-1 system conveys information regarding metabolic state to the centers governing reproductive function through a putative leptin–kisspeptin–GnRH pathway.

Ghrelin. The novel stomach hormone ghrelin is an endogenous agonist at the GHS receptor. In addition to its ability to stimulate GH secretion and gastric motility, ghrelin has a potent orexigenic effect mediated through hypothalamic neuropeptide Y (NPY) and Agouti-related peptide (AgRP), and increases respiratory quotient (VQ). Therefore, defective ghrelin signaling from the stomach could contribute to abnormalities in energy balance, growth, and associated gastrointestinal and neuroendocrine functions. However, paradoxically, in patients with chronic illness, such as inflammatory bowel disease (IBD), serum concentrations of ghrelin are increased, correlate with the severity of disease and show a negative correlation with IGF-1. These findings suggest that ghrelin resistance rather than deficiency may be characteristic of adaptation to chronic illness.

Chronic hypoxia. Chronic hypoxia is frequently associated with poor growth. Serum IGF-1 levels are lower and GH levels higher in patients with congenital heart disease than normal controls suggesting GH resistance. Moreover, serum IGF-1 levels are significantly lower in cyanotic CHD patients than those who are acyanotic. Many oxygen-sensitive regulatory mechanisms work through hypoxia inducible factor 1. Hypoxia-inducible factor 1 plays a pivotal role in the adaptation to chronic hypoxia by allowing energy production in anaerobic conditions, and is also involved in the development of anorexia through induction of the promoter of the leptin gene

Inflammation. The release of inflammatory cytokines and glucocorticoids, particularly in conditions characterized by wasting, lead to decreased protein synthesis in muscle and bone, development of GH and/or IGF-1 resistance, and enhanced protein degradation. Chronic inflammation, such as in JIA and inflammatory bowel diseases, is characterized by the production of cytokines, such as tumor necrosis factor and interleukin (IL)1 and IL6. In these disorders, growth retardation is strongly correlated with the severity and duration of the disease and serum concentrations of cytokines. High circulating IL6 levels in transgenic mice overexpressing the *IL6* gene induced a decrease in IGF-1 production and growth retardation. In addition, in patients with CD, either intestinal resection or enteral nutrition can induce catch-up growth in the early stages of puberty owing to remission of the inflammatory process and an early increase in IGF-1 levels preceding improvement in nutritional status.[43]

Abnormal Growth in Specific Disorders

In the past, abnormal growth and delayed puberty was a frequent consequence of chronic diseases. However, with modern treatment, severe short stature is no longer common. However in some specific situations, growth retardation remains a problem that is difficult to prevent and treat. In these cases, short adult stature will be a complication of the disease and will have an influence on the quality of life of the patient.

Diabetes

Clinical presentation. Extreme short stature was a component of diabetes in the past and part of the "historical" Mauriac syndrome. For example, in a study of identical twins discordant for diabetes, it was found that the diabetic twin was, on average, 5.8 cm shorter than the control twin. Although modern management of diabetes has eliminated severe growth alterations, some degree of growth impairment can be observed in poorly controlled diabetic patients. Furthermore, after a period of better metabolic control, an improvement in the growth velocity has been described, an observation that can be used as an incentive for a better glycemic control by the young patient. Longer disease duration and poorer metabolic control are factors associated with a shorter adult height. This loss in height is, to a large extent, caused by a decrease in the pubertal growth spurt, particularly in girls.

Elevated plasma concentration of GH and decreased concentration of IGF-1 have been shown in diabetes and this apparent GH resistance may explain, in part, the abnormal growth observed in some patients; improved metabolic control has been associated with an increase in IGF-1. However, one should keep in mind that autoimmune disorders frequently associated with type 1 diabetes, such as hypothyroidism and celiac disease, may be present and be a major cause of growth retardation. These disorders should be excluded in any diabetic patients with abnormal growth velocity.

Treatment. There is no specific treatment of short stature in children with diabetes. Improved compliance and metabolic control will result in increased growth rate and catch-up growth.

Chronic renal faliure

Immense progress has been made in the treatment of chronic renal faliure (CRF) but growth retardation remains a difficult problem in 30% to 60% of patients.

Clinical presentation. There is no single cause of growth failure in CRF and the underlying renal disease is important to consider when analyzing the mechanism of growth retardation. Congenital renal dysplasia is one of the most frequent causes of CRF during infancy and childhood. Children usually show a constant decline in renal function over time and renal insufficiency is frequently associated with electrolyte and water loss, which contribute to growth failure. Malnutrition owing to inadequate caloric intake and frequent vomiting may further exacerbate the poor growth. Children with glomerulopathies may also have growth retardation. The nephrotic state and glucocorticoid therapy in glucocorticoid-dependent nephrotic syndrome are both known causes of growth retardation in these patients.

In patients with tubular or interstitial nephropathies, the tubular dysfunction characterized by electrolyte, bicarbonate, and water loss can lead to severe growth retardation. The Fanconi syndrome is an example of complex tubular disorder that can be associated with severe stunting of growth. Cystinosis is another example of a disorder with severe short stature of complex etiology. Growth is compromised in infancy before alteration in glomerular function and the decreased growth velocity observed at this age is mainly because of tubular dysfunction. Generalized deposition of cystine crystals, particularly in the growth plate and several endocrine glands, further aggravate the growth failure that is one of the most severe observed in children with CRF.

Although the uremic state is corrected by dialysis treatment, dialysis usually has a weak impact on growth. Renal transplantation will improve the growth rate; however, the amplitude of the growth catch up varies widely. Catch up growth is influenced by glucocorticoid administration, a strong argument for using alternate day steroid treatment, decreasing the steroid dosage, and using alternative immunosuppressants to allow withdrawal of steroid therapy. Another factor is the age and glomerular function at transplantation. Indeed several studies have shown a negative association between age at transplantation and pubertal height gain. Since the total pubertal height gain is reduced in children with end stage renal disease, early transplantation will have a positive influence on pubertal height gain and adult height.

Treatment. General measures, such as adequate caloric intake, alkaline supplementation for the treatment of metabolic acidosis, and supplementation of water and electrolytes have a strong influence on growth in infants and young children. Since the impact of dialysis and transplantation on growth is far from optimal, the best strategy is to avoid the development of a growth deficit prior to transplantation. This means early transplantation, efficacious immune-suppressive therapy, and reduction (or avoidance) of steroids use. The efficacy of GH treatment in improving growth velocity and adult height has been widely recognized and this treatment has been approved in several countries. The effect of GH treatment on growth velocity is illustrated in Figure 2-24. The growth response is positively associated with residual renal function, duration of GH treatment, and target height and inversely associated with age at start of treatment. Long-term GH administration results in increased adult height but response is diminished in patients on dialysis and who have delayed puberty.[44] Whether induction of puberty and intensified dialysis will improve outcomes needs more investigation. The safety of GH therapy in this indication seems to be comparable to that shown for other indications.

Chronic inflammation
Clinical presentation. Poor growth and short stature is a characteristic feature of chronic inflammation, particularly in juvenile inflammatory arthritis. Although rare

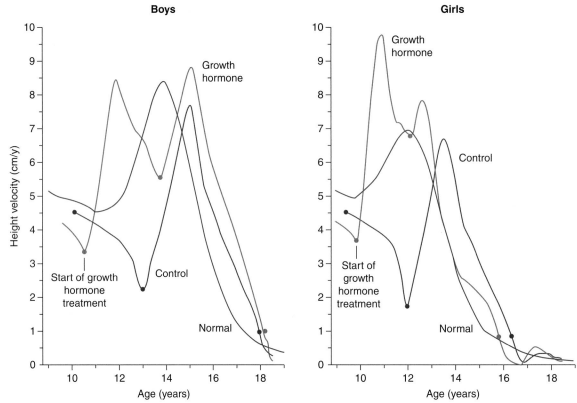

FIGURE 2-24 ■ Mean height velocity curves in 32 boys and 6 girls with CRF during treatment with GH (green circles) as compared with 50 children with renal failure not treated with GH (red circles) and 232 normal children (thin lines). The dots indicate three key moments in the follow-up: Start of treatment with GH, minimum prepubertal growth velocity, and end of the pubertal growth spurt. The cumulative height gain in the GH-treated children was twice that of the untreated controls. (*Redrawn from Haffner D, Schaefer F, Nissel R, et al. Effect of growth hormone treatment on the adult height of children with chronic renal failure. German study group for growth hormone treatment chronic renal failure. N Engl J Med. 2000; 343:923-930.*)

in the mono or polyarticular forms, stunting of growth is part of the clinical picture in the severe systemic forms. As shown in Figure 2-25, decreased growth rate and short stature occur very early in the course of the disease and will lead to severe adult short stature. Chronic inflammation and glucocorticoid administration are the main causes of growth impairment.

Treatment. Decrease steroid dosage and alternative therapy, such as anti-TNF-α may positively affect the growth rate of these patients. Moreover, it has been shown that GH administration will induce catch-up growth, improves final height and, when given at onset of the disease, will prevent the deleterious action of the disease on growth.[45,46] The safety of GH in this setting seems to be excellent and, in the few studies reported so far, glucose tolerance seems only moderately affected. The positive effect of GH on body composition, decreasing the fat mass and increasing the lean mass, is probably responsible for the modest anomalies of carbohydrate metabolism in these patients despite receiving glucocorticoids and GH, two drugs that induce insulin resistance.

Gastrointestinal diseases

Clinical presentation. Several intestinal disorders may cause growth failure and decreased growth velocity may precede any specific signs of malabsorption or inflammation. Gastrointestinal disorders should therefore be considered in a child with unexplained growth failure. Celiac disease may lead to a failure of statural growth, although short stature is probably not a frequent manifestation in this disease. After institution of a gluten-free diet, the symptoms will disappear rapidly and most patients will exhibit complete catch-up growth.

Growth failure is one of the major complications in children with inflammatory bowel disease. Although rare in children with ulcerative colitis, poor growth is a frequent manifestation in children with CD; short stature has been reported in 15% to 40% of adult patients with CD of pediatric onset. This large variation is probably explained by heterogeneity—extension of the lesions, degree of inflammation—of the cases included in the studies. The onset of puberty may be delayed and pubertal progression is frequently abnormal. Age at menarche is frequently late.

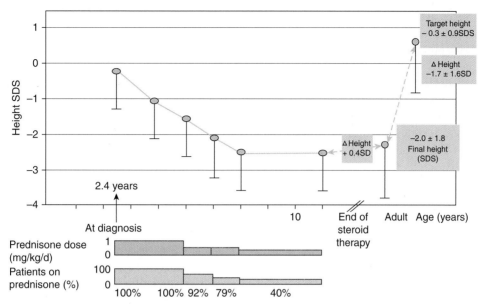

FIGURE 2-25 ■ Change in height SDS throughout follow-up in a group of 24 patients suffering from JIA. Note the marked loss in height occurring immediately after onset of the disease and glucocorticoid therapy and the partial catch-up growth after end of glucocorticoid treatment. However, the catch-up is incomplete and will result in adult short stature. (*Redrawn from Simon D, Prieur AM, Quartier P, Charles Ruiz J, Czernichow P. Early recombinant human growth hormone treatment in glucocorticoid-treated children with juvenile idiopathic arthritis: a 3-year randomized study.* J Clin Endocrinol Metab. *2007 Jul;92(7):2567-2573.*)

Treatment. There is no specific treatment of the short stature caused by chronic inflammatory disease. Improving nutrition and decreasing the inflammatory state, however, will usually induce rapid catch-up growth. In CD, for example (Figure 2-26), it has been shown that constant enteral nutrition and partial intestinal resection will quickly decrease inflammatory indices, increase plasma IGF-1, and ultimately increase growth velocity.

Chronic disease and corticosteroid therapy

Glucocorticoids (GCs) interfere with the GH-IGF-1 axis at the hypothalamic, pituitary, and target organ levels, affecting hormone release, receptor abundance, signal transduction, gene transcription, pre-mRNA splicing and mRNA translation.[39] In addition GCs disturb normal calcium balance at the intestine and kidney and have direct effects at the growth plate, including the suppression of gene expression, chondrocyte proliferation and matrix proteoglycan synthesis, sulfation, release, and mineralization as well as the augmentation of hypertrophic cell apoptosis. In addition pharmacological doses of GC can induce a decrease in LH secretion.

The role of steroid in CRF and JIA has been described earlier but there are several other situations where glucocorticoids are the key component of the treatment of a chronic disease and will be responsible for decreased growth and short stature. The severity of growth retardation mainly depends on the age at onset and severity of the disease and the duration and dose of glucocorticoid therapy. In asthma, for example, the

growth retardation is generally modest and the adult height is normal. This is mainly caused by improved use of inhaled steroid and decreased systemic glucocorticoid exposure. On the other hand, in children with

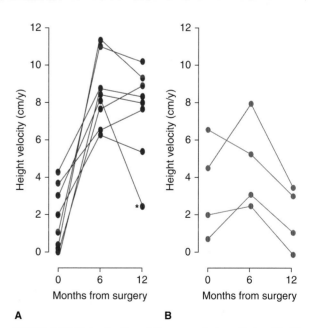

FIGURE 2-26 ■ Acceleration of linear growth in patients with CD after intestinal resection. In the pre- and early pubertal patients, growth velocity increased dramatically in the postoperative period compared with preoperative growth (**[A]** pre- and early puberty and **[B]** red dots and green dots mid- and late puberty). (*From Lipson AB, Savage MO, Davies PS, et al. Acceleration of linear growth following intestinal resection for Crohn's disease. Eur J Pediatr. 1990; 49:687-690.*)

Diamond-Blackfan anemia for example, short stature is present in one-third of the patients receiving prednisone, while being observed in only 5% of patients who were off treatment.

Glucocorticoid administration not only has an impact on growth. Major changes in body composition such as muscle wasting, increased fat mass, and bone demineralization frequently develop and will have long-term deleterious effects in adults.

Treatment. Decreasing steroid exposure, when possible, is the best way to diminish the consequences of treatment. The efficacy of GH administration on linear growth has been reported in patients with steroid-induced growth retardation. However, except for a few specific indications, evidence for a long-term effect of GH on adult height is still lacking.

NON-STATURAL GROWTH EFFECTS OF GH

Metabolic Effects of GH in Children

Linear growth requires an anabolic state of protein synthesis and utilization of stored energy in fat. The enhancement of protein synthesis occurs, not surprisingly, in bone, cartilage, and skeletal muscles, but also in the erythropoietic system, and other major organs (Figure 2-27). GH produces positive nitrogen balance, increases amino acid transport into cells, increases intracellular ribonucleic acid (RNA), and decreases urea production and blood urea nitrogen levels. A high-normal or mildly elevated blood, urea, nitrogen (BUN) level and low serum phosphorus and alkaline phosphatase level are usually observed in GH deficiency and reverse with GH treatment. Markers of bone mineral metabolism are also improved. GHD children on GH therapy have better bone density and 1,25-dihydroxyvitamin D levels.

GHRs and expression of GH receptor mRNA have been demonstrated both in preadipocyte cultures and in mature adipocytes. Some actions of GH in adipose tissue are mediated directly through interaction with the GH receptor, while others are mediated indirectly through IGF-1. These actions include: (1) inhibition of differentiation of immature adipocytes to mature adipocytes; (2) enhancement of lipolysis and site-specific FFA release from adipose tissue; and (3) inhibition of lipoprotein lipase and stimulation of hormone sensitive lipase. Consequently, GH-deficient children tend to demonstrate increased, predominantly abdominal, subcutaneous fat, which lessens and becomes more peripheral during therapy with exogenous GH. Non-GH-deficient children also display reduction in overall body fat during GH therapy.

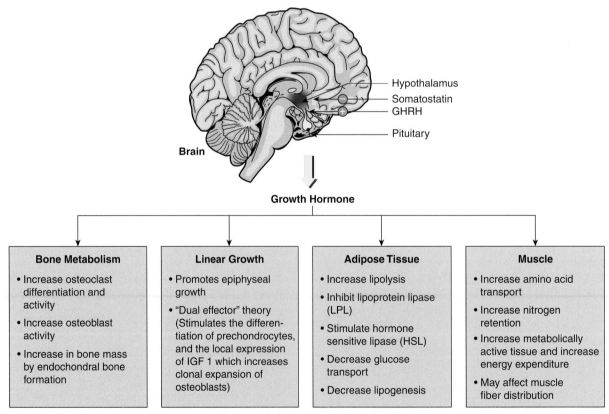

FIGURE 2-27 ■ Multiple sites of GH action. GH influences four major areas of development: bone metabolism, linear growth, adipose tissue, and development of muscle.

The effects of GH on carbohydrate metabolism are complex. GH is pivotal for maintenance of normal glucose homeostasis in infants, but this critical role is markedly diminished in older children and adults. In a child with GH deficiency, insulin secretion is diminished (related in part to pancreatic islet cell hypoplasia) and insulin sensitivity is heightened. Nearly all studies of GH therapy in children and adults show an increase in fasting and postprandial insulin levels. However, glucose homeostasis is generally not impaired. A theoretical concern is that normal levels of blood glucose and glycosylated hemoglobin during GH therapy are preserved by compensatory hyperinsulinemia, which when persistent can be associated with atherosclerosis and hypertension. Higher levels of insulin (which do not correlate closely with GH dose) usually return to normal when GH therapy is discontinued. Reports of diabetes occasionally appear, but large pharmaco-epidemiological databases do not indicate an increase in diabetes incidence. Continued careful prospective follow-up of individuals during and after GH therapy is needed to resolve this issue.

Potential Adverse Effects of GH Therapy

Recombinant biosynthetic GH preparations are highly purified and free of contaminants. The possibility of infectiuos transmission through GH has been virtually eliminated. However, surveillance of patients who received pituitary-derived GH for development of Creutzfeldt-Jacob remains important. Antigenicity of GH preparations is also low, although GH antibodies can be detected in 10% to 30% of treated children. With rare exceptions (< 0.1%), these antibodies do not impede effects of GH. Nevertheless, current dosages of GH therapy commonly result in pharmacological, rather than replacement therapy, prompting concerns about long-term effects of exposure to various degrees of GH excess during childhood.

Thyroid dysfunction

The GH administration to healthy subjects acutely increases serum T_3 and reciprocally decreases free thyroxine (T_4). Similarly, transient laboratory indications of hypothyroidism may be seen in as many as 25% of GH-deficient children treated with GH, with declines in serum T_4 levels reflecting increased peripheral conversion of T_4 to T_3. GHD patients who display subnormal nocturnal TSH surges, signifying a pre-existing central hypothyroidism, are more likely to display subnormal T_4 and free T_4 levels during GH therapy, and do benefit from thyroid replacement. Most studies, however, indicate that children with normal thyroid function before treatment do not develop significant perturbations in thyroid hormone metabolism during GH therapy.

Disproportionate growth

Concerns of disproportional growth have also risen in the context of children treated with higher than GHD replacement doses. The IGF-1 levels in some patients can approach those found in acromegaly, and development of acromegaloid features (eg, large hands and feet) during GH therapy has been reported, particularly when higher-than-conventional doses are used toward the final stages of treatment.

Malignancy concerns

Perhaps the greatest concern regarding GH therapy is the theoretical possibility that GH could facilitate the development of cancers. Growth hormone is mitogenic, and there is evidence in animals of a cause and effect relation between supra-physiological doses of GH and development of leukemia. There are three clinical settings which have raised concern: (1) GH-treatment induced new malignancy; (2) GH-treatment induced recurrent malignancy; and (3) GH-treatment induced second malignancy in those already treated for one tumor. In 1988, reports from Japan describing leukemia in GH-treated children raised concern about new malignancy. Subsequent analyses, based on much larger total patient-years of GH treatment, indicate that the rates of new leukemia in (non-Japanese) patients without pre-existing risk factors who are treated with GH is not greater than expected for the general population.[47] This lack of increased risk in children without preexisting risk factors has been confirmed in the Japanese population. Any possible increased incidence of leukemia appears limited to those patients with known risk factors, and owing to the small numbers of events in such patients, it remains impossible to determine any contribution of GH therapy. With regard to nonleukemia cancers, a retrospective analysis of large postmarketing database found no evidence of an increased risk of developing an extracranial, nonleukemia neoplasm in GH-treated patients.[48]

With regard to recurrent malignancy, no report has associated GH therapy with an increased incidence of tumor recurrence. Assessing the risk for recurrence of CNS tumors is more complicated by lack of reliable knowledge about the natural history of this heterogeneous group of tumors. Numerous studies report that the relative risk of recurrence or death is similar in GH-treated and untreated patients with prior malignancy.[49] However, a cautious interpretation of such data is still appropriate. Most recurrences occur within the first 2 years of treatment, and most endocrinologists defer institution of treatment until a year of stable remission has passed. While this may result in some lost growth for the child, it also avoids the inevitable association of GH therapy and tumor recurrence during this high-risk period.

With regard to second malignancy, GH therapy does not appear to increase the risk of disease recurrence or death in survivors of childhood cancer. The increased number of second neoplasms, particularly in survivors of acute leukemia, is of concern, but the data need to be interpreted with caution given the small number of events.

Pseudotumor cerebri

Edema and sodium retention rarely occurs early in the course of GH therapy (particularly in older, heavier children and adolescents), attributable to a direct antinatriuretic effect of GH and/or IGF-1 on the renal tubule and minor elevations in plasma renin activity and aldosterone. Occasionally, fluid shifts within the CNS are sufficient to cause benign intracranial hypertension (pseudotumor cerebri) and its symptoms of headache, visual loss, vomiting, and papilledema. It is speculated that direct fluid retaining properties of GH and/or action of locally produced IGF-1 on cerebrospinal fluid (CSF) production are causative. Most instances have occurred during early (though not invariably) treatment of patients with severe GHD or other risk factors for this condition (eg, chronic renal insufficiency, Prader-Willi syndrome). Cessation of GH therapy reverses symptoms, and resumption of GH treatment can be successfully accomplished with reinitiation at a lower dose and gradual return to the initial dose. It is recommended that fundoscopic examination be performed on all patients before initiation of GH therapy and periodically thereafter.

Slipped capital femoral epiphysis

The GH treatment causes an increase in both the proliferative and hypertrophied zones of the growth plate that may reduce the force needed to shear it. An increased frequency of SCFE has been reported during treatment with GH, but is also associated with both hypothyroidism and (untreated) GHD. This rare complication is more common in children with organic causes of severe GHD, who tend to exhibit the most marked increase in growth rates with GH replacement. These children require close monitoring for limp and hip or knee pain. Whether it is GH therapy or simply rapid growth per se that plays a role in SCFE is difficult to determine, particularly because the incidence of SCFE varies widely (2-140 cases per 100,000) depending on age, sex, race, and geographic location.

Miscellaneous side effects

Concerns raised regarding other potential adverse effects of GH therapy (eg, reduced testicular volume, gynecomastia, deterioration of renal function in CRF patients, cardiac ventricular hypertrophy in Turner and Noonan syndrome) have, to date, either not been realized or considered to be of sufficient clinical significance to alter prescribing.

In summary, nearly two decades of experience with recombinant GH has proven this therapy to be remarkably safe when used in conventional substitution doses for GH deficiency. Higher-dose therapy for other indications also appears to be safe, but continued surveillance of its metabolic effects is indicated. There appear to be very few medical contraindications to GH therapy. Nevertheless, a recent cohort study of 1848 patients treated during childhood and early adulthood with human pituitary GH between 1959 and 1985 suggested (based upon a small number of cases) increased risk of colorectal cancer incidence and mortality, and of Hodgkin disease mortality.[50] These data, and the experience of transmission of Creutzfeldt-Jakob via pituitary GH are poignant reminders that a farsighted view must be taken of the potential ramifications of long-term hormonal therapy.

ETHICAL CONSIDERATIONS IN GH THERAPY FOR SHORT STATURE

Limited availability of GH once provided a barrier to expanding its use beyond children who were unequivocally GHD. Today, increased supply of GH has been matched by increased demand. Ten years ago in the United States, there was one approved indication for GH, two GH manufacturers, and approximately 10,000 children receiving treatment at a cost ranging between $5000 and $40,000 per year. Today, we have eight FDA-approved indications for GH (Table 2-5), multiple US and international manufacturers, and well over 40,000 active patients treated in the United States. Nevertheless, GH therapy remains expensive. Relaxed diagnostic criteria have obliterated any clear boundary between GH deficiency and sufficiency, allowing many partially affected children access to treatment.

Widespread distribution of GH has been partially deterred by high drug costs. Prescribing GH requires a difficult and often uncomfortable balancing of responsible use of medical resources with an obligation to do the best for each individual patient. Concern about psychological harm is invoked as a primary rationale for treating short stature yet data confirming the efficacy of GH therapy in alleviating the psychosocial consequences of short stature are scarce.[51] If the ultimate goal of GH therapy is not tall stature but, rather, an improved quality of life, documentation of psychosocial impairment caused by stature prior to therapy and improvement following GH therapy ought to play an important role in the initiation of GH therapy and evaluation of its efficacy. To date, however, growth rate and final adult height remain the measures by which therapeutic success is judged.

Determining an appropriate end-point for GH therapy for short stature remains controversial. Attainment of genetic potential for height, a realistic possibility with optimal diagnosis and treatment, remains a goal for many. Consistent adherence to the goal of alleviating disabling short stature, on the other hand, implies that GH therapy for stature (ie, not for GH replacement in severely GH-deficient individuals) be discontinued when each treated child reaches an adult height and is no longer considered a disability. While no policy regarding GH therapy will ever eliminate the first percentile, the second strategy has as its goal bringing children into the normal opportunity range for height without further enhancing those who have achieved a height within the normal adult distribution.[10]

TALL STATURE AND OVERGROWTH DISORDERS

Tall stature and overgrowth disorders are relatively rare occurrences in pediatric endocrinology but like worrisome growth related to short stature, these disorders also warrant careful evaluation. Pathologic conditions can present with excessive growth, reflecting effects of intrauterine factors, genetic factors, and hormonal stimulation of growth, including GH excess.

Intrauterine Overgrowth

An infant born with a length and weight above the 90th percentile for gestational age (excessive intrauterine growth) is defined "large for gestational age (LGA)". This condition is most commonly caused by maternal diabetes mellitus and should prompt maternal evaluation even in the absence of a positive clinical history. In the postnatal period, blood sugars should be careful monitored as intravenous infusions of glucose may be necessary to prevent severe insulin-induced hypoglycemia.

Beckwith-Wiedemann syndrome is the next most common cause of intrauterine overgrowth. The complex molecular genetics involves multiple alterations to imprinted gene function on chromosome 11p15 region. Hypoglycemia frequently occurs and is secondary to islet cell hyperplasia and subsequent hyperinsulinemia. Clinical features include excessive somatic and organ overgrowth, macroglossia, umbilical abnormalities (omphalocele, umbilical hernia, diastasic recti), craniofacial abnormalities (midface hypoplasia, prominent occiput, flat nasal bridge, high arched palate), and earlobe abnormalities. Over-expression of the paternally derived gene for IGF-2 may account for fetal overgrowth, but no postnatal abnormality of the GH-IGF

axis has been identified. Various alterations in the growth regulatory genes in the 11p15 region may also account for somatic asymmetry and the syndrome's association with increased risk for various cancers such as Wilm tumor, adrenocortical carcinoma, hepatoblastoma, and rhabdomyosarcoma.

Children with Sotos syndrome are also usually born LGA and demonstrate abnormally rapid growth during the first 3 to 4 years of life. Body proportions are abnormal with arm span exceeding height by as much as 5 cm (normally this difference is negative up to age 12). Phenotypic features include prominent forehead, dolichocephaly and macrocephaly, high arched palate, hypertelorism with an unusual slant to the eyes, prominent ears, jaw, and chin, and enlarged hands and feet with thickened subcutaneous tissue. These children also have a nonprogressive neurological disorder associated with mental retardation and delayed motor milestones. Growth velocity remains rapid in childhood but with advancement in BA and early puberty resulting in early maturation of the growth plates resulting in a final height that is normal range. Multiple different mutations in the NSD1 (nuclear receptor SET domain-containing protein 1) gene on chromosome 5q35 have been identified and some are being correlated with variable phenotypes in this syndrome.

Constitutional Tall Stature

As with constitution short stature and delay of maturation, constitutional tall stature is a variant of normal childhood growth. By definition height is between 2 and 4 SD above the mean height for age. Birth length is usually normal, but accelerated growth during the first 12 to 15 months leads to crossing of percentiles toward a genetically determined (usually the mid-parental height) height percentile. Tall stature is evident by age 3 and subsequent growth is usually parallel to but above the 95th percentile. Body proportions are normal and the timing of puberty reflects familial characteristics. Genetic and familial factors, often from both parents, can explain the growth pattern of most children with tall stature. GH secretion and levels of IGF-1 and IGFBP-3 can be (but are not invariably) in the high-normal range, and elevated ratios of IGF-1/IGFBP-3 suggest greater bioavailability of IGF-1 for target tissue.

Because of societal definitions of normal height, cultural acceptance of tall stature and lack of parental concerns over a tall child cloud the true "incidence" of this growth pattern. Fortunately tall stature in females has become less stigmatizing and women are finding value in athletic and professional opportunities in which tall stature confers an advantage. Traditionally, treatment to attenuate height has relied on administration of gonadal steroids (usually estrogen) to hasten epiphyseal maturation. Discussion about therapy should be reserved for extreme cases (eg, boys with predicted height > 203 cm and girls > 186 cm). Even in those cases, clinically meaningful benefit depends on early and aggressive hormone therapy, and potential risks must be weighed against uncertain clinical benefit.

Growth Hormone Excess

The GH excess is a well-described but rare cause of tall stature and rapid growth in childhood. The etiology is usually a functioning pituitary adenoma driven by a constitutively activated G-protein reducing GTPase activity, increasing cAMP, and promoting excess GH secretion. While usually an isolated finding, GH producing tumors can occur in association with McCune-Albright syndrome (multiorgan G-protein activation), neurofibromatosis, and tuberous sclerosis. When prolonged GH excess occurs prior to epiphysial fusion or in the context of delayed puberty or absent gonadotrophs, adult heights typically exceeds MPH, and can be well above the normal range.

Diagnosis is suggested by accelerated growth diverging from the expected familial pattern. Skeletal age is normal or mildly advanced, yielding excessively tall adult height predictions. Basal serum GH levels may be normal or increased; given the pulsing nature of normal GH secretion, reliance on random samples can lead to both false-positive and false-negative impressions. Additional information suggesting the diagnosis includes lack of suppression of GH levels in response to a glucose load. Normally, a glucose load prompts insulin secretion, suppression of IGFBP-1 resulting in an increase in free IGF-1 levels and subsequent negative feed back to GH release. IGF-1 and IGFBP-3 levels are useful screening tests given their correlation to 24 hour GH secretion but are not always present in excess of values expected in normal puberty. Suggestive clinical and laboratory findings should prompt imagining of the hypothalamic/pituitary region with MRI.

Treatment is aimed at restoring the GH/IGF-1 axis to normal while preserving function of other pituitary hormones. Transsphenoidal resection can be curative for well-circumscribed adenomas but a transcranial approach may be necessary for more extensive adenomas. Adjunctive medical and radiation may be indicated for tumors not completely resected. The effects of radiation are typically delayed by several months to years (ie, GH levels decreased to 50% of initial levels by 2 years, 75% by 5 years, and 90% by 15 years) and loss of other pituitary function is common. Somatostatin analogues (octreotide) can be used to suppress GH levels and normalize IGF-1 as an alternative to surgical or radiation treatment. In children octreotide is given subcutaneously daily. Continuous subcutaneous pumps have also been utilized. Long-acting preparations are available and have been effective in the adult patients. Bromocriptine, a dopamine agonist, also leads to the reduction in GH secretion but most patients do not achieve normal IGF-1 levels and side effects (nausea, abdominal pain, fatigue, orthostatic hypotension) are common. In addition an analogue of GH that functions as a GH receptor antagonist has shown to be effective and approved for use of treatment of GH excess caused by pituitary tumors or ectopic GHRH hypersecretion. Long-term and pediatric studies are needed.

Other Genetic Syndromes Associated with Tall Stature

Klinefelter syndrome results from the presence of two or more X chromosomes in a male; 47, XXY is most common, with mosaic karyotypes (eg, XY/XXY) and other aneuploid karyotypes (eg, XXXY) occurring much less frequently. It occurs in between 1:500 and 1:1000 live male births. The presence of extra X chromosomes leads to testicular hyalinization and fibrosis, impaired testosterone production, and infertility. Depending on the severity of early testicular hypofunction, genital abnormalities such as unusually small testes, microphallus, cryptorchidism, and hypospadias may be present in the newborn period. Other clinical manifestations include abnormal body proportions (ie, long legs and low upper/lower segment ratio), mild mental retardation (reduced verbal IQ) and/or behavioral difficulties, learning disabilities, delayed or (more commonly) incomplete puberty, and gynecomastia. The clinical diagnosis is confirmed by demonstration of extra X chromosomes in the karyotype. Excessive growth in this syndrome may reflect dosage effects of the *SHOX* gene located on the X chromosome.

Therapeutic considerations for Klinefelter syndrome are focused on androgen replacement therapy. During puberty, laboratory evidence for hypergonadotropic hypogonadism becomes manifest, with abnormalities in FSH levels typically exceeding those in LH, and testosterone levels that are low for age during puberty and rarely rising above the low normal adult male range. It should be noted, however, that most patients with KS demonstrate transition to gonadal puberty without reliance on exogenous androgens. When androgen deficiency and evidence for testicular failure are severe, gradual introduction of long-acting intramuscular testosterone to a full replacement dosage of 200 mg q2 weeks will restore testosterone levels to the normal range. Gynecomastia (caused by aromatization of exogenous or endogenous androgens) can be severe, and may require surgical therapy. Rarely, concerns about excessive stature prompt discussion of height reduction therapy, but no data regarding the efficacy or advisability of early introduction of androgen therapy for this purpose is available. Recent studies have demonstrated residual foci of spermatogenesis in testicular biopsies of prepubertal boys with Klinefelter syndrome despite the characteristic extensive fibrosis and hyalinization of the seminiferous tubules. Novel sperm extraction techniques have allowed nonmosaic KS males to father children.[52] Since it appears possible that exogenous androgen treatment may negatively affect chances for later sperm extraction, reevaluation of criteria for androgen replacement therapy for adolescents with KS is underway.

The presence of an **extra Y chromosome,** which occurs in between 1:500 and 1:1000 live male births, also predisposes to tall stature. The incidence is markedly increased in males whose height exceeds 183 cm (6 ft). Other reported findings in affected individuals include hypospadias, cryptorchidism, severe acne, and variable degrees of mental retardation. However, broader studies indicate that predictions of behavior problems cannot be accurately made based upon the finding of an XYY karyotype.

Marfan syndrome is an autosomal dominant disorder of collage metabolism characterized by hyperextensible joints, dislocation of the lens, kyphoscoliosis, and aortic root dilatation. It is caused by mutations in the fibrillin gene located on chromosome 15, leading to a deficiency of elastin-associated microfibrils. Height is increased and body proportions are abnormal owing to excessive arm and leg length. Arm span is greater than height, and the upper/lower segment ratio is diminished. Long fingers and toes (arachnodactyly), pectus excavatum, and scoliosis are observed in most patients. Life expectancy is reduced primarily because of cardiovascular manifestations such as aortic regurgitation and dissection.

A similar body habitus and tendency toward tall stature is observed in **homocystinuria,** an autosomal recessive disorder caused by deficiency of cystathionine β-synthase. This enzyme catalyzes the combination of homocystine and serine to form cystathionine; a deficiency leads to elevations of homocystine in blood and urine. Patients usually appear normal at birth, but mental retardation, downward dislocation of the lens, and marked myopia and/or astigmatism are noted in early childhood. Osteoporosis, scoliosis, and thromboembolic phenomenon (arterial and venous) can also occur. Treatment includes dietary methionine restriction, and in responsive patients, pyridoxine administration. In some states, newborn screening for this rare disorder facilitates very early diagnosis.

REFERENCES

1. Nilsson O, Marino R, De Luca F, Phillip M, Baron J. Endocrine regulation of the growth plate. *Horm Res.* 2005; 64(4):157-165.

2. Greulich WPS, ed. Radiographic atlas of skeletal development of the hand and wrist. Stanford: Standford University Press; 1959.

3. Tanner Oshman D, Lindgren G, et al. Reliability of computer-assisted estimates of Tanner-Whitehouse skeletal maturity [CASA]: Comparison with manual method. *Horm Res.* 1994;42:288-294.

4. Biller BM. Concepts in the diagnosis of adult growth hormone deficiency. *Horm Res.* 2007;68(5):59-65.

5. Eugster EA, Pescovitz OH. New revelations about the role of STATs in stature. *N Engl J Med.* 2003 Sep 18; 349(12):1110-1112.

6. Cohen P. Overview of the IGF-I system. *Horm Res.* 2006; 65(1):3-8.

7. Allen DB, Fost N. hGH for short stature: ethical issues raised by expanded access. *J Pediatr.* 2004 May;144(5): 648-652.

8. Cohen P. Consensus statement on ISS. ISS Consensus Conference. Santa Monica, CA; 2007.

9. Allen DB. Growth hormone therapy for short stature: is the benefit worth the burden? *Pediatrics.* 2006 Jul;118(1): 343-348.

10. Moreira-Andres MN, Canizo FJ, de la Cruz FJ, Gomez-de la Camara A, Hawkins FG. Bone mineral status in prepubertal children with constitutional delay of growth and puberty. *Eur J Endocrinol.* 1998 Sep;139(3):271-275.

11. FDA approves humatrope for short stature. In: Administration FaD, ed: *Fed Regist.* 2003. pp. 24003-24004.

12. Quigley CA. Growth hormone treatment of non-growth hormone-deficient growth disorders. *Endocrinol Metab Clin North Am.* 2007 Mar; 36(1):131-186.

13. van Gool SA, Kamp GA, Visser-van Balen H, et al. Final height outcome after three years of growth hormone and gonadotropin-releasing hormone agonist treatment in short adolescents with relatively early puberty. *J Clin Endocrinol Metab.* 2007 Apr; 92(4):1402-1408.

14. Shulman DI, Francis GL, Palmert MR, Eugster EA. Use of aromatase inhibitors in children and adolescents with disorders of growth and adolescent development. *Pediatrics.* 2008 Apr;121(4):e975-983.

15. de Zegher F, Ong KK, Ibanez L, Dunger DB. Growth hormone therapy in short children born small for gestational age. *Horm Res.* 2006;65(3):145-152.

16. Saenger P, Czernichow P, Hughes I, Reiter EO. Small for gestational age: short stature and beyond. *Endocr Rev.* 2007 Apr; 28(2):219-251.

17. Ibanez L, Lopez-Bermejo A, Diaz M, Marcos MV, de Zegher F. Metformin treatment for four years to reduce total and visceral fat in low birth weight girls with precocious pubarche. *J Clin Endocrinol Metab.* 2008 May; 93(5):1841-1845.

18. Saenger P, Wikland KA, Conway GS, et al. Recommendations for the diagnosis and management of Turner syndrome. *J Clin Endocrinol Metab.* 2001 Jul; 86(7):3061-3069.

19. Rosenfeld RG, Attie KM, Frane J, et al. Growth hormone therapy of Turner's syndrome: beneficial effect on adult height. *J Pediatr.* 1998 Feb;132(2):319-324.

20. Stephure DK. Impact of growth hormone supplementation on adult height in Turner syndrome: results of the Canadian randomized controlled trial. *J Clin Endocrinol Metab.* 2005 Jun; 90(6):3360-3366.

21. Bondy CA. Care of girls and women with Turner syndrome: a guideline of the Turner Syndrome Study Group. *J Clin Endocrinol Metab.* 2007 Jan; 92(1):10-25.

22. MacFarlane CE, Brown DC, Johnston LB, et al. Growth hormone therapy and growth in children with Noonan's syndrome: results of 3 years' follow-up. *J Clin Endocrinol Metab.* 2001 May; 86(5):1953-1956.

23. Deng C W-BA, Shou R, Kuo A Leder P. Fibroblast growth factor receptor 3 is a negative regulator of bone growth. *Cell.* 1996; 84:911-921.

24. Horton WA, Rotter JI, Rimoin DL, Scott CI, Hall JG. Standard growth curves for achondroplasia. *J Pediatr.* 1978 Sep; 93(3):435-438.

25. Mullis PE, Patel MS, Brickell PM, Hindmarsh PC, Brook CG. Growth characteristics and response to growth hormone therapy in patients with hypochondroplasia: genetic linkage of the insulin-like growth factor I gene at chromosome 12q23 to the disease in a subgroup of these patients. *Clin Endocrinol (Oxf).* 1991 Apr; 34(4):265-274.

26. Carrel AL, Myers SE, Whitman BY, Allen DB. Benefits of long-term GH therapy in Prader-Willi syndrome: a 4-year study. *J Clin Endocrinol Metab.* 2002 Apr; 87(4):1581-1585.

27. Eiholzer U, Nordmann Y, L'Allemand D. Fatal outcome of sleep apnea in PWS during the initial phase of growth hormone treatment. A case report. *Horm Res.* 2002; 58(3):24-26.

28. Wit JM, Kamp GA, Rikken B. Spontaneous growth and response to growth hormone treatment in children with growth hormone deficiency and idiopathic short stature. *Pediatr Res.* 1996 Feb; 39(2):295-302.

29. Tauber M, Moulin P, Pienkowski C, Jouret B, Rochiccioli P. Growth hormone (GH) retesting and auxological data in 131 GH-deficient patients after completion of treatment. *J Clin Endocrinol Metab.* 1997 Feb; 82(2):352-356.

30. Laron Z. Disorders of growth hormone resistance in childhood. *Curr Opin Pediatr.* 1993 Aug; 5(4):474-480.

31. Buckway CK, Selva KA, Pratt KL, Tjoeng E, Guevara-Aguirre J, Rosenfeld RG. Insulin-like growth factor binding protein-3 generation as a measure of GH sensitivity. *J Clin Endocrinol Metab.* 2002 Oct; 87(10):4754-4765.

32. Woods KA, Camacho-Hubner C, Bergman RN, Barter D, Clark AJ, Savage MO. Effects of insulin-like growth factor I (IGF-I) therapy on body composition and insulin resistance in IGF-I gene deletion. *J Clin Endocrinol Metab.* 2000 Apr; 85(4):1407-1411.

33. Blum WF, Ranke MB, Kietzmann K, Gauggel E, Zeisel HJ, Bierich JR. A specific radioimmunoassay for the growth hormone (GH)-dependent somatomedin-binding protein: its use for diagnosis of GH deficiency. *J Clin Endocrinol Metab.* 1990 May;70(5):1292-1298.

34. Rosenfeld RG, Buckway C, Selva K, Pratt KL, Guevara-Aguirre J. Insulin-like growth factor (IGF) parameters and tools for efficacy: the IGF-I generation test in children. *Horm Res.* 2004;62(1):37-43.

35. Cohen P, Bright GM, Rogol AD, Kappelgaard AM, Rosenfeld RG. Effects of dose and gender on the growth and growth factor response to GH in GH-deficient children: implications for efficacy and safety. *J Clin Endocrinol Metab.* 2002 Jan;87(1):90-98.

36. Geffner ME. The growth without growth hormone syndrome. *Endocrinol Metab Clin North Am.* 1996 Sep; 25(3):649-663.

37. Mauras N, Attie KM, Reiter EO, Saenger P, Baptista J. High dose recombinant human growth hormone (GH) treatment of GH-deficient patients in puberty increases near-final height: a randomized, multicenter trial. Genentech, Inc., Cooperative Study Group. *J Clin Endocrinol Metab.* 2000 Oct; 85(10):3653-3660.

38. Collett-Solberg PF, Misra M. The role of recombinant human insulin-like growth factor-I in treating children with short stature. *J Clin Endocrinol Metab.* 2008 Jan;93(1):10-18.

39. Hochberg Z. Mechansims of steroid impairment of growth. *Hormone Res.* 2002;58(1):33-38.

40. Huiming Y, Chaomin W. Recombinant growth hormone therapy for X-linked hypophosphatemia in children. *Cochrane Database Syst Rev.* 2005(1):CD004447.

41. Van den Berghe G. Neuroendocrine pathobiology of chronic critical illness. *Crit Care Clin.* 2002 Jul;18(3):509-528.

42. Mahesh S, Kaskel F. Growth hormone axis in chronic kidney disease. *Pediatr Nephrol.* 2008 Jan; 23(1):41-48.

43. Simon D. Puberty in chronically diseased patients. *Horm Res.* 2002;57(2):53-56.

44. Nissel R, Lindberg A, Mehls O, Haffner D. Factors predicting the near-final height in growth hormone-treated children and adolescents with chronic kidney disease. *J Clin Endocrinol Metab.* 2008 Apr; 93(4):1359-1365.

45. Bechtold S, Ripperger P, Dalla Pozza R, et al. Growth hormone increases final height in patients with juvenile idiopathic arthritis: data from a randomized controlled study. *J Clin Endocrinol Metab.* 2007 Aug; 92(8):3013-3018.

46. Simon D, Prieur AM, Quartier P, Charles Ruiz J, Czernichow P. Early recombinant human growth hormone treatment in glucocorticoid-treated children with juvenile idiopathic arthritis: a 3-year randomized study. *J Clin Endocrinol Metab.* 2007 Jul; 92(7):2567-2573.

47. Allen DB, Rundle AC, Graves DA, Blethen SL. Risk of leukemia in children treated with human growth hormone: review and reanalysis. *J Pediatr.* 1997 Jul;131(1 Pt 2): S32-36.

48. Tuffli GA, Johanson A, Rundle AC, Allen DB. Lack of increased risk for extracranial, nonleukemic neoplasms in recipients of recombinant deoxyribonucleic acid growth hormone. *J Clin Endocrinol Metab.* 1995 Apr; 80(4): 1416-1422.

49. Swerdlow AJ, Reddingius RE, Higgins CD, et al. Growth hormone treatment of children with brain tumors and risk of tumor recurrence. *J Clin Endocrinol Metab.* 2000 Dec; 85(12):4444-4449.

50. Swerdlow AJ, Higgins CD, Adlard P, Preece MA. Risk of cancer in patients treated with human pituitary growth hormone in the UK, 1959-85: a cohort study. *Lancet.* 2002 Jul 27; 360(9329):273-277.

51. Sandberg DE, Bukowski WM, Fung CM, Noll RB. Height and social adjustment: are extremes a cause for concern and action? *Pediatrics.* 2004 Sep;114(3):744-750.

52. Wikstrom AM, Dunkel L. Testicular function in Klinefelter syndrome. *Horm Res.* 2008; 69(6):317-326.

CHAPTER 3

Posterior Pituitary and Disorders of Water Metabolism

Abhinash Srivatsa, Joseph A. Majzoub, and Michael S. Kappy

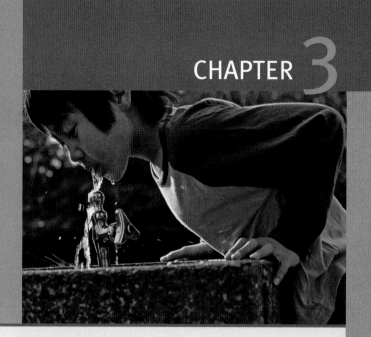

REGULATION OF WATER HOMEOSTASIS

Maintenance of the tonicity of extracellular fluids within a very narrow range is crucial for proper cell function, because extracellular osmolality regulates cell shape, as well as intracellular concentrations of ions and other osmolytes.[1,2] Furthermore, proper extracellular ionic concentrations are necessary for the correct function of ion channels, action potentials, and other modes of intercellular communication. Normal blood tonicity is maintained over a tenfold variation in water intake by a coordinated interaction among the vasopressin, thirst, and renal systems. Dysfunction in any of these systems can result in abnormal regulation of blood osmolality, which if not properly recognized and treated, may cause life-threatening hyperosmolality or hypo-osmolality.

Vasopressin

The control of plasma osmolality and intravascular volume involves a complex integration of endocrine, neural, and paracrine pathways. Plasma osmolality is regulated principally via vasopressin release from the posterior pituitary, or neurohypophysis, while volume homeostasis is determined largely through the action of the renin-angiotensin-aldosterone system, with contributions from both vasopressin and the natriuretic peptide family. The nine amino acid vasopressin consists of a six amino acid disulfide ring plus a three amino acid tail, with amidation of the carboxy-terminus (Figure 3-1). Vasopressin has both antidiuretic and pressor activities, actions caused by the hormone binding to different receptors, as discussed subsequently. A synthetic analog of vasopressin, dDAVP (desamino-D-arginine vasopressin,

desmopressin) with twice the antidiuretic potency and 100 times the duration of action of vasopressin, and no pressor activity, is routinely used to treat vasopressin-deficient patients (Figure 3-1).[3]

Synthesis and secretion

Vasopressin is synthesized in hypothalamic paraventricular and supraoptic magnocellular neurons, whose axons transport the hormone to the posterior pituitary, its primary site of storage and release into the systemic circulation (Figure 3-2). The bilaterally paired hypothalamic paraventricular and supraoptic nuclei are separated from one another by relatively large distances (approximately 1 cm). Their axons course caudally and converge at the infundibulum, before terminating at different levels within the pituitary stalk and posterior pituitary gland.[4] This anatomy has important clinical implications, as will be discussed. Vasopressin is also synthesized in the parvocellular neurons of the paraventricular nucleus, where it may have a role in regulating the hypothalamic-pituitary-adrenal axis, and in the hypothalamic suprachiasmatic nucleus, where it may participate in the generation of circadian rhythms.

Synthesis. During its synthesis and perhaps after secretion into the bloodstream, vasopressin is bound to neurophysin, a 10,000 Da (dalton) molecular weight protein, which may function to protect vasopressin against degradation during intracellular storage, or to promote more efficient packaging or posttranslation processing of vasopressin within secretory granules (Figure 3-3). Vasopressin and neurophysin are made from a common gene which consists of three exons. Exon 1 encodes the signal and vasopressin peptides and the aminoterminal 9 amino acids of neurophysin, exon 2 encodes the majority of neurophysin, and exon 3 codes

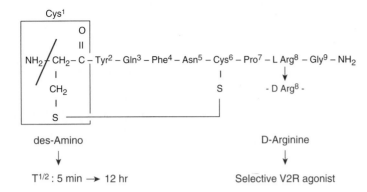

FIGURE 3-1 ■ Molecular structure of vasopressin and desmopressin. Substitution of the 8th amino acid L-Arginine of the nonapeptide vasopressin with D-Arginine confers selective agonist activity on the V2 receptors. Removal of the amino group from the 1st amino acid cysteine prolongs the half-life significantly since vasopressinase attacks vasopressin from this end of the molecule.

for the carboxyterminal end of neurophysin followed by an additional 39 amino acid-long glycopeptide.

Osmotic regulation. Water balance is regulated in two ways: vasopressin secretion stimulates water reabsorption by the kidney, thereby reducing future water losses, and thirst stimulates water ingestion, which restores past water losses (Figure 3-4). Ideally, these two systems work in parallel to efficiently regulate extracellular fluid tonicity. However, each system by itself can maintain plasma osmolality in the near-normal range. For example, in the absence of vasopressin secretion but with free access to water, thirst drives water ingestion up to the 5 to 10 L/m^2 of urine output seen with vasopressin deficiency. Conversely, an intact vasopressin secretory system can compensate for some degree of disordered thirst regulation. However, when both vasopressin secretion and thirst are compromised, either by disease or iatrogenic means, there is great risk for the occurrence of life-threatening abnormalities in plasma osmolality. In evaluating any disorder of water balance, the clinician should ask whether abnormalities exist in vasopressin secretion, in thirst, or in both systems.

Vasopressin secretion is stimulated by a rise in the plasma concentrations of osmotically active substances (ie, those that are not freely permeable across cell membranes) principally sodium chloride and glucose (with insulin deficiency). Normal blood osmolality ranges between 280 and 290 mOsm/kg (milli-osmoles per kilogram) H_2O, with the threshold for vasopressin release being approximately 283 mOsm/kg. Above this threshold, an osmosensor located outside the blood–brain barrier near the anterior hypothalamus, which can detect as little as a 1% to 2% change in blood osmolality, signals for posterior pituitary secretion of vasopressin.[5] Vasopressin rises in proportion to plasma osmolality, up to a maximum concentration of about 20 pg/mL (picogram per milliliter), when the blood osmolality is approximately 320 mOsm/kg (Figure 3-5).

Nonosmotic regulation. Separate from osmotic regulation, vasopressin is secreted in response to a decrease

in intravascular volume or pressure. Afferent baroreceptor pathways arising from the right and left atria, and aortic arch (carotid sinus) are stimulated by increasing intravascular volume and stretch of vessel walls, and send signals to the hypothalamic paraventricular nucleus (PVN) and supra-optic nucleus (SON) to inhibit vasopressin secretion. The pattern of vasopressin secretion in response to volume as opposed to osmotic stimuli is markedly different. While minor changes in plasma osmolality above 280 mOsm/kg evoke linear increases in plasma vasopressin, no change in vasopressin secretion is seen until blood volume decrease by approximately 8%. With intravascular volume deficits exceeding 8%, vasopressin concentration rises exponentially, such that when blood volume pressure decreases by approximately 25%, vasopressin concentrations rise to 20- to 30-fold above normal[6] (Figure 3-5), vastly exceeding those required for maximal antidiuresis, and high enough to cause vasoconstriction via V1 vascular receptors (see later in the chapter).

Nausea, pain, hypoglycemia, psychological stress, ethanol, and chlorpropamide are also clinically important triggers for vasopressin release (Figure 3-6). On the other hand, vasopressin secretion is inhibited by glucocorticoids, and because of this, loss of negative regulation of vasopressin secretion occurs in the setting of primary and secondary glucocorticoid insufficiency. Cortisol deficiency both enhances hypothalamic vasopressin production as well as directly impairs free water excretion, important considerations in the evaluation of the patient with hyponatremia, as subsequently discussed.

Metabolism

Once in the circulation, vasopressin has a half-life of only 5 to 10 minutes, due to its rapid degradation by a cysteine amino terminal peptidase, termed vasopressinase. The synthetic analog of vasopressin, dDAVP, is insensitive to amino terminal degradation, and thus has a much longer half-life of 8 to 24 hours. During pregnancy, the placenta secretes increased amounts of this vasopressinase, resulting in a fourfold increase in the

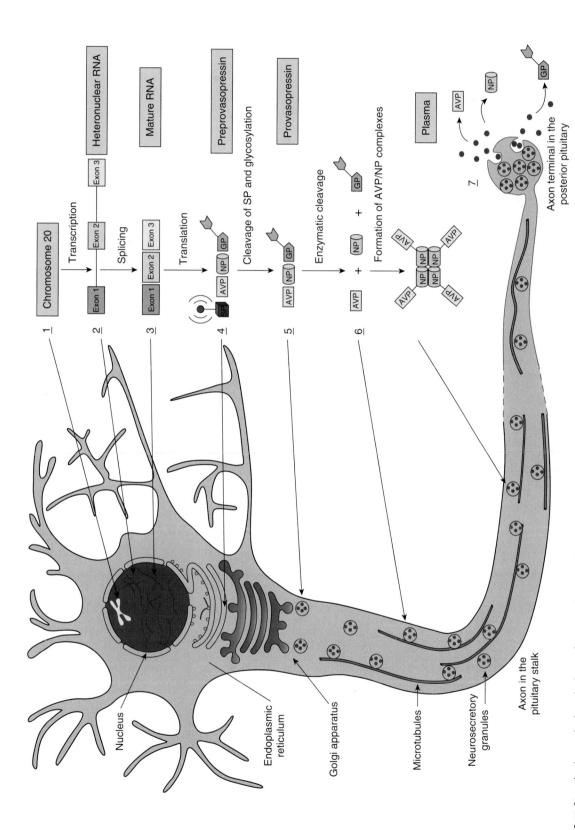

FIGURE 3-2 ■ Steps in the synthesis and release of vasopressin. **1. Nucleus:** Transcription of the vasopressin gene (Chromosome 20) to heteronuclear ribonucleic acid (RNA). **2. Nucleus:** Synthesis of the mature RNA by removal of the introns and the splicing of exons A, B, and C and its subsequent passage into the cytoplasm. Attachment of the mRNA to ribosomes in the endoplasmic reticulum (ER). **3. Endoplasmic Reticulum (ER):** Translation of the exons to pre-provasopressin. Exon 1 encodes the 19 amino acid (AA) signal peptide (SP), the 9-AA vasopressin (AVP) and the amino terminal of the 93–95-AA neurophysin (NP), Exon 2 encodes the middle portion of neurophysin and Exon 3 encodes the carboxyl terminal of neurophysin and a 39 AA glycopeptide (GP). **4. Endoplasmic Reticulum (ER):** Glycosylation of the glycopeptide portion of the preprovasopressin and cleavage of the signal peptide. **5. Golgi Complex:** Entry of provasopressin into the Golgi complex and its packaging into neurosecretory granules. Attachment to and the subsequent transport of the granules along microtubules to the site of storage in the posterior pituitary gland. **6. Neurosecretory Granules:** Enzymatic cleavage of provasopressin to vasopressin, neurophysin, and glycopeptide during the transport within the acidic granules. Amidation of the vasopressin, formation of complexes consisting of one vasopressin molecule with either a dimer or a tetramer of neurophysin. **7. Neurosecretory Granules:** Fusion of the granule with the plasma membrane as a result of an action potential and the release of vasopressin, neurophysin, and the glycopeptide into the extracellular space and plasma. *(Modified with permission from Alan Robinson, M.D, UCLA)*

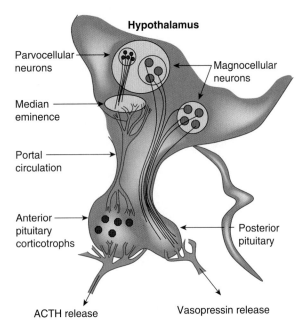

Hypothalamus

Parvocellular neurons

Magnocellular neurons

Median eminence

Portal circulation

Anterior pituitary corticotrophs

Posterior pituitary

ACTH release

Vasopressin release

FIGURE 3-3 ■ Anatomy of vasopressin-producing neurons. The bilaterally paired paraventricular nucleus (PVN) and the supra-optic nucleus (SON) of the hypothalamus synthesize vasopressin. The PVN contains magnocellular and parvocellular neurons while the SON contains only magnocellular neurons. The magnocellular neurons of the PVN and SON synthesize vasopressin in their soma and carry it through their long axons to the posterior pituitary gland through the pituitary stalk to eventually secrete it from their terminals in the neurohypophysis. Vasopressin released from magnocellular neurons is primarily involved in water balance. The parvocellular neurons which synthesize vasopressin along with corticotrophin-releasing hormone (CRH) have shorter axons that terminate on capillaries of the hypothalamic-hypophyseal portal system in the median eminence of the hypothalamus. Vasopressin secreted here is carried in the portal circulation directly to the anterior pituitary corticotrophs that secrete adrenocorticotropic hormone (ACTH). Vasopressin from the parvocellular neurons, along with CRH, regulates ACTH production and release. The suprachiasmatic nucleus also produces vasopressin which is thought to regulate circadian rhythms (not shown).

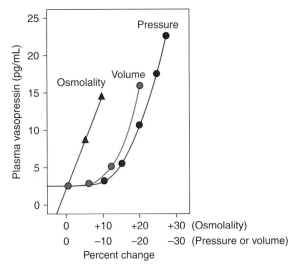

FIGURE 3-5 ■ Vasopressin secretion in response to osmotic and nonosmotic stimuli. Comparison in humans, of the percentage change in osmolality (increase) and pressure or volume (decrease) required to stimulate vasopressin release. While as little as a 1% increase in osmolality results in vasopressin secretion, greater than a 10% to 15% change in volume and pressure are required to stimulate release of vasopressin. However the magnitude of the vasopressin response to decreases in the volume or pressure is several folds greater than that in response to changes in osmolality. (*Kronenberg HM, Melmed S, Polonsky KS, Larsen PR*. William's Textbook of Endocrinology, *11th edition. Philadelphia: W.B. Saunders; 2008.*)

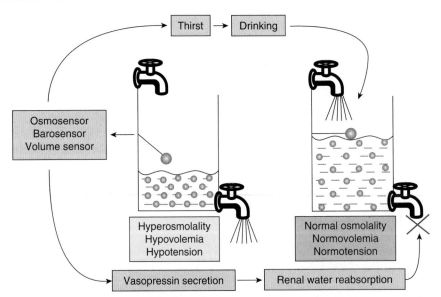

FIGURE 3-4 ■ Regulation of water balance. Hyperosmolality, hypovolemia, or hypotension are sensed by osmosensors, volume sensors, or barosensors, respectively, which stimulate the release of vasopressin and the sensation of thirst. Vasopressin acts on the V2 receptor in the kidney to increase water reabsorption and minimize further water loss in the urine. Thirst leads to increased intake of water and the replenishment of the body's water content. The results of these dual negative feedback loops cause a reduction in hyperosmolality and/or hypotension/hypovolemia.

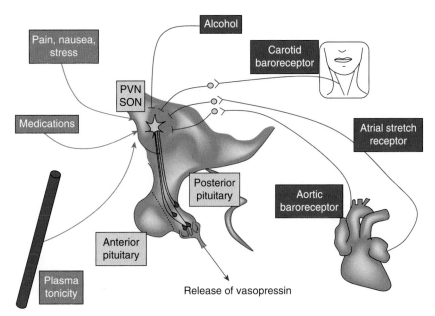

FIGURE 3-6 ■ Regulation of vasopressin secretion. Vasopressin is controlled by osmotic and nonosmotic factors. Osmotic regulation occurs through osmosensors in the organum vasculosum of the lamina terminalis (OVLT). An increase in plasma osmolality stimulates secretion of vasopressin. Several non-osmotic factors regulate vasopressin secretion. Blood pressure–controlled regulation of vasopressin is mediated by afferents from baroreceptors in the aorta and the carotid sinus via the cranial nerves IX and X with relays within the brainstem nuclei. Hypovolemia stimulates the secretion of vasopressin via stretch receptors in the atria and pulmonary veins. Nausea is a potent stimulator of vasopressin secretion. While pain, stress, and several medications stimulate the secretion of vasopressin, alcohol inhibits its release. All these factors ultimately act upon the magnocellular vasopressinergic neurons of the PVN and the SON nuclei of the hypothalamus to regulate the synthesis and secretion of vasopressin.

metabolic clearance rate of vasopressin. Normal women compensate with an increase in vasopressin secretion, but women with preexisting deficits in vasopressin secretion or action, or those with increased concentrations of placental vasopressinase associated with liver dysfunction or multiple gestation, may develop diabetes insipidus (DI) in the last trimester, which resolves in the immediate postpartum period. As expected, this form of DI responds to treatment with dDAVP (which is resistant to degradation by vasopressinase) but not with vasopressin.

Action

Vasopressin released from the posterior pituitary and median eminence affects the function of several tissue types by binding to three G protein–coupled cell surface receptors, designated V1, V2, and V3 (or V1b) (Table 3-1). The major sites of V1 receptor expression are on vascular smooth muscle and hepatocytes, where receptor activation results in vasoconstriction and glycogenolysis, respectively. The concentration of vasopressin needed to significantly increase blood pressure is several folds higher than that required for maximal antidiuresis. The V3 receptor is present on corticotrophs in the anterior pituitary, and acts to increase ACTH secretion.

Modulation of water balance occurs through the action of vasopressin upon V2 receptors located primarily on the blood (basolateral) side of cells in the renal

Table 3-1.

Vasopressin Receptors

Receptor	Target Tissue	Function
V1	Vascular smooth muscle, platelets and hepatocytes	Vasoconstriction, hemostasis, and glycogenolysis
V2	Distal tubule and collecting duct of the kidney	Aquaporin–2 mediated water reabsorption
V3 (V1b)	Anterior pituitary corticotrophs	ACTH release

collecting tubule. The human V2 receptor gene is located on the long arm of the X chromosome, at the locus associated with congenital, X-linked vasopressin-resistant nephrogenic DI. Vasopressin-induced increases in intracellular cAMP mediated by the V2 receptor trigger a complex pathway of events resulting in increased permeability of the collecting duct to water and efficient water transit across an otherwise minimally permeable epithelium (Figure 3-7). Activation of a cAMP-dependent protein kinase causes the insertion of aggregates of a water

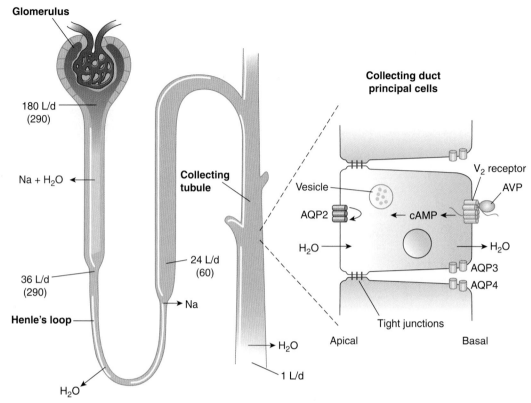

FIGURE 3-7 ■ Antidiuretic effect of vasopressin in the regulation of urine volume. In a typical 70-kg adult, the kidney filters approximately 180 L/day of plasma. Of this, approximately 144 L (80%) is reabsorbed isosmotically in the proximal tubule and another 8 L (4%-5%) is reabsorbed without solute in the descending limb of Henle loop. The remainder is diluted to an osmolarity of approximately 60 mmol/kg by selective reabsorption of sodium and chloride in the ascending limb. In the absence of AVP, the urine issuing from the loop passes largely unmodified through the distal tubules and collecting ducts, resulting in a maximum water diuresis. In the presence of AVP, solute-free water is reabsorbed osmotically through the principal cells of the collecting ducts, resulting in the excretion of a much smaller volume of concentrated urine. This antidiuretic effect is mediated via a G protein–coupled V2 receptor that increases intracellular cyclic AMP, thereby inducing translocation of aquaporin-2 (AQP-2) water channels into the apical membrane. The resultant increase in permeability permits an influx of water that diffuses out of the cell through AQP-3 and AQP-4 water channels on the basal-lateral surface. The net rate of flux across the cell is determined by the number of AQP-2 water channels in the apical membrane and the strength of the osmotic gradient between tubular fluid and the renal medulla. Tight junctions on the lateral surface of the cells serve to prevent unregulated water flow. (*Redrawn from Harrison's Online with permission from The McGraw-Hill Companies, Inc.*)

channel, termed aquaporin-2, into the apical (luminal) membrane. Insertion of aquaporin-2 causes up to 100-fold increase in water permeability of the apical membrane, allowing water movement from the tubule lumen along its osmotic gradient into the hypertonic inner medullary interstitium and excretion of a concentrated urine[7] (Figure 3-7).

Thirst

The sensation of thirst is determined by hypothalamic neurons anatomically distinct from those which make vasopressin. It makes physiologic sense that the threshold for thirst (~293 mOsm/kg) is slightly higher than that for vasopressin release (Figure 3-8). Otherwise, during the development of hyperosmolality, the initial activation of thirst and water ingestion would result in polyuria without activation of vasopressin release, causing a persistent diuretic state.

DISORDERS CAUSING HYPERNATREMIA

Hypernatremia along with hyponatremia constitutes the commonest electrolyte abnormality in children.

Hypernatremia

Hypernatremia usually occurs when free water loss exceeds salt loss from the body.

Definition and classification of hypernatremia

Hypernatremia is defined as a serum sodium concentration greater than 145 mmol/L. It occurs most often in the setting of dehydration: either due to pure water loss or due to water loss which exceeds salt loss. Hypernatremia can occur either due to free water loss or due to excessive intake of sodium. The latter usually causes transient

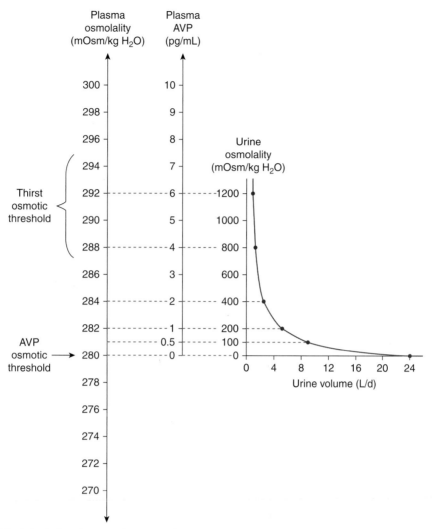

FIGURE 3-8 ▪ Physiological relations between plasma osmolality, plasma AVP concentrations, urine volume, and urine osmolality in healthy humans.[8] Note that the osmolality at which the secretion of vasopressin is stimulated is below that at which thirst is stimulated. (*With permission from National Kidney Foundation Inc.*)

hypernatremia. In the presence of intact thirst mechanism, the ability to drink water and intact renal function, it is followed by water intake leading to volume expansion and natriuresis, thus normalizing the serum sodium levels. Similarly excessive loss of free water is usually compensated by increased intake driven by the intact thirst mechanism. Inability to drink water freely as seen in infants and neurologically impaired children can thus lead to hypernatremia from either excessive ingestion of sodium or from excessive free water loss. Infants in particular also have a limited ability to excrete the osmotic solute load from their kidneys and hence can have persistent hypernatremia from accidental or deliberate inclusion of excessive amounts of salt in their food.

Clinical presentation and diagnosis

Children with significant hypernatremia progress from irritability to lethargy and coma. Neurological signs such as nuchal rigidity, hypertonia, and hyperreflexia may be present. Seizures and rhabdomyolysis can occur. Shrinkage of cells in the brain in acute hypernatremia can lead to the rupture of bridging veins causing intracranial hemorrhage. Venous infarcts from venous sinus thrombosis can also be seen. A mortality rate of 15% has been reported in children with hypernatremia.[9]

A diagnostic algorithm for hypernatremia (Figure 3-9) in most children with a normal thirst mechanism and a normal ability to drink water is thus most often limited to the identification of the source of the free water loss. The presence of polyuria with dilute urine confirms renal loss of free water. The diagnostic approach for polyuria will be discussed subsequently in this chapter. Free water may be lost relatively in excess to sodium loss through nonrenal routes such as the skin as in burns and excessive sweating, the respiratory tract or the gastrointestinal tract as occurs with diarrhea, or through fistulae. Since hypernatremia causes intracellular dehydration due to osmotic shift of intracellular fluid to the

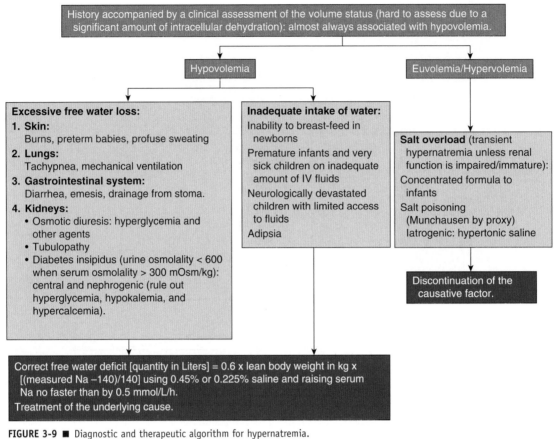

FIGURE 3-9 ■ Diagnostic and therapeutic algorithm for hypernatremia.

extracellular compartment, the extent of dehydration is often underestimated during physical examination. In addition to other signs of dehydration, the skin has been classically described as having a "doughy" consistency in hypernatremic dehydration. Laboratory investigations should include serum sodium, osmolality, blood urea nitrogen, creatinine, urine osmolality, and sodium level.

Treatment

The goals of treating hypernatremia should be to correct the hypovolemia and to normalize the serum sodium level. The management of hypernatremia should involve identification of the underlying cause and the duration of the hypernatremia. Treatment is directed at the underlying cause where one can be identified. An estimation of the free water deficit is made using the formula:

$$\text{Free H}_2\text{O deficit (L)} = [(\text{Serum sodium level} - 140) \div 140] \times \text{weight (kg)} \times 0.6$$

This free water deficit is best corrected with oral or nasogastric free water over a period of 24 to 48 hours. Ongoing losses should be replaced simultaneously while closely monitoring the clinical status and the serum electrolytes. In children who are unable to receive free water through the enteral route, a parenteral solution containing either 5% Dextrose, or 0.45% to 0.225% saline can be used.

The brain cells adapt to hypernatremia over a period of days, by increasing the intracellular osmolyte concentration in order to prevent intracellular dehydration and cell shrinkage (Figure 3-10). They do so by increasing the levels of electrolytes, amino acids like taurine, and glutamine and other osmotically active substances such as myoinositol, and betaine.[10] While this process is protective during chronic hypernatremia, rapid lowering of the serum sodium can cause swelling of the brain cells. The brain being enclosed within the cranial vault, which is nonexpandable after the closure of the fontanelles, can herniate infratentorially. Seizures, coma, and even death can occur with rapid lowering of chronically elevated serum sodium levels. Hence it is widely accepted that the serum sodium level should be corrected at least over a period of 48 hours. It should not be lowered more rapidly than by 15 mmol/L/day.

Deficiencies of Vasopressin Secretion or Action

Central diabetes insipidus

Causes and clinical presentation. Central (hypothalamic, neurogenic, or vasopressin-sensitive) DI in children is most often the result of surgical or accidental

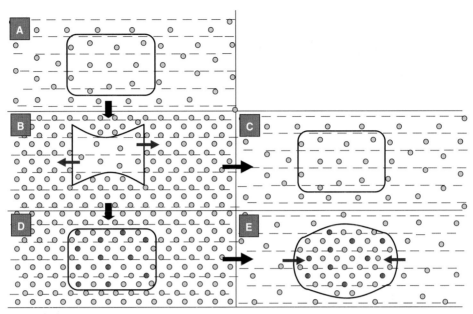

FIGURE 3-10 ▨ The effects of hypernatremia and its rapid correction on intracellular osmolality and size of the brain cell. The shape and size of cell are normal in the eunatremic state **(A)** in which the osmolality within and outside the cell are equal. Acute hypernatremia **(B)** causes an osmotic fluid shift out of the cell (blue arrows) leading to cell shrinkage. Rapid correction of the acute extracellular hypernatremia **(C)** once again equalizes the osmolality within and outside the cell and thus restores the cell shape and size. If hypernatremia persists uncorrected beyond 24 hours **(D)**, the cell tries to regain its original shape and size by generating new osmolytes (green circles) to equilibrate its osmolality with that of the outside. Rapidly lowering the serum sodium and extracellular osmolality at this stage **(E)** causes cell swelling due to osmotic flow of water into the cell (blue arrows). The cell is unable to eliminate some of its osmolytes rapidly enough to once more equilibrate the intracellular and extracellular osmolalities.

trauma to vasopressin neurons, congenital anatomical hypothalamic or pituitary defects, or neoplasms. It can also be caused by infiltrative, autoimmune, and infectious diseases affecting vasopressin neurons or fiber tracts, and least commonly, by disorders of vasopressin gene structure (Table 3-2). In approximately 50% of children with central DI, the etiology is not apparent.[11]

The most common cause of central DI is the neurosurgical destruction of vasopressin neurons following pituitary-hypothalamic surgery. It is important to distinguish polyuria associated with the onset of acute postsurgical central DI from polyuria due to the normal diuresis of fluids given during surgery. In both cases, the urine may be very dilute and of high volume, exceeding 200 mL/m²/h. However, in the former case, serum osmolality will be high, whereas in the latter case it will be normal. A careful examination of the intra-operative record should also help distinguish between these two possibilities. The axons of vasopressin-containing magnocellular neurons extend uninterrupted to the posterior pituitary over a distance of approximately 10 mm. These axons terminate at various levels within the stalk and gland (Figure 3-3). Since surgical interruption of these axons can result in retrograde degeneration of hypothalamic neurons, lesions closer to the hypothalamus will affect more neurons and cause greater permanent loss of hormone secretion. Not infrequently, a "triple phase"

response is seen (Table 3-3). Following surgery, an initial phase of transient DI is observed, lasting 1.5 to 2 days, and possibly due to edema in the area interfering with normal vasopressin secretion. If significant vasopressin cell destruction has occurred, this is often followed by a second phase of syndrome of inappropriate antidiuretic hormone (SIADH), which may last up to 10 days, and is due to the unregulated release of vasopressin, by dying neurons. A third phase of permanent DI may follow if more than 90% of vasopressin cells are destroyed. Usually, a marked degree of SIADH in the second phase portends significant permanent DI in the final phase of this response. In patients with coexisting vasopressin and cortisol deficits (eg, in combined anterior and posterior hypopituitarism following neurosurgical treatment of craniopharyngioma), symptoms of DI may be masked because cortisol deficiency impairs renal free water clearance, as discussed subsequently. In such cases, institution of glucocorticoid therapy alone may precipitate polyuria, leading to the diagnosis of DI.

Trauma to the base of the brain can cause swelling around or severance of these axons, resulting in either transient or permanent DI. Permanent DI can occur after seemingly minor trauma. Approximately one-half of patients with fractures of the sella turcica will develop permanent DI, which may be delayed by up to 1 month following the trauma, during which time neurons of

Table 3-2.

Causes of Central Diabetes Insipidus

Congenital:
  Septo-optic dysplasia
  Ectopia/hypogenesis of the pituitary
  Holoprosencephaly
  Other midline cranio-facial defects
  Familial:
    Autosomal dominant
    Autosomal recessive
    Wolfram syndrome (DIDMOAD)—AR
Acquired:
  Postoperative: with or without triple phase response
  Traumatic: transection of the stalk
  Septic shock (infarction)
  Hypoxic brain injury
  Neoplasms:
    Craniopharyngioma
    Germinoma
    Pinealoma
    Optic glioma
    Metastatic tumors: leukemias
  Infiltrative:
    Langerhans cell histiocytosis
    Sarcoidosis
    Pulmonary granulomatous diseases
  Autoimmune: lymphocytic hypophysitis
  Drugs: ethanol, phenytoin, opiate antagonists, α-adrenergics
  Infectious: (meningitis/encephalitis)
    Cryptococcus neoformans, Listeria monocytogenes
    Mycobacterium tuberculosis, Toxoplasmosis, congenital CMV
  Aneurysm and cysts
  Pregnancy: placental vasopressinase
  Sheehan syndrome (postpartum hemorrhage)
  Idiopathic

Table 3-3.

Triple Phase Response (After Surgical Damage to Vasopressin Neurons)

Phase	Condition	Underlying Cause	Duration
First	Transient diabetes insipidus	Impaired secretion: local edema	0.5-2 d
Second	SIADH	Release of VP from dying neurons	1-10 d
Third	Permanent diabetes insipidus	Cell loss	Permanent

severed axons may undergo retrograde degeneration. Septic shock and postpartum hemorrhage associated with pituitary infarction (Sheehan syndrome) may involve the posterior pituitary with varying degrees of DI. It is seen that DI is never associated with cranial irradiation of the hypothalamic-pituitary region.

Midline brain anatomic abnormalities such as septo-optic dysplasia with agenesis of the corpus callosum holoprosencephaly, and familial pituitary hypoplasia with absent stalk may be associated with central DI, which usually presents in the first month of life, often with signs of anterior pituitary dysfunction, such as jaundice, and in boys, microphallus. Central DI due to midline brain abnormalities may be accompanied by defects in thirst perception.

Because hypothalamic vasopressin neurons are distributed over a large area within the hypothalamus, tumors which cause DI must either be very large, be infiltrative, or be strategically located at the point of convergence of the hypothalamo-neurohypophyseal axonal tract in the infundibulum. Germinomas and pinealomas typically arise near the base of the hypothalamus where vasopressin axons converge prior to their entry into the posterior pituitary, and for this reason are among the most common primary brain tumors associated with DI. Germinomas causing the disease can be very small and undetectable by magnetic resonance imaging (MRI) for several years following the onset of polyuria. For this reason, quantitative measurement of the β subunit of human chorionic gonadotropin, often secreted by germinomas and pinealomas, and regularly repeated MRI scans should be performed in children with idiopathic or unexplained DI.

Empty sella syndrome, possibly due to unrecognized pituitary infarction, can be associated with DI in children. Craniopharyngiomas and optic gliomas, when very large, can also cause central DI, although this is more often a postoperative complication of the treatment for these tumors. Hematologic malignancies can cause DI. In some cases, such as with acute myelocytic leukemia, the cause is infiltration of the pituitary stalk and sella.

Langerhans cell histiocytosis and lymphocytic hypophysitis are the most common types of infiltrative disorders causing central DI. Approximately 10% of patients with histiocytosis will have DI. These patients tend to have more serious, multisystem disease for longer periods of time than those without DI, and anterior pituitary deficits often accompany posterior pituitary deficiency. MRI characteristically shows thickening of the pituitary stalk. Radiation treatment to the pituitary region within 14 days of onset of symptoms of DI may result in return of vasopressin function. Lymphocytic infundibulo-neurohypophysitis may account for over one-half of patients with "idiopathic" central DI. This entity may be associated with other autoimmune diseases. Image analysis discloses an enlarged pituitary and thickened stalk, and biopsy of the posterior pituitary reveals lymphocytic infiltration of the gland, stalk, and magnocellular hypothalamic nuclei. A necrotizing form of this entity has been described which also causes anterior pituitary failure and responds to steroid treatment. DI can also be associated with pulmonary granulomatous diseases including sarcoidosis.

Infections involving the base of the brain, such as meningococcal, cryptococcal, *Listeria*, and toxoplasmosis meningitis, congenital cytomegalovirus infection, and nonspecific inflammatory disease of the brain can cause central DI. The disease is often transient, suggesting that it is due to inflammation rather than destruction of vasopressin-containing neurons.

Familial, autosomal dominant central DI is manifest within the first half of the first decade of life. Vasopressin secretion, initially normal, gradually declines until DI of variable severity ensues. Patients respond well to vasopressin replacement therapy. The disease has a high degree of penetrance, but may be of variable severity within a family. Several different single nucleotide mutations in the vasopressin structural gene have been found to cause the disease, with most occurring in the neurophysin region. Endoplasmic reticulum stress from misfolding of the aberrant protein has been hypothesized to be the possible cause for the premature loss of the magnocellular vasopressin neurons seen in this disease.[12] Vasopressin deficiency is also found in the **DIDMOAD** syndrome, consisting of **D**iabetes **I**nsipidus, **D**iabetes **M**ellitus, **O**ptic **A**trophy, and **D**eafness. This syndrome complex, also known as Wolfram syndrome, is caused by recessive mutations in a recently identified gene, wolframin, located on chromosome 4p16. The normal function of this gene, which is expressed in several tissues including brain and pancreas, is unknown.

Whereas normal children have a nocturnal rise in plasma vasopressin associated with an increase in urine osmolality and a decrease in urine volume, those with primary enuresis have a blunted or absent rise in vasopressin, and excrete a higher urine volume of lower tonicity. This has suggested that enuretic children have a primary deficiency in vasopressin secretion, although the same outcome could be caused solely by excessive water intake in these children. The use of the V2 agonist, dDAVP, is highly effective in abolishing bed wetting episodes, although relapse is high once therapy is stopped. Fluid intake must be limited while a child is exposed to the antidiuretic action of dDAVP to guard against water intoxication.

Treatment. Patients with otherwise untreated DI crave cold fluids, especially water. With complete central DI, maximum urine concentrating ability is approximately 200 mOsm/kg. An average 10-year child with a body surface area of 1 m^2 would then require a urine output of 2.5 L of urine to excrete an average daily solute load of 500 mOsm/m^2. Insensible (nonrenal) fluid losses in this child would amount to 500 mL/day (500 mL/m^2/day). In order to maintain normal plasma tonicity, this child's fluid intake must match his/her fluid loss of 3 L/day. With an intact thirst mechanism and free access to oral fluids, a person with complete DI can maintain plasma osmolality and sodium in the high normal range, although at great inconvenience. Furthermore, long standing intake of these volumes of fluid in children can lead to hydroureter, and even hyperfluorosis in communities that provide fluoridated water.

There are two situations in which central DI is sometimes treated solely with high levels of fluid intake, without vasopressin. Vasopressin therapy coupled with excessive fluid intake (usually greater than 1 L/m^2/day as discussed subsequently) can result in unwanted hyponatremia. Because neonates and young infants receive all of their nutrition in liquid form, the obligatory high oral fluid requirements for this age (3 L/m^2/day), combined with vasopressin treatment are likely to lead to this dangerous complication.[13] Such neonates may be better managed with fluid therapy alone. The use of breast milk or Similac 60/40 formula reduces the renal solute load by 20% to 30%. This in turn reduces the urine volume in infants with DI by 20% to 30%. Chlorothiazide (oral dose 5 mg/kg twice daily) is a diuretic that increases the urine osmolality and decreases the urine output through mechanisms that are unclear. The latter two therapeutic options significantly reduce the amount of free water supplementation needed in infants with both forms of DI. However, supplementation with 20 to 30 mL of free water for every 120 to 160 mL of formula might still be required.[14] Infants with CDI have also been successfully treated with subcutaneous injections of dDAVP (initial dose 0.002-0.1 ug/kg once daily, titrated upwards and given twice daily if needed) until they are eating solid food. Therapy in infants with subcutaneous injections of dDAVP has been associated with far fewer episodes of hyponatremia and hypernatremia than with either intranasal or oral dDAVP.[15]

In the acute postoperative management of central DI occurring after neurosurgery in young children, vasopressin therapy may be successfully employed, but extreme caution must be exerted with its use. While under the full antidiuretic effect of vasopressin, a patient will have a urine osmolality of approximately 1000 mOsm/kg and become hyponatremic if she/he receives an excessive amount of fluids, depending on the solute load and nonrenal water losses. With a solute excretion of 500 mOsm/m^2/day, normal renal function, and nonrenal fluid losses of 500 mL/m^2/day, fluid intake of greater than 1 L/m^2/day will result in hyponatremia. In addition, vasopressin therapy will mask the emergence of the SIADH phase of the "triple phase" neurohypophyseal response to neurosurgical injury (as discussed earlier). For these reasons, it is often best to manage acute postoperative DI in young children with fluids alone, avoiding the use of vasopressin. This method consists of matching input and output hourly using between 1 and 3 $L/m^2/day$ (40-120 $mL/m^2/h$). If intravenous therapy is used, a basal 40 $mL/m^2/h$ should be given as 5% dextrose (D5) in 1/4 normal saline (normal saline = 0.9% sodium chloride) and the remainder, depending on the urine output, as 5% dextrose in water (D_5W). Potassium chloride (40 mEq/L) may be added if oral intake is to be delayed for several days. No additional fluid should be administered for hourly urine volumes under 40 $mL/m^2/h$. For hourly urine volumes above 40 $mL/m^2/h$, the additional volume should be replaced with D_5W up to a total maximum of 120 $mL/m^2/h$. For example, in a child with a surface area of 1 m^2 (~30 kg), the basal infusion rate would be 40 mL/h of D5 in 1/4 normal saline. For an hourly urine output of 60 mL, an additional 20 mL/h D_5W would be given, for a total infusion rate of 60 mL/h. For urine outputs above 120 mL/h, the total infusion rate would be 120 mL/h. In the presence of DI, this will result in a serum sodium in the 150 mEq/L range and a mildly volume contracted state, which will allow one to assess both thirst sensation as well as the return of normal vasopressin function or the emergence of SIADH. Patients may become mildly hyperglycemic with this regimen, particularly if they are also receiving postoperative glucocorticoids. However, this fluid management protocol, because it does not use vasopressin, prevents any chance of hyponatremia.

Intravenous therapy with synthetic aqueous vasopressin (Pitressin) is useful in the management of central DI of acute onset. If continuous vasopressin is administered, fluid intake must be limited to 1 $L/m^2/day$ (assuming normal solute intake and nonrenal water losses as described above). The potency of synthetic vasopressin is still measured using a bioassay and is expressed in bioactive units, with one milliunit (mU) equivalent to approximately 2.5 ng of vasopressin. For intravenous vasopressin therapy, 1.5 mU/kg/h results in a blood vasopressin concentration of approximately 10 pg/mL, twice that needed for full antidiuretic activity. Vasopressin's effect is maximal within 2 hours of the start of infusion. Patients treated with vasopressin for postneurosurgical DI should be switched from intravenous to oral fluid intake at the earliest opportunity, since thirst sensation, if intact, will help regulate blood osmolality, as discussed above. Intravenous dDAVP (Desmopressin) should not be used in the acute management of postoperative central DI, for it offers no advantage over vasopressin, and its long half-life (8-12 h) compared with that of vasopressin (5-10 min) is a distinct disadvantage, since it may increase the chance of causing water intoxication.

In the outpatient setting, treatment of central DI in children beyond infancy should begin with oral dDAVP tablets[16] (Table 3-4). Young children may respond to 25 or 50 μg (micrograms) at bedtime. If the dose is effective, but has too short a duration, it should be increased further or a second, morning dose should be added. Patients should escape from the antidiuretic effect for at least 1 hour before the next dose, to insure that any excessive water will be excreted. Otherwise, water intoxication may occur. dDAVP is also available for intranasal administration via a rhinal tube (10 μg/0.1 mL) or as a nasal spray (10 μg/spray). The initial dose is 0.025 mL (2.5 μg) given by the rhinal tube at bedtime. When switching patients from nasal to oral dDAVP, the equivalent oral dose is 10- to 20-fold greater. (Dose equivalence of dDAVP: 1 mcg subcutaneously = 10 mcg intranasally = 100 to 200 mcg orally.)

A special problem arises when a patient with central DI on chronic dDAVP treatment is to undergo an

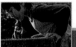

Table 3-4.

Treatment of Central Diabetes Insipidus

1. dDAVP (Desmopressin acetate)
   Oral: 100, 200 mcg tablets
   Dose: 100-400 mcg, every 12 hours
   10-20 times the nasal dose of dDAVP
   Onset of action: ~30 minutes
   Duration: 8 to 12 hours
   May become tachyphylactic
   Intranasal: rhinal tube (10 mcg/0.1 mL, 0.025 mL/squirt); nasal spray (10 mcg/0.1 mL, 0.1 mL/spray)
   Dose: ~10-20 mcg/dose, every 12 hours
   Onset of action: 15-30 minutes
   Duration: 8-12 hours
   Advantage: can be used when vomiting
   Disadvantages: some discomfort, variable absorption with rhinitis
   Subcutaneous (used in infants, not FDA-approved): 4 mcg/mL
   Initial dose: 0.02-0.1 mcg/kg/dose
   One-tenth of the intranasal dose
   Much lower incidence of hypo- and hypernatremia
2. Vasopressin
   Intravenous (IV) route: 20 units/mL (1 unit = 2.5 mcg)
   Dose: 1-10 mU/kg/h
   Onset of action:
   Half-life: 5-10 minutes
3. Chlorothiazide (in infants)
   5 mg/kg orally every 8-12 hours
   Increases the urinary concentration and decreases urine volume
   Can rarely cause hypokalemia and hyperuricemia
4. Low solute formula (in infants)
   Breast milk or Similac 60/40 (20%-30 % lower solute load than regular formula)

elective surgical procedure requiring general anesthesia (Table 3-5). Two options are possible. The patient can receive their usual regimen of dDAVP on the morning of surgery; alternatively dDAVP can be held the evening before and the morning of surgery. In either case, intra-operative and postoperative intravenous fluids must be limited to 1 L/m²/24 h as described previously, until the antidiuretic effect of dDAVP wanes, and the patient should be switched to oral fluid intake as soon as possi-ble, to allow thirst to guide replacement. Another special situation arises when a patient with established central DI must receive a high volume of fluid for therapeutic reasons, for example accompanying cancer chemother-apy. Such patients can either be managed by discontin-uing antidiuretic therapy and increasing fluid intake to 3 to 5 L/m²/day (rendering the patient moderately hypernatremic), or by using a low dose of intravenous vasopressin (0.1 mU/kg/h, approximately one-eighth of the full antidiuretic dose), with which the partial antid-iuretic effect allows the administration of higher amounts of fluid without causing hyponatremia.[17]

Table 3-5.

The Perioperative Management of Central Diabetes Insipidus

1. Ambulatory surgery or minor procedure:
   - The patient can receive the regular dose of dDAVP on the morning of the procedure
   - Restrict total fluid intake to 1 L/m²/day using normal saline containing IV fluids
2. More major procedures:
   - Discontinue dDAVP the night before the procedure, allow for urinary breakthrough
   - Procedure should be first case of the d
   - Once in diuretic phase of DI, IV vasopressin infusion starting at 1 mU/kg/h, maximum rate of 5 mU/kg/h
   - Titrate the rate to keep the urine osmolality >600 mOsm/kg
   - Total IV fluids: 1 L/m²/day = 40 mL/m²/h
3. Major surgery/procedures involving significant blood loss or fluid shifts:
   - Patient receives no vasopressin
   - Start IV fluids: 5% Dextrose with 0.225% saline at 1 L/m²/d
   - Replace urinary losses every hour if over 40 mL/m²/h (1 L/m²/d)
   - Maximal replacement of urinary losses: 3-5 L/m²/d = 120-200 mL/m²/h
4. Postoperative DI following injury to the hypothalamus, or the pituitary
   - Use option 2 or option 3.
   - Do not treat with the long-acting dDAVP for the first 48-72 hours as it can worsen the fluid overload if patient develops SIADH (triple-phase response)

Box 3-1. When to refer

Diabetes Insipidus:

■ History of polydipsia > 2 L/m²/day after ruling out dia-betes mellitus.
■ History of polyuria > 2 mL/kg/h or nocturia associated with polydipsia (when urine output can be measured) or secondary enuresis after ruling out diabetes mellitus
■ Dilute urine (SG < 1.010 or urine osmolality < 300) in the presence of hemoconcentration (serum osmolality > 300 mOsm/kg and Na > 145)
■ Following any surgery involving the hypothalamus and/or the pituitary gland
■ Any patient known to have DI who is hospitalized or in the emergency room (ER)
■ Any patient without an intact thirst mechanism who is hospitalized or in the ER

SIADH:

■ Hyponatremia (serum Na < 130 mmol/L) not associated with clinical evidence of volume depletion or decreased effective volume (CHF, cirrhosis, nephrotic syndrome, etc.)
■ Serum osmolality < 270 mOsm/kg in the presence of urine osmolality > 200 mOsm/kg
■ Following any surgery involving the hypothalamus and/or the pituitary gland
■ Any patient known to have SIADH who is hospitalized or in the ER
■ Any patient without an intact thirst mechanism who is hospitalized or in the ER

Box 3-1 lists the circumstances in which a patient with DI should be referred to a pediatric endocrinologist.

Nephrogenic diabetes insipidus

Causes and clinical presentation. Nephrogenic (vasopressin-resistant) DI can be due to genetic or acquired causes (Table 3-6). Genetic causes are less common but more severe than acquired forms of the disease, although genetic etiologies are more common in children than in adults.[18]

Congenital, X-linked nephrogenic DI is caused by inactivating mutations of the vasopressin V2 receptor. Due to its mode of transmission, it is a disease of males. Because of vasopressin resistance in congenital nephro-genic DI, the kidney elaborates large volumes of hypo-tonic urine with osmolality ranging between 50 and 100 mOsm/kg. Manifestations of the disease are usually present within the first several weeks of life, but may only become apparent after weaning from the breast. The predominant symptoms are polyuria and polydip-sia. Thirst may be more difficult to satisfy than in cen-tral DI. Many infants initially present with fever, vomit-ing, and dehydration, often leading to an evaluation for infection. Growth failure in the untreated child may be secondary to the ingestion of large amounts of water, which the child may prefer over milk and other higher

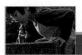

Table 3-6.

Causes of Nephrogenic Diabetes Insipidus

Congenital:
  X-linked: V2 receptor mutation
  Autosomal dominant: Aquaporin-2 mutation
  Autosomal recessive: Aquaporin-2 mutation
Acquired:
  Metabolic:
    Hypercalcemia
    Hypercalciuria
    Hypokalemia
  Renal disease:
    Polycystic kidney disease
    Medullary cystic kidney
    Sickle cell nephropathy (disease/trait)
    Chronic pyelonephritis
    Acute tubular necrosis
    Obstructive uropathy
  Primary polydipsia: washout of the gradient
  Drugs:
    Lithium
    Demeclocycline
    Amphotericin B
    Foscarnet
    Rifampin
    Methicillin
    Clozapine

caloric substances. Mental retardation of variable severity may result from repeated episodes of dehydration. Intracerebral calcification of the frontal lobes and basal ganglia is not uncommon in children with X-linked nephrogenic DI. Older children may present with enuresis or nocturia. They may learn to reduce food intake (and therefore solute load) to decrease polyuria, which may contribute to growth failure. After longstanding ingestion and excretion of large volumes of water, patients may develop nonobstructive hydronephrosis, hydroureter, and megabladder.

More than 30 mutations in the V2 receptor have been found to cause X-linked nephrogenic DI. In a family with a known mutation, prenatal or early postnatal DNA screening can unambiguously identify affected males, allowing the prompt institution of appropriate therapy. Several patients with autosomal recessive nephrogenic DI have been reported recently, who have mutations in the gene encoding the renal water channel, aquaporin-2. Aside from the mode of transmission (affecting both males and females), these patients have a clinical presentation similar to those with the X-linked disease.

Acquired causes of nephrogenic DI are more common and less severe than genetic causes. Nephrogenic DI may be caused by drugs such as lithium and demeclocycline. Approximately 50% of patients receiving lithium have impaired urinary concentrating ability, although only 10% to 20% of them develop symptomatic nephrogenic DI, which is almost always accompanied by a reduction in the glomerular filtration rate (GFR). The risk increases with duration of therapy. Treatment with demeclocycline, amphotericin, or rifampin can cause nephrogenic DI, as can hypercalcemia or hypokalemia. Osmotic diuresis due to glycosuria in diabetes mellitus, or to sodium excretion with diuretic therapy, will interfere with renal water conservation. Primary polydipsia can result in secondary nephrogenic DI because the chronic excretion of dilute urine lowers the osmolality of the hypertonic renal interstitium, thus decreasing renal concentrating ability.

Treatment. The treatment of acquired nephrogenic DI focuses on elimination, if possible, of the underlying disorder, such as offending drugs, hypercalcemia, or hypokalemia. Congenital nephrogenic DI is often difficult to treat. The main goals should be to ensure the intake of adequate calories for growth and to avoid severe dehydration. Foods with the highest ratio of caloric content to osmotic load should be ingested, to maximize growth and minimize the urine volume required to excrete urine solute. However, even with the early institution of therapy, growth and mental retardation are not uncommon. Thiazide diuretics in combination with amiloride or indomethacin are the most useful pharmacologic agents in the treatment of nephrogenic DI. The combination of thiazide and amiloride diuretics is the most commonly used regimen, because amiloride counteracts thiazide-induced hypokalemia, avoids the nephrotoxicity associated with indomethacin therapy, and is well tolerated, even in infants.[19] In addition, amiloride decreases the uptake of lithium by renal epithelial cells, and for this additional reason has been proposed in combination with thiazide as treatment for lithium-induced nephrogenic DI.

Differential Diagnosis of Polyuria and Polydipsia

In children, one must first determine if pathological polyuria or polydipsia, exceeding 2 L/m^2/day, is present, by asking the following questions: Is there a psychosocial reason for either polyuria or polydipsia? Can either be quantitated? Has either polyuria or polydipsia interfered with normal activities? Is nocturia or enuresis present? If so, does the patient also drink following nocturnal awakening? Does the history (including longitudinal growth data) or physical examination suggest other deficient or excessive endocrine secretion or an intracranial neoplasm?

If pathological polyuria or polydipsia is present, the following should be obtained in the outpatient setting: serum osmolality and concentrations of sodium, potassium, glucose, calcium, and blood, urea, nitrogen (BUN); and urinalysis, including measurement of urine osmolality, specific gravity, and glucose concentration. A serum osmolality greater than 300 mOsm/kg, with urine osmolality less than 300 mOsm/kg, establishes the diagnosis of DI (Figure 3-9). If serum osmolality is less than 270 mOsm/kg, or urine osmolality is greater than 600 mOsm/kg, the diagnosis of DI is unlikely. If upon initial screening, the patient has a serum osmolality less than 300 mOsm/kg, but the intake/output record at home suggests significant polyuria and polydipsia which cannot be attributed to primary polydipsia (ie, the serum osmolality is greater than 270 mOsm/kg), the patient should undergo a water deprivation test to establish a diagnosis of DI and to differentiate central from nephrogenic causes.

After a maximally tolerated overnight fast (based upon the outpatient history), the child is admitted to the outpatient testing center in the early morning of a day when an 8 to 10 hour test can be carried out, and deprived of water.[20] Physical signs (weight, pulse, blood pressure) and biochemical parameters (serum sodium, osmolality, urine volume, osmolality, specific gravity) are measured during the test, which may take up to 8 hours. If at any time during the test, the urine osmolality exceeds 1000 mOsm/kg, or 600 mOsm/kg and is stable over 1 hour, the patient does not have DI. If at any time the serum osmolality exceeds 300 mOsm/kg and the urine osmolality is less than 600 mOsm/kg, the patient has DI. If the serum osmolality is less than 300 mOsm/kg and the urine osmolality is less than 600 mOsm/kg, the test should be continued unless vital signs disclose hypovolemia. A common error is to stop a test too soon (especially in patients with primary polydipsia who are volume overloaded) based on the amount of body weight lost, before either urine osmolality has plateaued above 600 mOsm/kg or a serum osmolality above 300 mOsm/kg has been achieved. Unless the serum osmolality rises above the threshold for vasopressin release, a lack of vasopressin action (as inferred by nonconcentrated urine) cannot be deemed pathological. If the diagnosis of DI is made, aqueous vasopressin (Pitressin), 1 mU/m^2, should be given subcutaneously. If the patient has central DI, urine volume should fall and osmolality should at least double during the next hour, compared with the value prior to vasopressin therapy. If there is less than a twofold rise in urine osmolality following vasopressin administration, the patient probably has nephrogenic DI. dDAVP should not be used for this test, as it has been associated with water intoxication in small children in this setting.[21] Patients with longstanding primary polydipsia may have mild nephrogenic DI because of dilution of their renal medullary interstitium. This should not be confused with primary nephrogenic DI, since patients with primary polydipsia should have a tendency toward hyponatremia, rather than hypernatremia, in the basal state. Patients with a family history of X-linked nephrogenic DI can be evaluated for the disorder in the pre- or perinatal period by DNA sequence analysis, thus allowing therapy to be initiated without delay.

The water deprivation test should be sufficient in most patients to establish the diagnosis of DI, and to differentiate central from nephrogenic causes. Plasma vasopressin concentration may be obtained during the procedure, although they are rarely needed for diagnostic purposes in children. They are particularly helpful in differentiating between partial central and nephrogenic DI, in that they are low in the former and high in the latter situation. If urine osmolality concentrates normally, but only after serum osmolality is well above 300 mOsm/kg, the patient may have an altered threshold for vasopressin release, also termed a reset osmostat. This may occur following head trauma, neurosurgery, or with brain tumors. Magnetic resonance imaging is not very helpful in distinguishing central from nephrogenic DI. Normally, the posterior pituitary is seen as an area of enhanced brightness in T1-weighted images following administration of gadolinium. The posterior pituitary "bright spot" is diminished or absent in both forms of DI, presumably because of decreased vasopressin synthesis in central and increased vasopressin release in nephrogenic disease. In primary polydipsia, the bright spot is normal, probably because vasopressin accumulates in the posterior pituitary during chronic water ingestion, whereas it is decreased in SIADH, presumably because of increased vasopressin secretion.

In the inpatient, postneurosurgical setting, central DI is likely if hyperosmolality (serum osmolality over 300 mOsm/kg) is associated with urine osmolality less than serum osmolality. One must beware of intraoperative fluid expansion with subsequent hypoosmolar polyuria masquerading as DI.

Adipsic Hypernatremia

Causes and clinical presentation

Lesions in the anterior hypothalamus can affect the thirst mechanism causing adipsia. Hypernatremia with adipsia can occur even in the absence of associated DI because the free water intake maybe inadequate to match the obligatory renal and nonrenal losses. On the other hand, the lack of vasopressin despite causing significant polyuria, rarely causes significant hypernatremia when the osmosensor-thirst mechanism is intact. Disordered thirst mechanism is seen in about 10% of patients with DI. The vasopressin response to osmotic stimulation is often partially or completely deficient in this condition. However, the vasopressin response to nonosmotic stimuli-like hypotension may be intact.

Adipsic hypernatremia can potentially occur with a malformation of or any injury to the osmosensor for thirst. Malformations of the brain such as holoprosencephaly, hypoplasia of the corpus callosum including septo-optic dysplasia, vascular lesions such as anterior communicating artery aneurysms, neoplasms such as craniopharyngioma, suprasellar germinoma, and pinealoma have been associated with adipsia. Other associations include granulomatous diseases such as histiocytosis and sarcoidosis and miscellaneous conditions like hydrocephalus, arachnoidal cysts, and idiopathic hypothalamic dysfunction.

Patients with adipsic hypernatremia do not feel the urge to drink fluids even in the presence of hyperosmolar dehydration due to a disruption in the regulation of thirst by the osmosensor. The condition is characterized by chronic or recurrent hypernatremic dehydration usually accompanied by a deficient response of vasopressin to osmotic stimulation. The hypernatremia develops over time and is uncovered or accelerated by events such as gastroenteritis, fever, or excessive sweating, which increase renal or nonrenal fluid losses. Clinical manifestations of dehydration and hypernatremia may be seen. Laboratory manifestations include hypernatremia, azotemia, hypokalemia, and alkalosis. Complications such as acute renal failure, deep vein thrombosis, and rhabdomyolysis have been observed in this group of patients.

Treatment

In the presence of normal osmoregulation of vasopressin release, patients with adipsic hypernatremia are managed with controlled intake of daily fluids along with close monitoring of body weight, urine output, clinical symptoms, and serum sodium levels. While the patients should consume a minimum amount of fluids calculated from the renal and nonrenal losses, this amount may vary with events that increase these losses. The intact vasopressin response to osmotic stimulus should accommodate for variations in the fluid balance by regulating renal free water excretion. However, caution must be exercised in order to avoid fluid overloading, even in patients without significant polyuria because some of these individuals may be unable to fully suppress vasopressin release when faced with lower serum osmolalities.

Fluid management of adipsic hypernatremia is more difficult when it is associated with DI. There is the additional danger of hypo-osmolar overhydration with fluid intake in the presence of dDAVP. A practical method of managing these patients is to keep them antidiuresed on a fixed dose of dDAVP and then adjusting the controlled fluid intake based on changes in body weight, urine output, and the presence or absence of events associated with increased renal or nonrenal fluid

losses. A target body weight with the patient in a euvolemic state is identified. The intake of fluids for a particular day then could be adjusted to keep the daily weight close to this target weight.[22] Frequent revision of the target weight would be required for a growing child. Education of the family is vital in the management of this condition. Frequent monitoring of serum sodium levels using portable home analyzers maybe helpful in the management of children with this problem.

DISORDERS THAT CAUSE HYPONATREMIA

Hyponatremia is uncommon in children and it is usually associated with severe systemic disorders.

Hyponatremia

Hyponatremia is usually seen in the setting of salt loss that is in excess of water loss from the body. It is also seen when there is excessive intake of free water.

Definition and classification of hyponatremia

Hyponatremia (serum sodium less than 130 mEq/L) is uncommon in children. It is usually associated with severe systemic disorders. It is most commonly due to either intravascular volume depletion or excessive salt loss, as discussed subsequently, and is also encountered with hypotonic fluid overload, especially in infants. Hyponatremia can be broadly classified as that due to appropriately excessive or inappropriately excessive secretion of vasopressin and that which is associated with normal secretion of vasopressin. While hyponatremia in conjunction with hypovolemia from any cause is associated with an appropriately excessive secretion of vasopressin, inappropriately excessive secretion of vasopressin is one of the least common causes of hyponatremia in children, except following vasopressin administration for treatment of DI (Figure 3-11).

Clinical presentation and diagnosis

Because of cerebral edema, signs and symptoms when present are mostly neurological in nature. Headache, nausea, vomiting, and weakness are the most common symptoms. Behavioral changes and altered sensorium can be seen in more severe cases. Cerebral herniation can present with dilated pupils, bradycardia, hypertension, respiratory arrest, and a decorticate posture. In evaluating the cause of hyponatremia, one should first determine whether the patient is dehydrated and hypovolemic.[9] This is usually evident from the physical examination (decreased weight, skin turgor, central

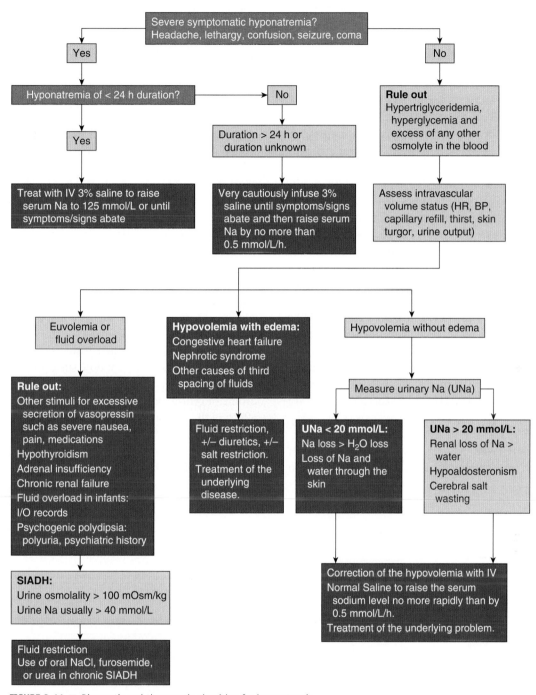

FIGURE 3-11 ■ Diagnostic and therapeutic algorithm for hyponatremia.

venous pressure) and laboratory data (high BUN, renin, aldosterone, uric acid). With a decrease in the GFR, proximal tubular reabsorption of sodium and water will be high, leading to urinary sodium less than 20 mEq/L. Patients with decreased "effective" intravascular volume due to congestive heart failure, cirrhosis, nephrotic syndrome, or lung disease will present with similar laboratory data, but also have obvious signs of their underlying disease, which often includes peripheral edema. Patients with primary salt loss will also appear volume depleted. When the salt loss is from the kidney (eg, diuretic therapy or polycystic kidney disease), urine sodium will be elevated, as may be urine volume. Salt loss from other regions (eg, the gut in gastroenteritis or the skin in cystic fibrosis) will cause urine sodium to be low, as in other forms of systemic dehydration. Cerebral salt wasting is encountered with central nervous system (CNS) insults, and results in high serum atrial natriuretic peptide concentrations leading to high urine sodium and urine excretion.

The syndrome of inappropriate vasopressin secretion exists when a primary elevation in vasopressin secretion is the cause of hyponatremia. It is characterized by hyponatremia and hypo-osmolality, a urine which is inappropriately concentrated given the degree of hypo-osmolality (>100 mOsm/kg), a normal or slightly elevated plasma volume, and a normal to high urine sodium (because of volume-induced suppression of aldosterone and elevation of atrial natriuretic peptide). Serum uric acid is low in patients with SIADH, whereas it is high in those with hyponatremia due to systemic dehydration or other causes of decreased intravascular volume. Measurement of plasma vasopressin is not very useful because it is elevated in all causes of hyponatremia except for primary hypersecretion of atrial natriuretic peptide. Because cortisol and thyroid deficiency cause hyponatremia by several mechanisms discussed subsequently, they should be considered in all hyponatremic patients. Drug-induced hyponatremia should be considered in patients on potentially offending medications, as discussed later in this chapter. In children with SIADH who do not have an obvious cause, a careful search for a tumor (thymoma, glioma, bronchial carcinoid) causing the disease should be considered.

Treatment

Most children with hyponatremia develop the disorder gradually, are asymptomatic, and should be treated with water restriction alone. However, the development of acute hyponatremia, or a serum sodium concentration below 120 mEq/L, may be associated with lethargy, psychosis, coma, or generalized seizures, especially in younger children. Acute hyponatremia causes cell swelling due to the entry of water into cells (Figure 3-12). If present for more than 24 hours, cell swelling triggers a compensatory decrease in intracellular organic osmolytes, resulting in the partial restoration of normal cell volume in chronic hyponatremia. The proper emergency treatment of cerebral dysfunction depends on whether the hyponatremia is acute or chronic. In all cases, water restriction should be instituted. If hyponatremia is acute, and therefore probably not associated with a decrease in intracellular organic osmolyte concentration, rapid correction with hypertonic, 3% sodium chloride administered intravenously may be indicated. Infusion of 1 to 2 mL/kg body weight of 3% sodium chloride will raise the serum sodium chloride concentration by approximately 1 to 2 mEq/L. If hyponatremia is chronic, hypertonic saline treatment must be undertaken with caution, since it may result in both cell shrinkage (Figure 3-12) and the associated syndrome of central pontine myelinolysis. This syndrome, affecting the central portion of the basal pons, is characterized by demyelination with sparing of neurons. It becomes evident within 24 to 48 hours following too rapid correction of hyponatremia, has a characteristic

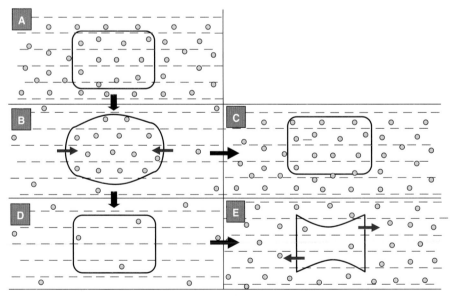

FIGURE 3-12 ■ The effects of hyponatremia and its rapid correction on intracellular osmolality and size of the brain cell. The shape and size of cell are normal in the eunatremic state **(A)** in which the osmolality within and outside the cell are equal. Acute hyponatremia **(B)** causes an osmotic fluid shift into the cell (blue arrows) leading to cell swelling. Rapid correction of the acute hyponatremia **(C)** once again equalizes the intracellular and extracellular osmolalities and restores the normal size and shape of the cell. If hyponatremia persists beyond 24 hours **(D)**, the cell tries to regain its original shape and size by extruding some of its osmolytes to equilibrate its osmolality with that of the outside. Rapidly raising the serum sodium and extracellular osmolality at this stage **(E)** causes cell shrinkage due to osmotic flow of water out of the cell (blue arrows). The cell is unable to generate new osmolytes rapidly enough to once more equilibrate the intracellular and extracellular osmolalities.

appearance by computed tomographic and magnetic resonance imaging, and often causes irreversible brain damage.[23] If hypertonic saline treatment is undertaken, the serum sodium should be raised only high enough to cause an improvement in mental status, and in no case faster than 0.5 mEq/L/h or 12 mEq/L/day. In the case of systemic dehydration, the rise in serum sodium may occur especially rapidly using this regimen. The associated hyperaldosteronism will cause avid retention of the administered sodium, leading to rapid restoration of volume and suppression of vasopressin secretion, resulting in a brisk water diuresis and a rise in serum sodium.

Hyponatremia with an Appropriate Increase in Vasopressin Secretion

Increased vasopressin secretion causing hyponatremia (serum sodium < 130 mEq/L) may either be an appropriate response or an inappropriate response to a pathological state. Inappropriate secretion of vasopressin, also termed the syndrome of inappropriate secretion of antidiuretic hormone (SIADH), is the much less common of the two entities. Whatever the cause, hyponatremia is a worrisome sign often associated with increased morbidity and mortality.

Causes

Systemic dehydration (water loss in excess of salt depletion) initially results in hypernatremia, hyperosmolality, and activation of vasopressin secretion, as discussed earlier in this chapter. In addition, the associated fall in the renal GFR results in an increase in proximal tubular sodium and water reabsorption, with a concomitant decrease in distal tubular water excretion. This limits the ability to form dilute urine, and along with the associated stimulation of the renin-angiotensin-aldosterone system and suppression of atrial natriuretic peptide secretion, results in the excretion of urine very low in sodium. As dehydration progresses, hypovolemia and/or hypotension become major stimuli for vasopressin release, much more potent than hyperosmolality (as discussed in a preceding section). This effect, by attempting to preserve volume, decreases free water clearance further and may lead to water retention and hyponatremia, especially if water replacement in excess of salt is given. Often, hyponatremia due to intravascular volume depletion is evident from physical and laboratory signs such as decreased skin turgor, low central venous pressure, hemoconcentration, and elevated blood urea nitrogen.

Congestive heart failure, cirrhosis, nephrotic syndrome, positive pressure mechanical ventilation, severe burns, and lung disease (bronchopulmonary dysplasia in neonates, cystic fibrosis with obstruction, and severe asthma) are all characterized by a decrease in "effective" intravascular volume. This occurs either because of impaired cardiac output, an inability to keep fluid within the vascular space, or impaired blood flow into the heart, respectively. As with systemic dehydration, in an attempt to preserve intravascular volume, water and salt excretion by the kidney is reduced, and decreased barosensor and volume sensor stimulation results in a compensatory, appropriate increase in vasopressin secretion, leading to an antidiuretic state and hyponatremia. Because of the associated stimulation of the renin-angiotensin-aldosterone system, these patients also have an increase in the total body content of sodium chloride and may have peripheral edema, which distinguishes them from those with systemic dehydration. In patients with impaired cardiac output and elevated atrial volume (such as with congestive heart failure or lung disease), atrial natriuretic peptide concentrations are elevated, which contributes to hyponatremia by promoting natriuresis (as discussed subsequently).

Treatment

Patients with systemic dehydration and hypovolemia should be rehydrated with salt-containing fluids such as normal saline or lactated Ringer solution. Because of activation of the renin-angiotensin-aldosterone system, the administered sodium will be avidly conserved, and a water diuresis will quickly ensue as volume is restored and vasopressin concentrations fall. Under these conditions, caution must be taken to prevent too rapid a correction of hyponatremia, which may itself result in brain damage, as discussed subsequently.

Hyponatremia due to a decrease in effective plasma volume caused by cardiac, hepatic, renal, or pulmonary dysfunction is more difficult to reverse. The most effective therapy is the least easily achieved: treatment of the underlying systemic disorder. Patients weaned from positive pressure ventilation undergo a prompt water diuresis and resolution of hyponatremia as cardiac output is restored and vasopressin concentrations fall. The only other effective route is to limit water intake to that required for the renal excretion of the obligate daily solute load of approximately 500 mOsm/m^2 and to replenish insensible losses. In a partial antidiuretic state with a urine osmolality of 750 mOsm/kg and insensible losses of 500 mL/m^2, oral intake would have to be limited to approximately 1200 mL/m^2/day. Because of concomitant hyperaldosteronism, the dietary restriction of sodium chloride needed to control peripheral edema in patients with heart failure may reduce the daily solute load and further limit the amount of water that can be ingested without exacerbating hyponatremia. However, hyponatremia in these settings is often slow to develop, rarely causes symptoms, and usually does not need treatment. If the serum sodium falls below 125 mEq/L, water restriction to 1 L/m^2/day is usually effective in preventing a further decline.

Hyponatremia with an Inappropriate Increase in Vasopressin Secretion

Causes

SIADH is uncommon in children. It can be seen with encephalitis, brain tumor, head trauma, in the postictal period following generalized seizures, following prolonged nausea, pneumonia, acquired immunodeficiency syndrome, and in association with drugs including chlorpropamide, vincristine, imipramine, and phenothiazines. Newer sulfonylurea agents, including glyburide, are not associated with SIADH. Although SIADH has been believed to be the cause of hyponatremia associated with viral meningitis, volume depletion is more commonly the etiology (Table 3-7). In the vast majority of children with SIADH, the cause is the excessive administration of vasopressin, whether to treat central DI,[13,21] or less commonly, bleeding disorders, or very rarely following dDAVP therapy for enuresis.

Treatment

Chronic SIADH is best treated by chronic oral fluid restriction to 1000 mL/m²/day to avoid hyponatremia, as discussed more fully in a preceding section. In young children, this degree of fluid restriction may not provide adequate calories for growth. In this situation, increasing the urine output by increasing the renal solute load or the creation of NDI using demeclocycline may be indicated to allow sufficient fluid intake for normal growth. This is not suitable in young children and pregnant women since tetracyclines are known to be extensively incorporated into the bones and enamel of children less than 8 years of age. The renal solute load is increased by treatment with sodium chloride alone or with a loop diuretic.[24] Oral therapy with urea has also been used safely and effectively in children with chronic SIADH.[25] Selective V2 receptor antagonists that could be used to treat SIADH and chronic disorders of decreased effective

volume associated with hyponatremia are not yet approved for use in children. Acute treatment of hyponatremia due to SIADH is only indicated if cerebral dysfunction is present. In that case, treatment is dictated by the duration of hyponatremia and the extent of cerebral dysfunction, as discussed previously.

Box 3-1 lists the circumstances in which a patient with SIADH should be referred to a pediatric endocrinologist.

Hyponatremia with No Increase in Vasopressin Secretion

Primary polydipsia

In primary polydipsia it is the excessive intake of water that drives the polyuria. In older children, with a normal kidney and the ability to suppress vasopressin secretion, hyponatremia does not occur unless water intake exceeds 10 L/m²/day, a feat which is almost impossible to accomplish. However neonates cannot dilute their urine as much as the older children, and are prone to develop water intoxication at levels of water ingestion above 4 L/m²/day (approximately 60 mL/h in a newborn). This may happen when concentrated infant formula is diluted with excess water, either by accident or in a misguided attempt to make it last longer. A primary increase in thirst, without apparent cause, leading to hyponatremia has been reported in infants as young as 5 weeks of age. Longstanding ingestion of large volumes of water will decrease the hypertonicity within the renal medullary interstitium, which will impair water reabsorption and guard against water intoxication.

Despite the presence of polyuria and polydipsia, this entity should not be confused with DI. Differentiating primary polydipsia from DI is important because treating primary polydipsia with dDAVP will abolish the protective diuresis, leading to potentially fatal fluid overload and profound hyponatremia. In primary polydipsia, although the urinary osmolality may be low, the serum osmolality and serum sodium levels are not elevated. Primary polydipsia may be classified as thirst driven (dipsogenic) or nonthirst driven as seen in the setting of psychiatric illnesses (psychogenic).

Psychogenic polydipsia. This nonthirst driven excessive intake of water, which is associated with schizophrenia and other psychiatric disorders, has a reported prevalence of 6% to 17% among psychiatric inpatients.[26] It may be a form of compulsive behavior, a means of stress reduction, or one of the "positive" symptoms of schizophrenia. Treatment options include controlled fluid intake, behavioral strategies, and pharmacotherapy. Patients do not complain of thirst when their fluid intake is restricted to the normal amount.

Table 3-7.

Causes of SIADH

Trauma/subdural hematoma/subarachnoid hemorrhage
Postoperative (triple phase response)
Meningitis, encephalitis, and brain abscess
Brain tumors
Pulmonary infections: pneumonias and empyema
Neonatal hypoxia
Tumors:
  ■ Mediastinal: thymoma, bronchogenic carcinoma
  ■ Other: leukemia

A Cochrane database review[27] of randomized controlled trials concluded that there was a lack of proper evidence to support the use of any of the medications described in case reports for the treatment of this condition. Therapy with dDAVP is not advised because the patient can have profound hyponatremia with impairment of the renal clearance of free water in the presence of unregulated fluid intake.

Dipsogenic polydipsia.

Unlike psychogenic polydipsia, the excessive water intake is driven by an altered thirst mechanism. Though this is seen in association with hypothalamic disease, quite often it is idiopathic. Normally, the threshold for the osmotic stimulation of thirst is approximately 10 mOsm/kg higher that for osmotic stimulation of AVP secretion (Figure 3-8). An individual's set plasma osmolality lies between these two thresholds.[28] If in the rare patient, thirst is activated below the threshold for vasopressin release, water intake and resulting hypo-osmolality will occur, suppressing vasopressin secretion, thus leading to persistent polydipsia and polyuria. Such individuals will drink plenty of fluids even as they are unable to concentrate their urine appropriately. However, when their plasma osmolality is allowed to rise to the threshold for vasopressin release by means of water deprivation, they are able to secrete vasopressin appropriately. The renal response to the vasopressin however may be blunted by the loss of the intra-renal concentration gradient due to the chronic polyuria. As long as daily fluid intake is less than 10 L/m², hyponatremia will not occur. Treatment of such a patient with dDAVP may lower serum osmolality below the threshold for thirst, suppressing water ingestion and the consequent polyuria.

Decreased renal free water clearance

Causes. Adrenal insufficiency, either primary or secondary in nature, has long been known to result in compromised free water excretion.[29] Both mineralocorticoids and glucocorticoids are required for normal free water clearance. By restoring the GFR through volume repletion, more free water is delivered to the distal tubule for excretion in the presence of mineralocorticoids. Glucocorticoid deficiency causes upregulation of aquaporin-2 expression in rodent kidney.[30] It is possible that glucorticoids may inhibit the activity of nitric oxide synthase in the collecting duct epithelium, decreasing the local production of nitric oxide which is known to lead to insertion of aquaporin-2 aggregates into the apical membrane.

Thyroid hormone is also required for normal free water clearance, and its deficiency likewise results in decreased renal water clearance and hyponatremia. Additionally, in severe hypothyroidism, hypovolemia is not present, and hyponatremia is accompanied by appropriate suppression of vasopressin.[31] This decrease in free water clearance may result from diminished GFR and delivery of free water to the diluting segment of distal nephron as suggested by both animal and human studies.

Given the often subtle clinical findings associated with adrenal and thyroid deficiency, all patients with hyponatremia should be suspected of these disease states and have appropriate diagnostic tests performed if indicated. Moreover, patients with coexisting adrenal failure and DI may have no symptoms of the latter until glucocorticoid therapy unmasks the need for vasopressin replacement.[32] Similarly, resolution of DI in chronically polyuric and polydypsic patients may suggest inadequate glucocorticoid supplementation or noncompliance with glucocorticoid replacement.

Some drugs may cause hyponatremia by inhibiting renal water excretion without stimulating secretion of vasopressin, an action that could be called nephrogenic SIADH. In addition to augmenting vasopressin release, both carbamazepine and chlorpropamide increase the cellular response to vasopressin. Acetaminophen also increases the response of the kidney to vasopressin, however, this has not been found to cause hyponatremia. High-dose cyclophosphamide treatment (15-20 mg/kg intravenous bolus) is often associated with hyponatremia, particularly when it is followed by a forced water diuresis to prevent hemorrhagic cystitis. Plasma vasopressin concentrations are normal, suggesting a direct effect of the drug to increase water resorption. Similarly, vinblastine, independent of augmentation of plasma vasopressin concentration or vasopressin action, and cisplatinum cause hyponatremia. These drugs may damage the collecting duct tubular cells, which are normally highly impermeable to water, or may enhance aquaporin-2 water channel activity and thereby increase water reabsorption down its osmotic gradient into the hypertonic renal interstitium.

Gain-of-function mutations in the V2 receptor have been described to cause hyponatremia in the absence of an elevation in blood vasopressin concentrations.[33] These patients may have a clinical presentation during infancy very similar to that of SIADH, except for the lack of elevation in vasopressin.

Treatment. Hyponatremia due to cortisol or thyroid hormone deficiency reverses promptly following institution of hormone replacement. Because the hyponatremia is often chronic, too rapid a rise in serum sodium should be avoided if possible, as has been discussed. When drugs that impair free water excretion must be used, water intake should be limited, as if the patient has SIADH to 1 L/m²/24 h, using the regimen discussed. Urea has been used to treat hyponatremia due to gain-of-function mutations in the V2 receptor. V2 antagonists may be useful in the future, if they are effective depending on the nature of the gene mutation and once they are FDA approved for this indication.

Miscellaneous Causes of True and Factitious Hyponatremia

Causes

Primary salt-losing disorders can cause hyponatremia. Salt can be lost from the kidney, such as in patients with congenital polycystic kidney disease, acute interstitial nephritis, and chronic renal failure. Mineralocorticoid deficiency, pseudohypoaldosteronism (sometimes seen in children with urinary tract obstruction or infection), diuretic use, and gastrointestinal disease (usually gastroenteritis with diarrhea and/or vomiting) can also result in excess loss of sodium chloride. Hyponatremia can also result from salt loss in sweat in cystic fibrosis, although obstructive lung disease with elevation of plasma vasopressin probably plays a more prominent role, as discussed above. With the onset of salt loss, any tendency toward hyponatremia will initially be countered by suppression of vasopressin and increased water excretion. However, with continuing salt loss, hypovolemia and/or hypotension ensue, causing nonosmotic stimulation of vasopressin. This, along with increased thirst, leads to ingestion of hypotonic fluids with low solute content, resulting in hyponatremia. Weight loss is usually evident, as is the source of sodium wasting.

Although atrial natriuretic peptide does not usually play a primary role in the pathogenesis of disorders of water metabolism, it may have an important secondary role. Patients with SIADH have elevated atrial natriuretic peptide concentrations, probably due to hypervolemia, which may contribute to the elevated natriuresis of SIADH and which decrease as water intake is restricted. However, hyponatremia in some patients, primarily those with CNS disorders including brain tumor, head trauma, and brain death, may be due to the primary hypersecretion of atrial natriuretic peptide. This syndrome, termed cerebral salt wasting (discussed subsequently in greater detail), is defined by hyponatremia accompanied by hypovolemia, elevated urinary sodium excretion (often exceeding 150 mEq/L), excessive urine output, suppressed vasopressin, and elevated atrial natriuretic peptide concentrations (>20 pmol/L).[34] Thus, it is distinguished from SIADH, in which euvolemia, normal or decreased urine output, only modestly elevated urine sodium concentration, and elevated vasopressin concentration occur. The distinction is important because the therapies of the two disorders are markedly different as shown is Table 3-13.

True hyponatremia is also associated with hyperglycemia, which causes the influx of water into the intravascular space. Serum sodium will decrease by 1.6 mEq/L for every 100 mg/dL increment in blood glucose above 100 mg/dL. Glucose is not ordinarily an osmotically active agent, and does not stimulate vasopressin release, probably because it is able to equilibrate freely across plasma membranes. However, in the presence of insulin deficiency and hyperglycemia, glucose becomes osmotically active, and can stimulate vasopressin release. Rapid correction of hyponatremia may follow soon after the institution of fluid and insulin therapy. Whether this contributes to the pathogenesis of cerebral edema occasionally seen following treatment of diabetic ketoacidosis is not known. Elevated concentrations of triglycerides may cause factitious hyponatremia, as can obtaining a blood sample downstream from an intravenous infusion of hypotonic fluid.

Treatment

In general, patients with hyponatremia due to salt loss require ongoing supplementation with sodium chloride and fluids. Initially, intravenous replacement of urine volume with fluid containing sodium chloride, 150 to 450 mEq/L depending on the degree of salt loss, may be necessary. Oral salt supplementation may be required subsequently. This treatment contrasts with that of SIADH, where water restriction without sodium supplementation is the mainstay.

Cerebral Salt Wasting

Definition

Cerebral salt wasting (CSW) is a condition of profound salt-wasting (natriuresis) that follows CNS insults, for example, infection, trauma, or tumor, and is thought to be due to an inappropriate secretion of atrial natriuretic hormone (ANH) following these insults.

Pathophysiology

ANH is a highly significant product of atrial tissue, as 2% to 3% of all atrial messenger ribonucleic acid (RNA) codes for it. It (and brain natriuretic peptide [BNP]) are synthesized in the hypothalamus and other regions of the CNS involved in cardiovascular regulation, as well as in many other tissues, suggesting *paracrine* functions for ANH and BNP. The majority of circulating ANH is derived from the atria, and its plasma concentration is highly dependent on and directly proportional to plasma volume. Some studies suggest however, that brain-derived ANH could account for significant amounts of the total circulating ANH under some circumstances.

High affinity receptors for ANH are found in a wide variety of tissues, including general vascular smooth muscle, renal glomerular arterioles, juxtaglomerular (JG) cells and tubules, the adrenal gland, heart, lung, and others. This explains the wide-ranging effects of ANH in the regulation of the body's salt and water metabolism, plasma volume, and blood pressure.

>   **Cardiovascular effects of ANH**—ANH acts on the heart and vascular smooth muscle and endothelium to produce significant decreases in heart rate, stroke volume, and mean arterial blood pressure (Table 3-8). Furthermore, ANH inhibits and reverses vasoconstriction mediated by angiotensin-II or norepinephrine. The net effect of ANH on the cardiovascular system, therefore, is hypotension, and (potentially) a reversal of essential and other forms of hypertension. Effects of intravenously administered BNP on the hemodynamics are similar.
>
>   **Renal effects of ANH**—ANH binds primarily to receptors in the glomerulus and JG cells, and, to a lesser extent, in the tubules and collecting ducts. ANH's main effects in the glomerulus are dilatation of the afferent arterioles and constriction of the efferent arterioles, leading to greatly increased GFR and sodium excretion. ANH also inhibits sodium resorption in the tubules, primarily that which is due to the effects of the angiotensin-II/aldosterone axis. In addition, ANH inhibits arginine vasopressin (antidiuretic hormone)-mediated resorption of free water. BNP's effects in the kidney are similar to those of ANH.

The net result of the actions of the natriuretic peptides in the kidney, therefore, are profound natriuresis and diuresis (Table 3-8 and Figure 3-13), which result in clinically significant hyponatremia and hypovolemia.

>   **CNS effects of ANH[35]**—When administered intraventricularly in pharmacologic amounts, ANH and BNP cause reductions in water intake. ANH in physiologic amounts also decreases salt intake and inhibits secretion of antidiuretic hormone. Thus the net local (paracrine) CNS effects of the natriuretic peptides complement their peripheral endocrine effects (see "Endocrine effects of ANH" section) by inhibiting the conservation of water and salt and thereby potentiating hyponatremia and hypovolemia. Insults to the CNS (eg, trauma, tumor, infection, etc.), therefore, could potentiate an "inappropriate" local secretion of ANH as well as a peripheral (cardiac) oversecretion of ANH to produce a "cerebral" salt wasting (CSW) seen in adults and children under these circumstances.

Table 3-8.

Systemic Effects of ANH

Cardiovascular Effects
   Relaxation of arterial smooth muscle
   Inhibition of and reversal of vasoconstriction due to
      angiotensin-II and norepinephrine
   Negative chronotropic and inotropic effects
      Net effects: Hypotension/reversal of hypertension
Renal Effects
   Dilatation of afferent arterioles
   Constriction of efferent arterioles: *Increase in glomerular
      filtration rate*
   Decrease in JG cell renin secretion
   Inhibition of angiotensin-II-induced, aldosterone-mediated
      sodium resorption: *Decrease in tubular sodium resorption*
   Inhibition of antidiuretic hormone-induced water resorption
      *Net effects: Increased urine and sodium excretion (true
      natriuresis) and diuresis/hypovolemia*
Central Nervous System Effects
   Inhibition of antidiuretic hormone secretion
   Inhibition of water and salt intake
      Net effects: Diuresis/hyponatremia

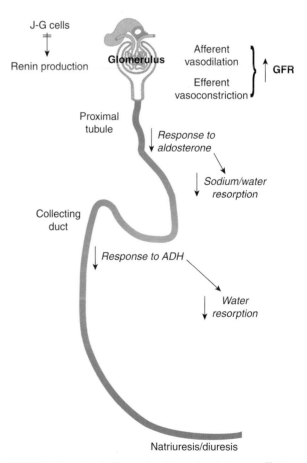

FIGURE 3-13 ■ Renal effects of atrial natriuretic hormone.[35] (The horizontal hash marks indicate inhibitory actions of ANH.)

Table 3-9.

Endocrine Effects of ANH on Water and Salt Balance

Inhibition of renin secretion
Inhibition of renin activity (PRA) on angiotensin-I generation
Inhibition of angiotensin-II mediated aldosterone secretion
Inhibition of antidiuretic hormone secretion and action
   Net effects: Increased sodium and water excretion (natriuresis/ diuresis)

Endocrine effects of ANH (see Table 3-9)—ANH inhibits renin secretion, its enzymatic action on angiotensinogen, and basal and angiotensin-II-mediated aldosterone synthesis and secretion. BNP is as effective in causing these changes as is ANH. ANH is also a potent inhibitor of the secretion and action of antidiuretic hormone.

   Inhibitory effects of ANH (and BNP) on the renal and endocrine regulation of salt and water metabolism/conservation are summarized in Figures 3-13 and 3-14, respectively. It is apparent that these peptides provide a counterbalancing influence to the renin-angiotensin-aldosterone axis in the regulation of blood pressure and blood volume. Thus, an oversecretion of ANH and/or BNP could account for the observed natriuresis and diuresis seen in patients with CNS injury, infection, or tumor.

ANH in disease states—ANH secretion is stimulated by atrial stretch and is therefore increased in conditions characterized by increased plasma volume, whereas its secretion is suppressed by plasma volume contraction (Table 3-10). Disease states characterized by plasma volume depletion, such as dehydration from any cause, including DI (see Figure 3-16A)[36] and diabetic ketoacidosis are associated with decreased plasma concentrations of ANH.

   Conditions associated with increased plasma ANH concentrations of ANH are usually characterized by increased plasma volume (eg, hypertension; Figure 3-16A). The increase in ANH concentrations in SIADH is most likely due to the increase in plasma volume, and there is speculation that CSW may be an inappropriate response to SIADH in acute CNS insults (see "Etiologic role of ANH in CSW" section).

Etiologic role of ANH in CSW—The SIADH secretion has, until recently, been thought to be responsible for most occurrences of hyponatremia developing after CNS insult. It has become

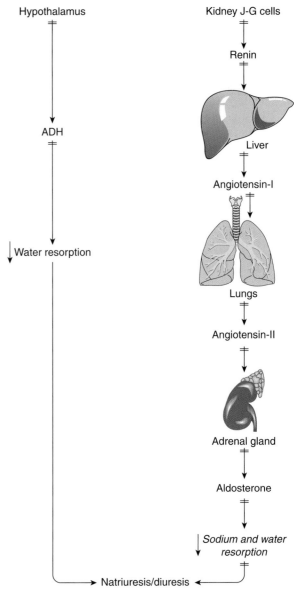

FIGURE 3-14 ■ Effects of ANH on the endocrine control of salt and water metabolism. (The horizontal hash marks indicate inhibitory actions of ANH.)

evident, however, that SIADH cannot account for all cases, particularly when the patient exhibits polyuria and dehydration. A true "salt wasting" associated with cerebral disease is now recognized as a distinct clinical entity. Because the treatments of CSW and SIADH are very distinct and potentially harmful if incorrectly applied, proper understanding of the cause of hyponatremia in a CNS-injured child is essential.

   The salt wasting syndrome associated with CNS pathology was first defined by Peters in 1950[38] as the inability to prevent salt loss in the urine despite hyponatremia in individuals with cerebral disease, or a "cerebral" salt wasting.[39]

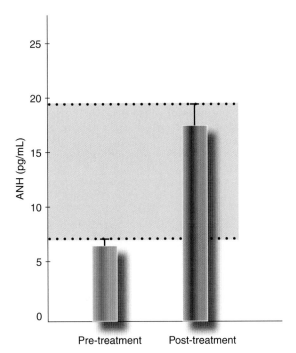

FIGURE 3-15 ■ Plasma ANH concentrations before and after treatment in patients with diabetes insipidus.[36] The horizontal lines represent the 95% confidence limits of plasma ANH concentrations in 108 normal subjects. (*Modified from Kamoi K, Ebe T, Kobayashi O, et al. Atrial natriuretic peptide in patients with the syndrome of inappropriate antidiuretic hormone secretion and with diabetes insipidus. J Clin Endocrinol Metab. 1990;70(5):1385-1390.[36]*)

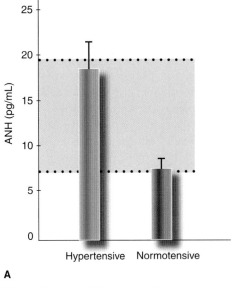

A

FIGURE 3-16A ■ Plasma ANH concentrations in normotensive vs hypertensive adults. (*Modified from Sagnella GA, Markandu ND, Shore AC, MacGregor GA. Raised circulating levels of atrial natriuretic peptides in essential hypertension. Lancet. 1986;1(8474):179-181.[37]*)

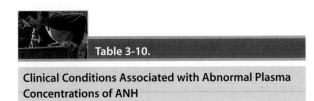

Table 3-10.

Clinical Conditions Associated with Abnormal Plasma Concentrations of ANH

Conditions (Hypovolemic) with Decreased Plasma Concentrations of ANH
    Diabetes insipidus (DI)
    Diabetic ketoacidosis (DKA) with dehydration
Conditions (Hypervolemic) with Increased Plasma Concentrations of ANH
    CSW
    SIADH
    Cushing syndrome/hyperaldosteronism
    Hypertension
    Congestive heart failure

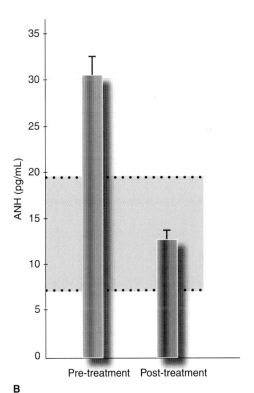

B

FIGURE 3-16B ■ Plasma ANH concentrations before and after treatment in patients with SIADH.[36] The horizontal lines represent the 95% confidence limits of plasma ANH concentrations in 108 normal subjects. (*Modified from Kamoi K, Ebe T, Kobayashi O, et al. Atrial natriuretic peptide in patients with the syndrome of inappropriate antidiuretic hormone secretion and with diabetes insipidus. J Clin Endocrinol Metab. 1990;70(5):1385-1390.[36]*)

An etiologic role for ANH in CSW is proposed, and its plasma concentration is elevated in some children and adults with various types of CNS injury.[40-43] In the acute period (eg, 1-4 days post subarachnoid hemorrhage) plasma antidiuretic hormone concentrations can be elevated and cause water retention and transient hyponatremia. In patients with persistent hyponatremia, plasma ANH levels are usually elevated.[44] This suggests that *CSW may follow SIADH in some patients if ANH secretion remains high after their CNS insult.*

Clinical presentation in CSW

CSW can occur in adults and children after CNS insults, including trauma, infection, tumor, and surgery. The diagnosis is suggested by marked salt wasting, as evidenced by hyponatremia accompanied by high urine volumes and excessive urine sodium concentrations (80-480 mEq/L). Renal salt losses up to 10 to 20 times predicted basal requirements can occur. Plasma ANH concentrations when measured are usually inappropriately elevated, given the hypovolemic state. CSW usually develops in the first week after surgery, but the range in presentation can be from 1 to 28 days. Its duration is usually between 3 and 11 days, but rarely can persist much longer when the causative CNS insult cannot be corrected. Key diagnostic components include evidence of net salt wasting (hyponatremia, high urine volumes with excessive urine sodium concentrations), elevated plasma ANH concentrations, and (inappropriately) suppressed plasma renin activity and aldosterone concentrations (Tables 3-11 and 3-12).[41-43,45] General characteristics of adults and children with CSW are shown in Table 3-11. While an occurrence rate of approximately

Box 3-2.
Measurements that distinguish between CSW, SIADH, and DI
■ Plasma volume status
■ Plasma sodium concentration
■ Plasma osmolality
■ Urine output (mL/kg/h) compared to fluid input
■ Urine sodium concentration
■ Urine osmolality
■ *Net urinary sodium loss: urine sodium concentration × urine volume*

1% after surgery for CNS injury has been reported,[45] too few studies of CSW in adults or children have been done to fully define its prevalence.

Differential diagnosis

Laboratory tests and other means of monitoring the overall plasma volume and electrolyte status in children who present with CNS insult (pre- or postoperatively) are shown in Box 3-2. Clinical and simple, readily available laboratory assessments provide the cornerstone of diagnosis, since other entities such as plasma renin activity and hormones such as ANH, aldosterone, and ADH that can help to distinguish between CSW and SIADH usually require "send outs" to regional reference laboratories and are not immediately available to the practicing physician.

The similarities and differences between CSW and SIADH are shown in Table 3-12. Hyponatremia is usually detected during the course of routine monitoring of serum electrolytes in CNS "at-risk" patients, and the

Table 3-11.

Characteristics of Cerebral Salt Wasting[41,42,45]

Prevalence: 11.3/1000 (1%) postoperative CNS-related
    abnormalities[45]
Onset within the first week of general CNS insult
Laboratory Findings
    Plasma sodium concentration: 95-130 mEq/L
    Urine Osmolality: 280-1100 mOsm/kg
    Urine sodium concentration (maximum): 100-310 mEq/L
    Urinary excretion rate: 3-15 mL/kg/h (average 6 mL/kg/h)
Acute, intermittent excessive fluid and salt loss 10-20 times
    maintenance
Duration variable: Usually 1-3 weeks, but may be months

Table 3-12.

Characteristics of CSW and SIADH[41,46,47]

	CSW	SIADH
Plasma volume	Decreased	Increased
Clinical evidence of volume depletion	Yes	No
Plasma sodium concentration	Low	Low
Urine sodium concentration	High	High
Urine output	Very high	Low
Plasma renin activity	Suppressed	Suppressed
Net sodium loss (urine Na+ × urine volume)	Very high	Normal
Plasma aldosterone concentration	Suppressed	Normal/high
Plasma antidiuretic hormone concentration	Suppressed	High

urine sodium concentration may be found to be inappropriately high for the observed low serum sodium concentration in both CSW and SIADH. In CSW however, there is a net negative water and sodium balance, as estimated by multiplying urine sodium concentration by urine volume. Thus a true and sustained net natriuresis is characteristic of CSW in contrast to SIADH. Furthermore, there is usually evidence of plasma volume depletion (eg, hypotension) in patients with CSW, while patients with SIADH may have at least a modest plasma volume expansion initially.

Plasma renin activity may be suppressed in both CSW and SIADH, but plasma antidiuretic hormone concentrations are usually suppressed in CSW in contrast to SIADH, by definition. Plasma ANH concentrations may be increased in both CSW and SIADH, but water restriction results in a return of plasma ANH concentrations to normal in SIADH despite little change in antidiuretic hormone. Thus, although antidiuretic hormone is known to stimulate ANH secretion, the plasma volume expansion in SIADH is a more likely stimulus for ANH release, and is possibly etiologic in CSW,[44] if ANH oversecretion persists "inappropriately" after SIADH resolves.

The differentiation of DI from CSW and/or SIADH is not usually difficult, since the polyuria in DI most often results in hypernatremia, and the urine sodium concentration and urine osmolality are low. It is imperative that the distinctions be made, however, since the treatment of each of these conditions is quite different, and the potential for increased morbidity/mortality exists if inappropriate treatment is given.

Treatment of CSW[41,43,46]

Treatments of CSW and SIADH are outlined in Table 3-13. It is critical to distinguish between SIADH and CSW as the cause of hyponatremia, since fluid restriction (indicated in SIADH) could be potentially disastrous in CSW.

Aggressive replacement of urine salt and water losses using 0.9% NaCl (or 3% NaCl if necessary) is the cornerstone of treatment of CSW. Administration of

parenteral antidiuretic hormone (as aqueous pitressin or dDAVP) does not usually provide any beneficial effect on urine output in CSW. Similarly, since CSW is characterized by a functional mineralocorticoid deficiency and resistance (hyporeninemic hypoaldosteronism), mineralocorticoid supplementation in the form of fludrocortisone has only been shown to be of benefit in a few patients.[41,48]

Summary

CSW is a clinical entity distinct from SIADH, although both may present with hyponatremia following an insult to the CNS. It is critical to distinguish between CSW and SIADH, since the treatment of the former would be deleterious to patients with the latter, and vice versa. A large body of evidence suggests that the oversecretion of brain- or cardiac-derived ANH is etiologic in CSW. Insults to the CNS could result in a direct oversecretion of ANH with resultant natriuresis and diuresis leading to hyponatremia and hypovolemia, that is, CSW. Alternatively, the CNS insult could lead to SIADH, which, in turn, could stimulate ANH secretion directly by antidiuretic hormone or indirectly by plasma volume expansion. The heightened secretion of ANH does not abate when plasma volume has returned to normal, and CSW results. It is also possible that the mechanism of the development of CSW varies between patients, and that a direct CNS insult and/or a secondary response to SIADH are possible antecedents in different patients. CSW is a potentially serious entity, which may result in life-threatening hyponatremia and severe plasma volume depletion, and must be distinguished from SIADH for optimal patient care.

Table 3-13.

Treatment of CSW and SIADH[41,43,46,48]

	CSW	SIADH
Fluids	Replacement	Restriction
Sodium	Replacement with 0.9% or 3% saline	Maintenance
Other	Fludrocortisone[41,47]	Demeclocycline, lithium

REFERENCES

1. Strange K. Regulation of solute and water balance and cell volume in the central nervous system. *J Am Soc Nephrol.* 1992;3(1):12-27.
2. Vokes TJ, Robertson GL. Disorders of antidiuretic hormone. *Endocrinol Metab Clin North Am.* 1988;17(2):281-299.
3. Vavra I, Machova A, Holecek V, Cort JH, Zaoral M, Sorm F. Effect of a synthetic analogue of vasopressin in animals and in patients with diabetes insipidus. *Lancet.* 1968;1(7549):948-952.
4. Brownstein MJ, Russell JT, Gainer H. Synthesis, transport, and release of posterior pituitary hormones. *Science.* 1980;207(4429):373-378.
5. Robertson GL, Shelton RL, Athar S. The osmoregulation of vasopressin. *Kidney Int.* 1976;10(1):25-37.
6. Arnauld E, Czernichow P, Fumoux F, Vincent JD. The effects of hypotension and hypovolaemia on the liberation of vasopressin during haemorrhage in the unanaesthetized monkey (Macaca mulatta). *Pflugers Arch.* 1977;371(3):193-200.

7. Harris HW Jr, Strange K, Zeidel ML. Current understanding of the cellular biology and molecular structure of the antidiuretic hormone-stimulated water transport pathway. *J Clin Invest.* 1991;88(1):1-8.

8. Pham PC, Pham PM, Pham PT. Vasopressin excess and hyponatremia. *Am J Kidney Dis.* 2006;47(5):727-737.

9. Moritz ML, Ayus JC. Disorders of water metabolism in children: hyponatremia and hypernatremia. *Pediatr Rev.* 2002;23(11):371-380.

10. Trachtman H. Cell volume regulation: a review of cerebral adaptive mechanisms and implications for clinical treatment of osmolal disturbances. I. *Pediatr Nephrol.* 1991;5(6):743-750.

11. Maghnie M, Cosi G, Genovese E, et al. Central diabetes insipidus in children and young adults. *N Engl J Med.* 2000;343(14):998-1007.

12. Russell TA, Ito M, Ito M, et al. A murine model of autosomal dominant neurohypophyseal diabetes insipidus reveals progressive loss of vasopressin-producing neurons. *J Clin Invest.* 2003;112(11):1697-1706.

13. Crigler JF Jr. Commentary: On the use of pitressin in infants with neurogenic diabetes insipidue. *J Pediatr.* 1976;88(2):295-296.

14. Rivkees SA, Dunbar N, Wilson TA. The management of central diabetes insipidus in infancy: desmopressin, low renal solute load formula, thiazide diuretics. *J Pediatr Endocrinol Metab.* 2007;20(4):459-469.

15. Blanco EJ, Lane AH, Aijaz N, Blumberg D, Wilson TA. Use of subcutaneous DDAVP in infants with central diabetes insipidus. *J Pediatr Endocrinol Metab.* 2006;19(7):919-925.

16. Boulgourdjian EM, Martinez AS, Ropelato MG, Heinrich JJ, Bergada C. Oral desmopressin treatment of central diabetes insipidus in children. *Acta Paediatr.* 1997;86(11): 1261-1262.

17. Bryant WP, O'Marcaigh AS, Ledger GA, Zimmerman D. Aqueous vasopressin infusion during chemotherapy in patients with diabetes insipidus. *Cancer.* 1994;74(9):2589-2592.

18. Knoers N, Monnens LA. Nephrogenic diabetes insipidus: clinical symptoms, pathogenesis, genetics and treatment. *Pediatr Nephrol.* 1992;6(5):476-482.

19. Alon U, Chan JC. Hydrochlorothiazide-amiloride in the treatment of congenital nephrogenic diabetes insipidus. *Am J Nephrol.* 1985;5(1):9-13.

20. Frasier SD, Kutnik LA, Schmidt RT, Smith FG Jr. A water deprivation test for the diagnosis of diabetes insipidus in children. *Am J Dis Child.* 1967;114(2):157-160.

21. Koskimies O, Pylkkanen J, Vilska J. Water intoxication in infants caused by the urine concentration test with vasopressin analogue (DDAVP). *Acta Paediatr Scand.* 1984;73(1):131-132.

22. Ball SG, Vaidja B, Baylis PH. Hypothalamic adipsic syndrome: diagnosis and management. *Clin Endocrinol (Oxf).* 1997;47(4):405-409.

23. Laureno R, Karp BI. Myelinolysis after correction of hyponatremia. *Ann Intern Med.* 1997;126(1):57-62.

24. Decaux G. Long-term treatment of patients with inappropriate secretion of antidiuretic hormone by the vasopressin receptor antagonist conivaptan, urea, or furosemide. *Am J Med.* 2001;110(7):582-584.

25. Huang EA, Feldman BJ, Schwartz ID, Geller DH, Rosenthal SM, Gitelman SE. Oral urea for the treatment of chronic syndrome of inappropriate antidiuresis in children. *J Pediatr.* 2006;148(1):128-131.

26. de Leon J, Verghese C, Tracy JI, Josiassen RC, Simpson GM. Polydipsia and water intoxication in psychiatric patients: a review of the epidemiological literature. *Biol Psychiatry.* 1994;35(6):408-419.

27. Brookes G, Ahmed AG. Pharmacological treatments for psychosis-related polydipsia. *Cochrane Database Syst Rev.* 2002(3):CD003544.

28. Robertson GL, Aycinena P, Zerbe RL. Neurogenic disorders of osmoregulation. *Am J Med.* 1982;72(2):339-353.

29. Boykin J, DeTorrente A, Erickson A, Robertson G, Schrier RW. Role of plasma vasopressin in impaired water excretion of glucocorticoid deficiency. *J Clin Invest.* 1978;62(4): 738-744.

30. Saito T, Ishikawa SE, Ando F, Higashiyama M, Nagasaka S, Sasaki S. Vasopressin-dependent upregulation of aquaporin-2 gene expression in glucocorticoid-deficient rats. *Am J Physiol Renal Physiol.* 2000;279(3):F502-F508.

31. Iwasaki Y, Oiso Y, Yamauchi K, et al. Osmoregulation of plasma vasopressin in myxedema. *J Clin Endocrinol Metab.* 1990;70(2):534-539.

32. Yamada K, Tamura Y, Yoshida S. Effect of administration of corticotropin-releasing hormone and glucocorticoid on arginine vasopressin response to osmotic stimulus in normal subjects and patients with hypocorticotropinism without overt diabetes insipidus. *J Clin Endocrinol Metab.* 1989;69(2):396-401.

33. Rosenthal SM, Feldman BJ, Vargas GA, Gitelman SE. Nephrogenic syndrome of inappropriate antidiuresis (NSIAD): a paradigm for activating mutations causing endocrine dysfunction. *Pediatr Endocrinol Rev.* 2006;4(1): 66-70.

34. Ganong CA, Kappy MS. Cerebral salt wasting in children. The need for recognition and treatment. *Am J Dis Child.* 1993;147(2):167-169.

35. Huang CL, Lewicki J, Johnson LK, Cogan MG. Renal mechanism of action of rat atrial natriuretic factor. *J Clin Invest.* 1985;75(2):769-773.

36. Kamoi K, Ebe T, Kobayashi O, et al. Atrial natriuretic peptide in patients with the syndrome of inappropriate antidiuretic hormone secretion and with diabetes insipidus. *J Clin Endocrinol Metab.* 1990;70(5):1385-1390.

37. Sagnella GA, Markandu ND, Shore AC, MacGregor GA. Raised circulating levels of atrial natriuretic peptides in essential hypertension. *Lancet.* 1986;1(8474):179-181.

38. Peters JP, Welt LG, Sims EA, Orloff J, Needham J. A salt-wasting syndrome associated with cerebral disease. *Trans Assoc Am Physicians.* 1950;63:57-64.

39. Cort JH. Cerebral salt wasting. *Lancet.* 1954;266(6815): 752-754.

40. Yamamoto N, Miyamoto N, Seo H, Matsui N, Kuwayama A, Terashima K. Hyponatremia with high plasma ANP level—report of two cases with emphasis on the pathophysiology of cerebral salt wasting. *No Shinkei Geka.* 1987;15(9):1019-1023.

41. Kappy MS, Ganong CA. Cerebral salt wasting in children: the role of atrial natriuretic hormone. *Adv Pediatr.* 1996;43:271-308.

42. Donati-Genet PC, Dubuis JM, Girardin E, Rimensberger PC. Acute symptomatic hyponatremia and cerebral salt

wasting after head injury: an important clinical entity. *J Pediatr Surg.* 2001;36(7):1094-1097.

43. von Bismarck P, Ankermann T, Eggert P, Claviez A, Fritsch MJ, Krause MF. Diagnosis and management of cerebral salt wasting (CSW) in children: the role of atrial natriuretic peptide (ANP) and brain natriuretic peptide (BNP). *Childs Nerv Syst.* 2006;22(10):1275-1281.

44. Morinaga K, Hayashi S, Matsumoto Y, et al. Serum ANP and ADH after subarachnoid hemorrhage and hyponatremia. *No To Shinkei.* 1991;43(2):169-173.

45. Jimenez R, Casado-Flores J, Nieto M, Garcia-Teresa MA. Cerebral salt wasting syndrome in children with acute central nervous system injury. *Pediatr Neurol.* 2006;35(4):261-263.

46. Palmer BF. Hyponatremia in patients with central nervous system disease: SIADH versus CSW. *Trends Endocrinol Metab.* 2003;14(4):182-187.

47. Sterns RH, Silver SM. Cerebral salt wasting versus SIADH: what difference? *J Am Soc Nephrol.* 2008;19(2): 194-196.

48. Taplin CE, Cowell CT, Silink M, Ambler GR. Fludrocortisone therapy in cerebral salt wasting. *Pediatrics.* 2006; 118(6):e1904-e1908.

CHAPTER 4

Thyroid

Stephen A. Huang

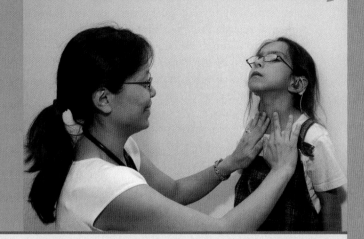

INTRODUCTION

Thyroid hormone is a potent regulator of metabolic rate and is essential to the function of most organ systems. In addition, the maintenance of normal thyroid status through childhood is necessary for normal growth and neurodevelopment. Best outcome in pediatric thyroid disease requires early detection as well as appropriate therapy with careful monitoring. These tasks are generally accomplished through successful collaboration between primary care providers and endocrine specialists. With an appropriate index of suspicion, pediatric thyroid disease can be detected in early stages and outcome is usually excellent. This chapter begins with a review of thyroid physiology and clinical testing. We then present diagnostic approaches to common pediatric thyroid disorders, grouped into the categories of hypothyroidism, thyrotoxicosis, and nodular thyroid disease.

THYROID PHYSIOLOGY

Embryonic Development

The fetal thyroid begins as a thickening of the pharyngeal floor which forms a diverticulum that descends caudally into the resting position of the mature thyroid gland. During this migration, a track called the thyroglossal duct is formed which connects the pharyngeal floor to the thyroid bed. This thyroglossal duct normally involutes and, by embryonic day 50, the thyroid primordium has fused with the ventral aspect of the fourth pharyngeal pouch and formed a bilobed structure. The cells of this primordium differentiate into thyroid follicular cells which synthesize thyroid hormone. In contrast, thyroid

C-cells, which instead produce calcitonin, are derived from the ultimobranchial glands.

By 11 to 12 weeks of gestation, the fetal thyroid is capable of concentrating iodine and synthesizing thyroxine. Prior to this, the human fetus is dependent upon maternal thyroid hormone. Even in later pregnancy, transplacental passage remains an important source of fetal thyroid hormone evidenced by the fact that thyroxine is detectable in the serum of infants born with complete thyroid agenesis.

Analyses of serum obtained through cordocentesis indicate that the fetal thyrotropin, also called thyroid stimulating hormone (TSH), to T_4 relationship matures throughout gestation. Compared to maternal serum, fetal serum is characterized by low concentrations of both thyroxine (T_4) and triiodothyronine (T_3). Birth is associated with a transient and robust peak in both serum TSH and T_4 (referred to as the neonatal surge), followed by rapid changes in the metabolism of thyroid hormone in peripheral tissues. This normal neonatal thyroid surge typically lasts about 1 to 2 days and this is the rationale for delaying newborn screening until 2 days after birth.

From a clinical standpoint, deviation from the normal anatomic development of the fetal thyroid is the most common cause of congenital hypothyroidism. These conditions are termed thyroid dysgenesis and, as described below, the study of affected patients has provided valuable insight into the molecular biology of normal thyroid development.

Thyroid Hormone Synthesis

The sole physiologic function of the thyroid gland is to synthesize T_4 and T_3. Dietary iodine is a critical nutritional precursor of both these active thyroid hormones.

Endemic cretinism is a term used to describe the clinical consequence of dietary iodine deficiency, which is characterized by thyroid enlargement and neurodevelopmental retardation from thyroid hormone insufficiency. The pathophysiology of endemic cretinism is fully prevented by supplementation of dietary iodine.

Iodine is absorbed from the small intestine via a TSH-independent mechanism. Once in the circulation, iodine is transported into thyroid follicular cells via the sodium-iodine symporter, oxidized, and finally organified onto tyrosyl residues of thyroglobulin, a large glycoprotein which resides in thyroid colloid. These iodinated tyrosyl residues couple to form T_4 and T_3, which are eventually released into the bloodstream after the proteolysis of thyroglobulin. Each step in the synthesis of thyroid hormone is catalyzed by enzymes which, when deficient, may lead to goiter and/or hypothyroidism. Naturally occurring autosomal recessive mutations in many of the genes which encode these enzymes have been shown to cause dyshormonogenic congenital hypothyroidism.

Regulation of the Hypothalamic Pituitary Axis

The hypothalamus produces thyrotropin releasing hormone (TRH) which stimulates pituitary thyrotrophs to secrete thyrotropin. TSH then stimulates the thyroid to secrete thyroid hormone. Both active thyroid hormones, T_4 and T_3, exert negative feedback upon the hypothalamus and pituitary (Figure 4-1). This inverse relationship between free T_4 and TSH is log-linear, so that small changes in serum T_4 produce large compensatory changes in serum TSH (Figure 4-2). Because of this, serum TSH is the most sensitive single test in the diagnosis of primary thyroid dysfunction. When persistent, laboratory results which document deviation from this normal serum free T_4 to TSH relationship warrant an investigation for "central" thyroid disease due to abnormalities at the level of the hypothalamus and/or pituitary (Table 4-1).

Thyroid Hormone Action

The effects of thyroid hormone are mediated by the binding of T_4 and T_3 to thyroid hormone receptors in the nuclei of target cells. Thyroid hormone receptors are encoded by two distinct genes, TRα and TRβ, which encode four distinct receptors (TRα1, TRβ1, TRβ2, and TRβ3) via alternative splicing. Three of these thyroid hormone receptor (TR) isoforms, TRα1, TRβ1, TRβ2, are functional and each has a unique tissue distribution. Binding of either T_4 or T_3 to one of these three functional receptors leads to the formation of a transcriptional complex which then stimulates or represses the expression of target genes.

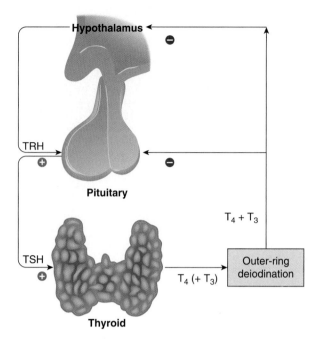

FIGURE 4-1 ■ Hypothalamic-pituitary-thyroid axis. The hypothalamus and pituitary stimulate thyroid secretion, primarily in the form of the prohormone T_4, which is then converted into T_3 by outer-ring deiodination in peripheral tissues. Both T_4 and T_3 feedback negatively on the hypothalamus and pituitary.

While both T_4 and T_3 can bind TRs and signal thyroid hormone action, T_3 is more potent and binds TR with 15-fold greater affinity than T_4. Most thyroid hormone secreted from the thyroid gland is in the form of T_4 that is subsequently converted into the more active T_3 by enzymatic outer-ring deiodination in peripheral

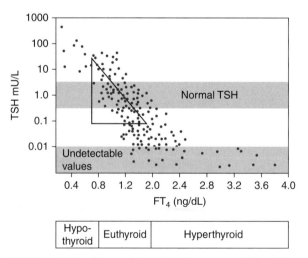

FIGURE 4-2 ■ Log/linear relationship between serum TSH and free T_4. Small changes in serum T_4 produce large deviations in serum TSH. (Redrawn from: Larsen P, Davies T, Schlumberger M, Hay I. Thyroid physiology and diagnostic evaluation of patients with thyroid disorders. In: Kronenberg HM, Melmed S, Larsen PR, Polonsky KS, eds. *Williams Textbook of Endocrinology,* 11th ed. Philadelphia, PA: Saunders/Elsevier; 2007.)

Table 4-1.

Serum Thyroid Test in Common Thyroid Disorders

	Serum TSH	Serum Free T_4 (or Free T_4 Index)	Serum Free T_3 (or Free T_3 Index)
Primary hypothyroidism	High	Normal or low	Normal or low
Central hypothyroidism	Low/medium/high	Low	Normal or low
Resistance to thyroid hormone	Normal/high	High	High
Consumptive hypothyroidism	High	Normal or low	Normal or low
Hyperthyroidism	Low	Normal or high	Normal or high
Thyrotoxicosis without hyperthyroidism	Low	Normal or high	Normal or high
TSH-secreting pituitary adenoma	Normal/high	High	High

tissues (Figure 4-3). Because of this, T_4 is often referred to as a "prohormone."

Thyroid Hormone Metabolism

The main pathway of thyroid hormone metabolism is sequential deiodination, catalyzed by a family of enzymes called the deiodinases. There are three members of this family, named type 1 (D1), type 2 (D2), and type 3 (D3) deiodinase. Removal of a single iodine group from the outer-ring of T_4 converts it into the more active T_3 and this "outer-ring deiodination" is catalyzed by types 1 and 2 deiodinases (D1 and D2). Together, D1 and D2 activity produce 80% of the T_3 in the circulation and this explains why hypothyroid patients treated with T_4 monotherapy have normal serum T_3 levels. Conversely, "inner-ring deiodination" of either T_4 or T_3 leads to substrate inactivation, pro-

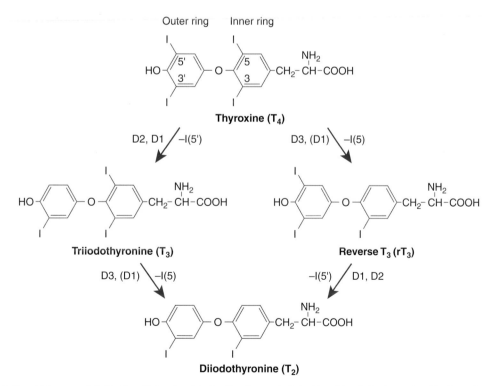

FIGURE 4-3 ■ Thyroid hormone deiodination. Outer-ring deiodination (removal of the 5' position iodine), catalyzed by D1 and D2, activates the T_4 prohormone into T_3. Inner-ring deiodination (removal of the 5 position iodine), primarily catalyzed by D3, inactivates T_4 and T_3. (Redrawn and modified from: Larsen P, Davies T, Schlumberger M, Hay I. Thyroid physiology and diagnostic evaluation of patients with thyroid disorders. In: Kronenberg HM, Melmed S, Larsen PR, Polonsky KS, eds. *Williams Textbook of Endocrinology*, 11th ed. Philadelphia, PA: Saunders/Elsevier; 2007.)

ducing the metabolites of rT_3 and T_2, respectively. Type 3 deiodinase (D3) is the major inactivating pathway for both T_4 and T_3 (Figure 4-3).

Free Hormone Hypothesis

The vast majority of thyroid hormone in the circulation is bound to serum proteins which include thyroglobulin-binding protein (TBG), transthyretin, and albumin. In euthyroid individuals, only 0.02% of T_4 and 0.3% of T_3 is unbound or "free" and immediately available to enter cells and mediate thyroid hormone signaling. An understanding of this is helpful in the interpretation of serum thyroid function tests because individuals with normal thyroid status (and normal free thyroid hormone concentrations) but abnormal binding proteins can have deranged serum measurements of total T_4 and/or total T_3. Recognizing this is important to avoid the false diagnose of thyroid disease in such individuals (Table 4-1).

THYROID TESTING

While many tests are available to evaluate thyroid disorders, most patients can be accurately diagnosed by a focused history and physical examination, combined with standard serum thyroid tests (Table 4-1). In a minority of thyrotoxic patients, quantification of thyroid radioiodine uptake (RAIU) can be useful to distinguish transient thyroiditis from early Graves hyperthyroidism. Anatomic imaging can generally be reserved for patients with thyroid nodules.

Physical Examination

The normal thyroid is located in the midline of the neck, between the thyroid cartilage and the suprasternal notch. Physical examination should begin with visual inspection of the neck to look for gross enlargement or asymmetry, followed by palpation of the gland. The examiner may palpate the thyroid while standing behind the patient, or alternatively the examiner can face the child and palpate the thyroid with his or her thumbs (Figure 4-4). In the author's opinion, the latter approach is more sensitive in the detection of small nodules and offers the benefit of visual correlation during palpation. Because the thyroid is encased by pretracheal fascia, it moves with swallowing and this feature is critically helpful to distinguish the gland from adjacent structures. Accordingly, the patient should be provided a cup of water and asked to intermittently take small sips while the examiner palpates the gland, beginning at midline and then moving laterally to define the lateral borders of the gland. Infants who are too small to stand or sit may be examined in the supine position. One hand should be placed under the infant's

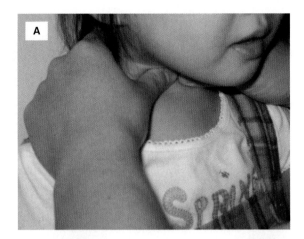

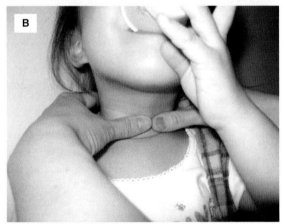

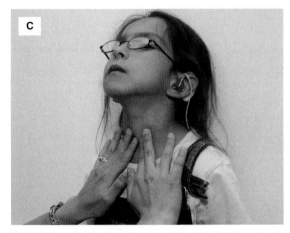

FIGURE 4-4 ■ Physical examination of the thyroid. Thyroid palpation in a toddler (**A** and **B**) and a school-age child (**C**).

shoulders and then slowly raised until the neck gently falls into mild hyperextension. The anterior neck can then be palpated with the opposite hand.

Thyroid size and the presence of any nodules should be noted. If a thyroid nodule is present, the cervical lymph node chains should be carefully palpated to assess the possibility of local metastasis from thyroid cancer. The normal thyroid grows during childhood and a helpful "rule of thumb" is to remember that each major thyroid lobe should be about the same size as the distal segment of the patient's own thumb. With practice, one should be able to feel the normal thyroid gland of nearly all school age children or adults.

Serum Thyroid Tests

Clinical testing to accurately measure serum TSH, T_4, and T_3 is widely available. Because variations in thyroid hormone binding proteins can occur, it is important to include an index of hormone binding, such as a thyroid hormone binding ratio (also called a T_3-resin uptake), when measuring total thyroid hormone concentrations. Alternatively, free T_4 and free T_3 concentrations may be assayed directly. While highly sensitive methods to accurately measure the picomolar serum concentrations of free thyroid hormone exist, they are generally available only in reference laboratories. The less expensive free T_4 assays which have become popular in most clinical laboratories indirectly estimate free T_4 concentrations without physically separating free from bound hormone. These estimates are inaccurate in patients with binding abnormalities or intercurrent nonthyroidal illness, but can be useful so long as the interpreting clinician is aware of their limitations. These issues are discussed in detail in various consensus guidelines (http://www.aacc.org/members/nacb/LMPG/Online Guide/PublishedGuidelines/ThyroidDisease).[1]

Because of the log-linear relationship between TSH and free T_4, serum TSH is the most sensitive single test to screen for primary thyroid disease (Figure 4-2). If central thyroid disease is being considered or the index of suspicion for thyroid dysfunction is high, serum free T_4 (or a calculated free T_4 index) should be added. While several adjunctive tests may be helpful after thyroid dysfunction is diagnosed, the combination of serum TSH and free T_4 is a sufficient initial screen as the combination of both a normal TSH and a normal T_4

effectively rules out thyroid dysfunction (Table 4-1). It is important to apply age-specific normal ranges (Table 4-2).[2] At several pediatric ages, both the upper and lower limits of free T_4 extend past the standard adult reference range. Failure to consider this can lead to the false diagnosis of central thyroid disease. Clinicians must also take into account other preanalytic factors which alter serum thyroid tests in the absence of thyroid pathology. The most common of these is nonthyroidal illness, a term used to describe the fact that up to 75% of hospitalized patients exhibit transient derangement of their serum thyroid function tests in the absence of true thyroid disease. Certain medications, including amiodarone and common anticonvulsants such as phenytoin and carbamazepine, can also confound the interpretation of serum thyroid tests by altering the normal serum T_4:T_3 ratio.

Thyroid Radioiodine Uptake

This test permits a direct assessment of thyroid function by quantifying the ability of an individual's thyroid gland to concentrate iodine. Thyroid radioiodine uptake (RAIU) is calculated by measuring thyroidal radioactivity 4 or 24 hours after oral radioiodine administration. While both I-131 and I-123 can be used, I-123 is preferred in children because radiation exposure is much lower with this isotope. Because RAIU depends upon dietary iodine intake, normal ranges vary from one geographic region to another. High RAIU values are characteristic of all hyperthyroid conditions and this feature is useful to distinguish hyperthyroid patients from those with thyrotoxicosis from exogenous thyroid hormone or transient thyroiditis. While RAIU can be low in certain forms of hypothyroidism, its measurement is not useful to diagnose hypothyroidism in iodine-supplemented populations such as North America because even euthyroid individuals can have RAIU values as low as 4%.

Table 4-2.

Age-Specific Normal Ranges for Serum Thyroid Tests in Children

Age	Free T_4 (ng/dL)	T_4 (μg/dL)	Free T_3 (pg/dL)	T_3 (ng/dL)	TSH (mLU/L)
Cord blood	0.9-2.2	7.4-13.0		15-75	1.0-17.4
1-4 d	2.2-5.3	14.0-28.4	180-760	100-740	1.0-39.0
2-20 wk	0.9-2.3	7.2-15.7	185-770	105-245	1.7-9.1
5-24 mo	0.8-1.8	7.2-15.7	215-720	105-269	0.8-8.2
2-7 y	1.0-2.1	6.0-14.2	215-700	94-241	0.7-5.7
8-20 y	0.8-1.9	4.7-12.4	230-650	80-210	0.7-5.7
21-45 y	0.9-2.5	5.3-10.5	210-440	70-204	0.4-4.2

Modified from DeBoer MD, Lafranchi SH. Pediatric thyroid testing issues. Pediatr Endocrinol Rev. 2007;5(1):570-577.

Thyroid Sonography

Sonography of the thyroid is a noninvasive tool which can accurately quantify thyroid size. In the hands of an experienced user, it is also an ideal modality to confirm the presence of thyroid nodules and, when appropriate, to monitor the size of thyroid nodules over time. Sonography is also critically helpful to guide the fine needle aspiration of the thyroid, optimizing both diagnostic accuracy and patient safety.

Thyroid Scintigraphy

Images may be obtained with a pinhole gamma camera after oral I-123 administration to define the location of functional thyroid tissue. This can identify sites of ectopic thyroid tissue or determine the functional status of thyroid nodules (Figure 4-5). Thyroid scintigraphy can also be used to detect avid metastases in patients with differentiated thyroid cancers of follicular cell origin. Like RAIU testing, thyroid scintigraphy is affected by dietary iodine intake and high pharmacologic doses of iodine (from sources such as iodinated computed tomography [CT] contrast) can compromise I-123 imaging.

HYPOTHYROIDISM

Definitions and Epidemiology

Hypothyroidism is defined as thyroid insufficiency. It is the most common thyroid disorder, with an estimated population prevalence in childhood of 0.14% and a female to male ratio of 3:1.[3] Autoimmune thyroiditis is the most common etiology.

Pathogenesis

Hypothyroidism can arise from secretory defects at any level of the hypothalamic-pituitary-thyroid axis (central or primary hypothyroidism), from decreased tissue responsiveness (resistance to thyroid hormone [RTH]), or from the accelerated degradation of circulating thyroid hormone at rates which exceed the synthetic capacity of the normal thyroid gland (consumptive hypothyroidism).

Clinical Presentation and Diagnosis

Common signs and symptoms of hypothyroidism are listed in Table 4-3. Of note, *none is completely specific or sensitive for hypothyroidism,* and symptom severity can vary greatly between patients with similar degrees of biochemical derangement. The clinician's history should include inquiry into energy level, sleep pattern, cold intolerance, and weight gain. In addition to thyroid palpation,

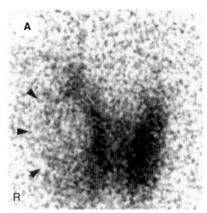

Anterior view
Right-sided cold nodule

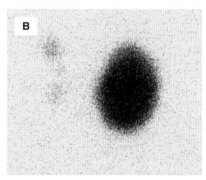

Anterior view
Left-sided hot "toxic" nodule

FIGURE 4-5 ■ Thyroid scintigraphy of cold versus hot nodules. Anterior views of two different patients with thyroid nodules are shown. Panel A shows a photopenic defect (marked by arrow-heads) in a euthyroid patient with a right-sided thyroid nodule, demonstrating that the nodule is hypofunctioning or "cold." Panel B shows focal I-123 uptake into the large left-sided nodule of a hyperthyroid patient, demonstrating that the nodule is hyperfunctioning or "hot." (Reproduced with modifications from: Huang SA. Thyroid. In: Treves ST, ed. *Pediatric Nuclear Medicine/PET,* 3rd ed. New York, NY: Springer; 2007:57-73, with kind permission of Springer Science and Business Media.)

Table 4-3.

Signs and Symptoms of Hypothyroidism

Goiter
Growth retardation
Delayed skeletal maturation
Abnormal pubertal (delay or pseudoprecocity)
Slowed mentation
Fatigue
Bradycardia (decreased cardiac output)
Constipation
Cold intolerance
Hypothermia
Fluid retention and weight gain (impaired renal free water clearance)
Dry, sallow skin
Delayed deep tendon reflexes

the physical examination should include an assessment of fluid status, muscle strength, heart rate, and deep tendon reflexes. Because autoimmune hypothyroidism can be the first presentation of an autoimmune polyglandular syndrome (see Chapter 5), symptoms of coexisting autoimmune disorders such as diabetes mellitus and Addison disease should be directly questioned.

Longstanding hypothyroidism causes growth retardation which disproportionately impairs linear progression more than weight gain. Prolonged hyperthyrotropinemia from untreated primary hypothyroidism can also cause pseudopubertal changes such as testicular enlargement and premature breast development due to cross-reactivity of TSH with the follicular stimulating hormone receptor. These changes may be distinguished from true puberty by the absence of growth acceleration and advanced skeletal maturation.

Algorithm

Serum thyroid tests are a sensitive screen to diagnose hypothyroidism and sufficient to identify the common subtypes (Table 4-1). Growth data and the review of systems can provide insight into the duration of thyroid insufficiency.

Diagnostic Tests

Serum TSH and free T_4 should be measured when hypothyroidism is suspected (Table 4-1). Serum TSH is elevated in all patients with primary hypothyroidism and, in more severe cases, serum free T_4 is low. If serum free T_4 is low with an inappropriately normal or low serum TSH, central hypothyroidism should be considered. Conversely, if serum TSH and serum free T_4 are both persistently high, the diagnosis of thyroid hormone resistance should be investigated. Due to compensatory increases in thyroidal T_3 secretion and peripheral T_4 to T_3 conversion, serum T_3 remains normal in many hypothyroid patients and its measurement is not a helpful diagnostic test.

Differential Diagnosis

This section will review the major causes of hypothyroidism in children. While identifying the specific cause of a child's hypothyroidism rarely changes initial therapy, the information is still useful to predict the patient's long-term course and to counsel parents appropriately.

Primary Hypothyroidism

The term primary hypothyroidism refers to disorders of the thyroid gland itself which reduce its production of T_4 and T_3. As serum T_4 and T_3 fall, loss of inhibitory feedback results in TSH hypersecretion. Elevation of serum TSH is the first abnormality detected in primary hypothyroidism. As the severity of primary hypothyroidism progresses, serum T_4 and then serum T_3 fall below normal range.

Autoimmune hypothyroidism

Autoimmunity is the most common cause of acquired hypothyroidism in both children and adults (Figures 4-6 and 4-7). Two forms of chronic autoimmune thyroiditis are associated with persistent hypothyroidism, type 2A (goitrous, classic Hashimoto disease) and type 2B (nongoitrous, atrophic thyroiditis). Both are characterized by lymphocytic infiltration of the thyroid parenchyma, destruction of follicular thyroid cells, and high serum concentrations of antithyroid autoantibodies. Documenting high serum titers of either anti-thyroid peroxidase antibodies or antithyroglobulin antibodies is sufficient to diagnose chronic autoimmune thyroiditis as the cause of a patient's hypothyroidism. Antithyroid peroxidase antibodies are the more sensitive test and should be measured first, but antithyroglobulin antibodies may be added if antithyroid peroxidase antibodies are not elevated. The combined sensitivity of both tests is approximately 95%.

The prevalence of autoimmune hypothyroidism increases with age, with a 3:1 female to male ratio.[3] Presentation under 3 years of age is rare, but cases have

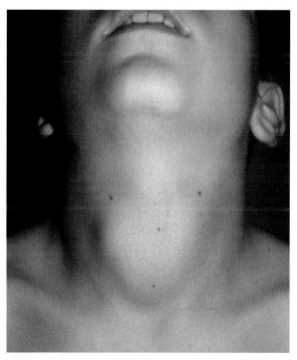

FIGURE 4-6 ■ Thyroid gland enlargement in a 10-year-old girl with documented autoimmune (Hashimoto) thyroiditis and hypothyroidism. Her initial TSH was >1000 mU/L.

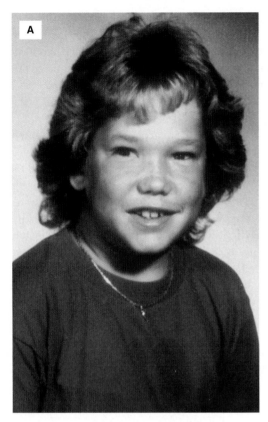

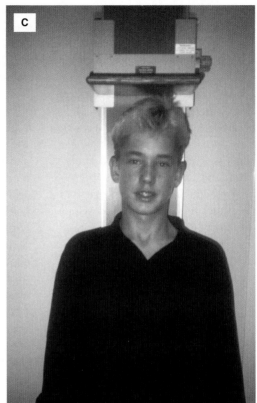

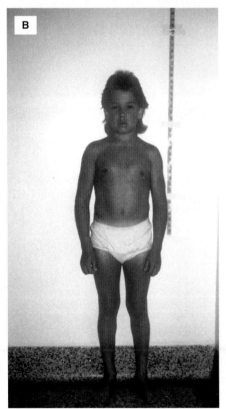

FIGURE 4-7 ▪ **(A)** A 14-year-old juvenile-appearing boy with long-standing autoimmune hypothyroidism. He was as tall as the average 8.5-year-old and had a skeletal maturation of 7.5 years. **(B)** The boy's general physically immature appearance. The fifth percentile of height for age is shown as the black line above his head. **(C)** The boy's appearance after 3.5 years of replacement thyroid hormone treatment. The stadiometer is set at the fifth percentile of height for age. Note that before leuprolide treatment was available, many children with long-standing hypothyroidism would undergo rapid pubertal development and skeletal maturation once started on treatment and would fail to reach "expected" adult height, as was the case in this child.

been described even in infancy. While the pathophysiology of thyroid autoimmunity is incompletely understood, there is a strong familial component. Individuals with Down syndrome, Klinefelter syndrome, and Turner syndrome are at increased risk.[4]

Upon diagnosis, families should be counseled that autoimmune hypothyroidism is usually lifelong but that replacement therapy is effective. On levothyroxine treatment, children should be followed carefully to ensure consistent euthyroidism. Because autoimmune thyroiditis may be the initial presentation of an autoimmune polyglandular syndrome (see Chapter 5), the review of systems should include direct inquiry into symptoms concerning for other autoimmune endocrinopathies such as Type 1 diabetes and Addison disease.

Congenital hypothyroidism

One in every 3000 to 4000 children is born with permanent hypothyroidism. Approximately 85% of these cases are sporadic and due to thyroid dysgenesis (abnormalities in the anatomic development of the thyroid gland such as agenesis, hypoplasia, and ectopy). Another 10% are due to dyshormonogenesis (inborn defects in thyroid hormone synthesis which are often inherited in an autosomal recessive pattern). A small percentage of congenital hypothyroidism is due to central hypothyroidism. Rarely, transient hypothyroidism occurs in the newborn period secondary to the transplacental passage of maternal medications or antithyroid autoantibodies.

Optimal levels of thyroid hormone are required for normal neurodevelopment and the brain is especially vulnerable to hypothyroidism in the first year of life. Untreated congenital hypothyroidism can produce profound somatic and neurologic injury (Figures 4-8 and 4-9), and treatment delay of congenital hypothyroidism remains one of the most common preventable causes of mental retardation in the world. Despite this, outcome is excellent when adequate replacement is initiated early in the newborn period, ideally within the first 2 weeks of life. Normal development, including cognitive outcome, is observed even in children with complete thyroid agenesis, illustrating the protective effects of maternal thyroid hormone to the fetus *in utero*.

Because even severe hypothyroidism is typically clinically silent in infants, newborn blood screening is universally recommended. Screening specimens should be obtained in all newborns prior to discharge from the hospital, ideally between 2 and 4 days of age to avoid the TSH elevation associated with the normal neonatal TSH surge.[5] Infants with high TSH and low T_4 should be considered to have congenital hypothyroidism until proven otherwise. Such screening results warrant immediate medical attention and the initiation of high-dose levothyroxine (10-15 μg/kg/day) to normalize thyroid status as soon as possible. Abnormal newborn screening results

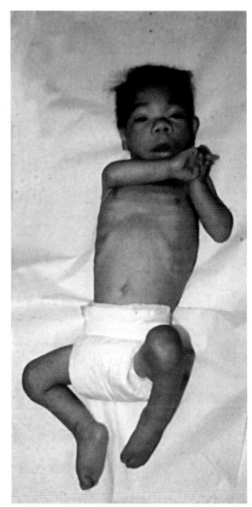

FIGURE 4-8 ■ A 17-year-old female with untreated congenital hypothyroidism. The patient is the average height of a 3-year-old and her estimated bone age is 9 months. *(From Brent G, Davies T, Larsen P. Hypothyroidism and thyroiditis. In: Kronenberg HM, Melmed S, Larsen PR, Polonsky KS, eds. Williams Textbook of Endocrinology, 11th ed. Philadelphia, PA: Saunders/Elsevier; 2007.)*

should be confirmed by the formal measurement of TSH and free T_4 in serum drawn prior to starting levothyroxine. Because factors such as prematurity, neonatal illness, and the transplacental transfer of maternal TSH-receptor blocking autoantibodies can delay TSH elevation, serum thyroid tests should be drawn in infants who develop clinical symptoms of hypothyroidism, even if their newborn screening was normal.

Radiographic studies such as neck sonography and radionuclide scintigraphy may be performed to characterize the subtype of an individual child's congenital hypothyroidism but, since these findings rarely alter acute management, they can be considered optional. Expert consensus guidelines for the therapy of congenital hypothyroidism are available (www.aap.org).[5] The goals of therapy are to normalize serum TSH and to maintain serum free T_4 in the upper half of normal range. Serum

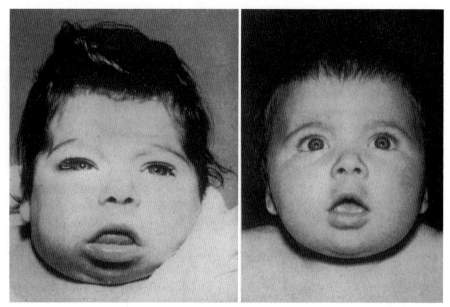

FIGURE 4-9 ■ A 1-year-old child with undiagnosed/untreated congenital hypothyroidism who was born before national screening programs for this condition. She was treated with replacement thyroid hormone, and 6 months later had a more normal facial appearance but significant developmental delays due to delay in diagnosis and treatment.

thyroid tests should be measured 2 to 4 weeks after treatment is begun, every 1 to 2 months in the first 6 months of life, every 3 to 4 months between 6 months and 3 years of age, and regularly thereafter. Parents should be counseled that neurologic outcome will be normal with early and consistent treatment. A trial off levothyroxine therapy may be offered after 3 years of age to assess the possibility that congenital hypothyroidism was transient.

Naturally occurring mutations in several of the genes that are important in thyroid hormone synthesis (including those that encode thyroperoxidase, thyroglobulin, thyroid oxidase 2, iodotyrosine deiodinase, and the sodium-iodine symporter) have been found to cause congenital hypothyroidism.[6] Because such kindreds represent a very small minority of patients with congenital hypothyroidism, the relevance of these findings to genetic testing and counseling is limited, but these examples have provided important insight into our understanding of thyroid hormone synthesis. Interestingly, milder mutations in several of these genes can result in less severe enzymatic deficiency and present not as congenital hypothyroidism but instead as acquired hypothyroidism or euthyroid goiter in later childhood or adolescence.

Other forms of acquired primary hypothyroidism

Incomplete descent of the thyroid gland (sublingual thyroid—Figure 4-10) or complete lack of descent of the gland (lingual thyroid—Figure 4-11) may lead to

hypothyroidism in the first decade of life, due, in part, to anatomical "entrapment" of the gland that makes it unable to keep up with the need for thyroid hormone as the child grows.

Primary hypothyroidism can develop after exposure to environmental goitrogens such as resorcinol or to medications with antithyroid effect such as lithium, iodine, amniodarone, and the thionamide derivatives

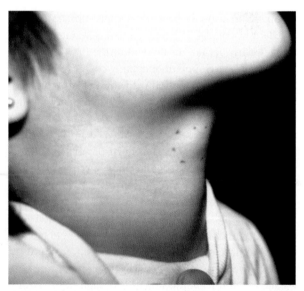

FIGURE 4-10 ■ An 8-year-old hypothyroid girl with a sublingual thyroid outlined.

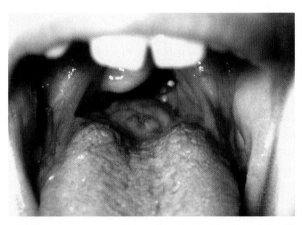

FIGURE 4-11 ■ A 9-year-old hypothyroid girl with a lingual thyroid, visible as a "goiter" at the base of the tongue.

used to treat hyperthyroidism. Hypothyroidism can also occur as a consequence of thyroid surgery or thyroid irradiation, including both I-131 radioiodine ablation and the external-beam radiation used to treat Hodgkin disease and other pediatric cancers.

Hypothyroidism may also develop in some patients after painful subacute thyroiditis or painless sporadic thyroiditis (see the "Thyrotoxicosis" section later in this chapter). This possibility should be considered in hypothyroid patients with normal serum antithyroid autoantibody titers, especially if there are recent symptoms of thyroid pain or transient thyrotoxicosis. While hypothyroidism is usually transient in these cases, levothyroxine may be offered if symptoms are significant and a trial off levothyroxine performed later.[7]

Central Hypothyroidism

Central hypothyroidism refers to disorders which decrease the production or biologic activity of TRH or TSH. In these diseases, serum free T_4 is low and serum TSH is usually inappropriately normal or low (Table 4-1). While provocative testing with TRH was used as a diagnostic tool in the past, unstimulated serum thyroid tests are now accepted as sufficient to diagnose central hypothyroidism. It is important to recognize that the pattern of serum tests seen in central hypothyroidism is also present transiently in preterm infants and also in older children during nonthyroidal illness, so serologies must be interpreted with caution in these settings. Because central hypothyroidism often occurs in combination with other pituitary endocrinopathies, its diagnosis warrants pituitary imaging and biochemical assessment for other hormone deficiencies.

Central hypothyroidism occurs congenitally in about 1 in 50,000 newborns. Congenital central hypothyroidism can occur in isolation, for example, due to mutations in the TRH or TSH genes, but it more commonly occurs in combination with other pituitary hormone deficiencies. The presence of hypoglycemia, microphallus, polyuria, visual abnormalities, or midline anatomic abnormalities in a newborn should raise the suspicion of panhypopituitarism.[5]

More often, central hypothyroidism is acquired. Pituitary adenomas or craniopharyngiomas (as well as the surgery and radiation therapy used to treat pituitary adenomas or craniopharyngiomas) are common causes, but central hypothyroidism can also occur in association with other brain tumors, Langerhans-cell histiocytosis, and sarcoidosis.[7]

Resistance to Thyroid Hormone

Resistance to thyroid hormone (RTH) is a tissue-specific syndrome of decreased thyroid hormone responsiveness due to genetic defects in the thyroid hormone receptor. Approximately 600 cases have been reported and virtually all are due to autosomal dominant mutations in the TRβ gene.[8] Affected individuals have high serum concentrations of T_4 and T_3 with inappropriately normal or even high serum TSH concentrations (Table 4-1). This pattern indicates defective feedback inhibition of the hypothalamic-pituitary-thyroid axis and is presumably due to impaired pituitary responsiveness to thyroid hormone. Despite these high circulating levels of thyroid hormone, tissues which express the mutant TRβ gene are functionally hypothyroid. Interestingly, because TRβ is expressed in a limited number of tissues, affected individuals can manifest signs and symptoms of hypothyroidism (such as growth delay and hearing impairment) and hyperthyroidism (such as tachycardia and anxiety) simultaneously.

For reasons that are not understood, thyroid status and symptoms vary greatly between affected individuals, even amongst those who carry exactly the same TRβ mutation. Patients may appear clinically hypothyroid, euthyroid, or hyperthyroid. Symptoms often change with time and may improve spontaneously with age. Therapies directed to the symptoms of RTH (such as β-blockers for palpitations and anxiolytics for nervousness) can be helpful but treatments to directly alter thyroid status are generally avoided. The high levels of circulating thyroid hormone in patients with RTH are considered to be an adaptive response to their tissue resistance, so antithyroid medications are contraindicated. Treatment with exogenous thyroid hormone may be considered in young children with RTH for the relative indications of seizure; developmental delay; extreme hyperthyrotropinemia; failure to thrive that cannot be explained on the basis of another illness or defect; and a history of growth or mental retardation in affected siblings.[8] For such patients, levothyroxine is typically used and the dose titrated to the normalization of serum TSH. The benefit of this intervention is unclear.

When considering the diagnosis of RTH, one must recognize that the pattern of serum thyroid tests (simultaneously high serum free T_4 and TSH), often referred to as inappropriate TSH secretion, is also characteristic of TSH-secreting pituitary adenomas (Table 4-1). This pattern can also be observed transiently in patients without thyroid disease during nonthyroidal illness or while taking certain medications such as amiodarone. It may also be due to laboratory artifact. Because both RTH and TSH-secreting pituitary adenomas are extremely rare, the discovery of suspicious thyroid function tests should be addressed first by a complete medication history and by repeating thyroid serologies 1 to 2 weeks later. If the pattern resolves, it was most likely due to nonthyroidal illness. If the pattern persists, an aliquot of the same serum should be assessed for possible artifact by repeating thyroid function tests on an alternate assay platform (from another institution) and by performing serial dilutions to confirm linearity. These simple maneuvers are important to avoid inappropriate testing and treatment.

Once the serum pattern of inappropriate TSH secretion is confirmed and shown to be persistent, the diagnostic evaluation should focus on distinguishing RTH from a TSH-secreting pituitary adenoma. This is critical because therapy is dramatically different for these two conditions. Obtaining thyroid function tests in the patient's first degree relatives is a good screen as documentation of the same pattern in other family members strongly supports the diagnosis of RTH. While a number of specialized biochemical tests such as TRH stimulation testing and measurement of the TSH alpha subunit can be considered to help distinguish RTH from TSH-secreting adenomas, pituitary imaging with MRI is usually required and is reasonable to do as a first-line test.

Consumptive Hypothyroidism

Consumptive hypothyroidism is a rare condition caused by the accelerated degradation of circulating thyroid hormones. Several tumors, including infantile hemangiomas, express high levels of the thyroid hormone-inactivating enzyme D3 and, in individuals with both high specific D3 activity and large tumor burden, systemic hypothyroidism can develop due to the rapid degradation of circulating T_4 and T_3 at rates that exceed the synthetic capacity of the normal thyroid. Unlike other forms of hypothyroidism, thyroid gland function is normal to increased. The index case of consumptive hypothyroidism was a 3-month-old infant with massive hepatic hemangiomas, but other D3-expressing tumor types including hemangioendotheliomas and solitary malignant fibrous tumors can also cause hypothyroidism, even in adults. Because hemangiomas proliferate during the first year of life when the brain is critically dependent upon thyroid hormone, infants with large hemangiomas should be screened for thyroid dysfunction with monthly serum TSH measurements until 1 year of age. Outside of infantile hemangiomas, acquired hypothyroidism in a patient with a large tumor should also raise the suspicion of consumptive hypothyroidism.

Standard thyroid function tests are identical to those seen in patients with primary hypothyroidism (Table 4-1), but evidence of increased thyroid hormone inactivation (such as serum rT_3 elevation or supernormal requirements for thyroid hormone) and increased thyroid hormone production (goiter, high RAIU, serum thyroglobulin elevation) will also be present. Severity of hypothyroidism is variable, with some patients responding adequately to conventional doses of levothyroxine and others requiring massive doses. Due to the shortened half-life of circulating thyroid hormone, frequent monitoring is required and daily doses may be divided bid or tid to minimize excursions in serum T_4. In some patients, the reduction of serum T_3 is disproportionately greater than the fall in serum T_4, presumably due to the differences in D3's substrate affinities. In such cases, if serum TSH remains elevated despite a high-normal serum T_4, liothyronine (T_3) can be administered in combination with levothyroxine therapy. Communication between caregivers is critical as thyroid hormone therapy must be adjusted in response to changes in tumor mass. Tumor proliferation warrants more frequent monitoring for the possibility of increased requirements. Conversely, clinicians must be prepared to taper or discontinue thyroid hormone therapy upon tumor involution or resection to avoid iatrogenic thyrotoxicosis.

Treatment

Levothyroxine (L-T_4) is the ideal therapy for hypothyroidism. While reactions to manufacturer-specific tablet binders or dyes may occur, the medication itself is universally tolerated and its long serum half-life of 5 to 7 days permits the convenience of once daily dosing. While pseudotumor cerebri has been reported in a small number of school age children upon the initiation of levothyroxine therapy, this complication is rare and resolves with temporary dose reduction.

Age-specific guidelines exist for the initiation of levothyroxine in children (Table 4-4).[9] While on therapy, serum thyroid tests should be obtained every 3 to 6 months in growing children and also 6 to 8 weeks after any dose adjustment. Because thyroid hormone is critically important to infant neurodevelopment, more frequent monitoring is recommended in the first year of life.[5] In patients with primary hypothyroidism, therapy should be adjusted to a serum TSH in the middle of the normal range (0.5-3.0 µU/mL). Patients with central hypothyroidism should be dosed to achieve a serum free T_4 concentration within the upper half of normal range.[10] To maximize intestinal absorption, it is generally recommended that levothyroxine be administered 30 to

Table 4-4.	
Recommended Doses of Levothyroxine, Based on Body Weight	

Recommended L-T$_4$ Treatment Doses	
Age	L-T$_4$ Dose (mcg/kg)
0-3 mo	10-15
3-6 mo	8-10
6-12 mo	6-8
1-3 y	4-6
3 to 10 y	3-4
10-15 y	2-4
>15 y	2-3
Adult	1.6

Modified from Lafranchi S. Thyroiditis and acquired hypothyroidism. Pediatric Ann. 1992;21(1):29, 32-39.

60 minutes prior to food or other medications but, from a practical standpoint, it is more important that it be given the same way every day. Parents should be counseled that consistent medication compliance is important but, should 1 day's dose be inadvertently missed, they should double their dose on the following day to compensate.

As described earlier in this chapter's "Thyroid Hormone Metabolism" section, the normal thyroid primarily secretes T$_4$ and the vast majority of circulating T$_3$ is derived from the peripheral conversion of T$_4$ into T$_3$ by outer-ring deiodination (Figure 4 3). This explains why serum T$_3$ is normal with adequate levothyroxine monotherapy for primary or central hypothyroidism.[10] While one recent study of hypothyroid adults reported improved mood and cognitive function with a combined levothyroxine/liothyronine regimen compared to levothyroxine alone, subsequent studies have failed to confirm this finding or show other benefit and levothyroxine monotherapy remains the preferred treatment for children with primary or central hypothyroidism. Combined therapy with supernormal doses of both levothyroxine and liothyronine has been used specifically to treat infants with severe consumptive hypothyroidism, where the peripheral metabolism of thyroid hormone is by definition deranged.

Several common conditions can alter a patient's levothyroxine requirements. Oral iron supplements, calcium carbonate, sucralfate, or even soy-based infant formula can bind intestinal levothyroxine and reduce its absorption. Other drugs such as phenytoin, carbamazepine, and rifampin can increase levothyroxine requirements by enhancing its hepatic metabolism. Even normal pregnancy increases thyroid hormone

requirements by an average of 47%.[11] Because this increase typically occurs in early pregnancy, adequately treated hypothyroid females can be counseled to increase their prepregnancy levothyroxine dose by 29% (by taking extra two extra daily doses each week) if pregnancy is discovered and access to full serum testing will not be immediate.[10,11]

THYROTOXICOSIS

Definitions and Epidemiology

The yearly incidence of childhood hyperthyroidism is cited to range from 1 to 8 per 100,000 children.[12] In adolescence, there is a high female to male ratio of over 6:1 and Graves disease is the most common etiology.[13] While the terms of thyrotoxicosis and hyperthyroidism are often used interchangeably, they are not synonyms. Thyrotoxicosis is a general term that refers to any condition that elevates circulating thyroid hormones while hyperthyroidism refers only to the subset of thyrotoxic disorders that are due to increased function of the thyroid gland itself. This distinction is clinically important because the antithyroid therapies used to treat hyperthyroidism have no role in the management of thyrotoxicosis without hyperthyroidism.

Pathogenesis

Etiologies of thyrotoxicosis can be divided into those which are caused by hyperthyroidism (thyroid gland hyperfunction) and those which are not (Table 4-5). Hyperthyroidism can result from the excessive stimulation of normal thyroid tissue (Graves disease, TSH-secreting pituitary adenomas) or from the presence of abnormal thyroid tissue which is intrinsically hyperfunctioning or "autonomous" (toxic thyroid nodules). In addition, thyrotoxicosis *without* hyperthyroidism can

Table 4-5.

Causes of Thyrotoxicosis

	Thyroid RAIU	Examples
Hyperthyroidism	High	Graves Disease
		Toxic thyroid nodules
		TSH-secreting pituitary adenoma
Thyrotoxicosis without hyperthyroidism	Low	Transient thyroiditis
		Painless sporadic thyroiditis
		Painful subacute thyroiditis
		Thyrotoxicosis factitia

result from glandular injuries which release excessive amounts of preformed hormone (transient thyroiditis) or from the over-administration of exogenous thyroid hormone (thyrotoxicosis factitia).

Clinical Presentation and Diagnosis

Common signs and symptoms of thyrotoxicosis are described in Table 4-6. The clinical history should include inquiry into energy level, sleep pattern, heat intolerance, weight loss, decreased school performance, skin changes, visual complaint, and the acceleration of linear growth. In addition to thyroid palpation, the physical examination should include careful assessment of heart rate, extraocular movements, skin, and whether a tremor is present. Because autoimmune hyperthyroidism

can be the presenting component of an autoimmune polyglandular syndrome (see Chapter 5), symptoms of potential coexisting autoimmune disorders such as diabetes mellitus or Addison disease should be directly questioned in the history.

Serum thyroid function tests are a sensitive screen to confirm (or refute) the presence of thyrotoxicosis (Table 4-1). A focused history and physical examination will usually identify the cause, but adjunctive testing with I-123 can be helpful in selected cases.

Algorithm

Serum TSH and free T_4 should be measured if thyrotoxicosis is suspected. In patients with normal hypothalamic-pituitary feedback, serum TSH will suppress to less than 0.1 μU/mL during thyrotoxicosis. If serum TSH is less than 0.1 μU/mL and serum free T_4 is high, significant thyrotoxicosis is present and the diagnostic evaluation should then focus on determining the cause. Because the normal thyroid gland contains a finite amount of preformed hormone (about a 30-60 day supply), thyrotoxicosis from transient thyroiditis is short-lived and the duration of a patient's thyrotoxicosis is an important diagnostic clue to its cause (Figure 4-12).

If signs and symptoms of thyrotoxicosis have been present for more than 8 weeks, hyperthyroidism is likely. If a diffuse goiter is noted with orbitopathy or dermopathy, Graves disease can be diagnosed clinically and no further tests are required. If instead the examiner palpates a large thyroid nodule, the possibility of a toxic adenoma should be considered and I-123 thyroid scintigraphy should be performed to address this (Figure 4-5).

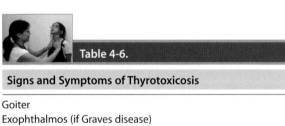

Table 4-6.

Signs and Symptoms of Thyrotoxicosis

Goiter
Exophthalmos (if Graves disease)
Acceleration of linear growth
Nervousness
Irritability
Decreased school performance
Palpitations/tachycardia
Increased pulse pressure
Polyphagia
Weight loss
Heat intolerance
Tremor

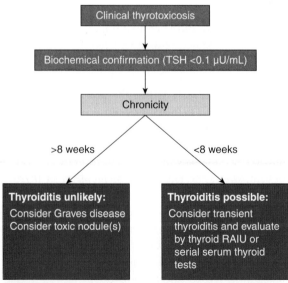

FIGURE 4-12 ■ Suggested algorithm for the evaluation of thyrotoxicosis.

If sign and symptoms of thyrotoxicosis have been present for less than 8 weeks, the possibility of transient thyroiditis should be addressed before offering antithyroid therapy, especially if thyromegaly is subtle. In patients with negligible symptoms, serum thyroid tests may be followed monthly without therapy with the reasoning that thyrotoxicosis which resolves spontaneously over the subsequent 2 months can be attributed to painless thyroiditis. In patients with more significant biochemical derangement or bothersome clinical symptoms, thyroid RAIU should be measured and antithyroid therapy offered if it is elevated (Figure 4-12).

Rarely, serum thyroid tests reveal the unusual pattern of high free T_4 with a simultaneously normal or high TSH (Table 4-1). When this pattern of inappropriate TSH secretion is persistent, the rare disorders of TSH-secreting pituitary adenomas and RTH should be evaluated. As described earlier in this chapter's "Resistance to Thyroid Hormone" section, preanalytic factors and laboratory artifact must be ruled out as the cause of abnormal serum testing to avoid unnecessary tests and the risk of inappropriate therapy.

Diagnostic Tests

Measuring serum TSH and free T_4 is an adequate screen for thyrotoxicosis. Serum free T_3 (or a free T_3 index) should be added only if serum TSH is low and free T_4 is normal. Thyroid palpation should focus on thyroid size and whether there is a discrete nodule.

While a focused history and physical examination will accurately diagnose the cause of thyrotoxicosis in most patients, measurement of thyroid RAIU can be helpful to distinguish early Graves disease from painless sporadic thyroiditis in those rare patients who present without prolonged symptoms or obvious thyromegaly. Documenting high serum titers of thyrotropin-receptor autoantibodies can also be used to support the diagnosis of Graves disease, but this is rarely necessary in clinical care.

Differential Diagnosis

This section reviews the major causes of thyrotoxicosis in children. Unlike hypothyroidism, where knowing the specific cause of a patient's hypothyroidism rarely affects treatment, optimal management of thyrotoxicosis requires the accurate identification of its etiology.

Graves disease

Graves disease is a form of autoimmune thyroiditis caused by the production of autoantibodies which bind and stimulate the thyrotropin receptor and lead to thyroid gland hyperfunction (Figure 4-13). Like other forms of autoimmune thyroiditis, lymphocytes infiltrate the thyroid parenchyma and circulating antithyroid

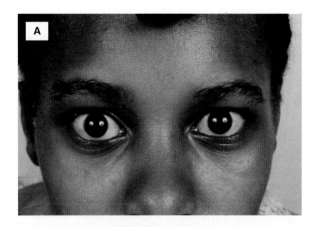

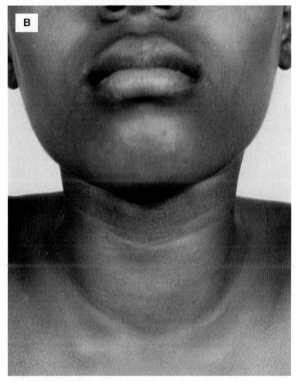

FIGURE 4-13 ■ A 14-year-old girl with Graves disease ophthalmopathy **(A)** and goiter **(B)**.

autoantibodies (including antithyroid peroxidase, antithyroglobulin, and antithyrotropin receptor antibodies) are often detectable. In addition to hyperthyroidism, the classic clinical triad of Graves disease also includes orbitopathy and dermopathy. These extrathyroidal manifestations, caused by lymphocytic infiltration and glycosaminoglycan accumulation in the periorbital tissues and skin, are less common in children than adults.

Controversy exists amongst experts regarding the optimal therapy for childhood Graves disease.[14,15] As in adults, a significant minority of affected children (about 30%) experience remission of their hyperthyroidism after several years of treatment with antithyroid medication. While several studies have associated young age and more severe hyperthyroidism with lower rates of remission, it is not currently possible to reliably predict the likelihood of remission in individual patients.[16] Because of this unpredictability and also concerns related to the risks of definitive therapy in children, most pediatric centers offer antithyroid medication as first-line therapy.

Of note, all standard treatments for Graves hyperthyroidism (see the "Definitive Therapy" section later in this chapter) are directed against the thyroid gland and not to the autoimmune cause of Graves disease itself. Accordingly, extrathyroidal features such as orbitopathy and dermopathy may persist or even progress despite the successful treatment of hyperthyroidism.

Rarely, Graves hyperthyroidism can occur in the fetal or neonatal period due to the transplacental passage of maternal stimulating TSH-receptor autoantibodies (Figure 4-14). Women with a history of Graves hyperthyroidism who have undergone definitive therapy or who have a history of a prior affected offspring should have maternal TSH-receptor autoantibody titers measured in the second trimester and, if these are elevated, an endocrinologist should be consulted to collab-

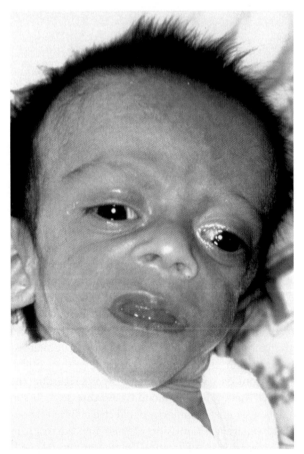

FIGURE 4-14 ■ A newborn with congenital (transplacentally acquired) Graves disease.

orate with obstetrics and monitor thyroid status through gestation. In high risk mothers, serum thyroid tests should be performed on cord blood upon birth and then measured monthly in the offspring until 3 months of age. An extra set of thyroid function tests should be drawn at 7 days of life if the infant's mother received antithyroid medications during the third trimester of pregnancy.

Toxic thyroid nodules

A small minority of thyroid nodules (<5%-10%) are "autonomous" in that they produce thyroid hormone even in the absence of TSH. Autonomous nodules are as a rule benign, but treatment may be required if they grow large enough to cause hyperthyroidism. In this setting, autonomous nodules are also referred to as hyperfunctional, "toxic," or "hot." The presence of a thyroid nodule in a hyperthyroid patient should raise the suspicion of a toxic nodule. The diagnosis of autonomy requires confirmation by thyroid scintigraphy performed when serum TSH is low (<0.1 µU/mL) and documentation of I-123 uptake into the nodule (Figure 4-5) despite the absence of serum TSH. Autonomous nodules must be large, about 2 to 3 cm in diameter, to cause hyperthyroidism so scintigraphy should be reserved for patients with palpable abnormalities.

Because hyperthyroidism from toxic nodules rarely remits, definitive therapy with either I-131 radioiodine ablation or surgical lobectomy is the standard initial treatment in adults. I-131 therapy should not however be used in children with toxic nodules because it delivers a subcytotoxic radiation dose to the rim of normal thyroid parenchyma surrounding the nodule and this increases thyroid cancer risk in the very young. Surgical resection may be considered instead, or antithyroid medications may be used until the patient becomes an adult and I-131 therapy can be offered.

Transient thyroiditis

Various forms of thyroiditis can cause transient thyrotoxicosis due to the release of preformed hormone from the gland. As discussed earlier, because the normal thyroid contains a finite amount of preformed hormone, these forms of thyrotoxicosis are self-limited and generally last less than 8 weeks. Both painless sporadic thyroiditis and painful subacute thyroiditis can cause transient thyrotoxicosis. These types of thyroiditis should be distinguished from acute suppurative thyroiditis, which typically presents with symptoms of infection and a painful thyroid mass, rather than with thyroid dysfunction.[17]

Mild thyromegaly is present in about half of patients with painless sporadic thyroiditis and care must be taken to avoid misdiagnosing Graves disease. Measurement of thyroid RAIU can be helpful, as it is low in painless sporadic thyroiditis and high in Graves hyperthyroidism (Table 4-5). No therapy is required for thyroiditis-associated transient thyrotoxicosis, other than the provision of reassurance and the potential treatment of symptoms such as tachycardia and thyroid pain with β-blockers and nonsteroidal anti-inflammatory drugs respectively. Some patients develop hypothyroidism after the thyrotoxic phase of transient thyroiditis. This hypothyroidism is generally transient, but a short course of levothyroxine replacement can be offered if symptoms are significant.

Thyrotoxicosis factitia

Thyrotoxicosis can occur in patients who take large doses of exogenous thyroid hormone, either intentionally or by accident. A careful history is usually sufficient to diagnose this. On physical examination, the thyroid will be normal or decreased in size. Because endogenous thyroid function is suppressed, serum thyroglobulin and thyroid RAIU will be low, rather than high as in hyperthyroid patients (Table 4-5).

TSH-secreting pituitary adenoma

TSH-secreting pituitary adenomas are an extremely rare cause of hyperthyroidism. The characteristic pattern of serum thyroid tests is a high free T_4 with an inappropriately normal or high TSH (Table 4-1). As discussed earlier in this chapter in "Resistance to Thyroid Hormone" section, it is important to rule out medication use and laboratory artifact as the explanation for this pattern. Pituitary imaging is helpful to distinguish TSH-secreting pituitary adenomas from RTH. The therapy of patients with TSH-secreting pituitary adenomas is to decrease TSH secretion, either by surgical removal of the adenoma or medical suppression of thyrotropin secretion with dopaminergic agonists or somatostatin analogs.

Subclinical hyperthyroidism

A subset of hyperthyroid patients present with mild serum TSH suppression and normal serum concentrations of free T_4 and free T_3. When persistent, this pattern is termed subclinical hyperthyroidism and it reflects a state of mild thyroid hormone excess. Patients are generally asymptomatic. While subclinical hyperthyroidism is associated with an increased risk of atrial fibrillation in the elderly, similar risks have not been identified in children.[18] Accordingly, it is reasonable to monitor children with subclinical hyperthyroidism without antithyroid therapy. This approach avoids the risks of antithyroid medication. In the absence of symptoms, serum thyroid tests may be obtained every 3 to 6 months, monitoring for both progression to overt hyperthyroidism (when therapy can be initiated) and the alternative possibility of spontaneous remission.

Treatment

As described earlier, the first critical step in the management of thyrotoxic patients is to determine whether or not hyperthyroidism is present, as antithyroid therapies have no benefit in its absence. Graves disease is the most common cause of hyperthyroidism and is therefore the focus of this section. Treatment can be divided into the two categories of antithyroid medication and definitive therapy. Debate exists amongst experts regarding the optimal treatment for childhood Graves disease.[14,15] Because all standard therapies are directed toward the patient's hyperthyroidism and not toward the autoimmune cause of Graves disease itself, physicians must be aware that extrathyroidal manifestations such as orbitopathy and dermopathy can persist or progress even after successful antithyroid treatment.

Antithyroid medications

The thionamide derivatives, Tapazole and propylthiouracil (PTU), are the mainstay of medical therapy. Both decrease thyroid hormone synthesis and, when used at high doses (over 400 mg/day), PTU has the additional benefit of decreasing T_4 to T_3 conversion. Tapazole's longer half-life usually permits the convenience of once daily maintenance dosing and, outside of early pregnancy (because in utero Tapazole exposure has been associated with the rare congenital defect of aplasia cutis), it is generally favored over PTU, This preference for Tapazole over PTU was strongly supported by two meetings this year where data from the Food and Drug Administration's Adverse Event Reporting System and the United Network for Organ Sharing indicated that the risk of life-threatening liver failure is categorically higher with PTU[19] and that this risk is disproportionately greater in children.[20] Based upon these data, the Endocrine Society has endorsed the recommendation that PTU no longer be used as first-line treatment for hyperthyroid children.

Because rare but potentially serious adverse reactions can occur with either thionamide derivative, risks must always be explained to parents and to referring physicians before starting antithyroid medications. Families should be provided written instructions to immediately discontinue antithyroid medication and page the treating physician if they develop signs or symptoms of neutropenia (fever greater than 101°F, sore throat, mouth lesions, other concerning symptoms of infection) or hepatitis (right upper quadrant pain, jaundice). Blood tests (a complete blood count with differential and/or liver function tests) should be obtained urgently in such cases to address the possibility of a life-threatening idiosyncratic reaction. This patient education and physician communication is especially important in pediatrics, where febrile illness is common and,

Table 4-7.	
Recommended Starting Doses of Tapazole for Adolescent Patients, Based on Severity of Hyperthyroidism	
Serum Free T$_4$	**Starting Tapazole Dose**
<1.5 × upper limit of normal	10 mg po qd
1.5-2.0 × upper limit of normal	10 mg po bid
>2.0 × upper limit of normal	20 mg po bid

due to the relative rarity of hyperthyroidism, primary care pediatricians are often unfamiliar with the risks of thionamide administration.

Despite the above, antithyroid medications are well tolerated in most children and play an important role as first line therapy at most pediatric centers. Weight-based guidelines have been recommended for the initiation of Tapazole in children (0.5-1.0 mg/kg/day). However, it is logical to consider the severity of hyperthyroidism and the author recommends the following rule of thumb for starting Tapazole in adolescents and young adults (Table 4-7). Graves hyperthyroidism alone can cause mild pancytopenia, so a baseline white blood cell count should be obtained prior to starting antithyroid medications.

In patients with severe hyperthyroidism, inorganic iodine can speed the fall in serum thyroid hormones and is a helpful adjunct to the thionamides. Saturated saluation of potassium iodide (SSKI), administered at the dose of 3 drops by mouth three times daily has a potent and rapid antithyroid effect. Clinicians must remember that patients can escape from SSKI's antithyroid effect after about 2 weeks, so it cannot be relied upon as chronic monotherapy. Furthermore, SSKI is contraindicated if radioiodine ablation is desired in the near future as even its brief administration will compromise thyroidal uptake of radioiodine for months.

Because the serum half-life of T$_4$ is long (5-7 days), biochemical correction takes time and patients should be counseled that symptoms generally take 3-4 weeks to improve. While on antithyroid medication, serum thyroid tests should be obtained every 3 months and also 3 weeks after any dose adjustment. After prolonged hyperthyroidism, serum TSH may remain suppressed for many months so serum free T$_4$ is the best initial test to guide therapy. Once serum free T$_4$ falls into the upper half of normal range, the starting dose of Tapazole should be reduced by one-half to one-third to avoid iatrogenic hypothyroidism. After TSH secretion recovers, normalization of serum TSH is the best index to guide maintenance therapy.

Some experts advocate a "block-and-replace" approach that consists of high doses of antithyroid med-

ication to "block" endogenous secretion combined with a full replacement dose of levothyroxine. While one study reported higher remission rates with this strategy, all subsequent attempts to reproduce this finding have failed and so this theoretical benefit should be discounted.[21] For simplicity, the author favors monotherapy, titrated to the lowest Tapazole dose required to maintain euthyroidism. If euthyroidism is maintained for 6-12 months on a very low Tapazole dose (2.5 or 5 mg/day), a trial-off medication can be offered. Serum TSH should be measured every 3-4 weeks after the thionamide is discontinued. If TSH remains normal, the patient is in remission. If TSH falls below normal range, Tapazole should be restarted or, if appropriate, definitive therapy offered. In the author's opinion, because the risks of definitive therapy in the pediatric population are incompletely defined, it is appropriate to offer prolonged courses of Tapazole to children until they become adults.

Definitive therapy

In children, definitive therapy is typically used after an adverse reaction to antithyroid medication has occurred or when thionamide therapy has failed to achieve consistent euthyroidism. Two options, subtotal thyroidectomy and radioiodine, are available.[14,15] Both definitive therapies are administered with the goal of ablating as much thyroid tissue as possible and parents should be counseled that the desired outcome of either treatment is lifelong hypothyroidism. Both definitive therapies carry some risk of failure or later relapse. Like antithyroid medication, definitive therapy is directed only against the thyroid and not the autoimmunity which causes Graves disease so extrathyroidal manifestation such as orbitopathy and dermopathy may progress even after successful ablation.

Surgery. Surgery was historically the first definitive therapy used to treat hyperthyroidism. Today, its use in adults is generally reserved for rare patients who have massive goiters (more than 8 times normal size) or coexisting cytologically abnormal thyroid nodules. Outcome studies are limited in children, but subtotal thyroidectomy is cited to achieve lasting hypothyroidism in 84% to 99% of pediatric cases.[14] If thyroidectomy is considered, parents should be fully informed of the risks of both surgery (which include vocal cord paralysis and permanent hypoparathyroidism) and anesthesia. The risk of serious operative complications is greatly reduced by referral to a surgeon with extensive personal experience in subtotal thyroidectomy and, in such hands, complication rates may be as low as 2%.[14]

Radioiodine ablation. Radioiodine ablation with I-131 is the default definitive therapy in adults with hyperthyroidism. In the past, I-131 therapy was avoided in children due to concerns of radiation exposure, but recent reports of high-dose I-131 regimens have been reassuring. Unlike older dosing guidelines which were intended to leave behind a functional thyroid remnant, full ablative doses are now recommended with the rationale that this minimizes the risks of both treatment failure and secondary thyroid cancer. Therapeutic I-131 doses should be adjusted on the basis of estimated thyroid size and RAIU to deliver approximately 200 µCi/g of thyroid tissue.[12]

Antithyroid medications should be discontinued 3 to 5 days before radioiodine administration to optimize radioiodine uptake. Thyroid RAIU should be measured with I-123 before I-131 ablation to facilitate dose determination. Thionamide derivatives can be restarted 7 days after I-131 administration and thyroid function tests measured monthly thereafter to monitor for response. Parents should be counseled that the response to I-131 is delayed and that an interval of 6 months should pass before the option of a second I-131 dose is considered.

THYROID NODULES AND CANCER

Definitions and Epidemiology

A thyroid nodule is a discrete mass within the gland that is distinct from the surrounding parenchyma. The frequency of thyroid nodules increases with age and in contrast to adults, where sonographically detectable nodules are reported in 19% to 67% of randomly selected patients,[22] the estimated frequency of nodules in children is 0.05% to 1.8%.[23,24] While early pediatric series cited high rates of cancer in thyroid nodules, recent studies of children estimate a much lower cancer

prevalence of 5% to 33%, which is similar to the rates observed in adults. Like thyroid nodules, thyroid cancers are also relatively rare in childhood, with a reported frequency of 0.2 to 5 cases per million children per year.[25] The vast majority of differentiated thyroid cancers are of follicular cell origin, with papillary thyroid cancer being the most common subtype.

Pathogenesis

Childhood neck irradiation increases the risk of thyroid neoplasia, and experience with both external radiation and the Chernobyl accident indicates that this risk is inversely proportional to the child's age at the time of exposure. While neck irradiation is no longer performed for benign conditions, it is still performed in young children as therapy for lymphoma and other malignancies so the risk remains clinically relevant today. Beyond the environmental risk factor of childhood neck irradiation, certain familial disorders also predispose to the development of thyroid neoplasia. It should however be noted that the vast majority of children (and adults) who present with thyroid neoplasia have no history of either neck irradiation or familial thyroid cancer.

Clinical Presentation and Diagnosis

Thyroid nodules can present as a neck mass noted by the patient or be discovered by palpation on a clinician's physical examination. Nodules may also be revealed as incidental findings on radiographic studies performed for unrelated indications. Regardless of how a nodule is detected, all nodules of significant size should be evaluated for the risk of thyroid cancer.

Algorithm for the Evaluation of Thyroid Nodules

As with most other solid cancers, the prognosis of thyroid carcinoma depends in part upon tumor size. Accordingly, the primary goal in the evaluation of nodular thyroid disease is the timely identification of the minority of patients who have malignant nodules so that therapy can begin. The following is a suggested approach to the evaluation of thyroid nodules.

When a thyroid nodule is detected, serum thyroid tests should be obtained. If serum TSH is low, I-123 thyroid scintigraphy should be performed to address the possibility of a toxic nodule. As described earlier in this chapter's "Thyrotoxicosis" section, such nodules are rare and as a rule benign. If serum TSH is normal or high, the patient should instead be referred to sonography and nodules which are greater than or equal to 1 cm in diameter should be biopsied by ultrasound-guided fine needle aspiration (Figure 4-15).

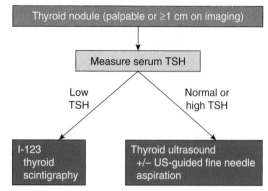

FIGURE 4-15 ■ Evaluation of thyroid nodules.

Diagnostic Tests

Thyroid scintigraphy can diagnose toxic thyroid nodules, but clinicians should recognize that such nodules are extremely rare and that scintigraphy must be performed during TSH suppression to confirm autonomy. For these reasons, serum TSH should be measured in all patients upon the discovery of a thyroid nodule and scintigraphy reserved only for the subset of children whose serum TSH is low. For the vast majority of patients who present with a normal to high serum TSH concentration, thyroid ultrasound is the optimal imaging modality to confirm or refute the presence of a thyroid nodule.

If a thyroid nodule greater than or equal to 1 cm in size is documented by sonography in a child with a normal or high serum TSH concentration, it should be biopsied. Ultrasound-guided fine needle aspiration is the preferred method as it is minimally invasive and easily detects the nuclear changes that are pathognomonic of papillary thyroid cancer.[22] When reviewed by an experienced cytopathologist, benign cytology is highly accurate and surgery can usually be deferred. Cytology that is positive for papillary thyroid cancer is also highly predictive (over 98% accuracy at our center) so near-total thyroidectomy is an appropriate response to this finding. For patients with unilateral disease and intermediate cytologic abnormalities which predict a less than 50% likelihood of cancer, thyroid lobectomy (removal of the ipsilateral lobe and isthmus) is recommended. Completion thyroidectomy (removal of the contralateral lobe) can be performed as a second operation for the minority of such patients who are confirmed to have cancer by lobectomy.

Differential Diagnosis

This section will review the common types of benign and malignant thyroid nodules.

Benign thyroid nodules

The majority of thyroid nodules are benign and, in the absence of associated hyperthyroidism or compressive symptoms, no therapy is required. As described above, benign cytology has high negative predictive value and usually permits the deferral of surgery. Such patients should be carefully monitored by annual sonography to address the unlikely possibility of a false-negative result. If a nodule is over 4 cm in size, the author recommends thyroid lobectomy even with benign cytology.

About 5% to 10% of thyroid nodules are autonomous and, if they reach significant size and/or number, they can cause hyperthyroidism. While exceptions have been reported, autonomous nodules are as a rule benign and, if an I-123 thyroid scan documents focal uptake in the nodule during TSH suppression (Figure 4-7), biopsy can be deferred. As described earlier in the "Thyrotoxicosis" section, autonomous nodules may warrant treatment for hyperthyroidism or local compressive symptoms despite their low cancer risk.

Thyroid cancers of follicular cell origin

Over 95% of childhood thyroid cancers are of follicular thyroid cell origin.[26] Of the two subtypes, papillary and follicular carcinoma, papillary is the most common. Compared to adults, childhood thyroid cancer is characterized by high rates of regional and distant metastases and by high rates of recurrence. Despite this, the outcome of pediatric thyroid cancer is generally referred to as favorable. Estimates of cause-specific mortality in children vary widely from 0% to 18%.[27] While several of these estimates approximate the general statistics for adults with thyroid cancer, the direct comparison of pediatric and adult outcome studies is problematic because pediatric series generally follow patients for much shorter periods of time.

Most thyroid cancers are characterized by slow tumor growth (relative to other common solid cancers). This slow progression contributes to the favorable short-term outcome observed in most patients but is also believed to be responsible for the observation that late recurrences can occur, even more than 30 years after initial treatment. Thyroid cancers are refractory to conventional chemotherapy. However, adjunctive therapies such as TSH suppression and radioiodine treatment which exploit similarities between malignant and benign thyroid tissue have been shown to improve outcome. For this reason, specially trained endocrinologists, rather than oncologists, typically serve as the continuity physicians for thyroid cancer.

While thyroid cancer usually occurs sporadically, several familial syndromes are known to be associated with an increased risk of thyroid neoplasia, including Cowden syndrome (characterized by mucocutaneous lesions, breast cancer, macrocephaly, and endometrial carcinoma) and familial adenomatous polyposis (characterized by the progressive development of numerous adenomatous colon polyps). In addition, there are other families where thyroid cancer alone clusters in an autosomal dominant pattern. Accordingly, the evaluation of a new thyroid nodule should include a complete family history and direct inquiry into whether extrathyroidal symptoms suspicious for Cowden syndrome and familial adenomatous polyposis are present.

Medullary thyroid cancer and multiple endocrine neoplasia type 2

Medullary thyroid cancer is a rare form of thyroid cancer. In contrast to papillary and follicular carcinoma which arise from the thyroid follicular cells, medullary thyroid cancers arise from the parafollicular C-cells which produce calcitonin. For this reason, the adjunctive therapies of TSH suppression and radioiodine are of no benefit in medullary thyroid cancer and treatment is primarily surgical.

Medullary thyroid cancer can occur sporadically or in the context of a familial syndrome. The autosomal dominant disorders of familial medullary thyroid cancer (FMTC) and multiple endocrine neoplasia syndromes type 2A (MEN-2A) and type 2B (MEN-2B) are all associated with germline mutations in the RET proto-oncogene. The component endocrine neoplasia of MEN-2A are medullary thyroid cancer, hyperparathyroidism, and pheochromocytoma. MEN-2B is comprised of medullary thyroid cancer and pheochromocytoma (without hyperparathyroidism) with concomitant development of mucosal neuromas. All these disorders must be distinguished from multiple endocrine neoplasia type 1 which is not associated with thyroid cancer and instead is characterized by neoplastic transformation of the parathyroid glands, pancreatic islets, and pituitary.

The careful study of families with FMTC and MEN-2 has allowed risk stratification for the most common RET mutations. Medullary thyroid cancer is highly penetrant in all forms of MEN-2 and a primary determinant of mortality so prophylactic thyroidectomy is recommended to prevent it. Knowing an individual child's specific RET mutation allows not only the confirmation of carrier state but prediction of thyroid cancer aggressiveness. Consensus guidelines categorize germline RET mutations into three risk levels which correspond to specific recommendations for the timing of prophylactic thyroidectomy: before 6 months of life for level 3 (highest risk); before 5 years of age for level 2 (high risk); and before the 5 to 10 years of age for level 1 (least high risk).[28] In addition to prophylactic thyroidectomy, the care of individuals with MEN-2A and MEN-2B should include chronic biochemical surveillance for the other associated endocrine neoplasia of

pheochromocytoma (measurement of plasma free metanephrines) +/− hyperparathyroidism (measurement of serum calcium).

Treatment

This section discusses general concepts in the treatment of thyroid cancer, focusing on cancers of follicular cell origin (papillary carcinoma and follicular carcinoma) because these represent over 95% of childhood thyroid cancers and because they are treated with the adjunctive endocrine therapies of radioiodine and TSH suppression.[26] Medullary thyroid cancer, which arises from parafollicular C-cells, is typically treated with surgery alone. While a detailed discussion of the management of thyroid cancer is beyond the scope of this chapter, consensus guidelines from organizations such as the American Thyroid Association are regularly updated and freely accessible on the internet at http://cancer.thyroidguidelines.net.[22]

Surgery

Surgery is the initial therapy for all primary thyroid cancers. The optimal operation is near-total thyroidectomy as it removes occult microscopic disease which may reside in the contralateral lobe; lowers recurrence risk for patients who present with advanced disease; and increases the sensitivity of the diagnostic tests used to monitor for disease progression. While lobectomy may be appropriate for certain individuals with unifocal microcarcinomas, such patients are rare in childhood and, in practice, near total thyroidectomy is the most common operation performed in both adults and children.

In addition to the general risks of surgery and anesthesia, thyroid surgery is associated with the specific operative risks of vocal cord paralysis (due to injury of the recurrent laryngeal nerve) and permanent hypoparathyroidism (due to inadvertent injury or removal of the parathyroid glands). These risks are greatly reduced by referral to a surgeon with extensive experience in thyroid surgery and a low personal complication rate. As described earlier in the "Diagnostic Tests" section, we recommend a staged approach where nodule cytology is used to triage patients to lobectomy versus near-total thyroidectomy. Because most nodules are benign, this staged approach avoids the risks of bilateral surgery in the majority of children who present with nodules. Hypothyroidism is the expected consequence of thyroidectomy and, as it is readily treated, it should not affect decisions regarding operative strategy.

About one third of children successfully treated for thyroid cancer experience disease recurrence and this is most often local. If recurrent regional lymph node metastasis is macroscopic (palpable or easily visualized by sonography), surgical neck dissection should be considered. As with nodules, neck sonography and ultrasound-guided fine needle aspiration should be performed preoperatively to confirm the presence of metastatic disease and to plan the surgical approach.

Radioiodine therapy

Even after near-total thyroidectomy, radioiodine uptake usually persists in the thyroid bed due to a microscopic residuum of normal thyroid tissue. Postoperative radioiodine ablation of this remnant with I-131 has been shown to lower recurrence rates, presumably due to the destruction of malignant thyroid cells within the macroscopically normal remnant, and to improve the sensitivity of the surveillance tests used to monitor for disease progression. Separate from remnant ablation, higher I-131 doses may be used to treat thyroid cancer foci which are not amenable to surgical resection, including distant metastases.

I-131 doses are calculated to deliver therapeutic activity without exceeding safe radiation exposures to normal tissues such as the bone marrow and gonads. Pediatrician must be aware that the absorbed radiation dose to normal tissues is higher in young children secondary to their smaller organ volumes and increased cross radiation so administered doses must be adjusted accordingly. An interval of 12 months between I-131 treatments is generally recommended to minimize the risk of radiation-induced leukemia.

To optimize radioiodine uptake into thyroid cells, patients should be prepared with a low iodine diet and hyperthyrotropinemia should be induced by levothyroxine withdrawal. Children may become nauseous with I-131 administration so antiemetics such as ondansetron and lorazepam should be used as needed (or given prophylactically to children who have vomited with prior I-131 doses). Oral hydration, frequent urination, regular stooling, and sialogogs should be encouraged for 2 to 3 days after I-131 administration to minimize radiation exposure to the intestinal tract, bladder, gonads, and the salivary glands. Levothyroxine therapy and a normal diet can be reinstituted 2 days after I-131 administration and a posttherapy whole body scan should be performed 4 to 7 days post treatment.

TSH suppression

Thyrotropin (TSH) stimulates thyroid follicular cell growth so the suppression of serum TSH is recommended in children with papillary or follicular thyroid cancers. Levothyroxine should be titrated to a goal serum TSH concentration of less than or equal to 0.1 µU/mL. As a rule, this can be achieved without hyperthyroxinemia or thyrotoxic symptoms. When used to an adjunct to surgery, TSH suppression reduces recurrence risk and

---

> **Box 4-3. When to Refer**
>
> Thyroid Nodules and Cancer
>
> ■ The discovery of a thyroid nodule of significant size warrants immediate referral to a center with expertise in ultrasound, fine needle aspiration, and thyroid surgery. How a nodule is detected has no impact on cancer risk, so all nodules of significant size warrant evaluation. Our center uses the size criteria of 1 cm as the threshold for biopsy.
>
> ■ Because the progression of thyroid cancer is slow, parents should be reassured that taking time to identify expert consultants is safe and provides the most efficient path to optimal therapy (and the avoidance of unnecessary treatment).
>
> ■ Because thyroid cancers are rare in childhood but extremely common in adult medicine, collaboration between pediatric caregivers and adult thyroid centers can be invaluable. The care of children with thyroid cancer should be transferred to an adult thyroid cancer center by the age of 18 years.

can improve survival in patients with advanced disease. The parents of children with thyroid cancer should be counseled that levothyroxine is important not only as hormone replacement but as a means of suppressing cancer progression, and that consistent medication compliance is critical for this reason.

Monitoring for disease progression

Pediatric thyroid cancer can recur more than 30 years after initial surgery and all children with thyroid cancer warrant lifelong surveillance. The timely detection of cancer recurrence provides the greatest opportunity to eradicate disease in its early stages.

Serum thyroglobulin is produced exclusively by thyroid follicular cells and is routinely employed as a tumor marker. Because thyroglobulin is also produced by normal thyroid tissue, its greatest utility as a cancer marker is realized only after surgical thyroidectomy and radioiodine ablation. Surveillance should also include serial neck imaging. In the hands of an experienced operator, thyroid sonography is extremely sensitive and, when coupled with ultrasound-guided fine needle aspiration, it becomes a highly specific modality to screen for local recurrence. Institutions with less experience in neck sonography may consider MRI or CT instead. Given the high rates of distant metastasis associated with childhood thyroid cancer, I-123 diagnostic whole body scans should be performed regularly.

REFERENCES

1. Demers LM, Spencer CA. Laboratory medicine practice guidelines: laboratory support for the diagnosis and monitoring of thyroid disease. *Clin Endocrinol.* 2003;58(2):138-140.

2. DeBoer MD, Lafranchi SH. Pediatric thyroid testing issues. *Pediatr Endocrinol Rev.* 2007;5(1):570-577.

3. Hunter I, Greene SA, MacDonald TM, Morris AD. Prevalence and etiology of hypothyroidism in the young. *Arch Dis Child.* 2000;83(3):207-210.

4. Hanna CE, LaFranchi SH. Adolescent thyroid disorders. *Adolesc Med.* 2002;13(1):13-35, v.

5. Rose SR, Brown RS, Foley T, et al. Update of newborn screening and therapy for congenital hypothyroidism. *Pediatrics.* 2006;117(6):2290-2303.

6. Kopp P. Perspective: genetic defects in the etiology of congenital hypothyroidism. *Endocrinology.* 2002;143(6):2019-2024.

7. Roberts CG, Ladenson PW. Hypothyroidism. *Lancet.* 2004;363(9411):793 803.

8. Weiss RE, Refetoff S. Treatment of resistance to thyroid hormone—primum non nocere. *J Clin Endocrinol Metab.* 1999;84(2):401-404.

9. Lafranchi S. Thyroiditis and acquired hypothyroidism. *Pediatric Ann.* 1992;21(1):29, 32-39.

10. Mandel SJ, Brent GA, Larsen PR. Levothyroxine therapy in patients with thyroid disease. *Ann Intern Med.* 1993; 119(6):492-502.

11. Alexander EK, Marqusee E, Lawrence J, Jarolim P, Fischer GA, Larsen PR. Timing and magnitude of increases in levothyroxine requirements during pregnancy in women with hypothyroidism. *N Engl J Med.* 2004;351(3):241-249.

12. Huang SA. Thyroid. In: Treves ST, ed. *Pediatric Nuclear Medicine.* New York, NY: Springer; 2007:57-73.

13. Forssberg M, Arvidsson CG, Engvall J, Lindblad C, Snellman K, Aman J. Increasing incidence of childhood thyrotoxicosis in a population-based area of central Sweden. *Acta Paediatr.* 2004;93(1):25-29.

14. Lee JA, Grumbach MM, Clark OH. The optimal treatment for pediatric Graves' disease is surgery. *J Clin Endocrinol Metab.* 2007;92(3):801-803.

15. Rivkees SA, Dinauer C. An optimal treatment for pediatric Graves' disease is radioiodine. *J Clin Endocrinol Metab.* 2007;92(3):797 800.

16. Kaguelidou F, Alberti C, Castanet M, Guitteny MA, Czernichow P, Leger J. Predictors of autoimmune hyperthyroidism relapse in children after discontinuation of antithyroid drug treatment. *J Clin Endocrinol Metab.* 2008;93(10):3817-3826.

17. Pearce EN, Farwell AP, Braverman LE. Thyroiditis. *N Engl J Med.* 2003;348(26):2646-2655.

18. Biondi B, Cooper DS. The clinical significance of subclinical thyroid dysfunction. *Endocr Rev.* 2008;29(1):76-131.

19. Cooper DS, Rivkees SA. Putting Propylthiouracil in Perspective. *J Clin Endocrinol Metab.* 2009;94:1881-1882.

20. Rivkees SA, Mattison DR. Ending propylthiouracil-induced liver failure in children. *N Engl J Med.* 2009;360: 1574-1575.

21. Cooper DS. Antithyroid drugs. *N Engl J Med.* 2005;352(9): 905-917.

22. Cooper DS, Doherty GM, Haugen BR, et al. Management guidelines for patients with thyroid nodules and differentiated thyroid cancer. *Thyroid.* 2006;16(2):109-142.

23. Rallison ML, Dobyns BM, Keating FR Jr, Rall JE, Tyler FH. Thyroid nodularity in children. *JAMA.* 1975;233(10): 1069-1072.

24. Trowbridge FL, Matovinovic J, McLaren GD, Nichaman MZ. Iodine and goiter in children. *Pediatrics.* 1975;56(1):82-90.

25. Zimmerman D, Hay ID, Bergstralh E. Papillary thyroid carcinoma in Children. In: Robbins J, ed. *Treatment of Thyroid Cancer in Childhood.* Springfield, VA: US Department of Commerce, Technology Administration, National Technical Information Service; 1992:3-11.

26. LiVolsi VA. Pathology of pediatric thyroid cancer. In: Robbins J, ed. *Treatment of Thyroid Cancer in Childhood.* Springfield, VA: National Technical Information Service; 1992:11-22.

27. Landau D, Vini L, A'Hern R, Harmer C. Thyroid cancer in children: the Royal Marsden Hospital experience. *Eur J Cancer.* 2000;36(2):214-220.

28. Brandi ML, Gagel RF, Angeli A, et al. Guidelines for diagnosis and therapy of MEN type 1 and type 2. *J Clin Endocrinol Metab.* 2001;86(12):5658-5671.

CHAPTER 5

Adrenal Disorders

Patricia A. Donohoue

OVERVIEW

Disorders of adrenal function occur at all ages. Adrenal dysfunction may be an isolated problem or in conjunction with multiple organ involvement in certain syndromes. The chapter below details many aspects of the pathogenesis, diagnosis, and treatment of various forms of adrenal disease. Principles that are helpful in evaluating the most common pediatric clinical situations in which an adrenal disorder is suspected include:

1. Patients with early pubic hair development (premature pubarche) will have in order of frequency:
   a. Premature adrenarche
   b. Precocious puberty
   c. Late-onset congenital adrenal hyperplasia (CAH)
   d. Adrenal or gonadal tumor
2. Patients with "simple" obesity are distinguished from those with Cushing syndrome by the following clinical features:
   a. Cushing syndrome often develops rapidly
   b. Cushing syndrome patients do not grow well in height, but patients with obesity generally have accelerated height growth
   c. Cushing syndrome patients often have signs of androgen excess
3. Patients with adrenocortical insufficiency will have either:
   a. Primary adrenal failure, usually with symptoms of both glucocorticoid or mineralocorticoid (ie, salt loss) deficiency. Most commonly seen:
      i. Congenital adrenal hyperplasia (ambiguous genitalia in females)
      ii. Autoimmune Addison disease (often associated with other endocrinopathies)
      iii. Adrenoleukodystrophy
   b. Lack of adrenocorticotropic hormone (ACTH) stimulation of cortisol secretion, with symptoms of glucocorticoid deficiency alone. Most commonly seen:
      i. ACTH deficiency associated with multiple pituitary hormone deficiencies
      ii. Suppression of the hypothalamic-pituitary-adrenal axis because of recent discontinuation of corticosteroid treatment

GENERAL PRINCIPLES OF ADRENAL FUNCTION

The adrenal cortex secretes three classes of biologically active steroid hormones. These are glucocorticoids (cortisol), which are controlled by the hypothalamic-pituitary-adrenal axis; mineralocorticoids (aldosterone), which are controlled through the renin-angiotensin system; and androgens (dehydroepiandrosterone [DHEA] and androstenedione), which are controlled by an as yet uncharacterized trophic hormone.

Metabolic effects of steroid hormones are mediated by the interaction of each class of steroids with a specific cellular receptor. The ligand activated steroid-receptor complex dimerizes, enters the nucleus of target cells, and binds to various transcription factors. These form stable complexes at the site of a specific "steroid response elements." This bound complex then acts to modulate the transcription of specific target genes to exert the hormone effects.

The adrenal medulla secretes catecholamines, mainly epinephrine (adrenaline). Epinephrine secretion is stimulated by the sympathetic nervous system and by high cortisol levels from the adrenal cortex. The effects of epinephrine are mediated through adrenergic receptors, which produce tissue-specific effects.

THE ADRENAL GLAND

Anatomy

The human adrenal gland is made up of two embryologically and functionally distinct endocrine organs, the adrenal cortex and the adrenal medulla. The adrenal glands lie at the upper pole of each kidney. Ectopic nodules (rests) of adrenocortical tissue may be located in the broad ligaments of the female or in the testes or spermatic cords of the male. The location of adrenal rests is determined by the location of the embryonic mesenchymal cells that develop into the adrenal cortex, gonad, kidney, and liver.

The size of the adrenal glands varies with age, and this variation is due almost entirely to changes within the adrenal cortex (Figure 5-1). During gestation and at birth, the adrenal glands are much larger relative to body size than during adulthood, and at birth the weight of the glands is nearly that of adult glands. During the first year of life, the adrenal cortex undergoes involution of its fetal component reducing its size by more than 50%. The adrenal glands then gradually increase in size throughout childhood and adolescence. In adults, the average weight of the glands is 8 to 12 g.

The adrenal glands are supplied by arteries that form a subcapsular plexus, which sends arterial branches toward the adrenal medulla, from which capillary loops return into the cortex. Because of the structure of adrenal circulation, the medulla is exposed to high glucocorticoid concentrations from the venous drainage of the cortex. Cortisol stimulates adrenal medullary epinephrine secretion.

Histology

The adult adrenal cortex is divided into three histologically distinct zones, the outer zona glomerulosa, the middle zona fasciculata, and the inner zona reticularis. The zona fasciculata is the largest, comprising up to 75% of the cortex. The zona glomerulosa is site of mineralocorticoid synthesis. There is a gradual transition to the zona fasciculata, where the cells function in cholesterol storage. There is a clear transition to the zona reticularis, which contains cells with relatively lipid-free cytoplasm. The cells of the zona reticularis and the clear cells at the interface between the zona fasciculata and zona reticularis are the site of synthesis of glucocorticoids and androgens. The three zones of the adult cortex are mature by 18 to 20 years of age, and show regression associated with aging by 41 to 50 years.

The adrenal medulla is a component of the sympathoadrenal-neuroendocrine system with chromaffin cells (pheochromocytes) arranged in nests and cords. Sympathetic ganglion cells are also present. The chromaffin cells are surrounded by a rich vascular network, and their abundant cytoplasm contains catecholamine storage granules. Epinephrine is the major synthesized and stored catecholamine of the adrenal medulla. It is not synthesized in significant amounts in other tissues.

Embryology

The adrenal cortex is derived from mesodermal tissue, the medulla from neuroectoderm. During the 5th week

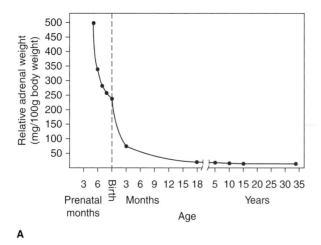

A

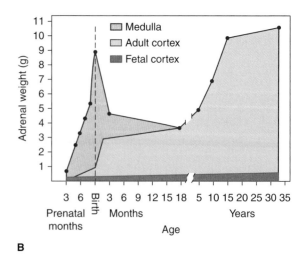

B

FIGURE 5-1 ▪ Adrenal gland size at different stages of life. **(A)** Relative adrenal weight at various ages. **(B)** Absolute adrenal gland weight at various ages. The relative contributions of the fetal zone (cortex), adult zone (cortex), and medulla are shown. (*Redrawn from Bethune JE. The Adrenal Cortex. A Scope Monograph. Kalamazoo, The Upjohn Company, 1975.*)

of gestation, mesothelial cells migrate into the underlying mesenchyme (near the developing gonad) and form the fetal zone of the adrenal cortex. A second migration of mesothelial cells arrive to form the smaller definitive (adult) zone. The adrenal cortex is actively synthesizing and secreting steroid hormones during the first trimester in response to tropic hormone stimulation. This is evidenced by androgen overproduction and subsequent ambiguity of the external genitalia in female infants with steroid 21-hydroxylase (CYP21) deficiency. During late fetal life, the adrenal cortex is relatively larger than that of adults, and consists mostly of the fetal zone that involutes rapidly after birth (Figure 5-1).

During the 7th week of gestation, primitive sympathetic nerve cells differentiate into pheochromoblasts and migrate into the adrenal gland. By the 20th week, these cells have formed clusters of chromaffin cells within the adrenal medulla which does not become a distinct organ until the fetal cortex undergoes atrophy. However, it is functioning at birth as evidenced by the presence of both epinephrine and norepinephrine in the plasma and urine of newborns.

Mechanisms that lead to the differentiation of the adrenal cortex include major effects of transcription factors known as steroidogenic factor 1 (SF-1) and dosage-sensitive sex reversal adrenal hypoplasia congenital on the X chromosome gene 1 (DAX-1). SF-1, a member of the nuclear hormone receptor family of zinc finger transcription factors, first was described as a regulator of the tissue-specific expression of steroidogenic enzymes, the ACTH receptor, the steroidogenic acute regulatory protein (StAR), and Müllerian inhibiting substance (MIS). During embryogenesis, SF1 transcripts are present in the gonads, adrenals, anterior pituitary, and hypothalamus. SF1 regulates the expression of hormones that are critical for both adrenal functional development and male sexual differentiation, as well as other levels of the endocrine axis such as pituitary and hypothalamic function. SF-1 defects are known to cause congenital adrenal insufficiency as well as disorders of sex development (DSD).

DAX-1 encodes an atypical member of the nuclear receptor family. DAX-1 was isolated initially by positional cloning of the gene responsible for X-linked adrenal hypoplasia congenita (AHC), in which there is impaired development of the definitive (adult) zone of the adrenal cortex and hypogonadotrophic hypogonadism. Animal studies have shown that both SF-1 and DAX-1 genes are expressed in many of the same sites during embryogenesis, including the gonads, adrenal cortex, pituitary gonadotropes, and the ventromedial hypothalamus, and that DAX-1 is stimulated by SF-1.[1]

ADRENOCORTICAL STEROIDS

Nomenclature

The precursor for all adrenal and gonadal steroid hormones is cholesterol. All steroids, therefore, have the same basic structural backbone, the cyclopentanophenanthrene molecule (Figure 5-2). The C18 derivative of this molecule is estrane, C19 is androstane, and C21 is pregnane. Adrenal steroids are derived from the 21- and 19-carbon rings. In general, the C19 steroids are androgens, and when there is a ketone group added at carbon 17 during metabolism, they are excreted in the urine as 17-ketosteroids. The C21 steroids are the mineralocorticoids and

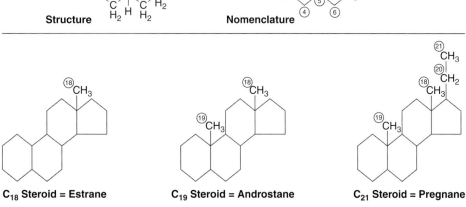

FIGURE 5-2 ■ The steroid nucleus and its derivatives. The structure and ring nomenclature of cyclopentanophenanthrene are shown in the upper panel. The structures of the C_{18} (estrane), C_{19} (androstane), and C_{21} (pregnane) derivatives are presented in the lower panel.

glucocorticoids. When a hydroxyl group is added at carbon 17, they are excreted in the urine as 17-hydroxycorticosteroids.

Biosynthesis of Adrenocortical Steroids

The stepwise conversion of cholesterol to adrenal steroid hormones involves a series of enzymes (Figure 5-3), all but one of which belong to the cytochrome P450 family of mitochondrial and microsomal proteins. The adrenal P450s require nicotinamide adenosine dinucleotide phosphate (NADPH) as an electron donor, but have differing cofactor requirements. In the mitochondria they require both an iron-sulfur protein and a flavoprotein as electron-transport intermediates, but the microsomal P450s require only the flavoprotein intermediate. The regulation of P450 enzymatic activities within the zones of the adrenal cortex depends on tropic hormone stimulation, activity of SF-1, physiological demands (eg, intravascular volume, serum sodium concentration, blood glucose), and the gradients of oxygen and steroids across the capillary bed as it passes through the three cortical zones.[2]

   Conversion of cholesterol to pregnenolone—This is the first and rate-limiting step in adrenal steroidogenesis. This step is mediated by CYP11A (P450scc, side-chain cleavage), a single enzyme that mediates the three chemical reactions that convert cholesterol to pregnenolone: 20α-hydroxylation, 22-hydroxylation, and cleavage of the cholesterol side-chain bond at position 20-22 (Figure 5-3). All three reactions occur at the same active site on the CYP11A molecule. CYP11A is under the tropic stimulation of ACTH from the anterior pituitary gland. Optimal stimulation of CYP11A expression by ACTH requires an intermediate protein, StAR, which is essential for access of cholesterol to the enzyme. StAR is expressed in the adrenal cortex and gonads, but not in the placenta (see in the section "Control of Adrenal Steroid Secretion").

   3β-Hydroxysteroid dehydrogenase—3β-Hydroxysteroid dehydrogenase (3β-HSD) mediates the conversion of pregnenolone to progesterone and of 17-hydroxypregnenolone to 17-hydroxyprogesterone (Figure 5-3). This enzyme system requires NAD and is located within the microsomes (endoplasmic reticulum). It is the only steroidogenic enzyme that is not a cytochrome P450, and it is required for the synthesis of glucocorticoids, mineralocorticoids, and sex steroids. There are two highly homologous human 3β-HSD isoenzymes, type 1 and type 2. It is the function of the type 2 3β-HSD enzyme that

is altered in 3β-HSD-deficiency CAH, as type 2 is the isoform that localizes to the adrenal cortex and gonad. The type 1 isoform is present in the placenta, skin, and mammary gland.

17α-Hydroxylase and 17,20-lyase reactions—The enzymatic conversions of pregnenolone to 17-hydroxypregnenolone and of progesterone to 17-hydroxyprogesterone require hydroxylation at the 17α-position. The subsequent conversion of these two 17-hydroxylated compounds to dehydroepiandrosterone (DHEA and androstenedione, respectively, require 17,20-lyase activity (Figure 5-3). Both 17α-hydroxylase and 17,20-lyase are enzymatic activities of the same protein, CYP17 or P450c17. CYP17 is required for glucocorticoid and sex steroid synthesis, but not for mineralocorticoid synthesis. CYP17 is a microsomal cytochrome P450 found in both the human adrenal cortex and testis. The contribution of ACTH to physiologic CYP17 transcription remains unclear.

21-Hydroxylase—The conversion of 17-hydroxyprogesterone to 11-deoxycortisol and of progesterone to 11-deoxycorticosterone (DOC) is mediated by the steroid CYP21 enzyme (P450c21) (Figure 5-3). CYP21 is required for the synthesis of both glucocorticoids and mineralocorticoids, but not for the synthesis of androgens. CYP21 activity was the first biological function attributed to a cytochrome P450. CYP21 is a microsomal cytochrome, and immunohistochemical studies have demonstrated CYP21 peptide in all three zones of the normal adrenal cortex. ACTH stimulation results in increased concentrations of CYP21 mRNA, but additional factors control CYP21 transcription within the functionally different zonae glomerulosa and reticularis, including SF-1.[3]

11β-Hydroxylase, 18-hydroxylase, and 18-oxidase—Within the zona glomerulosa DOC undergoes hydroxylation at the 11β-position by CYP11B1 (P450c11) to form corticosterone, which is then converted by 18-hydroxylase (corticosterone methyl oxidase I or CMOI) to form 18-hydroxycorticosterone. This product is subsequently converted by 18-oxidase (CMOII) to form aldosterone, the major circulating mineralocorticoid. CMOI and CMOII activities reside within the enzyme CYP11B2 or aldosterone synthase. Within the zona fasciculata, 11-deoxycortisol is converted by CYP11B1 to form cortisol (Figure 5-3). CYP11B1 and CYP11B2 are mitochondrial cytochromes. As with the above P450s (scc, c17, and c21), CYP11B1 activity and transcription are stimulated *in vitro* by ACTH and by SF-1.

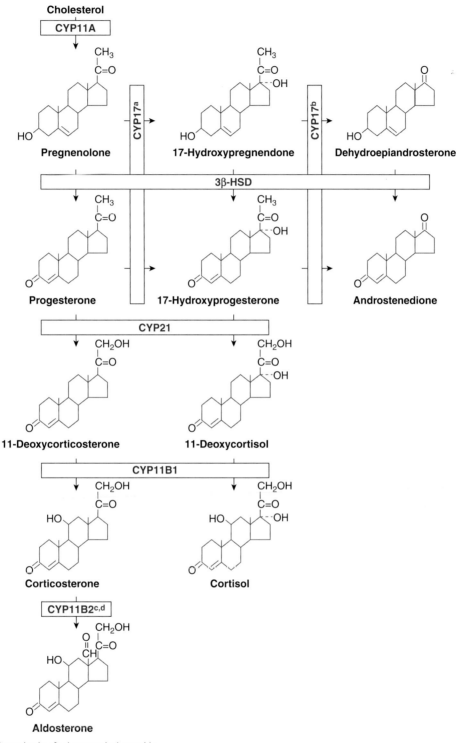

FIGURE 5-3 ▪ Biosynthesis of adrenocortical steroids.
Enzyme names:
CYP11A1= P450scc; activities: 20-hydroxylase, 22-hydroxylase, 20,22-lyase
CYP17 = P450c17; activities: a 17a-hydroxylase;[b] 17,20-lyase
3bHSD; activities: 3 beta-hydroxysteroid dehydrogenase (type 2); D⁵D⁴-isomerase
CYP21 = P450c21; activity: 21-hydroxylase
CYP11B1 = P450c11; activity: 11b-hydroxylase
CYP11B2 = P450 aldo; activities: c 18-hydroxylase (CMOI);[d] 18-dehydrogenase (CMOII)
CMOI = cortocosterone methyl oxidase type 1
CMOII = corticosterone methyl oxidase type 2
(*Adapted from: Donohoue PA. The Adrenal Gland and Its Disorders. In Kappy MS, Allen DB, Geffner ME (Ed)* Principles and Practice of Pediatric Endocrinology. *Springfield, IL: Charles C. Thomas Publishers Ltd.; 2005: 357-485.*)

ACTH Physiology and Control of Adrenal Steroid Secretion

In contrast to cells that secrete peptide or catecholamine hormones, steroidogenic cells do not maintain reservoirs of stored hormone. In addition, steroid hormones, once formed, are highly lipophilic and thus freely permeable to the cell membrane, and specific secretory processes have not been identified. As a result, *de novo* production of steroids from cholesterol is vital in controlling steroid hormone concentrations. The regulation of steroidogenesis can be viewed at two separate levels. First, adrenal steroid hormone production is controlled at the *level of the organism,* with input of complex feedback loops involving the hypothalamus, pituitary, and kidney. Production of steroids is also controlled by the specific biochemical events that regulate steroidogenesis at the *level of the adrenocortical cells.*

Steroid production in the intact organism

Secretion of glucocorticoid by the adrenal cortex is under the control of pituitary ACTH, a single peptide chain of only 39 amino acids. Its half-life in blood is only 7 to 12 minutes. The 1,24 N-terminal amino acid sequence of ACTH has the same steroidogenic activity as the native peptide, and is the peptide sequence of synthetic ACTH used for diagnostic testing. ACTH is one of the differentially spliced products of the proopiomelanocortin (*POMC*) gene, as described elsewhere.

The hypothalamic factor corticotropin releasing hormone (CRH) increases ACTH secretion. CRH is a 41 amino acid peptide. It is stimulated by multiple factors including a diurnal clock, low cortisol levels, and various stresses. CRH activity is located in discrete parts of the hypothalamus, particularly the median eminence. CRH is now known to be an important modulator of body size, not only through its control of ACTH and cortisol secretion, but also through its direct anorexigenic effects. Several other peptides homologous to CRH, called urocortins, act in the same manner to regulate food *intake.*[4]

Although CRH is the major factor controlling ACTH secretion, other secretagogues are known, such as arginine vasopressin, insulin-induced hypoglycemia, and pyrogen-induced fever Vasopressin and CRH have a synergistic effect on ACTH release. Chemical factors other than blood cortisol concentrations may control CRH secretion. These include an inhibitory effect by norepinephrine and a stimulatory role for serotonin.

Control at the cellular level

Temporally, ACTH stimulates steroidogenesis biphasically. The acute response occurs within seconds to minutes, and largely reflects increased delivery by StAR of cholesterol substrate to the mitochondria, where CYP11A carries out the initial rate-limiting reactions. The chronic phase requires hours to days and requires increased transcription of the cytochrome P450 steroid hydroxylases and other components of the steroidogenic apparatus.

Acute response. The primary event is the translocation of cholesterol to the inner mitochondrial membrane, where CYP11A carries out the initial steps in steroidogenesis.

This translocation system is induced by cAMP, the second messenger for most actions of ACTH, and requires ongoing protein synthesis, suggesting that a labile protein mediates the stimulation.

Chronic response. The chronic response of steroidogenic cells to trophic hormones largely reflects increased transcription of the steroid hydroxylases in two major areas of gene regulation: cell-selective and hormonally induced expression. Cell-specificity refers to distinct but overlapping patterns of P450 enzyme expression. CYP11A is expressed in all classic steroidogenic tissues (adrenal cortex, testicular Leydig cells, ovarian theca cells, and placenta). The CYP17 gene likewise is expressed in multiple steroidogenic tissues. In contrast, CYP21, CYP11B1, and CYP11B2 are expressed only in the adrenal cortex, with the latter two enzymes displaying zone-specific expression.

The second major level of regulation of the steroid hydroxylases is their response to trophic hormones. As noted above, the induction of steroid hydroxylase gene transcription is an essential component of the chronic response to trophic hormones, and several different promoter elements and transcriptional regulators have been proposed to confer responsiveness to ACTH.

Glucocorticoid Physiology and Action

Glucocorticoid secretion is controlled by the hypothalamic-pituitary-adrenal axis, as illustrated in Figure 5-4. The control of ACTH secretion is in part determined by the concentration of blood cortisol, the major circulating glucocorticoid. Cortisol in the circulation is 95% protein bound; 90% is bound to corticosteroid-binding globulin (CBG) or transcortin. Transcortin has a high affinity for cortisol as well as progesterone, and can bind prednisolone and aldosterone, but not dexamethasone. The free fraction of cortisol is biologically active, and is about 8% of the total cortisol when serum concentrations are normal. Compounds that bind to transcortin (eg, prednisone) will displace cortisol. At normal serum concentrations, the half-life of endogenous cortisol is 60 to 80 minutes; this may increase to up to 2 hours at higher concentrations. Cortisol, both free and bound, is

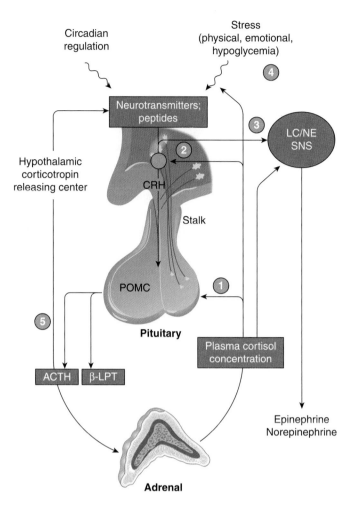

FIGURE 5-4 ■ The hypothalamic-pituitary-adrenal axis. The main sites for feedback control by plasma cortisol are the pituitary gland (1) and the hypothalamic corticotropin-releasing center (2). Feedback control by plasma cortisol also occurs at the locus coeruleus/sympathetic system (3) and may involve higher nerve centers (4) as well. There may also be a short feedback loop involving inhibition of corticotropin-releasing hormone (CRH) by adrenocorticotropic hormone (ACTH) (5). Hypothalamic neurotransmitters influence CRH release; serotoninergic and cholinergic systems stimulate the secretion of CRH and ACTH; α-adrenergic agonists and γ-aminobutyric acid (GABA) probably inhibit CRH release. The opioid peptides β-endorphin and enkephalin inhibit, and vasopressin and angiotensin II augment, the secretion of CRH and ACTH. β-LPT, β-lipotropin; POMC, proopiomelanocortin; LC, locus coeruleus; NE, norepinephrine; SNS, sympathetic nervous system. (*From Williams GH, Dluhy RG. Disorders of the adrenal cortex. In: Jameson JL, ed. Harrison's Endocrinology. New York, NY: McGraw-Hill; 2006:113-149.*)

distributed rapidly and widely throughout the body compartments, including the extracellular fluid.

The metabolism of all steroid hormones occurs mainly in the liver, a major site of their action. The sulfated and glucuronidated steroids are then returned to the circulation through the hepatic vein or excreted into the intestinal lumen through the bile. Glucocorticoids and their metabolites and conjugates are excreted mainly by the kidney (approximately 90%), and the remainder are excreted in the intestine. In addition, the kidney acts as a site of the inactivation of cortisol to cortisone. The tetrahydro metabolites are measured as urinary 17-hydroxycorticosteroids (17-OHCS).

The glucocorticoid actions are mediated by the interaction of steroid hormones with the glucocorticoid receptor (GR) or type 1 steroid hormone receptor. Steroids that interact with the GR or type 1 receptor are considered to be glucocorticoids, and may include both naturally occurring and synthetic (pharmacological) compounds. Genetic variation within the GR gene may confer increased or decreased glucocorticoid sensitivity.[5]

Glucocorticoid effects on carbohydrate metabolism are widespread (Table 5-1). At physiological concentrations, these effects are counterbalanced by the effects of

other hormones. The term "glucocorticoid" implies a major effect on carbohydrate metabolism, mainly the production and storage of glucose, so-called anti-insulin or glucose-sparing actions. Cellular glucose uptake and utilization are inhibited. Amino acid and free fatty acid substrates for gluconeogenesis are mobilized from plasma and muscle proteins, and from adipose tissue and plasma lipids. The metabolism of amino acids results in increased urinary nitrogen excretion and induction of urea cycle enzymes. Glycogen synthesis is also stimulated. In states of glucocorticoid excess, these effects may produce insulin resistance and hyperglycemia.

The glucocorticoid effects on fat metabolism are complex, and are also physiologically counterbalanced by those of other hormones. As discussed above, glucocorticoids exert a lipolytic action, which produces substrates for gluconeogenesis and glycogen synthesis. In hypercortisolemia, however, obesity is a common finding. This lipogenic effect is mediated by the combined actions of excess cortisol and insulin, which together produce both stimulation of appetite and the characteristic change in body fat distribution (central obesity, "buffalo hump").

In addition to metabolic effects, other glucocorticoid effects include anti-inflammatory and immunosuppressive

Table 5-1.

Glucocorticoid Effects in Humans

Biochemical Effects
Increased gluconeogenesis
Increased glycogen synthesis
Increased blood glucose concentration
*Negative nitrogen balance

Lipid Metabolism Effects
Increased sensitivity to lipid mobilizing agents
*Net mobilization of extremity fat and deposition of truncal fat

Gastrointestinal Effects
Increased production of gastric pepsin
Increased production of gastric HCl
Inhibition of Vitamin D-mediated calcium absorption

Reticuloendothelial System Effects
Granulocytosis (demargination)
Decreased production of inflammatory cytokines
*Involution of lymphatic and thymic tissue

Connective Tissue Effects
*Decrease in collagen content of skin, bone (osteoporosis)
*Decrease in collagen content of blood vessel walls (capillary fragility)
*Inhibition of granuloma formation

Vascular Effects
Increased renal plasma flow and GFR
Increased free water clearance

Neurologic Effects
Increased cardiac conduction velocity
Decreased electroconvulsive threshold
Inhibition of ACTH and CRH release
Inhibition of ADH release
*Sleep disturbances
*Stimulation of appetite
*Neuropsychiatric alterations (psychosis, depression)
*Euphoria

Other Effects
Requirement of normal growth
*Muscle weakness
*Inhibition of skeletal growth
*Inhibition of thyroid hormone release

These effects are seen in conditions of glucocorticoid excess.

actions via direct effect on cells of the immune system, inhibition of wound healing, skeletal growth retardation and loss of bone mineral, decreased vitamin D mediated calcium absorption from the gut, psychiatric disturbances such as depression and psychosis, and fluid and electrolyte disturbances that may be mediated through the mineralocorticoid or type 2 steroid hormone receptor.

Mineralocorticoid Physiology and Action

The control of aldosterone secretion by the renin-angiotensin system

Renin is a proteolytic enzyme that converts angiotensinogen in the liver to angiotensin I, which has mild vasopressor properties. Proteolytic cleavage of angiotensin I by angiotensin-converting enzyme (ACE) in the lungs produces the octapeptide angiotensin II which is a potent vasoconstrictor (Figure 5-5). It also stimulates production of the major adrenal salt-retaining steroid, aldosterone.

Renin secretion is indirectly controlled by negative feedback from aldosterone. Renin secretion from the renal juxtaglomerular cells is controlled by a baroreceptor system of the arterioles located in their proximity. An increase in aldosterone augments increased sodium and water retention with increased intravascular volume. The resultant stretching of the renal arterioles results in decreased secretion of renin. Inversely a decrease in blood volume as can occur in dehydration, hemorrhage, or low-salt diet will increase renin secretion.

Although angiotensin II is the major stimulator of aldosterone secretion, ACTH has a definite but temporary effect as well. By contrast, a constant intravenous (IV) infusion of ACTH through a prolonged period of time results in a sustained increase in plasma cortisol concentrations but a progressive fall of aldosterone concentrations. The temporary effect of ACTH on aldosterone secretion is owing to eventual suppression of the renin-angiotensin system after aldosterone release as well as the mineralocorticoid effect of the high cortisol levels.

Potassium can directly increase the secretion of aldosterone by the zona glomerulosa as evidenced in anephric patients who are maintained on dialysis. They show a progressive increment of potassium concentration in their blood that is directly correlated with an increase in aldosterone concentrations.

Although the most potent mineralocorticoid is aldosterone, some mineralocorticoid activity is found in 11-deoxycorticosterone (DOC). Circulating aldosterone is bound to transcortin with 10% of the affinity of cortisol. The plasma half-life of aldosterone is approximately 45 minutes. The liver catabolizes virtually all of the aldosterone, which enters the hepatic circulation, and the two primary metabolites are tetrahydroaldosterone and aldosterone-18-glucuronide, both of which are excreted in the urine.

The mineralocorticoid actions are mediated by the interaction of steroid hormones with the mineralocorticoid receptor (MR) or type 2 steroid receptor. In humans, the major natural mineralocorticoids are aldosterone and DOC. However the MR binds also glucocorticoids such as cortisol and corticosterone with affinities similar to aldosterone. Within the major

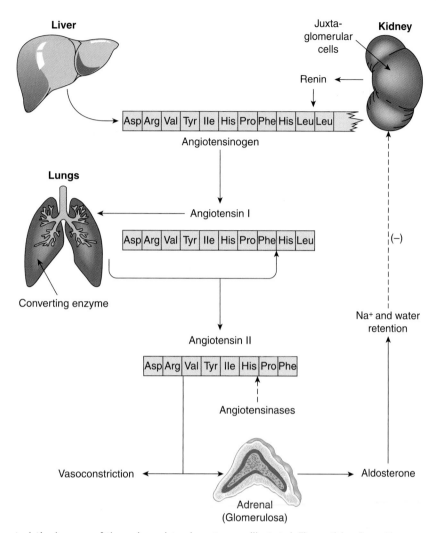

Liver

Asp|Arg|Val|Tyr|Ile|His|Pro|Phe|His|Leu|Leu
Angiotensinogen

Kidney

Juxta-
glomerular
cells

Renin ←

Lungs

Angiotensin I

Asp|Arg|Val|Tyr|Ile|His|Pro|Phe|His|Leu

Converting enzyme

(−)

Na⁺ and water
retention

Angiotensin II

Asp|Arg|Val|Tyr|Ile|His|Pro|Phe

Angiotensinases

Vasoconstriction ←   → Aldosterone

Adrenal
(Glomerulosa)

FIGURE 5-5 ■ The proteolytic cleavages of the renin-angiotensin system are illustrated. The partial amino acid sequence of angiotensinogen, and the complete sequences of angiotensin I and II are shown. The sites of formation and action of the various components of the renin-angiotensin-aldosterone system are also presented.

mineralocorticoid target site, the kidney, tissue-specific 11β-HSD type 1 promotes the efficient conversion of cortisol to inactive cortisone, thus removing cortisol as a significant ligand of the MR in that tissue.

Mineralocorticoids, as the name implies, control the excretion of electrolytes, mainly in the kidney. Aldosterone acts at the level of the cortical collecting duct to enhance the reabsorption of sodium. This effect is accompanied by chloride and water retention and results in expansion of extracellular volume. Within the outer portion of the medullary collecting duct, aldosterone acts to enhance proton excretion, particularly potassium ions. Aldosterone action on the collecting duct cells is mediated by the ligand-receptor complex stimulation of specific ion transport channels. These include several subtypes of chloride channels. Defects in these channels can cause pseudohypoaldosteronism.

The stimulation of potassium excretion is dependent upon sodium intake. Experimental animals receiving a diet deficient in sodium fail to exhibit an increase in urinary potassium excretion after aldosterone administration. The sodium conserving and potassium wasting effects of aldosterone are also present in the salivary and sweat glands, and in the gut.

Mineralocorticoid effects at supraphysiologic concentrations (eg, in primary hyperaldosteronism) include hypokalemia, metabolic alkalosis, and hypertension. Whereas hypokalemia and hypervolemia seem natural consequences of mineralocorticoid excess, the basis for metabolic alkalosis is unclear. It is postulated that severe potassium deficiency may alter normal acid excretion by the renal tubule.

Adrenal Androgen Physiology and Action

Several clinical observations demonstrated that the secretion rate of cortisol and adrenal androgens are divergent. Prepubertal children secrete cortisol at rate that is similar to that of adult subjects when the output is corrected for body size. Yet, the plasma concentrations of adrenal androgens are almost undetectable during childhood but increase gradually but markedly at puberty without any change in ACTH or cortisol secretion. Cortisol secretion also remains similar with adult aging, while the concentrations of adrenal androgens in blood fall. In premature adrenarche, when adrenal androgens prematurely reach adult concentrations resulting in appearance of pubic hair, the cortisol secretion remains normal for size. The identity of a peptide-regulating adrenal androgen secretion remains elusive.

The adrenal androgens are DHEA, its sulfate, and androstenedione. Androstenedione is the more potent androgen, however both compounds exert their biological effects through extra-adrenal conversion to the potent androgens testosterone and dihydrotestosterone (DHT), which then interact with the androgen receptor (AR) within androgen target tissues (Figure 5-6). Circulating androstenedione and DHEA bind to sex-hormone binding globulin (SHBG) to a much greater degree than to transcortin, but to a lesser degree than testosterone and DHT binding to SHBG. Adrenal androgens are metabolized to some degree in the liver; however a significant degree of production and interconversion of the sex steroids occurs in the gonads, skin, and adipose tissue.

The plasma half-life of DHEA is relatively brief at approximately 25 minutes. DHEA-sulfate (DHEA-S) is rapidly produced in both the liver and the adrenal cortex.

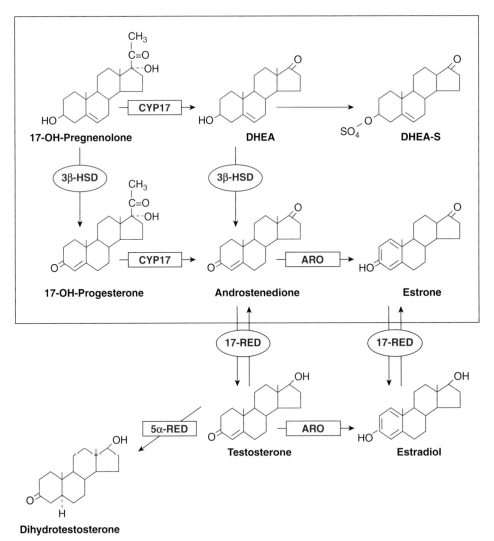

FIGURE 5-6 ■ General metabolism and distribution of adrenal steroids. Sex steroids secreted include dehydroepiandrosterone (DHEA) and its sulfate, androstenedione, and estrone. Androstenedione is metabolized peripherally to testosterone and dihydrotestosterone, whereas estrone is metabolized to estradiol. Enzyme activities: 3βHSD = 3β-hydroxysteroid dehydrogenase; CYP17 = 17α-hydroxylase/17,20-lyase; ARO = aromatase; 17RED = 17-ketoreductase; 5α-RED = 5α-reductase. (*Donohoue PA. The Adrenal Gland and its Disorders. In Kappy MS, Allen DB, Geffner ME (ED). Principles and Practice of Pediatric Endocrinology. Springfield, IL: Charles C. Thomas Publishers Ltd.; 2005: 357-485.*)

DHEA-S has a relatively long half-life of 8 to 11 hours, and undergoes very little hepatic extraction or renal clearance.

In adults, 15% of the circulating androstenedione is produced by peripheral conversion of DHEA and testosterone. The remainder is produced by relatively equal contributions from the adrenal and the gonad. Androstenedione is reversibly converted to testosterone by the enzyme 17-ketosteroid reductase. Androstenedione may also be converted to estrone by aromatase (Figure 5-6). The measurement of urinary 17-ketosteroids (17-KS) has long been used as an assessment of adrenal androgen production. This reaction measures conjugated and unconjugated C_{19},17-keto compounds; DHEA and androstenedione are the major precursors of the urinary 17-KS, whereas testosterone and its metabolites contribute very little.

Whether or not there are roles for adrenal androgens (DHEA and androstenedione) in their native state is a matter of controversy. Several studies have addressed DHEA treatment in various patient groups. It has not been shown to alter perimenopausal symptoms, or body composition in the elderly. In women with adrenal insufficiency, there can be improvement in sexual interest and overall sense of well-being. Other studies show differing and inconsistent effects on insulin sensitivity, body fat stores, lipid profiles, energy metabolism, and insulin-like growth factor levels.

ADRENOCORTICAL FUNCTION AT VARIOUS AGES OF LIFE

Fetal Life

The fetus produces cortisol by about 10 weeks of gestation. In the female fetus with congenital adrenal hyperplasia, masculinization of the external genitalia from excessive adrenal androgens starts at 8 to 10 weeks of gestation. However, the fetal adrenal is deficient in 3β-hydroxysteroid dehydrogenase (3β-HSD). As shown in Figure 5-7, 3β hydroxysteroids (and their sulfates) pass from the fetus to the placenta, which has abundant 3β-HSD and sulfatase. The progesterone and 17-hydroxyprogesterone produced in the placenta returns to the fetus and is converted to cortisol and aldosterone.

Cortisol preparations administered to the mother only minimally cross the placenta early in gestation because only the unbound cortisol can be transferred to the fetus. In addition, both placenta and fetus have 11β-hydroxysteroid dehydrogenase type 2 (11βHSD2) activity that forms inactive cortisone from cortisol. It has been estimated that the mother contributes approximately 20% of the total fetal cortisol, the balance being secreted by the placental-fetal unit. By contrast the mother contributes about 75% of fetal cortisone. As a consequence,

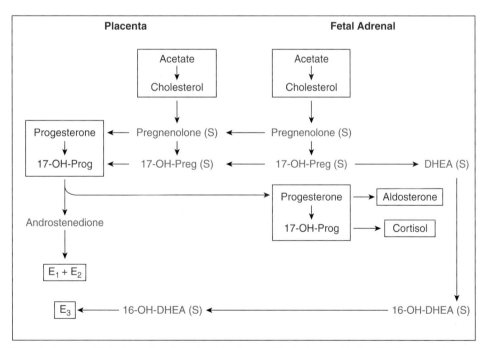

FIGURE 5-7 ■ Biosynthesis of steroids in fetal adrenal gland and in placenta. The fetal adrenal lacks 3β-hydroxysteroid dehydrogenase, and the placenta is rich in this enzyme. Fetal pregnenolone and 17-hydroxypregnenolone are converted to progesterone and 17α-hydroxyprogesterone in the placenta and then returned to the fetal adrenal where they serve as substrates for the formation of cortisol and aldosterone. Note that the substrate for placental estriol is fetal 16-OH DHEA. (S) = sulfate; 17-OHPreg = 17-hydroxypregnenolone; 17-OHProg = 17α-hydroxyprogesterone; DHEA = dehydroepiandrosterone; 16-OHDHEA = 16-hydroxyDHEA; E_1 = estrone; E_2 = estradiol; E_3 = estriol.

when glucocorticoid therapy of the fetus is considered for congenital adrenal hyperplasia, it is necessary to administer a steroid like dexamethasone that does not bind to transcortin and is not readily metabolized.

At mid-pregnancy and at term, the fetal plasma cortisol levels, in the range of 2 mcg/dL, are much lower than in the mother. In contrast, the newborn concentrations of aldosterone are about twice those of the mother.

The relative deficiency of 3β-HSD activity in normal fetal adrenals results in the formation of large amounts of DHEA-S and its 16-hydroxy derivative. The 16-OH-DHEA is transferred into the placenta where sulfatase and aromatase transform 16-OH-DHEA into estriol. Whereas estrone and estradiol arise mainly from placental synthesis, estriol has its main origin in the fetal adrenal (Figure 5-7). This explains why a drop in urinary estriol in pregnancy suggests either abnormal placental function, or poor fetal adrenal function.

Delivery, Birth, and Neonatal Period

Labor and vaginal deliveries are markedly stressful conditions that produce an elevation of maternal plasma cortisol concentrations. As with all forms of stress, the higher cortisol concentration results from both increased secretion and slower clearance. At elective cesarean section, there is little stress for the mother, at least until the infant is delivered. At that time, cortisol concentrations in the mother exceed concentrations of cortisone about tenfold, but in the cord blood and newborn plasma the concentrations are nearly equal. It is only after 3 or 4 weeks of life that the concentrations of cortisol increase in relation to those of cortisone. Furthermore, there is little or no diurnal variation of glucocorticoid concentrations in early infancy, both in preterm and full-term infants.

As noted above, the fetal adrenal cortex lacks sufficient activity of some of the enzymes required for efficient cortisol secretion, but rather functions to provide precursors for sex steroid, which are abundant during gestation. It is not surprising, therefore, that plasma cortisol concentrations in preterm infants, especially in response to stress and illness, are in the range considered "deficient" in full term and older infants. In preterm infants, there is a gestational age-related decrease in inactive cortisone concentrations relative to cortisol, and a lower cortisol and 17-hydroxyprogeterone response to ACTH at less than 30 weeks gestation, when compared to 30 to 33 weeks. The adrenal cortex of preterm infants continues to produce the major products of the fetal cortex, and without the placenta it lacks the substrates needed for sufficient cortisol secretion. The urinary excretion of "fetal zone" steroid metabolites persists until the postconceptual age approaches 40 weeks, thus involution of the fetal zone and

development of the definitive zone is not accelerated by premature birth. In sick preterm infants on ventilators, the cortisol response to ACTH stimulation is lower than in gestational age matched healthier infants.[6]

During the first 10 days of life in full-term infants, the cortisol secretion rate corrected for body size is about 1.5 to 2 times higher than it is later in infancy, childhood, and adulthood (Figure 5-8). In contrast, the aldosterone secretion is the same from infancy to childhood and adulthood. The concentrations of aldosterone in infancy tend to be higher than those observed later on in childhood (Figure 5-9).

Plasma adrenal androgens (DHEA, DHEA-S, androstenedione) and urinary 17-ketosteroids are relatively high shortly after birth but fall to low concentrations after 4 to 6 weeks of age. This decrease in adrenal androgen secretion parallels the involution of the fetal zone of the adrenal cortex. In addition, plasma levels of 17-hydroxyprogesterone are quite high at birth, and for the first 24 hours of life. It is important therefore to obtain a newborn screen sample after 24 hours of age to minimize the risk of a false-positive screen for CAH.

Childhood

During childhood, puberty, and adulthood, cortisol secretion rate corrected for body surface area remains constant, blood cortisol concentrations following their expected diurnal variation (Figure 5-8). Aldosterone secretion rate and plasma concentrations are similar in childhood, puberty, and adulthood (Figure 5-9). In childhood, adrenal androgen secretion is quite low, and urinary 17-ketosteroids are low.

Normal and Premature Adrenarche

In the few years prior to gonadal maturation and puberty, under the stimulation of an as yet uncharacterized CNS-derived substance, there is increased secretion of DHEA, DHEA-S, and androstenedione (Figure 5-10) and this state is called adrenarche. As is seen with the timing of puberty, adrenarche occurs 1 to 2 years earlier in girls than in boys. In both sexes the rise in plasma levels adrenal androgens that is characteristic of adrenarche occurs before physical evidence of androgen effects are noted. At the same time, there is no change in ACTH concentration in blood or cortisol secretion rate corrected for body size. In children with hypopituitarism, a lack of adrenarche is often noted. In some children, adrenal androgen maturation occurs much earlier than gonadal maturation, producing signs of androgen effect long before the expected age. This condition is known as premature adrenarche.

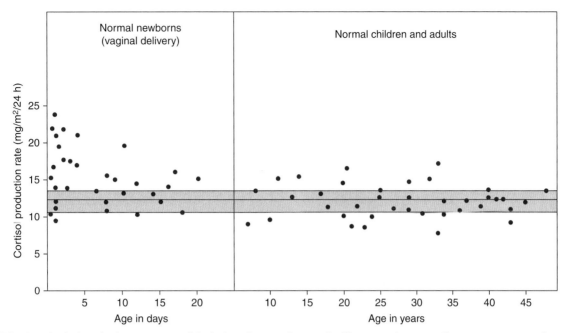

FIGURE 5-8 ■ Cortisol production rate corrected for body surface area in normal subjects at various ages. The rates are constant throughout life except shortly after birth when they are slightly higher. (*Redrawn from Kenny FM, Preeyasombat C, Migeon CJ. Cortisol production rate. II. Normal infants, children and adults. Pediatrics. 1966; 37:34.*)

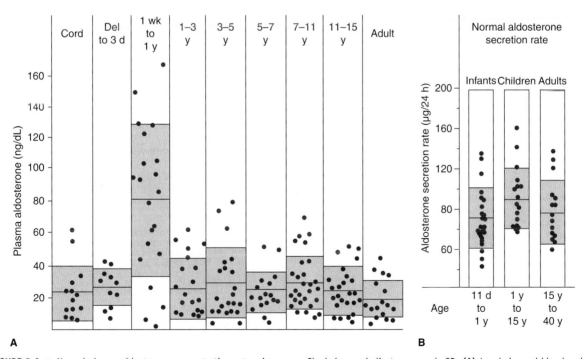

FIGURE 5-9 ■ Normal plasma aldosterone concentrations at various ages. Shaded areas indicate mean +/− SD. **(A)** Levels in cord blood and at delivery were obtained from infants whose mothers had received a normal sodium diet during pregnancy. **(B)** Aldosterone secretion rate in normal infants, children, and adults. In contrast to cortisol secretion rate, which increases with greater body size, aldosterone secretion rate is constant throughout life. (*(A) Redrawn from Kowarski A, Lacerda L, Migeon CJ. Integrated concentration of plasma aldosterone in normal subjects: correlation with cortisol. J Clin Endocrinol Metab. 1975;40:205.* **(B)** *Redrawn from Weldon VV, Kowarski A, Migeon CJ. Aldosterone secretion in normal subjects from infancy to childhood. Pediatrics. 1967;39:829.*)

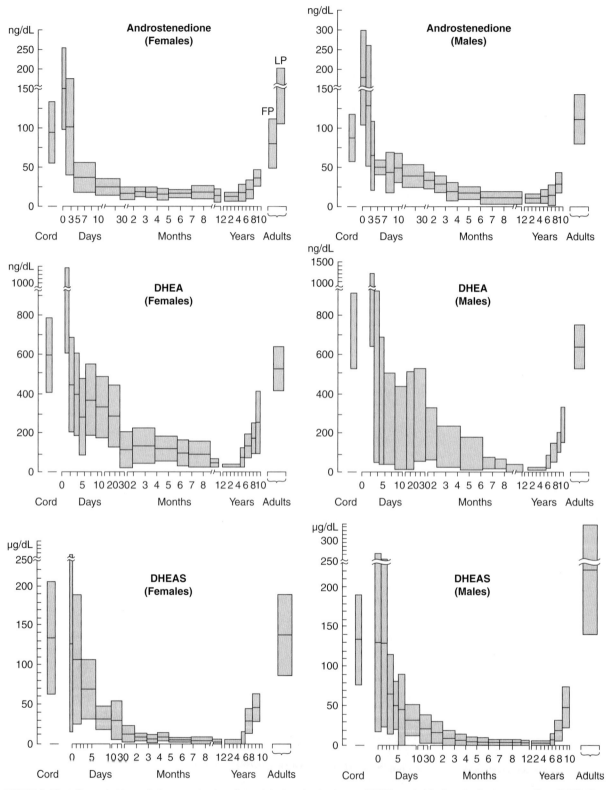

FIGURE 5-10 ■ Concentrations of plasma androstenedione, dehydroepiandrosterone (DHEA), and dehydroepiandrosterone sulfate (DHEA-S) at various ages in male and female subjects. Shaded areas are means ± SD. *(Redrawn from: Forest MG, dePeretti E, Bertrand J. Testicular and adrenal androgens and their binding to plasma proteins in the perinatal period. J Steroid Biochem. 1980;12:25. Forest MG, et al. Hypophysicogonadal function in human beings during the first year of life. J Clin Invest. 1974;53:819.dePeretti E, Forest MG. Unconjugated dehydroepiandrosterone plasma levels in normal subjects from birth to adolescence in humans: the use of a sensitive immunoassay. J Clin Endocrinol Metab. 1978;47:572.)*

Premature adrenarche occurs predominately in girls. It is characterized clinically by the appearance of pubic and/or axillary hair owing to premature adrenal androgen secretion before age 8 years in the absence of breast development. There remains controversy in the actual age that defines "premature" development. In the majority of children with premature adrenarche, the etiology is unknown. Premature sexual hair growth, body odor, and mildly increased height velocity and/or skeletal age are typical. While most children go on to experience normal puberty, some demonstrate abnormal laboratory findings consistent with the metabolic syndrome and (in girls) early signs of polycystic ovary syndrome (ovarian *hyperandrogenism*).[7] It is unknown at this time whether the premature adrenarche itself or its association with high body mass index (BMI) or certain ethnic groups confers the increased risk of insulin resistance and ovarian hyperandrogenism.

Box 5-1 lists the circumstances in which a patient with premature adrenarche should be referred to a pediatric endocrinologist.

Pregnancy

Cortisol—During pregnancy there is an estrogen-stimulated increase in transcortin concentration causing a greater binding capacity for cortisol and a rise in plasma concentrations of total cortisol, as well as an increase in the half-life of the steroid. The unbound cortisol concentrations are also elevated. At the same time, cortisol secretion is decreased during pregnancy, thus replacement therapy in pregnant women with hypoadrenocorticism consists of usual dosages. Labor and delivery, as well as many other types of stress, increase cortisol secretion and plasma cortisol concentrations. For this reason, at the time of labor, cortisol therapy must be increased to stress levels in pregnant women with hypoadrenocorticism.

Aldosterone—Pregnant women have increased plasma renin activity (PRA), plasma aldosterone concentrations, and aldosterone secretion rate. Perhaps the stimulation of the renin-angiotensin-aldosterone system is owing to a salt-losing tendency produced by abundant progesterone. Unlike cortisol, aldosterone does not have a specific binding protein; its binding does not increase significantly during pregnancy and its half-life in blood does not change markedly.

Androgens—It has been observed that maternal DHEA-S concentrations are decreased in pregnancy.

ADRENOCORTICAL FUNCTION IN STRESS

A number of stressful conditions are associated with an increase in adrenocortical secretion of cortisol, secondary to increases in CRH and ACTH output. The increase in cortisol levels with stress is a mediator of the adrenal medullary catecholamine response to stress.

Stress conditions can be classified into *surgical* (trauma, anesthesia, tissue destruction), *medical* (acute illness, infection, fever, hypoglycemia), and *emotional* (psychological). It is not clear whether the mechanism stimulating adrenal function is unique or different for each type of stress.

With regard to infection, hormones of the hypothalamic-pituitary-adrenal axis interact with components of the immune system in a complex manner. The cytokine interleukin-1 (IL-1) is secreted by macrophages in response to microbial invasion, inflammation, immunologic reaction, and tissue injury. IL-1 then activates and increases T cells, accelerates the transformation of B cells into plasma cells, which then produce antibodies. In addition, IL-1 activates the CRH-ACTH-cortisol system; the increased cortisol concentration in plasma results in a negative feedback on the macrophages. Other cytokines including tumor necrosis factor alpha and IL-6, as well as IL-1, stimulate CRH release but are inhibited by cortisol. The endocrine immune system interactions are influenced reciprocally by the autonomic nervous system.[8]

It has also been shown in multiple studies that the products of the *POMC* gene, collectively called melanocortins (ACTH, α-, β-, and γ-melanocyte stimulating hormone or MSH) interact with leukocytes, which contain their specific receptors. These receptors mediate both immunomodulatory and anti-inflammatory effects independent of production of cortisol. In addition, there are central neurogenic anti-inflammatory melanocortin-stimulated signals. These signals utilize both the adrenergic and cholinergic pathways.

Box 5-1.

When to refer: Premature pubic hair development

1. Children who are younger than the typical ages for premature adrenarche (eg, less than 6 years in girls or 8 years in boys).
2. Children who have advanced bone age or rapidly progressive signs of adrenarche.
3. Children who have abnormal elevations of sex steroid or cortisol precursor levels.
4. Children with a family history of congenital adrenal hyperplasia.

CONDITIONS THAT ALTER ADRENOCORTICAL FUNCTION

Obesity

Obesity related to high caloric intake is usually accompanied by an increase in cortisol secretion rate. However, a concomitant decrease in the half-life of cortisol results in normal plasma concentrations. The increased cortisol secretion is reflected in increased urinary 17-OHCS and urinary free cortisol. In most obese subjects correction of the cortisol secretion or urinary 17-OHCS for body surface area or creatinine normalize the values. About 20% of obese subjects have values that remain elevated after correction for body size, and tests to rule out Cushing syndrome may be necessary.

Investigation of cortisol/cortisone metabolism in obesity has resulted in new insights. As described above, the enzyme 11β-HSD type 2 converts cortisol to inactive cortisone mostly in the kidney. The enzyme 11β-HSD type 1 catalyzes the reactivation of cortisone to cortisol mostly in the liver and in adipose tissue. These two enzymes are functionally similar, but are encoded by two different genes on different chromosomes. Several lines of evidence support a role for elevated 11β-HSD type 1 activity as an etiologic factor in *obesity*.[9]

Malnutrition/Anorexia Nervosa

A low calorie or protein intake is associated with elevated plasma cortisol levels. Cortisol response to ACTH stimulation is normal, but response to CRH is blunted. There is probably some degree of cortisol resistance, as these patients are not Cushingoid. Following rehabilitation, plasma cortisol concentrations normalize.

Thyroid Disorders

In general, hypothyroidism results in slower metabolism and hyperthyroidism results in rapid metabolism, including the metabolism of cortisol. Patients with thyroid disorders tend to maintain normal plasma cortisol concentrations by either decreasing cortisol secretion in hypothyroidism or increasing it in hyperthyroidism. It should be noted that cortisol deficiency may be masked by hypothyroidism, and restoring such patients to the euthyroid state may precipitate symptoms of adrenal insufficiency.

Hepatic Disease

The liver extracts a large fraction of plasma steroids for metabolism, usually by reduction and by conjugation to glucuronic acid. Advanced hepatic failure results in decreased cortisol clearance and a prolonged half-life, thus plasma cortisol remains normal. The urinary excretion of 17-OHCS is usually decreased as the technique measures glucuronide metabolites.

Renal Disease

Since large fractions of cortisol and aldosterone metabolites are excreted in urine, renal failure causes lower excretion of steroid metabolites. However, the secretion of cortisol and its plasma concentration usually remains normal. As noted earlier, hyperkalemia in renal failure has a direct effect on increasing aldosterone secretion.

Critical Illness

In patients with normal adrenal responsiveness to the stress of severe infection, plasma cortisol levels will increase three- to tenfold, unless the sepsis has caused bilateral adrenal hemorrhage. In both adults and children with septic shock, an inadequate basal cortisol level and/or an inadequate cortisol response to IV ACTH correlates highly with poor outcome. This adrenal insufficiency during stress is believed to be maladaptive, and results in unchecked actions of cytokines (Figure 5-11). The lessons learned from septic shock have been expanded to include other forms of critical illness. Definite guidelines for diagnosis and treatment of cortisol deficiency in these settings have been established.[10]

Drugs

Dichlorodiphenyltrichloroethane (DDT), its -dichloroethane derivative (DDD) and related compounds such as o,p'-DDD can suppress adrenal cortical function. The latter substance is used in the treatment of adrenal carcinoma with some success, but the drug is often poorly tolerated because of nausea, anorexia, and protracted vomiting.

Another substance, *1,1 bis-(p-aminophenyl)-1-methyl-propanone*, called Amphenone B, can also suppress adrenal function. This compound as well as o,p'-DDD tend to produce a destruction of the cells of the adrenal cortex rather than to specifically inhibit its function.

Aminoglutethimide has been reported to affect both thyroid and adrenal function. In the adrenal cortex it appears to block CYP11A, thereby inhibiting transformation of cholesterol to pregnenolone. Aminoglutethimide also has some effects on CYP11B1.

Metyrapone, also called SU-4885 or metopirone, is a potent inhibitor of CYP11B1 with a milder effect or CYP11A. Metyrapone is used widely as a means of

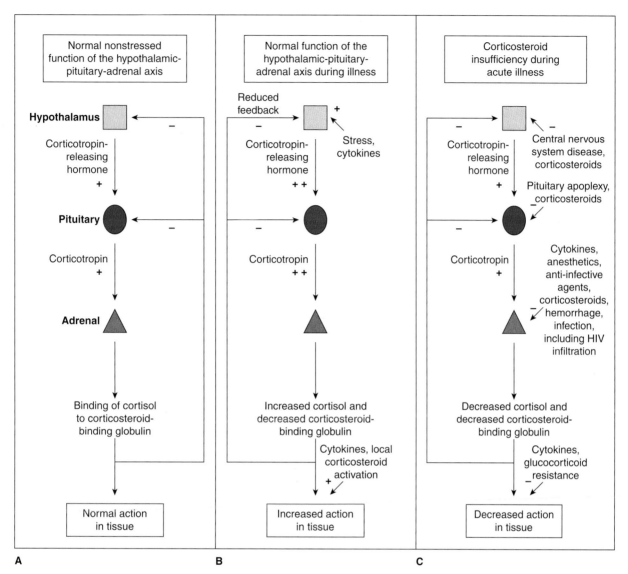

FIGURE 5-11 ■ Activity of the hypothalamic pituitary-adrenal axis under normal conditions **(A)**, during an appropriate response to stress **(B)**, and during an inappropriate response to critical illness **(C)**. A plus sign indicates a stimulatory effect and a minus sign an inhibitory effect. (*Redrawn from Cooper MS, Stewart PM. Corticosteroid insufficiency in acutely ill patients. N Engl J Med. 2003;348(8):727-734. Copyright © 2003 Massachusetts Medical Society. All rights reserved.*)

determining ACTH capacity of the pituitary gland (see "Test Of Anterior Pituitary ACTH Reserve"). It has also been used infrequently to treat Cushing syndrome.

In addition to compounds that have a direct effect on the enzymes involved in the biosynthesis of adrenal steroids, some compounds such as *spironolactone* are aldosterone antagonists at the target cell level. Their effect is related to their ability to compete for the mineralocorticoid receptor. Progesterone and 17-hydroxyprogesterone have similar properties and are therefore considered as mild salt-losing hormones. The antifungal agent ketoconazole is known to generally suppress cytochrome P450 enzyme activity. This is associated

with a blunted cortisol response to ACTH, and thus has a risk of inducing adrenal insufficiency. It has been used therapeutically to suppress adrenal androgen excess in patients with CAH, cortisol excess in Cushing syndrome, and gonadal androgen secretion in boys with precocious puberty.

The progestational agent *megestrol acetate* (Megace), a potent appetite stimulator used in patients with cachexia, may suppress adrenal function through its action at the GR. Through this mechanism, it can activate the negative feedback loop that inhibits ACTH and cortisol secretion. In a few patients on high doses, its interaction with the GR has caused Cushing syndrome.

DIAGNOSTIC EVALUATIONS

Disorders of deficient or excess adrenocortical function can be correctly identified with proper selection of tests of basal hypothalamic-pituitary-adrenal (HPA) function and dynamic tests of HPA axis capacity.

Tests of Glucocorticoid Secretion

Plasma cortisol

The plasma concentrations of total and free cortisol, the main human glucocorticoid, are determined accurately using immunoradiometric assays.

Pulsatile secretion and diurnal variation of cortisol: Because cortisol is secreted in a *pulsatile* manner, small variations can be observed when blood samples are collected at frequent intervals. Changes in the episodic secretion of cortisol with time result in the *diurnal or circadian variation* (rhythm) of plasma cortisol concentrations. There is a surge of secretion between 4 and 6 AM, then the concentrations decrease, being at their lowest in the evening and during the night. Blood ACTH concentrations have a similar diurnal variation. Thus it is important to obtain plasma samples for analysis of basal cortisol or ACTH secretion at standard times, usually 8 AM and/or 4 PM. Stressful situations are likely to raise the ACTH and cortisol concentrations, including anxiety and pain associated with phlebotomy.

The circadian rhythm is related to sleep-wake cycles. Modification of the sleep-wake distribution throughout a 24-hour period changes the profile of cortisol concentrations, as long as the modification is maintained for a sufficient time. The rhythm of cortisol can be altered by strict sleep reversal, but night workers with a variable schedule tend to maintain a normal diurnal rhythm. Blind subjects may also have disturbances of the normal diurnal pattern.[11]

Urinary 17-hydroxycorticosteroids (17-OHCS)

Urinary 17-hydroxycorticosteriods (17-OHCS) concentration is a measure of the excretion of glucocorticoid metabolites. Although the technique to measure 17OHCS is cumbersome and infrequently used at present, it is extremely reliable. The values in normal subjects tend to increase with body size and when these values are corrected for surface area the mean + SD is 2.9 ± 1.2 mg/m^2/24 h.

Urinary free cortisol

Unbound or free plasma cortisol is excreted by the kidney. As only free plasma cortisol is biologically available, the fraction of unbound plasma cortisol that is excreted in urine as free cortisol reflects glucocorticoid activity at the cellular level. Current assays show only 1% to 2% cross-reactivity with some steroids (cortisone, corticosterone, 11-deoxycortisol, and 17-hydroxyprogesterone), but prednisolone has about 30% cross-reactivity.

The range of urinary free cortisol for normal adults is 35 to 120 mcg/24 h. In children, the values are correlated with body size, the range corrected for body surface area being 25 to 65 mcg/m^2/24 h. In Cushing syndrome the concentrations are usually above 150, and in adrenal insufficiency less than 10 mcg/24 h.

Salivary cortisol

Salivary glands and sweat glands excrete only unconjugated, unbound (free) glucocorticoids. The samples can be collected at home in a nonstressful setting. The diurnal pattern of salivary cortisol concentration reflects those of total plasma cortisol, but concentrations are about 90% lower. This is due in part to the metabolism of cortisol to cortisone by the salivary glands. Nighttime salivary cortisol concentrations have been validated as a useful screening test for Cushing syndrome.[12]

Cortisol production rate

Knowledge of the cortisol production rates in normal subjects forms the basis for cortisol replacement dosage recommendations in patients with adrenal insufficiency. In normal subjects of various ages, cortisol production increases with body size. When the values were corrected for body surface area, the average $\pm$ SD was 12.1 ± 1.5/m^2/24 h (Figure 5-8). In the first week of life the values are somewhat greater than those of the children and adults, coming down to that range after 3 to 4 weeks of age. In children older than infants and toddlers, the cortisol production rate is estimated at 6.8 ± 1.9 mg/m^2/24 h.[13,14]

ACTH

Plasma ACTH can be measured accurately by immunoassay in plasma. As with cortisol, it is important to standardize the time at which blood samples are collected, usually at 8 AM and 4 PM. At 8 AM, normal individuals have concentrations ranging from 20 to 120 pg/mL. Plasma ACTH values in the evening range from 0 to 50 pg/mL. Because cortisol has a negative feedback on ACTH secretion, when cortisol concentrations are elevated those of ACTH tend to decrease, and reciprocally. For this reason, it is often helpful to measure simultaneously the cortisol and ACTH concentrations.

Dexamethasone, a potent glucocorticoid, when administered to normal subjects, will have a negative feedback on plasma ACTH and cortisol resulting in extremely low values. In contrast, the administration of metyrapone, an inhibitor of 11β-hydroxylase, results in a decrease of cortisol concomitant with a marked increase of plasma ACTH.

CRH

Assay techniques for the measurement of CRH concentration are available, but determining its concentration in plasma is not often useful. Since CRH reaches the anterior pituitary corticotrophs via a portal system of vessels, it is not surprising that studies of CRH in peripheral circulation have not been very fruitful. It is probable that there is a diurnal variation of CRH in the pituitary portal vessels, but a diurnal pattern has not been observed in plasma.

Tests of adrenocortical capacity[15]

ACTH stimulation tests. After prolonged loss of ACTH secretion, such as in Cushing syndrome or hypopituitarism, the adrenal cortex can become resistant to its stimulatory effect. The rapid IV ACTH test is often employed to screen for ACTH deficiency in such patients. In this setting, either a low dose (0.1-1 mcg) or high dose (250 mcg) test has been employed. The 250 mcg test is more widely employed, and the cortisol response 30 to 60 minutes after injection should peak at or above 20 mcg/dL to rule out adrenal insufficiency. The 1 mcg test, though, may be more sensitive in detecting milder degrees of adrenal gland function suppression. However, the cortisol response to insulin-induced hypoglycemia remains the gold standard.

In the intensive care setting, screening for relative adrenal insufficiency involves measurement of blood cortisol before and 30 to 60 minutes after 250 mcg of IV ACTH. In this stressful setting, basal levels of cortisol should normally exceed 30 mcg/dL; if less than 15 mcg/dL, and if the cortisol concentration does not rise by at least 9 mcg/dL over baseline values that are less than 30, then relative adrenal insufficiency is suspected.

Tests of anterior pituitary ACTH reserve

Metyrapone. Metyrapone (Metopirone) inhibits CYP11B1 activity in the adrenal cortex, resulting in decreased secretion of cortisol and corticosterone. This produces an increase of ACTH secretion. Then 11-deoxycortisol (Compound S) and 11-deoxycorticosterone (DOC) are produced in large quantities, and their levels can be directly measured in plasma, or their metabolites can be measured as urinary 17-OHCS. The blood levels are preferred. A single oral dose of Metyrapone (300 mg/m² per dose) is administered at midnight. The next day at 8 AM a plasma sample is obtained for the measurement of plasma 11-deoxycortisol (compound S; the normal response showing a value of 7-22 mcg/dL) and ACTH.

The administration of Metyrapone also reduces the secretion of aldosterone, which is partially corrected by increased DOC secretion. In contrast, cortisol deficiency is not compensated by 11-deoxycortisol, which is a very weak glucocorticoid. For this reason, it is recommended to avoid administrating Metyrapone to patients who are known to have primary hypoadrenocorticism, because of the risk of precipitating an adrenal crisis.

CRH stimulation test. Another method to determine the pituitary reserve is the IV administration of ovine CRH (100 mcg per dose). Following the dose, the plasma ACTH

increases from approximately 8 to 25 ng/dL with a concomitant increase of plasma cortisol. The ACTH response to CRH may be useful in the evaluation of patients with suspected Cushing disease, and may help in the differentiation of Cushing from pseudoCushing syndrome. Normative data now exist for ACTH response to CRH test in very low birth weight infants, in whom antenatal maternal corticosteroid treatment may induce adrenal suppression.

Insulin tolerance test. Hypoglycemia is a potent stimulus for ACTH secretion. At 8 AM after an overnight fast, 0.05 to 0.075 units/kg regular insulin is given by IV injection. Serum glucose and cortisol are measured at baseline and every 15 minutes for 1 hour. A normal response is seen if the 8 AM baseline cortisol concentration is within the expected reference range, and the level doubles or rises over 20 mcg/dL with hypoglycemia. Basal cortisol and the insulin tolerance test (ITT) are thought to be more accurate for detection of hypothalamic-pituitary-adrenal axis deficiency than is the CRH test or the low-dose (1 mcg) ACTH test; however it is contraindicated in some patients such as infants.[15]

The pituitary (dexamethasone) suppression test. The basis for this test is the negative feedback regulation of cortisol on ACTH secretion. Administration of a potent glucocorticoid, such as dexamethasone, suppresses ACTH secretion and secondarily decreases cortisol secretion. There are several types of dexamethasone suppression tests. One method uses a single nighttime dose followed by measurement of 8 AM cortisol. More prolonged "low dose" and "high dose" tests last several days and are followed by measurement of plasma ACTH and cortisol. The test is useful in the evaluation of patients with suspected Cushing disease (Table 5-2). Dexamethasone administration may also be useful in differentiating whether hyperandrogenemia in a female results from adrenal or gonadal secretion, the latter not being sensitive to ACTH suppression.

Tests of Mineralocorticoid Secretion

Nonspecific tests, such as electrolytes in serum and in urine, as well as occasionally in sweat and saliva, can be of importance in the diagnosis abnormalities in mineralocorticoid secretion or action. However, precise immunoassays for aldosterone and PRA provide a direct assessment of mineralocorticoid secretion.

Plasma aldosterone

Plasma concentrations of aldosterone follow a circadian variation that is similar to but less marked than that of cortisol. Aldosterone concentrations change slowly in relation to sodium intake (24-48 hours of low or high sodium intake). In contrast, changes in body position (standing versus lying down) bring about rapid but unsustained variation in aldosterone concentrations.

Table 5-2.

Dexamethasone Suppression Tests for the Evaluation of Hypercortisolism

Overnight Test:
20 mcg/kg dexamethasone PO (up to 1.0 mg[a]) at 2300, with
  serum cortisol level at 0800 the following morning
  Normal response: 0800 cortisol <5 mcg/dL rules against
    Cushing Syndrome[b,c]

Low Dose Test:
48 hour, 2 mg/d (0.5 mg PO q6 h)
  Normal response: 0800 cortisol level obtained 2 hours after
    the last dose of dexamethasone ≤1.8 mcg/dL rules against
    Cushing syndrome[d]
48 h, 2 mg/d test combined with CRH stimulation test at
  0800, 2 hours after the last dose of dexamethasone
  Normal response: serum cortisol <1.4 mcg/dL, 15 min
    after CRH 1 mcg/kg IV (or 100 mcg IV in adults) rules against
    Cushing syndrome

High Dose Test for Differential Diagnosis of ACTH-dependent Cushing Syndrome[e]:
48 hour, 8 mg/day (2 mg dexamethasone PO q6 hours)
  Suppression of urinary 17-OHCS by >50% consistent with
    pituitary source of ACTH
Overnight test (8 mg dexamethasone PO at 2300)
  Serum cortisol at 0800 the mornings before and after show
    suppression of serum cortisol by >50% suggests pituitary
    source of ACTH

[a] The use of a 1.5 or 2.0 mg dose offers no better discrimination between the presence and absence of Cushing syndrome.
[b] There are some patients with Cushing Syndrome whose serum cortisol will suppress to <5 mcg/dL. A cut-off of ≤1.8 mcg/dL effectively excludes all cases of Cushing syndrome.
[c] Some suggest simultaneous measurement of a dexamethasone level to assure compliance if the testing is performed as a outpatient.
[d] The original report of GW Liddle (Tests of pituitary-adrenal suppressibility in the diagnosis of Cushing syndrome. J Clin Endocrinol Metab. 20:1539, 1960) described suppression of urinary 17-hydroxycorticosteroid excretion as the expected outcome.
[e] This test is utilized after excess ACTH has been demonstrated. It has been largely replaced by high resolution radiologic studies, bilateral inferior petrosal sampling, and CRH stimulation testing.

In early infancy, plasma aldosterone concentrations are quite variable, but in general are elevated relative to older children and adults, as seen in Figure 5-9. After 1 year of age and up into adulthood, the mean values remain constant, although there are still large individual variations.

Aldosterone secretion rate

Aldosterone secretion rate is relatively constant throughout life, and this forms the basis for the recommended replacement doses of 9α-fluorocortisol in patients with mineralocorticoid deficiency being similar throughout childhood and adulthood. There are slighter lower values observed during the first 2 weeks after birth, but the blood levels of aldosterone are higher (Figure 5-9). Changes in sodium diet influence the aldosterone secretion rate as well as plasma concentrations of this steroid.

Plasma renin

Plasma renin activity. The PRA is measured by the rate of release of angiotensin II from the renin substrate angiotensinogen. The angiotensin II being formed is measured by immunoassay and the PRA is expressed as angiotensin II formed in pg/mL of plasma. PRA shows an episodic variation as well as a mild diurnal variation. On an average sodium intake in the PRA is 10 to 50 pg/mL/h. Concentrations increase markedly during a low sodium diet and are suppressed by a high sodium diet.

Direct renin measurement. Direct determination of renin concentration in the plasma is made with a specific immunoassay. The normal ranges vary based on sodium intake, posture, and age. There is some question as to whether this test is as useful as the PRA for many clinical applications.

Tests of Adrenal Androgen Secretion

Clinical signs may suggest hypersecretion of androgens, and lead to the measurement of their concentration in blood. In the prepubertal male, they include increase in size of the penis, appearance of pigmentation and thinning of the scrotum, presence of pubic, axillary, and facial hair, and deepening of the voice. In the female, they include premature pubarche, enlargement of the clitoris, deepening of the voice, disruption of menstrual cycling, and hirsutism.

Plasma androgens

As previously mentioned, the main adrenal androgens include androstenedione, DHEA and DHEA-S (Figure 5-6). These steroids do not bind to the androgen receptor and therefore have negligible biological activity. However, 5% to 10% of DHEA is converted to androstenedione, and a similar fraction of androstenedione is converted to testosterone.

Adrenal androgens have very little significance in adult males but they contribute about 75% of the testosterone in adult women. The life cycle of plasma concentrations of adrenal androgens is shown in Figure 5-10. The concentration of DHEA-S in plasma is the best indicator of adrenarche during pubertal maturation. As mentioned above, among hormonal steroids in human plasma DHEA-S has by far the highest concentrations, owing to its long half-life.

Urinary 17-ketosteroids

Androgens, whether secreted by the adrenals or the gonads, are partially metabolized into 19-carbon steroids with a 17-ketone and are excreted as urinary 17-ketosteroids. About one-third of testosterone produced in the body is excreted in the urine as 17-ketosteroids. The normal values are quite low before puberty (<2 mg/24 h), compared with adolescence and adulthood. Normal values in adults are higher in males than females (7-17 mg/24 h vs 4-13 mg/24 h). Although most providers prefer to measure specific plasma androgens, the determination of urinary 17-ketosteroids can still be useful in specific situations, such as when phlebotomy is not feasible or assessment of 24-hour integrated adrenal androgen production is warranted.

CLINICAL PRESENTATIONS AND MANAGEMENT

Hypoadrenocorticism

The syndromes of hypoadrenocorticism can be classified on the basis of whether the disorder is intrinsic to the adrenal cortex (primary hypoadrenocorticism), owing to CRH/ACTH deficiency (central or secondary hypoadrenocorticism), or owing to unresponsiveness to trophic or adrenocortical hormones (Table 5-3).

The signs and symptoms of adrenocortical insufficiency vary, depending upon the hormones that are deficient (Table 5-4), as well as those that are in excess (eg, androgens) in patients with synthetic defects of cortisol and aldosterone. The clinical features of chronic hypoadrenocorticism may be influenced by other symptoms resulting from the autoimmune polyglandular syndromes (Table 5-5).

The treatment of adrenal insufficiency consists of hormone replacement therapy. In primary adrenal insufficiency, both glucocorticoid and mineralocorticoid treatment is usually needed. This group of patients is at risk for a salt-losing crisis at the time of diagnosis or during times of stress. In isolated cortisol deficiency (eg, owing to ACTH deficiency or resistance), only glucocorticoid treatment is needed. In all patients, the dose of glucocorticoid must be increased during times of stress. A detailed description of treatment protocols is given below.

Primary hypoadrenocorticism

Based on physiology and embryology, these abnormalities can be classified as follows (Table 5-3). First, there may be lack of differentiation of adrenal cortex resulting in *congenital adrenal aplasia or hypoplasia.* An example of this is X-linked adrenal hypoplasia. Next, abnormalities of the membrane receptors for ACTH or Angiotensin II

Table 5-3.

Classification of Syndromes of Hypoadrenocorticism

Primary Adrenocortical Insufficiency
Congenital adrenal aplasia
X-linked adrenal hypoplasia congenita (AHC) due to DAX-1 defect
Adrenal hypoplasia due to SF-1 defect
Congenital adrenal hyperplasia owing to CYP21 deficiency
Congenital adrenal hyperplasia owing to CYP11B1 deficiency
Congenital adrenal hyperplasia owing to CYP17 deficiency
Congenital adrenal hyperplasia owing to 3βHSD 2 deficiency
Congenital adrenal hyperplasia owing to CYP11A or StAR deficiency
Congenital adrenal hyperplasia owing to P450 oxidoreductase (POR) deficiency
Adrenoleukodystrophy/adrenomyeloneuropathy
Wolman disease (acid lipase deficiency)
Steroid sulfatase deficiency (X-linked ichthyosis) Smith-Lemli Opitz Syndrome
Mineralocorticoid deficiency owing to CMOI or CMOII (CYP11B2) defect
Chronic hypoadrenocorticism (Addison disease)

Secondary to Deficient ACTH Secretion
Panhypopituitarism or multiple anterior pituitary hormone deficiencies
Isolated ACTH deficiency (eg, owing to TPIT or POMC defect)
Cessation of pharmacologic glucocorticoid treatment
Resection of unilateral cortisol-secreting tumor
Infants born to steroid-treated mothers

Secondary to End-Organ Unresponsiveness
Pseudohypoaldosteronism (mineralocorticoid resistance)
ACTH resistance
Cortisol resistance

may results in lack of adequate cortisol (eg, *congenital unresponsiveness to ACTH)* or aldosterone secretion, respectively. The next level of defects includes steroidogenic abnormalities, such as those affecting formation of cortisol (*congenital adrenal hyperplasia*) or aldosterone (*CMOI and CMOII deficiencies owing to aldosterone synthase defects*). Conditions altering the availability of cholesterol for steroidogenesis may also occur, and examples of these are *adrenoleukodystrophy, adrenomyeloneuropathy (AMN), Wolman disease, and steroid sulfatase deficiency or X-linked ichthyosis.* Finally, normal adrenal glands can be damaged or destroyed by extrinsic factors, such as is the case in *bilateral adrenal hemorrhage of the newborn, adrenal hemorrhage of acute infection, and Addison disease.*

Congenital aplasia or hypoplasia of the adrenal glands. This is a rare condition considered to be a congenital malformation owing to a developmental disorder of the adrenal anlage. Clinically it is manifested

Table 5-4.

Signs and Symptoms of Adrenal Insufficiency

Glucocorticoid Deficiency	Mineralocorticoid Deficiency	Adrenal Androgen Deficiency*
Fasting hypoglycemia	Weight loss	Decreased pubic and axillary hair
Increased insulin sensitivity	Fatigue	Decreased libido
Decreased gastric acidity	Nausea, vomiting, anorexia	
Nausea, vomiting	Salt-craving	
Fatigue	Hypotension	
Muscle weakness	Hyperkalemia, hyponatremia, metabolic acidosis with normal anion gap	

Increased Melanocyte Stimulating Hormone
Hyperpigmentation

Seen only in female patients at or after puberty

Table 5-5.

Features of Autoimmune Polyglandular Syndromes (APS) Associated with Chronic Hypoadrenocorticism

	Type I	Type II[a]
General		
Prevalence	Rare	Not as rare as type 1
Age at onset	Infancy/young childhood	Adolescence/adulthood
Inheritance	Autosomal recessive	Dominant
Gender predominance	None	Female
Cause	AIRE gene mutations	Polygenic/multifactorial
HLA association	None	HLA DR/DQ association
Hormonal Abnormalities		
Hypoparathyroidism	>80%	Rare
Addison disease	>60%	Common but variable[b]
Hypogonadism	>30%	<10%
Autoimmune thyroid disease	<10%	>70%
Type 1 diabetes	<20%	40%-50%
Hypopituitarism	Uncommon	Rare
Other Clinical Features		
Mucocutaneous candidiasis	80%-100%	Not seen
Ectodermal dysplasia	>75%	Not seen
Alopecia	25%-30%	<10%
Pernicious anemia	10%-15%	Variable
Autoimmune hepatitis	10%-15%	Rare
Intestinal malabsorption	10%-25%	Rare
Vitiligo	10%	<10%
Asplenism	Uncommon	Not seen
Keratoconjunctivitis	Uncommon	Rare

[a] *APS types 2, 3, and 4 have also been described. APS type 3 consists of autoimmune thyroid disease associated with one or more autoimmune diseases other than Addison disease. Its prevalence is increased in Down syndrome, Turner syndrome, and Klinefelter syndrome. APS type 4 consists of any two autoimmune-affected organ diseases in a combination not included in types 1, 2, or 3, or associated with nonorgan-specific autoimmune disease.*
[b] *The association of Addison disease with autoimmune thyroid disease is known as Schmidt syndrome. When type 1 diabetes is added, the triad is known as Carpenter syndrome.*

Data adapted from the following references:

Brown RS. The autoimmune polyglandular syndromes. Serono Symposia International, Inc. Curr Rev Pediatr Endocrinol. 2003;51-58.

Neufeld M, Maclaren NK, Blizzard RM. Two types of autoimmune Addison syndrome associated with different polyglandualr autoimmune (PGA) syndromes. Medicine. 1981; 60:355.

Schatz DA, Winter WE. Autoimmune polyglandular syndrome II: Clinical syndrome and treatment. Endocrinol Metab Clin N Am. 2002;31:937.

very early in life by vomiting and diarrhea with hyponatremia, hyperkalemia, and hypoglycemia. Shortly thereafter, the affected children present an acute shock with tachycardia, hyperpyrexia, apnea, cyanosis and eventually seizure, vascular collapse, and coma. It is difficult to differentiate this condition from septicemia, intracranial hemorrhage, or other serious illness. For this reason it is often diagnosed at autopsy. Careful pathological studies have often revealed small amounts of adrenal tissue either in its usual location or associated with the gonads, or scattered throughout the peritoneum. If some adrenal tissue is found, the condition may be attributed to one of the other syndromes described later on.

The *X-linked form of congenital adrenal hypoplasia* is also known as adrenal hypoplasia congenita (AHC). In this condition, both cortisol and aldosterone secretion are impaired. It is described as cytomegalic adrenal hypoplasia because of the histological appearance of the adrenal cortex in patients studied at autopsy. X-linked AHC most often presents in the newborn period (1-4 weeks) with signs and symptoms of a salt-losing crisis. However, affected patients may have variable degrees of adrenocortical development, therefore some patients may not have symptoms of adrenocortical insufficiency until later in childhood.

X-linked AHC generally occurs with hypogonadotrophic hypogonadism. Mutations of DAX-1 (dosage-sensitive sex reversal adrenal hypoplasia on the X chromosome gene 1) cause combined AHC and HH in affected males. In some patients, there is a contiguous gene syndrome owing to a deletion including DAX-1 (discussed later on in the chapter), dystrophin (causing Duchenne muscular dystrophy [DMD]) and the glycerol kinase gene (causing juvenile glycerol kinase deficiency [GKD]). The patients with this complex (DMD, AHC, and GKD) also have a characteristic phenotype that may include short stature, mental retardation, testicular abnormalities (cryptorchidism, hypogonadism), and peculiar facies (drooping mouth, wide-set eyes).

Congenital defects in adrenocortical development may also be due to mutations of the SF-1 gene. This syndrome may include male to female sex reversal, as is seen in SF-1 knockout mice. Females with primary adrenal failure and SF-1 mutations have normal genitalia. Mutations of SF-1 may also lead to DSD (disorders of sex development) without *adrenal insufficiency*.[16]

Treatment of congenital adrenal hypoplasia or aplasia consists of replacement therapy for both mineralocorticoid and glucocorticoid deficiencies (see the section "Principles of Treatment").

Adrenocortical unresponsiveness to ACTH. The pathogenesis of this disorder is an inability of the zona fasciculata and reticularis to produce cortisol in response to ACTH stimulation. By contrast the zona glomerulosa secretes aldosterone normally. The defect is owing to a genetic abnormality of the ACTH receptor (also known as the MC2R or melanocortin 2 receptor). This condition is distinct from adrenal unresponsiveness to ACTH owing to developmental, autoimmune, or infectious causes.

Clinically, the patients present early in life with feeding problems, vomiting and failure to thrive, and occasionally with hypoglycemia. There is also hyperpigmentation of the skin, as is seen in Addison disease. Laboratory evaluation reveals low glucose with normal electrolytes, and cortisol secretion is below normal but not absent. Aldosterone secretion is normal. Plasma ACTH levels are markedly elevated. There is evidence to suggest that there are two modes of inheritance of this disorder: X-linked recessive and autosomal recessive. Over 30 cases of what is also known as Migeon syndrome have been reported, but some of these patients probably had a different disease. Some had sodium loss suggesting primary adrenal disease, and others presented with neurological symptoms suggesting adrenoleukodystrophy (discussed later on in the chapter).

The association of ACTH-resistant cortisol deficiency with achalasia and absent lacrimation is known as the triple A syndrome. Patients present with hypoglycemia and severe feeding difficulties. There is also evidence of defects of both the sympathetic and the central nervous system (CNS). The defective gene in this autosomal recessive disorder is the *ALADIN* gene (**Al**acrima-**A**chalasia-**Ad**renal **I**nsufficiency **N**eurologic Disorder), a member of the WD-repeat family of regulatory proteins.[17]

Congenital adrenal hyperplasia
CAH owing to deficiency of CYP21. Of the many defects of adrenal steroidogenesis, the greatest progress has been made in our understanding of CYP21 deficiency. This reflects the fact that CYP21 deficiency is the most common cause of disorders of steroidogenesis, and that the location of its gene (CYP21) within the HLA complex on human chromosome 6 makes it highly susceptible to mutation through recombination. The molecular basis for the majority of cases of CYP21 deficiency is now established. Moreover, studies have provided a correlation between severity of the clinical disorder and the effect of specific mutations on enzymatic activity. The clinical management of this disease was the subject of an international consensus statement.[18]

CYP21 deficiency is often divided into three forms, depending on the initial presentation. Two of these forms, which reflect severe deficiencies in CYP21 activity, present early in life. The most severe impairment in enzyme activity results in the salt-losing form of CAH. Male patients with this form present with acute adrenal crisis in the neonatal period or early infancy and are designated as having the *salt-losing form*. Females with the salt-losing form are usually detected at birth due to ambiguity of the external genitalia. Female patients who have milder masculinization of the external genitalia but no evidence of acute adrenal crisis, or males who show signs of androgen excess early in life, are considered to have the *simple virilizing form*. The identification of cases by newborn screening has in many cases blurred the distinction between these two forms, as cases are often identified before the salt-losing process is clinically significant.

The *attenuated form* (also called "late-onset" or "nonclassical") is manifested essentially only in female patients. At puberty or shortly thereafter, evidence of mild androgen excess develops, including hirsutism, amenorrhea, and infertility. In males, the mild androgen excess is typically undetectable, as the effects of testicular testosterone far outweigh the masculinizing effects of adrenal androgens. Newborn screening will detect some of these cases, which may lead to confusion about the timing and necessity of treatment.

Individual patients with the various forms of CYP21 deficiency represent a continuum of clinical manifestations secondary to impaired adrenal production of cortisol which reflect the spectrum of underlying genetic mutation variability.[19]

Simple virilizing form of CYP21 deficiency

Pathogenesis

Decreased in cortisol secretion—A decrease in cortisol secretion reduces negative feedback at the hypothalamic-pituitary level, which leads to increased secretion of CRH and ACTH. High concentrations of plasma ACTH cause the adrenocortical hyperplasia characteristic of the syndrome. Since CYP21 deficiency is not complete in the simple virilizing form, the increased ACTH activity is capable of restoring cortisol secretion to an approximately normal rate.

Increased secretion of cortisol precursors—The increased ACTH concentration required to normalize cortisol secretion markedly elevates production of cortisol precursors. As shown in Figure 5-3, the immediate precursor, which reaches the highest plasma concentration, is 17-hydroxyprogesterone. There is also increased secretion of progesterone and 17-hydroxypregnenolone. The androgen synthetic pathway is not affected by the enzyme deficiency, thus androstenedione production is high because to the ample substrate availability.

Increased activity of the renin-angiotensin-aldosterone system—The major precursor of cortisol, 17-hydroxyprogesterone, has limited biologic activity in normal subjects. In excess, it produces sodium loss and potassium retention, and this is accompanied by water loss. To compensate, a greater amount of angiotensin II is formed. In salt-losing CAH, the marked deficiency in CYP21 does not permit the secretion of aldosterone. In the simple virilizing form of CAH, the partial deficiency permits increased secretion of aldosterone, which produces a normal sodium balance.

Increased secretion of androgens—In normal subjects, the concentration of ACTH in blood is inadequate to stimulate the secretion of adrenal androgens. In CAH, the ACTH hypersecretion, combined with the enzymatic block, causes an elevated secretion of androstenedione, DHEA, and DHEA-S. These adrenal androgens lack significant intrinsic biologic activity, as they do not bind to the androgen receptor. Androstenedione is metabolized peripherally into testosterone, as described earlier, and this is responsible for the symptoms of androgen excess characteristic of CAH.

Clinical manifestations. Patients with simple virilizing CAH have increased ACTH secretion resulting in normal plasma cortisol concentrations, and there are no symptoms of glucocorticoid deficiency. The salt-losing tendency caused by 17-hydroxyprogesterone is compensated by increased aldosterone levels. Therefore, these patients do not normally have electrolyte abnormalities.

Secretion of excess androgens produces different symptoms in males and females. Increased androgen production starts early in fetal life, between 6 and 10 weeks of gestation. In the female fetus, this results in variable degrees of posterior fusion of the labia, and hypertrophy of the clitoris. The labial fusion often results in formation of a urogenital sinus located at the base of the phallus. The degree of masculinization of the external genitalia of the female fetuses is usually classified as described by Prader (Figure 5-12). Despite the virilized appearance of the external genitalia, the uterus and fallopian tubes are normal. In the male fetus, testicular androgens carry out the normal masculinization of the external genitalia, and the addition of adrenal androgens has minimal or no effect.

Later in life, hypersecretion of androgens in either sex causes early appearance of pubic hair, usually between 6 months and 2 years of age. This is followed by early appearance of axillary hair between 2 and 4 years of age, and facial hair between 8 and 14 years of age. Acne and deepening of the voice will also occur. The anabolic effect of elevated adrenal androgens in infancy and early childhood causes rapid skeletal maturation.

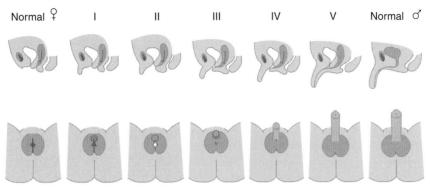

Normal ♀   I   II   III   IV   V   Normal ♂

FIGURE 5-12 ■ Typing of the degree of virilization of the external genitalia of females as proposed by Prader (1958). In type I, the only abnormality is a slight enlargement of the clitoris. In type V, there is a markedly enlarged phallus with a penile urethra. (*Redrawn from Prader A. Vollkommen mannliche usBere Genitalwickling und Salzverlustsyndrom bei Madchen mit kongenitalem adrenogenitalem Syndrom.* Helv Paediat Acta. 1958;13:5.)

Bone age and height age may become markedly advanced. Premature closure of the epiphyses will result in short adult stature in untreated or inadequately treated patients.

In males, the anabolic effects of adrenal androgens generally result in advanced somatic growth and skeletal age, enlargement of the penis, and development of pubic hair; however, the testes remain small. If a patient's skeletal age is advanced to that of a child of pubertal age, suppression of adrenal androgen secretion with glucocorticoid therapy may be followed by the onset of true gonadotropin-mediated precocious puberty. This would result in the need to treat both the CAH and the true precocious puberty.

In females, the hypersecretion of adrenal androgens interferes with the maturation of the hypothalamic-pituitary-ovarian axis. With complete suppression of adrenal androgen secretion patients may have normal puberty and menstruation. Females may also be at risk for the development of true precocious puberty if inadequate or delayed therapy results in significant advancement of skeletal age prior to the initiation of treatment.

In males, one can frequently observe hypertrophic adrenal rests located either in the body of the testes, near the epididymus, or in the spermatic cord. Such findings reflect the fact that adrenal rests are frequent in the normal population but are detected only when they are hypertrophic. These rests have been associated with infertility. Females also may have adrenal rests, usually in the broad ligament and, on occasion, in the ovary.

Laboratory diagnosis. Increased plasma concentrations of specific cortisol precursors and adrenal androgens are characteristic of CAH owing to CYP21 deficiency. As already noted, the main elevated cortisol precursor is 17-hydroxyprogesterone and to a lesser extent, progesterone, and 17-hydroxypregnenolone. In addition, androstenedione, DHEA, DHEA-S, and to a lesser degree, testosterone concentrations will be elevated. Urinary excretion of 17-ketosteroids, the metabolites of adrenal androgens, will be markedly elevated. The elevation of the plasma concentrations of ACTH is often difficult to demonstrate. As discussed secretion of cortisol is normal and that of aldosterone is increased in untreated patients.

Positive and differential diagnosis. In female patients, the diagnosis of simple virilizing CAH is made by the presence of ambiguous external genitalia with 46,XX karyotype and markedly increased concentrations of 17-hydroxyprogesterone and androstenedione that return to normal under glucocorticoid suppressive therapy. Ambiguous external genitalia and a 46,XX karyotype can also be seen in infants without CAH who have been masculinized either by maternal androgens (virilizing adrenal or ovarian tumor of the mother), by maternal ingestion of androgenic preparations, or by excessive gonadal secretion of androgen such as seen in patients with ovotestes.

In milder cases of simple virilizing CAH, the masculinization of the external genitalia of the newborn female can be minimal and unnoticed at birth. In such patients, the first symptom is usually the appearance of pubic hair between 6 months and 2 years of age. The differential diagnosis includes virilizing adrenal or ovarian tumor, and premature adrenarche if the child is older. In virilizing adrenal tumors, the main androgens secreted are DHEA and DHEA-S, and to a lesser degree, androstenedione; in contrast, 17-hydroxyprogesterone concentrations are normal or only slightly elevated. A dexamethasone-suppression test will fail to suppress the adrenal androgens from a virilizing tumor. The diagnosis is confirmed by a computed tomography (CT) or magnetic resonance imaging (MRI) scan of the abdomen showing a mass in one of the adrenal glands.

In premature adrenarche, one observes an increase of DHEA and DHEA-S as well as androstenedione above the low level expected in prepubertal children, but never above the concentration observed in normal adults. In addition, the concentration of 17-hydroxyprogesterone is normal in premature adrenarche.

In male infants, the diagnosis of simple virilizing CYP21 deficiency is usually missed at birth in the absence of a newborn screen for CAH. The diagnosis is considered only after premature appearance of pubic hair later in life, along with advanced bone and height ages. The testes remain prepubertal in size. The diagnosis of CAH is confirmed by high plasma concentrations of 17-hydroxyprogesterone and androstenedione, or by elevated urinary excretion of 17-ketosteroids. The differential diagnosis of early pubic hair in a boy includes complete central precocious puberty of idiopathic origin, or a benign or malignant gonadal or adrenal tumor. In sexual precocity, the androgen responsible for the masculinization is testosterone; the concentrations of androstenedione, DHEA, and DHEA-S, on the other hand, are only slightly elevated above the prepubertal concentration but not higher than the values found in normal adults. In true precocious puberty (gonadotropin-mediated), the testes enlarge as opposed to the small testes typical of CAH. Sexual precocity can also be related to a human chorionic gonadotropin-producing tumor such as a dysgerminoma or hepatoma, to a testosterone-secreting unilateral Leydig-cell tumor, or to a virilizing adrenal tumor. Leydig-cell tumors usually can be palpated in one of the testes; a sonogram of the scrotum confirms the presence of the lesion. Leydig-cell tumors produce mainly testosterone, in contrast to virilizing adrenal tumors, which produce DHEA-S and DHEA.

Salt-losing form of CYP21 deficiency

Pathogenesis. The pathogenesis of the salt-losing form of CAH owing to CYP21 deficiency is similar to that of the simple virilizing form. The only difference is that the CYP21 deficiency is more severe or even complete. Hence, secretion of cortisol may be very low. In addition, the adrenal cortex cannot secrete sufficient aldosterone to respond to the salt-losing tendency created by the overproduction of 17-hydroxyprogesterone. This results in an acute adrenal or salt-losing crisis, which will be described below. Simultaneously, the severe reduction of cortisol results in a maximal activity of the CRH-ACTH axis, inducing maximal secretion of adrenal androgens and near total masculinization of the external genitalia in females.

Clinical manifestations. In female infants, attention is attracted first to the markedly ambiguous genitalia. The degree of virilization is related to the severity of the enzyme defect. The masculinization may be so extreme

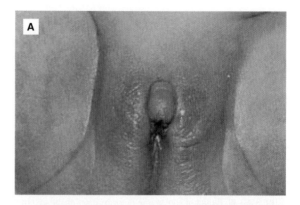
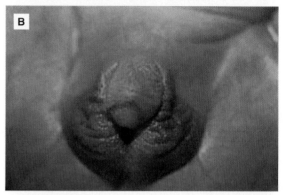
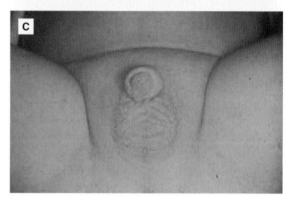

FIGURE 5-13 ■ (A) 2-week-old infant; positive newborn screen, abnormal genitalia missed; serum 17-OH progesterone = 30,690 ng/dL; electrolytes: Na = 133 meq/L , K = 7.1 meq/L. **(B)** 12-day-old "male with perineal hypospadius and cryptorchidism"; newborn screen 17-OH progesterone was normal; urology consultant suggested endocrine evaluation; high dose steroids for respiratory problem day of life 1-12; day 12: 17-OH progesterone 169 ng/dL, karyotype 46,XX; day 14: 17-OH progesterone 37,400 ng/dL. **(C)** 3-week-old infant; discharged after circumcision as bilateral cryptorchid male with follow-up appointment in urology clinic; presented near death with salt losing crisis; karyotype 46, XX.

that there is complete fusion of the labia and formation of a penile urethra (Figure 5-13). In such cases, the external genitalia are those of a normal male except that no gonads are descended. The elevated secretion of ACTH is often accompanied by excess melanocyte-stimulating hormone (MSH); in both male and female infants, this may cause hyperpigmentation of the external genitalia.

In infants not detected presymptomatically by newborn screening, the total or almost complete absence of cortisol and aldosterone secretion results in an acute adrenal crisis usually between the 4th and 15th days of life, but occasionally as late as 6 to 12 weeks of age. The infants feed poorly, have vomiting and diarrhea, and lose a significant amount of weight from dehydration. The serum electrolytes show an increase in serum potassium and a fall in sodium. In the absence of treatment, the acute adrenal crisis readily develops into cardiovascular collapse, cardiac arrest, and death.

On occasion, salt loss is first noted not in infancy but in early childhood, usually at the time of a major infection. These cases probably have degree of deficiency of CYP21 that is intermediate between that of the simple virilizing and salt-losing forms. In most patients, the salt-losing tendency seems to be somewhat less marked after 4 or 5 years of age and even less in late childhood and adulthood. Despite this, it has been shown that such patients cannot sustain a prolonged low-sodium diet without experiencing a major sodium and water loss. There are many patients with salt-losing CAH who tolerate discontinuation of their mineralocorticoid treatment in later life.[20]

Diagnosis. In areas that have a newborn screening test for CAH, the diagnosis is often made prior to the development of clinical symptoms, especially in affected males. The screening test can also speed the diagnostic evaluation of females with ambiguous genitalia.

In areas that do not employ a newborn screening test for CAH, in female infants with ambiguous external genitalia or with completely masculinized genitalia without palpable gonads, the diagnosis of the salt-losing form of CYP21 deficiency is made on the basis of a normal female karyotype of 46,XX, the characteristic pattern of serum electrolytes (hyponatremic, hypochloremic, hyperkalemic acidosis), and markedly elevated plasma concentrations of plasma 17-hydroxyprogesterone and androstenedione. Because of the dehydration, there is usually a decrease in plasma volume resulting in hemoconcentration. Low plasma concentration of aldosterone along with elevated PRA confirms the primary adrenal insufficiency.

In male infants the absence of ambiguous genitalia makes the diagnosis somewhat more difficult. The clinical symptoms can be confused with those of pyloric stenosis. The typical pattern of serum electrolytes of CAH will contrast with that of pyloric stenosis (hyponatremic, hypochloremic, hypokalemic alkalosis). The diagnosis is confirmed by demonstrating elevated concentrations of plasma 17-hydroxyprogesterone and androstenedione. The diagnosis is supported if there is a family history of an older sib with CAH, or one who died in the neonatal period from a syndrome of dehydration without a specific diagnosis.

Attenuated form of CYP21 deficiency. This form of CAH has the mildest degree of CYP21 deficiency. Because the symptoms in the female appear at puberty or later, it was formerly inappropriately called "acquired adrenal hyperplasia." The terminology "late-onset" has also been used. In the recent past, the term "nonclassical form" has been proposed to contrast with the "classical forms" (simple virilizing and the salt-losing). There also exists an asymptomatic or cryptic form of CYP21 deficiency manifested by the steroid pattern diagnostic of CAH in the complete absence of symptoms of the disorder.

Pathogenesis. The pathogenesis is similar to that of the other two forms except that the minimal CYP21 deficiency causes less change in steroidogenesis and therefore an attenuation of the symptoms of the disorder. The absence of masculinization of the female genitalia during fetal life reflects the low degree of fetal adrenal androgen secretion. Similarly, there are little or no signs of androgen effects during childhood. The effect of hypersecretion of adrenal androgens is noted only in females, usually at the time of adrenarche and puberty.

Clinical manifestations. There are essentially no symptoms of the attenuated or nonclassical form of CAH in males, since at puberty the testicular secretion of testosterone overrides the effects of increased adrenal androgen output. In females there is no abnormality of the external genitalia at birth. The virilization that occurs at puberty is probably triggered by the same mechanism that normally produces adrenarche, the difference in CAH being an excessive response of adrenal androgens. Most affected girls have normal breast development, but with hirsutism. The androgen excess causes either primary or secondary amenorrhea, and in some patients there are multiple, small ovarian cysts.

Laboratory diagnosis. In female patients of pubertal age, the baseline concentrations of plasma 17-hydroxyprogesterone and androstenedione are quite elevated, and administration of IV ACTH causes exaggerated increases of 17-hydroxyprogesterone and progesterone. Blood testosterone levels are often high.

Differential diagnosis of the attenuated form of CYP21 deficiency. The polycystic ovary syndrome (PCOS), also called Stein-Leventhal syndrome or ovarian hyperandrogenism, presents with symptoms that are similar to those found in the attenuated form of CAH. In both conditions, there are signs of excessive androgens, including hirsutism, acne, and menstrual abnormalities. In both PCOS and CAH the androgen effects are be quite marked, resulting in a slight enlargement of the clitoris, some increase in muscle mass, and deepening of the voice.

In PCOS, there are abnormal rises in plasma 17-hydroxyprogesterone and androstenedione in response to a gonadotropin-releasing hormone stimulation test, but not necessarily to ACTH. PCOS is more common than attenuated CAH, the latter being present in less than 10% of women with hirsutism and menstrual irregularities.

The IV ACTH test may be the best means to distinguish the two conditions. In PCOS, the rate of increase of 17-hydroxyprogesterone and progesterone is either normal or similar to that of obligate heterozygotes for CAH. In contrast, in attenuated CAH the rates of increase of 17-hydroxyprogesterone and progesterone are markedly above normal. To complicate the differential diagnosis further, ovarian cysts are found in both conditions and both may respond to glucocorticoid-suppressive treatment.

Long-term follow-up in CAH. Glucocorticoid therapy of CAH owing to CYP21 deficiency has been available since 1949, and several centers have now published the results of long-range treatment.

Adult male patients. In one of the earlier studies of adult male CAH patients adult height was significantly below the normal. Those not receiving treatment had no significant health complaints. Concentration of plasma testosterone was within the normal range in all, including patients who were off therapy. Concentrations of serum LH were significantly lower than normal. Using sperm count and reproductive history, all appeared to be fertile. Diagnosis at a later age correlates with reduction in adult height. Infertility has been described, and may in some cases be related to the presence of adrenal rests in the testes. For this reason, regular testicular examinations, and perhaps regular testicular ultrasounds, are recommended for sexually mature males with CAH.[18]

Adult female patients. In adult females, the height of those who started treatment later in life is shorter than those treated earlier. The age at pubarche is approximately 3 years earlier than normal, thelarche occurs at a normal age, and menarche is usually delayed by 2 or more years. Adult women with salt-losing CAH tend to have more severe problems related to genital surgery and infertility than those with the simple virilizing form. Reduced fertility is also reported in female CAH patient populations. In addition, among the women with CAH who become pregnant, there is increased risk of gestational diabetes, and an unexplained reduction in the number of male infants born (26% males vs 56% in controls).[18]

There are concerns about the risks of glucocorticoid therapy on the growth and development of patients with CAH. Studies point to increased fat mass, elevated plasma lipid levels, and growth inhibition during infancy and prepuberty. Adrenal medullary deficiency has also been shown.[21]

Genetic aspects of CYP21 deficiency

Inheritance. CAH owing to CYP21 deficiency is inherited as an autosomal recessive trait and is expressed clinically only in homozygous subjects. It was later discovered that there was a tight linkage between CYP21 deficiency and the HLA locus within the major histocompatibility complex (MHC) on chromosome 6.[22]

Genetic linkage disequilibrium. The CYP21 locus is in the HLA complex between the genes of the class III products of the MHC and the complement C4 genes. Isolation of the cytochrome P450 protein having CYP21 activity led to the cloning and sequencing of the duplicated CYP21 gene and CYP21P pseudogene.

The extended haplotype HLA-A3,Bw47,C6,DR7, GLO1/BfF,C2C,C4A1,C4BQO (so-called HLA-Bw47) was found to be linked to a large deletion including one of the CYP21 genes and one of the C4 genes; the remaining CYP21 gene was inactive and was the precursor of the CAH-linked HLA-Bw47 haplotype.

In the attenuated form of CYP21 deficiency, a genetic linkage disequilibrium occurs with the HLA-B14,DR1 haplotype. This haplotype includes three complement C4 genes (C4A2, C4B1, C4B2) in tandem with three CYP21 genes, two of them being pseudogenes and one being a CYP21 gene with a missense mutation in exon 7 (P281L).

Frequency of CYP21 mutations in the general population. Comparing the number of clinically diagnosed cases to the population base underestimates the frequency owing to deaths and unrecognized cases. Using the newborn screen to estimate frequency overestimates cases due to false positives.

Various surveys in Europe and North America reported an incidence of the disorder ranging from 1 in 10,000 to 1 in 25,000 births, giving a frequency of carriers for the mutant gene of 1:50 to 1:80. The incidence of CAH found in various newborn screenings showed incidences slightly higher than those obtained by case surveys with values between 1:10,000 and 1:18,000.[23] Much higher incidences were found in markedly inbred populations such as the Yupik Eskimo of Alaska (1:490 case survey, 1:684 by screening). Another example of the effect of inbreeding was found in the island of La Reunion in the Indian Ocean, where the incidence by screening was 1 in 2000 births. The frequency of the attenuated form of CYP21 deficiency is even more difficult to determine in view of the frequent complaint of hirsutism and virilism in female subjects.

Types of mutations

> **Deletions of the CYP21 gene**—The presence of highly homologous, tandemly arranged genes leads to meiotic mispairing and unequal crossing

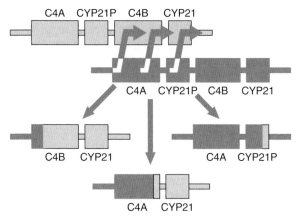

FIGURE 5-14 ■ Schematic representation of crossing-over events involving the C4/CYP21 genes. If transcription starts with the C4A gene, represented with green shading, and crosses over into the C4B gene, the patients end up with a normal phenotype, having received the CYP21 gene (arrow on the left). On the other hand, if the transcription includes the C4A, represented with green shading, and half of the CYP21P gene and ending with the CYP21 gene, the subject lacks the functional 21-hydroxylase.

over. This leads to gene duplication in one chromatid and deletion in the other (Figure 5-14). Abnormal numbers of CYP21 and CYP21P genes are found frequently both in the normal population and in patients with CYP21 deficiency. The average from a number of studies suggests that deletion events may account for approximately 20% to 25% of all CYP21-deficient chromosomes. Of these, the most frequent is deletion of a 30-kb region that includes the 3′ portion of CYP21P, all of C4B, and the 5′ end of CYP21. The 5′ end of the fusion gene contains sequences derived from CYP21P that include deleterious mutations that preclude enzymatic activity of the product may be owing to a previously undescribed large gene tandem deletion.

Gene conversion events—Gene conversion is another mechanism that frequently produces CYP21 mutations. It involves a nonreciprocal exchange of homologous genetic information; the sequence of one gene (the target) is "converted" to that of a related gene (the source). Gene conversion events probably involve incorrect meiotic alignment of the two CYP21 genes followed by mismatch repair converting a segment of the sequence of the CYP21 to that of the CYP21P pseudogene. The net result of such gene conversion events is the transfer of deleterious mutations from CYP21P to CYP21. These small gene conversions generate the full spectrum of clinical phenotypes of CYP21 deficiency, accounting for most mutations that alter the enzymatic activity of the CYP21 product.

The most common point mutation of CYP21 is in intron 2. It occurs normally in the CYP21P gene, and alters splicing. This is the presumed cause of CAH in the Yupik Eskimos. Genotype-phenotype correlations have been useful in the classification of patients at the time of diagnosis, and have been validated with long-term follow-up.

In some patients, the C4B/CYP21 tandem appears to be replaced by a C4A/CYP21P tandem, a so-called large gene conversion. This accounts for up to 15% of mutations in the salt-losing form and may have arisen as a result of two unequal crossing over events.

Rarely, de novo point mutations and mutations that were not transferred from CYP21P occur in CYP21 deficiency, and are associated with salt-losing and nonsalt-losing forms.

Detection of heterozygotes for the CAH trait. Determination of carrier status by hormonal testing was first performed using obligate CAH heterozygotes (parents of patients). Carriers showed normal basal concentrations of steroids but elevated cortisol precursors (17-hydroxyprogesterone, progesterone) in response to ACTH stimulation. Because the ovaries produce 17-hydroxyprogesterone and progesterone late in the menstrual cycle, it is necessary to perform the tests of adult females during the early follicular phase. Using a 30-minute test, an additive rate of increase of progesterone plus 17-hydroxyprogesteroone that is less than 7 ng/dL/min is found in subjects who have two normal CYP21 genes. Values of 9 to 30 ng/dL/min are found in heterozygotes for CAH. However, there is a 5% to 10% overlap between normals and carriers. When biochemical tests are compared with genotyping to determine carrier status in one study, the latter method is more reliable in families where the genotype of the index case is known. HLA-types, if known, can also help in the identification of carriers.[24]

Prenatal diagnosis of CYP21 deficiency. The prenatal diagnosis of CAH can be useful in preparing for appropriate postnatal therapy if the fetus is affected. A biopsy of chorionic villi can be obtained during the first trimester. This material can be used for karyotyping, characterization of CYP21 mutations, and HLA typing if needed. All of these methods imply that an index case has already been studied and the genotype is known. Sources of error can arise from recombination in the HLA locus, possibility of contamination of the fetal material by maternal tissue, and generation of unauthentic sequences by the PCR amplification used for the genotyping.

Amniocentesis can be performed at 15 to 18 weeks of gestation. Cells can be used for a karyotype, and HLA type and CYP21 genotype in some cases, whereas the fluid permits measurement of steroid concentrations, but the steroid levels can only be interpreted accurately if the mother is not receiving prenatal dexamethasone treatment (see in the section "Prenatal Therapy of CYP21 Deficiency"). In affected fetuses the levels of 17-hydroxyprogesterone and androstenedione are markedly elevated; the concentration of cortisol, progesterone, DHEA, and DHEA-S show no significant abnormalities.[25]

Prenatal therapy of CYP21 deficiency. The reason for treatment is to reduce the masculinization of the genitalia in affected female fetuses. Of major importance is the fact that surgery of the external genitalia is imperfect. If gender identity of female patients is impacted by fetal brain exposure to elevated concentrations of androgens, prenatal treatment could reduce this exposure.

Since cortisol does not cross the placenta readily, it is necessary to use dexamethasone. Because the masculinization of the external genitalia takes place between 5 and 12 weeks of gestation, for therapy to be maximally effective it must be started at 5 to 6 weeks. Treatment can normalize the external genitalia of affected females.[25] The dose of dexamethasone used is 20 mcg/kg of body weight/24 h with a daily dose varying between 1 and 1.5 mg/day. Treatment is monitored by study of the suppression of cortisol secretion (concentration of maternal plasma cortisol, measurement of urinary excretion of free cortisol). Full suppression of the fetal adrenal secretion results in suppression of estriol in maternal plasma and maternal urine. Hence, estriol measurement is also used for monitoring therapy.

Since the chances of heterozygous parents having an affected child is 1 in 4, and since half the fetuses will be male, the risk of an affected female fetus is only 12.5%, and dexamethasone therapy is given unnecessarily in 87.5% of pregnancies. Attempts to decrease the length of unnecessary therapy are made by prenatal karyotype and diagnosis of CAH. Treatment is discontinued in all male fetuses, and in heterozygous females or homozygous normal females. In general, few side effects of therapy have been observed, but abnormal weight gain, fluid retention, and hypertension may occur. The potential advantages of treatment may outweigh the possible risk of side effects, but informed consent for this treatment must include the fact that long-term studies have not verified its safety. This treatment should only be performed in centers with expertise and experience in this area.

Neonatal Screening. The concentration of 17α-hydroxyprogesterone can be determined on neonatal screening blood spots. Neonatal screening has prevented complications occurring when CAH is unrecognized and untreated. Specifically, the purpose of screening would be to treat appropriately prior to an acute adrenal crisis and to avoid potential death. At birth, females with the salt-losing form *should* attract attention because of their ambiguous genitalia. The major benefit has been the identification of affected males while they are still healthy. The pitfalls have been false positives in premature infants, false negatives (particularly in females), and difficulty in differentiating the salt-losing and nonsalt-losing forms in affected patients. Complementing the screening test with a second screen, or with genotyping in presumptive positive cases, has been helpful in some situations, including the evaluation of premature infants.[26]

CAH owing to deficiency of 11β-hydroxylase. Steroid 11β-hydroxylase (CY11B1) deficiency, a hypertensive form of CAH, accounts for approximately 5% of all cases of CAH.

Pathogenesis. In the zona fasciculata, CY11B1 deficiency impairs cortisol and corticosterone secretion. The consequent ACTH release increases the production of the steroid precursors 11-deoxycortisol, DOC, and 18-hydroxy DOC. The hypertension is as a result of the increased secretion of DOC, a mineralocorticoid. Secretion of 17-hydroxyprogesterone and progesterone are also increased, but to a lesser extent than in CYP21 deficiency. The mineralocorticoid effect of high DOC concentrations suppresses renin and angiotensin, resulting in very low aldosterone secretion. Thus, this disorder is thus a genetically defined cause of low renin hypertension.

Clinical manifestations. CY11B1 deficiency, like CYP21 deficiency, is characterized by masculinization of the female fetus and by early virilization postnatally. Females present at birth with ambiguity of the external genitalia. On occasion, the virilism is not evident until puberty or adulthood in a late-onset form of the disease generally diagnosed only in adolescent or adult females.

Male newborns have normal external genitalia with descended testes. As with CYP21 deficiency, it is not unusual in older patients to find nodules of hyperplastic ectopic adrenal tissue in the spermatic cord, epididymus, or testes. Gynecomastia can also develop prior to puberty. Deficient cortisol production and the consequent ACTH hypersecretion lead to significant increases in 11-deoxycortisol and DOC (Figure 5-3). Although 11-deoxycortisol has little biologic activity, DOC is a potent salt-retaining steroid and causes a high-mineralocorticoid, low-renin form of hypertension. This hypertension is usually moderate, but can occasionally be sufficiently severe to cause cardiomegaly and eventual cardiac failure.[27]

Diagnosis. The diagnosis is made by detecting increased levels of DOC and 11-deoxycortisol in blood and/or their tetrahydro derivatives in urine. These levels

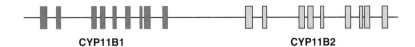

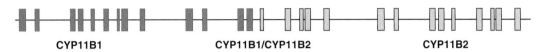

FIGURE 5-15 ■ Organization of CYP11B1 and B2 genes. The normal gene organization of the CYP11B1 and CYP11B2 genes is shown above. Below is the hybrid CYP11B1/CYP11B2 gene that results from meiotic mismatch and unequal crossing over. In all instances, the crossover is located 5′ to intron 4 of the CYP11B genes.*(Donohoue PA. The Adrenal Gland and its Disorders. In Kappy MS, Allen DB, Geffner ME (ED) Principles and Practice of Pediatric Endocrinology. Charles C. Thomas Publishers, Ltd. Springfield, IL, 2005; 357-485.)*

vary considerably even among sibs who are expected to have the same genotype. The diagnosis may be delayed in male infants as they have normal genitalia. Prenatal diagnosis of CY11B1 deficiency is now available, based on measurement of maternal urinary tetrahydro-11-deoxycortisol. This is of greatest benefit in populations at risk, such as Jews of Moroccan origin.

Genetics. CY11B1 deficiency is an autosomal recessive disorder. A gene encoding CY11B1 has been cloned and maps to chromosome 8q21-q22, a finding consistent with the functional and anatomical segregation of the CY11B1 isozymes discussed below.

Two homologous adjacent CY11B1 genes, designated CYP11B1 and CYP11B2, encode two distinct proteins (Figure 5-15). Although the two genes have 93% identity in their predicted amino acid sequences, they differ in their sites of expression and in the enzymatic activities of their protein products. The product of the CYP11B1 gene, termed "11β-hydroxylase," is expressed at high levels in the zonae fasciculata/reticularis where it converts 11-deoxycortisol (compound S) to cortisol. In the zona glomerulosa it converts DOC to corticosterone but not to aldosterone. Thus, this protein mediates 11β-hydroxylation but does not perform the terminal reactions required for aldosterone biosynthesis. The other gene, CYP11B2, encodes a protein called designated aldosterone synthase. It is expressed only in the zona glomerulosa, where mineralocorticoids are produced, and catalyzes all reactions needed for the conversion of deoxycorticosterone to aldosterone (11β-hydroxylation, 18-hydroxylation, and 18-dehydrogenation)(Figure 5-16). In patients with CYP11B1 deficiency, nonsense mutations, missense mutations, small insertions and deletions, as well as a 5 bp duplication have been identified. The duplicated CYP11B1/CYP11B2 gene arrangement confers a predilection for unequal crossing over and gene deletion, and such mutations have been noted in CY11B1 deficiency. This mutation mechanism, however, occurs much less frequently than in CYP21 deficiency.

Corticosterone

CMO I

18-Hydroxycorticosterone

CMO II

Aldosterone

FIGURE 5-16 ■ Biosynthesis of aldosterone from corticosterone. This pathway requires two enzymatic activities, corticosterone methyloxidase type I (CMO I) and corticosterone methyloxidase type II (CMO II). CMO I permits the 18-hydroxylation of corticosterone; CMO II permits subsequent 18-dehydrogenation.

Congenital adrenal hyperplasia owing to deficiency of 17α-hydroxylase. Steroid 17α-hydroxylase (CYP17) catalyzes more than one enzymatic conversion, both CYP17 and 17,20-lyase reactions. Patients with combined deficiencies of both activites are more common than those with isolated deficiency of 17,20-lyase. CYP17 is expressed both in the adrenal cortex and in the gonad.

Pathophysiology and clinical manifestations. Severe deficiency of CYP17 is relatively rare, although the reported number of patients now exceeds 120, at least 14 of which exhibited only 17,20-lyase deficiency. As with all forms of CAH, the underlying clinical manifestations result from the inability to produce normal levels of glucocorticoids, and the consequent increase in ACTH secretion. Although cortisol is not produced, patients with CYP17 deficiency can produce corticosterone, which binds with low affinity to the GR. DOC is also secreted in abnormally large amounts (Figure 5-3), thus patients with CYP17 deficiency present with hypertension. Although the biochemical pathways for aldosterone production in the zona glomerulosa are intact, the presence of high circulating concentrations of DOC suppress the renin-angiotensin system, thus leading to decreased aldosterone levels and low rennin hypertension.

Deficiency of 17,20-lyase causes inability to form androgens and estrogens. Since normal development of external genitalia in males requires testosterone biosynthesis in utero, affected males have incomplete genital development and present with ambiguous external genitalia and in some cases with completely female-appearing genitalia. Müllerian regression occurs normally, as production of testicular Müllerian inhibiting factor is not affected by the CYP17 deficiency. The external genitalia of affected females are normal at birth. In both females and males, the inability to produce sex steroids is manifested later in life at the time of puberty. Female patients usually present with primary amenorrhea and lack of breast development owing to ovarian estrogen deficiency. They also have scant or absent axillary and pubic hair owing to adrenal androgen deficiency. Males present with ambiguous genitalia and failure of masculinization at puberty.

Diagnosis. Increased levels of pregnenolone, progesterone, DOC, 18-hydroxy-DOC, and corticosterone are characteristic. Because of increased DOC, 18-hydroxy-DOC, and corticosterone, the renin and aldosterone levels are below normal in the face of hypertension. From 3 to 4 months of age until puberty, plasma concentrations of 17-hydroxyprogesterone and 17-hydroxypregnenolone are normally low; thus, demonstration of decreased concentrations in patients with CYP17 deficiency is not always possible. The same is true for concentrations of androgens (DHEA, DHEA-S, androstenedione, testosterone) and estrogens (estradiol).

The steroid patterns so far described apply to patients with combined CYP17 and 17,20-lyase deficiencies. In the rare patients with isolated 17,20-lyase deficiency, there is an increase in 17-hydroxyprogesterone and 17-hydroxypregnenolone concentrations. Thus, an adequate flow of precursors results in normal cortisol and aldosterone secretion, and the levels of corticosterone and DOC are approximately normal. They develop signs of gonadal steroid deficiencies in adolescence.

In newborn patients with 46,XY karyotype and ambiguous genitalia, the measurement of cortisol and androgen precursors elucidate the enzymatic defect. It must be noted that the diagnosis may be missed in infants with completely female-appearing genitalia whether the karyotype is 46,XX or 46,XY. At the age when puberty is expected, CYP17 deficiency will be detected because of elevated gonadotropin levels, low gonadal steroid concentrations, elevated levels of precursors, and low-renin hypertension.

Genetics. The gene encoding 17α-hydroxylase, CYP17, has been cloned and mapped to chromosome 10q24.3. Analyses of CYP17 in patients with CYP17 deficiency have defined the causal mutations in a number of patients. In contrast to CYP21 deficiency, large-scale deletions are not an important cause of CYP17 deficiency. Rather, the deleterious mutations include missense and nonsense mutations as well as small insertions or deletions that alter the reading frame or splice sites. Patients with isolated 17, 20-lyase deficiency have also had the causative mutations identified.[28]

Congenital adrenal hyperplasia owing to deficiency of 3β-hydroxysteroid dehydrogenase
Pathogenesis and clinical manifestations. CAH owing to 3β-HSD deficiency represents less than 1% of all CAH cases. In severe 3β-HSD deficiency there is a nearly total absence of secretion of biologically active glucocorticoids, mineralocorticoids, and androgens. The only accumulated precursors prior to the enzymatic blocks are pregnenolone and DHEA, and several of their metabolites (Figure 5-3). The mapping of a gene encoding 3β-HSD to chromosome 1 confirmed the clinical observation that it was an autosomal recessive trait.

The main androgens secreted in this form of CAH are DHEA and its 16-hydroxylated derivative. Neither binds to the androgen receptor, and thus neither has biologic activity. Regardless of this, patients with severe 3β-HSD deficiency exhibit some androgenic effects (females present with slight labial fusion and clitoral enlargement; males present with ambiguous genitalia). This suggests that the enzyme deficiency is not complete and that biologically active androgens are produced and cause mild masculinization of the external genitalia in females. On the other hand, there is inadequate androgen production to result in complete masculinization of the genitalia in males. As with CYP21 deficiency, the impaired corticosteroid production is manifested by signs and symptoms of adrenal insufficiency that may be fatal if left untreated in the neonatal period. Patients with less severe defects produce sufficient mineralocorticoid to avoid salt-wasting crises. 3β-HSD deficiency also prevents gonadal steroidogenesis, and patients exhibit abnormal genital development as discussed above. Analysis of steroid profiles, particularly following ACTH infusion, have suggested a mild defect in 3β-HSD activity in some older females presenting with hirsutism, oligomenorrhea, or infertility. However, studies of the various isoforms of 3β-HSD in these patients have not revealed mutations, and recent studies indicate that this hormonal phenotype is a variant of insulin resistant PCOS.[29,30]

Diagnosis. Deficiency of 3β-HSD may be diagnosed by demonstrating elevated serum levels of pregnenolone, 17-hydroxypregnenolone, DHEA, and DHEA-S. In patients with severe deficiency, ambiguous genitalia and evidence of salt loss are present. Normal newborn infants normally secrete relatively high amounts of DHEA, DHEA-S, and pregnenolone and its metabolites. Newborns with CYP21 deficiency may also secrete increased amounts of these steroids. Thus, the steroid concentrations must be interpreted with caution and sometimes it may be difficult to establish the diagnosis in milder deficiencies.

Genetics. Two distinct human genes that encode isozymes of 3β-HSD, designated types 1 and 2, map to chromosome 1p13. Although the products of these two genes differ slightly in the kinetics with which they metabolize steroids, both forms have similar enzyme activities arguing against distinct roles of the two isozymes in the production of glucocorticoids and androgens. The type 2 gene is expressed only in the typical steroidogenic tissues (adrenal and gonads), whereas the type 1 gene is expressed predominantly in placenta, skin, and mammary tissue.

The molecular defects responsible for salt-losing CAH in association with 3β-HSD deficiency have been identified in the type 2 3β-HSD gene, and are nonsense and frameshift mutations. As more patients with deficiency of 3β-HSD have been studied, structure-function relationships of mutations in the salt-losing and nonsalt-losing forms have been determined. Mutations of the type 2 3β-HSD gene have also been identified in a milder, nonsalt-losing form.

Congenital lipoid adrenal hyperplasia (StAR deficiency, CYP11A deficiency)

Pathogenesis, clinical manifestations, and diagnosis. The underlying defect in the rare disorder of lipoid CAH is an inability to convert cholesterol to pregnenolone, preventing the biosynthesis of all major steroid classes.

Because of a failure to produce androgens in utero, genetic males present with normal-appearing female external genitalia; because of unimpaired production of MIS, the internal ducts develop along male patterns. Females appear completely normal at birth. Because of their inability to produce glucocorticoids and mineralocorticoids, patients present with symptoms and signs of adrenocortical insufficiency and salt loss. In contrast to patients with salt-wasting 21-hydroxase deficiency, the age of presentation varies and patients may not be diagnosed until several months of age. Moreover, there are reports of genetic females (46,XX) with lipoid CAH who, at the time of puberty, underwent menarche, indicating capacity for gonadal steroidogenesis.[31]

The adrenal glands in these patients show marked hyperplasia, with cortical cells engorged with lipoid material. This histologic picture and the failure to produce significant amounts of any steroids led to the hypothesis that congenital lipoid adrenal hyperplasia results from a mutation in CYP11A, the enzyme required for the three steps to convert cholesterol to pregnenolone. However, most cases of lipoid CAH result from mutations in steroidogenic acute regulatory protein (StAR), required for cholesterol delivery to the mitochondria where CYP11A acts.

Genetics. CYP11A is encoded by a gene that maps to chromosome 15q23-q24. The StAR gene maps to chromosome 8p11.2. StAR mutations causing lipoid CAH include frameshift, nonsense, missense, and splicing mutations that interfere with StAR activity. StAR is expressed in the adrenal cortex and gonad, but not in the placenta or brain. Thus, patients with StAR mutations can have placental and gonadal pregnenolone synthesis. This explains why patients with lipoid CAH survive gestation as the placenta has active steroidogenesis without StAR, and some patients with lipoid CAH have gonadal steroid synthesis at the time of puberty.

Based on the known importance of placental steroids in the maintenance of human pregnancy, it has been proposed that mutations in CYP11A are incompatible with fetal survival in utero. The proposal that placentally-derived progesterone, and thus CYP11A, is essential to maintain human pregnancy suggested to some that occasional cases of recurrent miscarriage may result from mutations of CYP11A that preclude placental steroidogenesis. However, a number of patients with CYP11A deficiency as a result of CYP11A gene mutations have now been described.

P450 oxidoreductase deficiency. P450 oxidoreductase deficiency (POR deficiency) is rare and is caused by mutations in the gene encoding P450 oxidoreductase (an enzyme that transfers electrons to CYP21A2 and CYP17). This results in a partial deficiencies of the enzymes 21-hydroxylase and 17 alpha-hydroxylase. In many cases, this form of virilizing adrenal hyperplasia is associated with features of the skeletal dysplasia known as Antley-Bixler Syndrome.[32]

Adrenoleukodystrophy (Siemerling-Creutzfeldt disease; Schilder disease).

Adrenoleukodystrophy (ALD), adrenomyeloneuropathy (AMN), and closely related variants are peroxisomal disorders which affect the CNS, adrenal cortex, and at times other organs. The biochemical abnormality common to all forms is elevated plasma and tissue concentrations of very long chain fatty acids (VLCFA). These unbranched saturated VLCFA accumulate owing to a defect which inhibits their normal breakdown in the peroxisome.

ALD is of great importance to the endocrinologist because of the nearly constant occurrence of adrenocortical failure concomitantly with the irreversible degenerative neurologic defects seen in these patients. Adrenal failure may predate, occur simultaneously with or follow the onset of the neurologic deterioration. Descriptions of patients formerly thought to have Addison disease, who then were shown to have ALD or AMN, underscores the need to measure plasma VLCFA concentrations in all male patients with primary adrenal failure of unknown etiology.[33]

X-linked ALD/AMN.

There are several different phenotypes in X-linked ALD, and more than one phenotype may exist within a family. *Childhood ALD* was the first type described and is believed to be the most common. These boys develop normally in early childhood but then develop progressive neurologic disability by about age 7 years (range 2.75-10 years). Neurological deterioration progresses rapidly, often leading to the bedridden state within 2 years. *Adolescent ALD* occurs in boys whose illness presents between the ages of 10 and 21 years. The symptoms resemble those of childhood ALD, but the rate of neurologic deterioration may be slower. AMN occurs in men whose neurologic symptoms begin after the age of 21 years. The rate of neurologic deterioration is fairly slow, over 5 to 20 years. Primary gonadal failure is common among these patients, as it is in other forms of X-linked ALD. *Adult cerebral ALD* presents in men after the age of 21 years with cerebral neurologic defects such as dementia, seizures, or behavioral disturbances. *"Addison only" form of ALD* belongs to a subset of patients with adrenal failure and no symptoms of neurologic deterioration. At least 9% of ALD patients belong to this group. The time between the onset of adrenal failure and the onset of neurologic abnormalities may be decades. *Asymptomatic ALD* has been detected in some 100 individuals. These individuals have the biochemical abnormalities of ALD but none of the clinical features. *Symptomatic heterozygotes:* About 200 subjects have been identified among 1000 heterozygotes tested. These women have a clinical picture similar to AMN, but the

onset occurs later (~40 years of age) with a slower rate of progression, adrenocortical insufficiency being rare.

Neonatal (autosomal recessive) ALD.

In this form, neurologic abnormalities and adrenocortical insufficiency occur in the prenatal or neonatal period. The presentation is not preceded by a period of normal development, as is the case with X-linked ALD. It is an autosomal recessive disorder of the peroxisomes in which VLCFA accumulate, as in X-linked ALD. However, the peroxisomes are scant in number and smaller than normal in size. The biochemical defect is more extensive than in X-linked ALD, and more organ systems are generally involved. Neonatal ALD is similar to but less severe than the cerebro-hepato-renal syndrome of Zellweger, in which peroxisomes are totally absent. An intermediate severity form of ALD exists, known as Refsum disease.

Genetics of ALD.

The positional cloning of the Xq28 gene that is defective in X-linked ALD has lead to a greater understanding of the pathogenesis of the disorder. Rather than causing a single enzyme defect causing defective fatty acid oxidation and accumulation of VLCFA, this mutation prevents normal functioning of a peroxisomal membrane protein with an ATP-binding motif. The ALD gene encodes an ABC (**A**TP-**B**inding **C**assette) protein that shares homology with the cystic fibrosis transmembrane regulator (CFTR) and multidrug resistance (mdr1) proteins. It is thought to be involved in the transfer of VLCFA CoA synthase into the peroxisomal membrane. Mutations of this gene found in patients with ALD include missense, nonsense, frameshift, and splice sites defects.

In the autosomal recessive forms of ALD, defects in a gene required for peroxisomal biosynthesis, PEX1, are common. Patients with PEX1 gene defects include those with Zellweger syndrome, neonatal ALD, and infantile Refsum disease. Other patients with Zellweger syndrome have mutations in the gene encoding the 70K peroxisomal membrane protein (PMP70).

Acid lipase deficiency (Wolman disease).

Wolman disease is an autosomal recessive disorder caused by deficiency of lysosomal acid lipase, an enzyme that catalyzes the hydrolysis of cholesterol esters and triglyceride. Patients develop massive accumulation of esterified lipids, which produces multisystem failure at an early age. This disorder was first called "generalized xanthomatosis with calcified adrenals" or "primary familial xanthomatosis with adrenal calcification." Over 50 cases of this disease have been reported. Patients generally present within the first weeks of life with failure to thrive, vomiting, abdominal distention, and jaundice. They have anemia, hepatosplenomegaly, steatorrhea, and calcified enlarged adrenal glands. This is a rapidly progressive, untreatable disease, which usually results in death by 6 months of age. The diagnosis is made by demonstration of deficient cellular activity of acid lipase, usually in cultured skin fibroblasts or lymphocytes. Serum lipid profiles are characteristically normal. Storage of cholesterol esters and triglycerides occurs and produces foam cells in the liver, adrenal cortex, spleen, intestine, lymphnodes, circulating leukocytes, bone marrow, and CNS.

In patients tested with ACTH, a blunted adrenocortical response has been described. The adrenocortical insufficiency is explained on the basis of a lack of acid lipase, which is needed to free cholesterol from its esters in order to make it available for steroidogenesis.

The gene encoding acid lipase, which is defective in lysosomal acid lipase deficiency maps to chromosome 10. An allelic variant of Wolman disease, cholesterol ester storage disease, is a milder form of the disorder. The age of onset is later, the course is less rapidly progressive, and the adrenal glands are rarely calcified. However, hyperbetalipoproteinemia is common, and severe premature atherosclerosis may occur.

Steroid sulfatase deficiency (X-linked ichthyosis).
Steroid sulfatase (STS) deficiency is an X-linked recessive disorder of steroid metabolism in which the major clinical manifestation is ichthyosis. The enzyme deficiency results in accumulation of DHEA-S and cholesterol sulfate. It is believed that ichthyosis occurs because of cholesterol sulfate accumulation in the skin, and its interference with epidermal cohesion. The altered steroid metabolism does not produce adrenal insufficiency. However, it may erroneously suggest fetal adrenal insufficiency because of low maternal estriol levels.

Smith-Lemli-Opitz syndrome.
Smith-Lemli-Opitz syndrome is an autosomal recessive disorder of cholesterol biosynthesis caused by mutations in 7-dehydrocholesterol reductase, an enzyme required to convert 7-dehydrocholesterol to cholesterol. The syndrome includes microcephaly, facial typical feautres, and syndactyly. Affected males have either ambiguous genitalia or nearly normal female external genitalia. Adrenal insufficiency is not universal, but patients have presented with mineralocorticoid deficiency.[34]

Defects in aldosterone production.
Isolated defects in the steroidogenesis of mineralocorticoids do not cause the hyperplasia of the adrenal glands as seen with deficient glucocorticoid biosynthesis and consequent elevated ACTH secretion. There are three major genetic disorders of mineralocorticoid biosynthesis. Deficiencies in CYP11B2 are associated with two of these disorders. A third genetic disorder of this locus is a rare form of autosomal dominant hypertension caused by a hybrid CYP11B1/CYP11B2 gene.

Defects in aldosterone synthase. A genetic defect in the CYP11B2 gene impairs the production of mineralocorticoids without compromising glucocorticoid production. CYP11B2 carries out both 18-hydroxylase and 18-dehydrogenase reactions. Deficiencies of these two activities are clinically distinct—corticosterone methyloxidase I (CMO I) or 18-hydroxylase deficiency and corticosterone methyloxidase II (CMO II) or 18-dehydrogenase deficiency (Figure 5-16). In the zona glomerulosa, CYP11B2 also catalyzes the 11β-hydroxylation required for aldosterone production. As discussed above, the CY11B1 reaction in the glucocorticoid pathway is catalyzed by CYP11B1, which is stimulated by ACTH.

Pathophysiology, clinical features, and diagnosis. Deficiency of CMO I or CMO II causes aldosterone deficiency and elevated renin, accompanied by accumulation of steroid precursors prior to the biosynthetic block: DOC and corticosterone in CMO I deficiency; DOC, corticosterone, and 18-hydroxycorticosterone in CMO II deficiency (Figure 5-16). These precursors possess some mineralocorticoid activity, which compensates partially for the aldosterone deficiency. Thus, patients with CMO I or CMO II deficiency generally present with partial salt loss, rather than the typical salt-losing crisis of complete mineralocorticoid deficiency. Infants may present only with failure to thrive.

18-Hydroxylase (CMO I) deficiency. Renal salt-wasting and decreased growth velocity develop in these children. Laboratory evaluation reveals undetectable urinary aldosterone with elevated excretion of DOC and corticosterone. Postmortem histopathological specimens show poor development of the adrenal zona glomerulosa and hyperplasia of the renal juxtaglomerular apparatus. Treatment with mineralocorticoid supplementation results in resumption of normal growth along with decreased excretion of DOC and corticosterone.

Genetics. Molecular analyses of patients with CMO I deficiency show that CYP11B2 mutations obliterate all aldosterone synthase activity, rather than selectively impairing 18-hydroxylation.

18-Oxidase (CMO II) deficiency. This is more common than CMO I deficiency, based on the greater number of reported cases. Because of their selective inability to produce mineralocorticoids, patients with CMO II deficiency present with typical abnormalities of electrolyte and water metabolism. Severe electrolyte abnormalities can occur in the neonatal period, with potentially life-threatening hyponatremia and hyperkalemia. Although electrolyte abnormalities and poor growth persist throughout early childhood, symptoms later in life are attenuated and eventually disappear. At the time of diagnosis, there are increased concentrations of corticosterone and 18-hydroxycorticosterone in plasma, with low aldosterone and high renin.

Genetics. Like CMOI deficiency, CMOII deficiency is caused by CYP11B2 mutations.[35]

Adrenal hemorrhage of the newborn. This occurs usually after a prolonged labor and traumatic delivery. It is often associated with toxemic pregnancy. It occurs more often in males than in females. The bleeding results from injury to the subcapsular vascular plexus of the adrenal glands, thus causing separation of the parenchyma from the capsule. The adrenal insufficiency results from the lack of vascular supply to the adrenal cortex. In order to cause symptomatic adrenal insufficiency, the hemorrhage must be bilateral.

The clinical picture is similar to that of an acute adrenal crisis: the newborns commonly also show hyperpyrexia, tachypnea, twitching, or convulsion. Hypoglycemia, hyponatremia, and hyperkalemia are present. On physical examination the adrenals may be palpable. They can also be detected by sonography or radiography as a mass which displaces the kidneys downward. Bilateral adrenal hemorrhage can be confused with renal vein thrombosis, but in the latter condition there is normal adrenal function.

If the infant recovers there is often adrenal calcification as the hemorrhage resolves. The calcification can be visible on x-ray several months after the hemorrhage has occurred but with time the calcification tends to resolve and disappear.

Adrenal hemorrhage associated with infection. The normal adrenocortical response to acute infection is augmentation of cortisol production, as demonstrated by patients with meningitis. However, patients with serious bacterial infections develop acute adrenocortical insufficiency owing to bilateral adrenal hemorrhage as a result of the effects of bacterial endotoxin. The most commonly associated bacterial pathogen is *Neisseria meningitis.* The adrenal crisis resulting from acute meningococcemia is also known as the "Waterhouse-Frederickson syndrome." Other pathogens associated with septicemic adrenal hemorrhage include *Pseudomonas aeruginosa,* pneumococci, and streptococci.

Chronic hypoadrenocorticism (Addison disease). Chronic primary adrenal insufficiency is referred to as Addison disease. It is fairly rare in childhood. The most frequent etiology is autoimmune destruction of the adrenal cortex, as is seen in the autoimmune polyglandular syndromes (Table 5-5). This has replaced tuberculosis as the major etiology. Up to 45% of patients with autoimmune Addison disease will develop one or more other autoimmune endocrinopathies, most often thyroid disease (14%-25%). There is a slight preponderance of females, as is the case with autoimmune diseases in general. Type 1 APS is an autosomal recessive disorder as a result of mutations in the **AutoImmune REgulator gene (AIRE)**, located on chromosome 21q22.3. Over 40 mutations of this gene have been reported. This gene is expressed in thyroid, lymph nodes, spleen, and fetal liver. It probably regulates autoimmunity

by promoting the ectopic expression of peripheral tissue-restricted antigens to medullary cells of the thymus. There is not a close association between genotype and phenotype in this heterogeneous disorder.[34]

Pathogenesis in nonautoimmune Addison disease

Nonbacterial pathogens may produce chronic adrenocortical insufficiency as a result of infiltration and destruction of the gland. In these cases the adrenal insufficiency progresses chronically, and the adrenals may appear calcified on abdominal radiographs. The most common pathogen is tuberculosis, which was the etiology of adrenal insufficiency in Dr. Addison's first case description of the syndrome. Other rare causes are fungal infections such as histoplasmosis, coccidiomycosis, and blastomycosis.

Adrenocortical abnormalities have been described in association with HIV infection in patients with acquired immunodeficiency syndrome (AIDS) or AIDS-related complex. These abnormalities include either frank adrenal insufficiency, blunted cortisol response to acute ACTH stimulation, or decreased cortisol reserve after 3 days of ACTH stimulation. These blunted responses are accompanied by elevated basal levels of cortisol. In children with HIV infection, basal and ACTH-stimulated cortisol levels are increased, suggesting an effect of chronic stress.

Adrenocortical insufficiency may result from a number of iatrogenic causes. Anticoagulant therapy may produce bilateral adrenal hemorrhage and acute adrenal insufficiency, even in the absence of bleeding elsewhere. A number of drugs may inhibit cortisol synthesis, however if the inhibition is incomplete, it is usually compensated by increased ACTH secretion. These drugs include aminoglutethimide, ketoconazole, and etomidate. The drug o,p'-DDD, which is used in the treatment of Cushing syndrome, damages the mitochondria of the adrenocortical cells and may produce adrenal insufficiency.

Clinical features. In primary adrenal failure, there is decreased or absent production of one or all three groups of adrenal steroid hormones. In most cases, the signs and symptoms of adrenal insufficiency develop slowly (Table 5-4). Nearly all patients complain of fatigue, muscle pain, and weight loss. Orthostatic and gastrointestinal symptoms are frequent, as well. In children, there may be growth failure. The weight loss is partly related to anorexia and later, various GI problems such as nausea, vomiting, mild diarrhea. Patients may come to medical attention because of signs and symptoms of acute adrenal insufficiency precipitated by a febrile illness.

Hyperpigmentation is present in over 90% of patients, and may develop over a period of months to years. The typical distribution of hyperpigmentation is over the extensor surfaces of the extremities, particularly in sun-exposed areas. The mucous membranes (gingival borders, vaginal mucosa), axillae, and palmar creases are involved, and are hallmarks of Addison disease. The melanocytes are stimulated by excessively high levels of α-MSH, which is secreted concomitantly with ACTH from the anterior pituitary gland, as both are cleavage products of POMC.[35]

Diagnosis. The diagnosis is based on demonstration of elevated ACTH levels combined with decreased or absent cortisol and mineralocorticoid production. Fasting 8 AM cortisol levels are low and fail to rise with ACTH stimulation. Fasting glucose may be low, and hyponatremia and hyperkalemia with acidosis may be present. Aldosterone levels are low, and PRA is usually elevated. Adrenal androgen levels may be below normal in adolescent and adult patients. Anti-adrenal antibody levels should be measured, as well as antibodies to other endocrine glands. In addition, serum calcium, phosphorus, and thyroxine levels should be measured because of the possibility of associated parathyroid and thyroid insufficiency. Of particular importance are the features that may cluster in either of the two types of autoimmune polyglandular syndromes (Table 5-5).

Hypoadrenocorticism Secondary to Deficient ACTH Secretion

Hypopituitarism

This disorder is characterized by a deficiency of one, some, or all, of the peptide hormones secreted by the anterior pituitary gland. Considered here are cases that include deficient ACTH secretion. ACTH deficiency may also result from deficient CRH secretion by the hypothalamus. Causes of reduced ACTH secretion are listed in Table 5-3.

Pathophysiology. Congenital malformations of the brain, particularly midline defects, may result in hypothalamic insufficiency. Septo-optic dysplasia and its variants are such conditions. Congenital malformations of the pituitary can also occur, such as the hypoplastic pituitaries seen in some of the genetic defects in development of certain pituitary cell lineages. Trauma at delivery or later in life may result in infarction involving the hypothalamus and/or the pituitary. Infectious processes such as meningitis or encephalitis can result in hypopituitarism. Intracranial hemorrhage, as is seen in premature or very low birth weight infants, may also produce hypopituitarism.

Infiltrative disorders that destroy normal tissues such as hemochromatosis, sarcoidosis, Langerhans histiocytosis, or granulomatous formations can also cause the loss of pituitary function. Treatment for various neoplasias including radiation therapy often impairs the secretion of pituitary tropic hormones. Finally, tumors arising inside the sella turcica (such as craniopharyngioma) or in the hypothalamus will often result in hypopituitarism. When no specific pathology is detected the hypopituitarism is termed idiopathic.

Clinical manifestations. In congenital malformations of the brain or pituitary, the first symptom in the neonate of ACTH deficiency is usually hypoglycemia. When there is consistently low blood glucose, it is important to measure growth hormone, insulin and cortisol concentrations at the time of the hypoglycemia. In pituitary disorders, cortisol and growth hormone will be abnormally low and the insulin level will be suppressed. In contrast, hyperinsulinism will be characterized by high insulin as well as high growth hormone and cortisol. MRI of the head may demonstrate atrophy of the optic chiasm and absence of the septum pellucidum, classical signs of septo-optic dysplasia. In male infants, a concomitant gonadotropin deficiency can be manifested by small genitalia and/or cryptorchidism. Other congenital malformations (such as cleft lip and/or palate) can also be associated with hypopituitarism.

It is difficult to relate hypopituitarism to a trauma of delivery or to a traumatic accident, unless there is clear-cut evidence of hemorrhage in the hypothalamic-pituitary area. When infections result in hypopituitarism there are often concomitant signs of impaired mental development. Because of variation in the localization of brain tumors, the pattern of tropic hormone insufficiency is quite variable and it may vary further after neurosurgery. In general, there is no impairment of aldosterone secretion. However, antidiuretic hormone deficiency (diabetes insipidus), when it occurs, causes disturbance of electrolytes and water balance. It must also be noted that inappropriate ADH secretion can be seen in the postneurosurgical period, and this may result in electrolyte abnormalities as well.

In idiopathic panhypopituitarism, there is usually no abnormality of the posterior pituitary gland. However, various patterns of hormone deficiencies from the anterior pituitary can be observed. Approximately one-half of the patients have normal adrenocortical function. Most of the others have normal basal cortisol secretion but are unable to increase their secretion during mild stress. However, they can respond to acute, marked stress such as IV metyrapone test, IV insulin test, IV pyrogen test.[36]

A number of cases of idiopathic isolated ACTH deficiency have been reported in the literature. Such patients have normal thyroid function and normal growth hormone secretion as well as normal sexual maturation at puberty. However, pubertal girls may have no or scant pubic hair because of lack of adrenal androgens. Many patients demonstrate hypoglycemia in infancy, leading to the diagnosis. Mutations in the TPIT gene, which encodes a transcription factor required for fetal corticotroph development, is the cause of isolated congenital ACTH deficiency in some families.

Diagnosis. In patients with hypopituitarism, it is important to evaluate the functions of the various pituitary hormones in order to determine the extent of the insufficiencies. ACTH deficiency causes low cortisol levels at any time of day, inadequate response of cortisol to stimulation tests such as the insulin-induced hypoglycemia or rapid IV ACTH tests, and low morning ACTH levels.

Cessation of glucocorticoid therapy

Glucocorticoid doses that exceed replacement requirements potentially suppress CRH and ACTH through the negative feedback mechanism that normally exists for the regulation of cortisol secretion. The general rules about hypoadrenocorticism owing to withdrawal of steroid treatment are as follows:

    a. If the dose of glucocorticoid administered was less than replacement therapy, independent of the duration of the administration, there will be no major adrenocortical suppression.

    b. If the dose of glucocorticoid administered was greater than replacement then there may be adrenocortical suppression:

        i. If the duration of therapy was less than 4 weeks the suppression will be transient with prompt recovery.

        ii. If the duration of therapy was more than 4 weeks then the adrenocortical suppression can last from 1 week to 6 months. For these patients, it may be appropriate to resume glucocorticoid administration in cases of stress for up to 6 months following cessation of treatment. If there is a need to document adrenocortical recovery, then specific testing of the ACTH/cortisol axis may be necessary (Figure 5-17).

It must be noted that adrenocortical suppression can also occur after the cessation of topical steroid therapy such as inhaled corticosteriods nasal spray, eye drops, or dermal creams and lotions.

Removal of a cortisol-secreting adrenal tumor

In cases of unilateral adrenocortical tumor producing cortisol and resulting in Cushing syndrome, the high concentration of circulating cortisol will suppress the endogenous CRH/ACTH secretion resulting in atrophy of the contralateral adrenal. Following removal of the tumor, the situation is similar to the cessation of glucocorticoid therapy. It is therefore appropriate to consider stress therapy with hydrocortisone for up to 6 months.

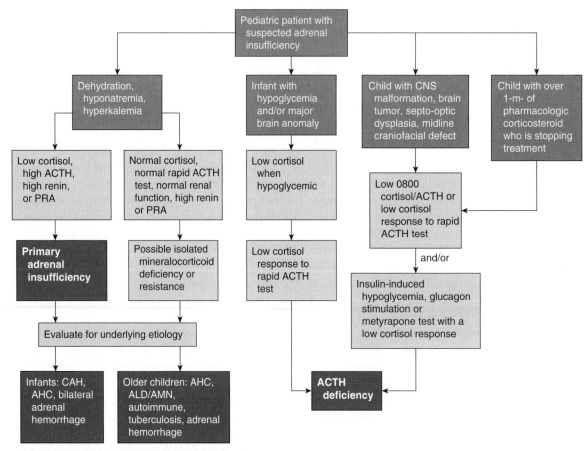

FIGURE 5-17 ■ Diagnostic algorithm for adrenal insufficiency.

Infants born of steroid-treated mothers

Usually, only a fraction of maternal cortisol crosses the placenta to reach the fetus, such that maternal cortisol contributes about 10% of the fetal concentrations. However, with therapeutic doses well above the physiologic levels, significant placental passage of steroids could result in suppression of the fetal adrenal. The cortisol secretion of 10 infants born of steroid-treated mothers was evaluated and found to be normal in cases where the mother was treated with prednisone at two to five times replacement doses. Nevertheless, it is appropriate to follow carefully the glucose concentrations of the infants, postnatally. This is especially true if the mother is treated with dexamethasone prior to delivery, as this crosses the placenta quite freely.

Hypoadrenocorticism Related to End-Organ Unresponsiveness

Unresponsiveness of the kidney to aldosterone

Unresponsiveness of the kidney to aldosterone is a heterogeneous disorder known as pseudohypoaldosteronism (PHA). PHA type 1 presents in infancy with dehydration, hyponatremia, hyperkalemia, despite marked elevations of plasma aldosterone and renin concentrations. Mineralocorticoid therapy is ineffective; patients respond only to sodium chloride supplementation.

PHA1 represents at least two disease entities, as both autosomal dominant and autosomal recessive modes of inheritance have been described. In the autosomal dominant form, there is isolated renal unresponsiveness to aldosterone. These patients typically respond to oral salt supplementation, and their clinical status improves with age. Mineralocorticoid receptor deficiency in PHA1 is as a result of mutations in the type 2 steroid hormone receptor or mineralocorticoid receptor gene

In autosomal recessive PHA1, there are multiple organs that contribute to the salt loss. These include the kidney, colon, salivary and sweat glands. In these patients, the clinical course is more severe, and correction of the life-threatening electrolyte abnormalities is quite difficult. These patients may develop a chronic lung disease similar to cystic fibrosis. The molecular defect in this type of PHA1 is now known to lie within subunits of the amiloride-sensitive epithelial sodium channel (EnaC).

In PHA type 2 (PHA2), there is hyperkalemia with metabolic acidosis, but, as opposed to PHA1, low renin hypertension is also present. These patients are effectively treated with diuretics. The molecular defect is within WNK 4 kinase.[37,38]

Obstructive uropathy may cause renal resistance to aldosterone , which is usually reversible as the obstruction is treated and renal function returns to normal.

Cortisol resistance

Cortisol resistance in humans is a rare autosomal dominant disorder that is typified by high plasma cortisol and ACTH levels, high urinary free cortisol levels, and absent suppression of cortisol and ACTH by dexamethasone. Yet, there are no clinical features of Cushing syndrome. Inheritance is reported as being autosomal dominant. Studies of the type 1 steroid hormone receptor or GR gene reveals a point mutation within the steroid-binding domain. In most families studied, cortisol resistance is partial and is compensated by elevated cortisol levels.

Naturally occurring variants of the human GR gene may confer increased or decreased sensitivity to cortisol. In addition, the GR itself has several different isoforms that mediate a wide variety of physiologic responses in a tissue-specific manner. Such variation may play a role in body fat stores and other biological responses.[39]

Approach to Clinical Management of Adrenal Insufficiency

Diagnosis of adrenal insufficiency

A proposed evaluation algorithm for patients with suspected adrenal insufficiency is shown in Figure 5-17. Different presenting signs will guide the evaluation. For example, a child with dehydration, hyponatremia, and hyperkalemia may have primary adrenal failure with symptoms related to both glucocorticoid and mineralocorticoid deficiencies. On the other hand, a patient with hypoglycemia and/or a midline craniofacial defect would need to be tested for cortisol deficiency owing to lack of ACTH effect.

The specific syndromes described above may have additional diagnostic features, such as abnormal levels of cortisol precursors or other unique laboratory test results. Please see the individual disease descriptions for these details.

The normal ranges for blood and urinary glucocorticoids, and blood ACTH are shown in Table 5-6. Protocols and normal responses for stimulation tests are shown in Table 5-7.

Treatment of adrenal insufficiency

Medical treatment. The goal of maintenance treatment is to administer a dose of cortisol equal to that normally secreted. The administered steroid produces a negative feedback on the hypothalamic-pituitary axis reducing CRH and ACTH secretion. This, in turn, suppresses the excessive secretion of cortisol precursors and adrenal androgens in CAH, and the excessive MSH secretion in Addison disease. In simple virilizing CAH, treatment replaces cortisol in amounts approximating the endogenous production, eliminates the mild salt-losing

Table 5-6.

Normal Blood and Urinary Hormone Values			
Test		**Values**[a]	
Serum cortisol[b]		μg/dL	
Premature infants (day 4)	26-28 wk	1-11 (6.0)	
	31-35 wk	2.5-9.1 (6.4)	
Full-term infants	3 d	1.7-14 (6.2)	
	7 d	2-11 (4.4)	
	31 d-11 mo	2.8-23 (9.4)	
Children	12 m-15 y (8:00 AM)	3-21 (9.8)	
Adults	8:00 AM	8-19 (11.0)	
	4:00 PM	4-11 (5.9)	
Urinary 17-hydroxycorticosteroids	(17-OHCS)	mg/g creatinine	mg/24 h
Prepubertal children	1-4 y	1.7-6.4 (4.1)	0.2-2.5 (0.8)
	5-9 y	2.2-6.0 (3.5)	0.5-2.5 (1.2)
Pubertal children and adults	Male	2.4-4.3 (3.2)	3-10 (6.4)
	Female	1.6-3.6 (2.3)	2-6 (2.8)
Urinary free cortisol		μg/g creatinine	μg/24 h
Prepubertal children		7-25 (15)	3-9 (5.2)
Adults	Male	7-45 (21)	11-84 (40)
	Female	9-32 (19)	10-34 (20)
	Pregnancy	14-59 (38)	16-60 (47)

[a] Normal ranges and means (in parentheses) are based on reference ranges from Esoterix Laboratories, Calabasas Hills, California, and are used with permission. In other laboratories, serum rather than plasma cortisol may be measured, but the reference ranges are similar.
[b] Stress (physiological or psychological) may cause elevation of cortisol levels above the reference range.

tendency, returns aldosterone secretion to normal, and suppresses androgen production and its virilizing effects.

Maintenance therapy. Based on the estimates of normal cortisol secretion rate a child with a body-surface area of 1 m² requires a dose of 5 to 16 mg/day of parenteral cortisol (mean of 12 mg or 7 mg, depending on the reference). Because of the short half-life of cortisol (hydrocortisone) given orally, and its partial destruction by gastric acidity, the optimal daily oral replacement dose may approximate 1.5 to 2 times normal daily cortisol secretion rate (ie, 14-24 mg/m²/24 h). The total daily oral dose of hydrocortisone should be divided in three fractions, given approximately every 8 hours. As the replacement dose is related to body surface area (as is the cortisol production rate), it is natural that the dose will need to be increased with growth.

Cortisol liquid for oral use (Cortef) can be compounded at a concentration of 2.5 mg/mL. If this service is not available, it may be necessary to divide the 5 mg tablets into pieces and crush the pieces to suspend in water. One can also use prednisolone syrup (Prelone 1 or 3 mg/mL, Pediapred 1 mg/mL, or Orapred 3 mg/mL). These steroids are at least five times more potent than cortisol (daily dose 3-5 mg/m²/24 h). In addition, they have a longer half-life than cortisol, which makes it possible to give the daily dose in two fractions, every 12 hours. Other synthetic glucocorticoid preparations even more potent than prednisolone, such as dexamethasone, are not often used for replacement therapy in pediatrics. Their great potency makes it difficult to titrate the appropriate dosage of each patient. Prednisolone, prednisone, and dexamethasone lack significant mineralocorticoid activity (Table 5-8). In addition, for stress dosing the longer-acting more potent corticosteroids may be less preferable to oral or injected hydrocortisone, which produces more rapid plasma cortisol peaks.

The data regarding normal cortisol production rates is helpful in estimating an initial replacement dose of cortisol; however the dose must be adjusted to the clinical courses of individual patients. In addition, the classical estimates of relative glucocorticoid potencies have come under scrutiny, leading to the suspicion that the more potent glucocorticoids may have greater therapeutic potency as glucocorticoids than as immunosuppressive agents. This would increase the risk of overtreatment and Cushingoid effects.

Therapy under stress conditions. In patients with primary or central adrenal insufficiency, there is an inadequate cortisol response to stress. In milder forms of CAH, after approximately 4 weeks of exogenous

Table 5-7.

Tests of Adrenal Capacity and ACTH Secretory Ability: Protocols and Normal Blood and Urinary Steroid Responses

Adrenal Capacity (ACTH Stimulation Tests)

Rapid IV ACTH test[a]:

Cortosyn 15 mcg/kg in neonates, 125 mcg up to 2 years, 250 mcg over 2 years of age infused IV over 1 minute. (a 1 mcg dose has been used to define more subtle degrees of adrenal insufficiency).[b]

Sample blood for serum cortisol and ACTH at baseline and for cortisol at 1 hour after infusion.

Normal response: serum cortisol at 1 hour is 7-10 mcg/dL over baseline level and >18 mcg/dL.

Prolonged ACTH test[a]: The response can either be measured as a change in urinary steroid concentrations or a change in serum cortisol levels.

Prior to starting ACTH, obtain baseline (8:00 AM) ACTH and cortisol levels, or obtain 2 consecutive days of 24-hour urine collections for 17-hydroxycorticosteroids (17OHCS) and free cortisol ending at 0800 on the morning of ACTH administration.

Give 20 U/m[2] Acthar gel (injectable ACTH that is a long-acting repository form) IM every 12 hours for 3 days, or give 250 mcg/1.73 m[2] Cortrosyn IV over 8-12 hours beginning at 8:00 AM for 3 consecutive days.

Measure serum cortisol at the end of the ACTH treatment (after 3 days of Acthar gel or once daily for 3 days at the end of the Cortrosyn infusion). If measuring urinary steroids, continue 24 hour urine collections for 17-OHCS and free cortisol during the 3 days of ACTH treatment.

Normal responses: Serum cortisol increases to >36 mcg/dL. Urinary 17-OHCS and free cortisol show a three- to fivefold increase over baseline.

ACTH Secretory Ability

Insulin-induced hypoglycemia[b]:

After fasting since midnight, the test is performed in the morning. Obtain baseline 8:00 AM serum cortisol and glucose levels. Give 0.05 units/kg of regular insulin IV, and measure cortisol and glucose levels at 15, 30, 45, and 60 minutes. If desired, samples for growth hormone can be obtained at the same time points to screen for growth hormone deficiency. Blood sugar levels should drop by 50% or to <45 mg/dL. If this does not occur by 45 minutes, the dose of insulin can be repeated.

Normal: The cortisol level should increase to twice the baseline level or above 20 mcg/dL.

Glucagon Stimulation test[c]:

After fasting since midnight, the test is performed in the morning. Obtain baseline 8:00 AM serum cortisol and glucose. Give glucagon 0.1 mg/kg IM and obtain blood samples at 15, 30, 45, 60, 90, 120, 150, and 180 minutes for glucose and cortisol levels. If desired, samples for growth hormone measurement can be obtained at the same time points to screen for growth hormone deficiency.

Normal response: the cortisol level normally decreases during the first 60-90 minutes, and then reaches a peak of >20 mcg/dL by 180 minutes. Hypoglycemia is a risk during the second half of the test.

Single dose Metyrapone Test[a] (this test should be performed in the hospital):

Obtain baseline blood sample for ACTH, cortisol, and 11-deoxycortisol levels at 8:00 AM

Give 30 mg/kg (up to 3.0 g) metyrapone PO at midnight with food.

Obtain blood for ACTH , cortisol and 11-deoxycortisol levels at 8:00 AM the following morning.

Normal response: ACTH level rises to over 100 pg/mL, 11-deoxycortisol rises to >7 mcg/dL, and cortisol drops to <5 mcg/dL if there has been adequate suppression of 11-hydroxylase activity.

Prolonged Metyrapone Test[a] (this test should be performed in the hospital):

Obtain baseline blood sample for ACTH, cortisol, and 11-deoxycortisol at 8:00 AM

Give 15 -mg/kg or 300 mg/m[2] every 4 hours for six doses at 8:00 AM, 12:00 noon, 4:00 PM, 8:00 PM, 12:00 midnight, and 4:00 AM.

Four hours after the last dose, at 8:00 AM, obtain blood for ACTH, cortisol, and 11-deoxycortisol.

Normal response: ACTH level rises to over 100 pg/mL, 11-deoxycortisol rises to >7 mcg/dL, and cortisol drops to <5 mcg/dL if there has been adequate suppression of 11-hydroxylase activity

[a] Normal ranges and protocols are from Esoterix Laboratories, Calabasas Hills, California, and are used with permission.

[b] References for insulin-induced hypoglycemia: Donohoue PA. The adrenal gland and its disorders. In: Kappy MS, Allen DB, Geffner ME, eds. Principles and Practice of Pediatric Endocrinology. Charles C. Thomas Publisher; Springfield, IL; 2005:381.

Schmidt IL, et al. Diagnosis of adrenal insufficiency: Evaluation of the corticotropin releasing hormone test and basal serum cortisol in comparison to the insulin tolerance test in patients with hypothalamic-pituitary-adrenal disease. J Clin Endocrinol Metab. 2003;88:4193.

[c] The glucagon stimulation test is described by Vanderschueren-Lodeweyckx M, et al. The glucagon stimulation test: effect on plasma growth hormone and on immunoreactive insulin, cortisol, and glucose in children. J Pediatr. 1974;85:182-187.

Table 5-8.

Relative Potency of Oral Corticosteroid Preparations

Generic Name	Trade Name	Glucocorticoid Effect Equivalent to 100 mg Cortisol PO	Sodium Retention Effect Equivalent to 0.1 mg Florinef PO
Cortisol (hydrocortisone)	Hydrocortone, Cortef	100	20
Cortisone	Cortone	125	20
Δ-cortisol (prednisolone)	Delta-cortef, Orapred, Pediapred	20	50
Δ-cortisone (prednisone)	Deltasone, Meticorten, Sterapred	25	50
6α-CH$_3$-Δ-prednisolone (methylprednisolone)	Medrol	15 (20[a])	No effect[a]
9α-Fluoro-16α-CH$_3$-prednisolone (dexamethasone)	Decadron, Hexadrol	1.5 (3.75[a])	No effect[a]
9α-Fluorocortisol acetate	Florinef acetate, Fludrocortisone acetate	6.5	0.1

All values in mg.
[a] *Values estimated by the respective pharmaceutical companies.*

cortisol therapy, the CRH-ACTH system is suppressed and unable to respond normally to stress. In all of these situations, it is necessary for the patient to increase their cortisol doses. Minor infection and/or low-grade fever (sore throat, runny nose, temperature up to 38°C) may not require a change in dosage. During conditions of moderate stress (severe upper respiratory infections) the dosage should be doubled, whereas in major stress, with temperature above 38°C and/or vomiting, the cortisol requirement may be three to four times the normal replacement.

Under stress conditions, infants and children are frequently unable to retain oral medications. In such cases, the parents are advised to administer an intramuscular injection of cortisol sodium succinate (SoluCortef). A simple age-based dose regimen can be used: less than 3 years, 25 mg; 3 to 12 years, 50 mg; 12 years and older, 100 mg. This treatment will provide up to 6 hours of coverage, and allow the family time to get medical treatment (Table 5-9). There is a growing experience with parenteral hydrocortisone in rectal suppositories. The dose is approximately 100 mg/m². This route is often better accepted by families and patients than intramuscular injection.[18]

Therapy during surgical procedures. During general anesthesia, with or without surgery, the cortisol secretion rate in normal subjects increases greatly. Similarly, in patients with adrenal insufficiency, the glucocorticoid requirement increases.

Although protocols vary, the following protocol from the consensus conference for congenital adrenal hyperplasia[18] is useful for surgical procedures that last longer than 30 to 45 minutes. The initial dose is given as an IV bolus followed by a continuous IV infusion. The stress doses of hydrocortisone are tapered rapidly according to the clinical improvement, generally by reducing the dose by 50% each day.

- 0 to 3 years: Hydrocortisone 25 mg IV, then 25 to 30 mg/day
- 3 years to 12 years: Hydrocortisone 50 mg IV, then 50 to 60 mg/day
- 12 years and older: Hydrocortisone 100 mg IV, then 100 mg/day

For procedures lasting longer than 30 to 45 minutes, we suggest using a protocol that includes a continuous infusion of glucocorticoid, such as the following[18]: A rapid injection of 25 mg/m² of hydrocortisone sodium succinate (eg, SoluCortef) is given IV just prior to anesthesia and is followed by a dose of approximately 50 mg/m² as a constant infusion for the period of the surgical procedure. If the patient will not be able to take oral hydrocortisone postoperatively, a third dose of approximately 25 to 50 mg/m² hydrocortisone is given as a constant IV infusion for the rest of the first 24 hours of the surgical day. This is followed the next day by three to four times replacement therapy hydrocortisone given by constant IV infusion or orally. These high doses will provide the needed extra glucocorticoid as well as mineralocorticoid coverage. Hydrocortisone 40 mg has approximately the same mineralocorticoid effect as 0.2 mg of 9α-fluoro cortisol. Stress dosing is generally continued until the patient can tolerate oral intake, is afebrile, and is hemodynamically stable. The timing is dictated by the nature of the surgery and expected recovery time.

Table 5-9.

Adrenal Crisis and Stress—Evaluation and Treatment

A. Stresses that may increase the risk of adrenal crisis:
Fever
Sepsis
Trauma
Anesthesia
Surgery

B. Signs and symptoms that may indicate adrenal crisis:
Hypotension or shock, particularly if disproportionate to apparent underlying illness.
Serum electrolyte abnormalities:
  Hyponatremia
  Hyperkalemia
  Hypoglycemia
  Metabolic acidosis
Vomiting and diarrhea, sometimes with severe abdominal pain or unexplained fever, weight loss, and anorexia.

C. Consider adrenal crisis in the following settings:
Any patient with known disorders of adrenal insufficiency (eg, congenital adrenal hyperplasia), especially if exposed to stress (illness).
Other patients presenting with the above signs, especially with hyperpigmentation or vitiligo.
Critically ill patients with septic shock, who are unresponsive to fluid resuscitation and inotropic medications (in this case, adrenal crisis is caused by bilateral adrenal hemorrhage).
Patients on or withdrawing from chronic treatment with steroids, especially if exposed to stress.
Patients with other autoimmune endocrine deficiencies, such as hypothyroidism or gonadal failure.
Neonates with the above symptoms and signs should prompt consideration of the diagnosis of congenital adrenal hyperplasia (CAH) owing to 21-hydroxylase deficiency, or (very rarely) other causes of adrenal insufficiency.

D. Evaluation:
If adrenal crisis is suspected, then patients should be treated empirically with stress doses of corticosteroids, as outlined below.
Baseline blood samples should be drawn for subsequent testing for cortisol, ACTH, and steroid precursors (if CAH is suspected) prior to the administration of corticosteroids.
Treatment should not be delayed pending results.

E. Treatment:
Fluids: give bolus of 5% Dextrose with 0.9% saline, without potassium (D5NS), 20 mg/kg over 1 hour
Stress steroids (parenteral): administer hydrocortisone succinate (SoluCortef) urgently at the following doses:
  Infants and toddlers, 0-3 years old: 25 mg IV
  Children 3-12 years: 50 mg IV
  Children and adolescents 12 years and older: 100 mg IV
Continue corticosteroids at the same dose given as a constant rate over the following 24 hours.
Electrolytes: if hyperkalemia is present or is suspected, perform ECG.
  ECG changes consistent with hyperkalemia: initially a tall peaked T wave with shortened QT interval, followed by progressive lengthening of the PR interval and QRS duration.
  If these changes are present, treat with insulin and glucose infusion, with or without other measures to treat hyperkalemia.
Monitor and treat other electrolyte abnormalities and fluid balance.

Box 5-2 lists the circumstances in which a patient with adrenal insufficiency should be referred to a pediatric endocrinologist.

Treatment of adrenal crisis

The rapid recognition and prompt electrolyte and fluid therapy of the salt-losing crisis are critical to survival of these patients, especially infants. In patients who do not have a specific diagnosis of adrenal insufficiency, appropriate blood samples must be obtained for the measurement of cortisol and ACTH, of steroid precursors (if suspicious for CAH), or VLCFAs if considering ALD. In patients with signs of adrenal insufficiency and ambiguous genitalia, a karyotype is needed.

Treatment of adrenal crisis is outlined in Table 5-9, and is initiated with a 1 hour bolus of 20 mL/kg of 5%

dextrose with normal saline. Although this will correct the plasma sodium and chloride concentrations, as well as hypoglycemia if present, the potassium concentration usually remains elevated and the acidosis may persist. Approximately 100 to 150 mL/kg of the same IV solution may be needed over the next 24 hours. In addition, therapy with glucocorticoid and mineralocorticoid is started. In newborn infants we advise an IV injection of 25 mg of Solu-Cortef. This is followed by another 20 to 25 mg of SoluCortef administered at a constant rate over the next 24-hour period. This 40 to 50 mg dose of cortisol is the equivalent of about 12 to 15 times replacement therapy for an infant with a normal body-surface area of approximately 0.25 m², and has a salt-retaining activity of approximately 0.2 mg of 9α-fluoro-cortisol. It may be necessary to use Kayexalate, or insulin and glucose, if the hyperkalemia is associated with electrocardiogram (ECG) changes. Throughout the treatment, electrolytes and water balance must be monitored very carefully in order to avoid hypernatremia, water retention, and possible pulmonary edema. Parenteral mineralocorticoid is not available, so as soon as the patient is able to tolerate oral medication, treatment is started with 9α-fluoro-cortisol, 0.1 to 0.2 mg/day.

Mineralocorticoid replacement therapy. The only medication currently available for this specific purpose is 9α-fluoro-cortisol given orally at a dose of 0.05 to 0.15 mg/24 h. In infancy, breast milk or prepared formula provides a very little salt (8-10 mEq of sodium per 24 hours). For this reason, 20 to 40 mEq sodium chloride is added to the regimen, divided into three or four daily doses. This can be prescribed as a 2 mEq/mL solution, or prepared by the parents. One-fourth of a teaspoon of table salt is about 20 meq of sodium. When the diet of the child becomes more varied and includes solid food, which is usually rich in sodium, the salt supplement is no longer required.

CAH—special considerations

The most common cause of adrenal insufficiency in pediatrics is CAH owing to CYP21 deficiency, thus a discussion relating to treatment of this specific disease is important.

The criteria for determining the appropriate cortisol dose in CAH owing to CYP21 deficiency include the concentration of 17-hydroxyprogesterone and androstenedione in plasma, or the excretion of 17-ketosteroids in urine, and the close follow-up of somatic growth (weight, bone age, and height and weight velocities). In affected children, levels of plasma androstenedione and urinary 17-ketosteroids should be in the prepubertal reference range. However, *normal prepubertal concentrations of 17-hydroxyprogesterone are usually indicative of over treatment.* Normal prepubertal 17-hydroxyprogesterone is 0 to 80 ng/dL; acceptable values for treated CAH are up to 500 ng/dL; concentrations of more than 1000 ng/dL usually indicate insufficient therapy. Patients with simple virilizing CAH have normal serum electrolytes, and do not have an absolute requirement for mineralocorticoid replacement therapy. However, in the clinical setting of difficulty in suppressing adequately the adrenal androgen excess, combined with an elevated PRA, mineralocorticoid treatment may be beneficial, and avoids the deleterious effects of higher cortisol replacement doses. The mechanism of this beneficial effect is not entirely clear. Perhaps the mineralocorticoid effect of increased intravascular volume suppresses vasopressin secretion and its stimulation of ACTH production. Another possibility is that the minor glucocorticoid effect of fludrocortisone enhances the effect of cortisol treatment. The use of antagonists of androgens and aromatase has been reported, and is still considered investigational.

During the growth period of the child, it is important to increase the glucocorticoid dose in relation to increasing body size as described for the simple virilizing form. It is also important to adjust the dose to individual requirements. It is of interest that even when dose is adjusted to body size, there appears to be a temporal variation of requirement (Figure 5-18); in infancy the average required dose is much higher than it is in childhood; then there is another increase at the time of puberty.

Surgery of the external genitalia of female CAH patients. Surgery to change the appearance of the external genitalia of female infants with the salt-losing form is available, just as it is for female infants with the simple virilizing form. Girls with the salt-losing form, in general, have more completely masculinized external genitalia, and in many there is no connection between the upper third of the vagina and the exterior of the perineum. In these patients, the vagina opens by a narrow passage into the posterior part of the urethra, sometimes at the neck of the bladder. In such cases, a two-step surgical repair is often advised, with the first step in the first year of life and the second step at the time of puberty.

Alternative therapies. In some females with salt-losing CAH, results of therapy are suboptimal, and androgen

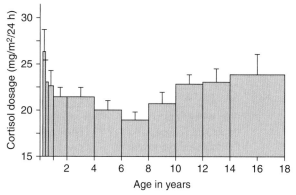

FIGURE 5-18 ■ Cortisol dosage variation in congenital adrenal hyperplasia. The shaded columns represent the mean dose and each bar is the standard error of the mean (SEM). The dosage, which was maximal very early in life, dropped rapidly by 1 year of age and was minimal between 6 and 8 years, before it returned to a higher adult level. *(Redrawn from Sandrini R, Jospe N, Migeon CJ. Temporal and individual variations in the dose of glucocorticoid used for the treatment of salt-losing congenital vitalizing adrenal hyperplasia owing to 21-hydroxylase deficiency. Acta Paediatr Suppl. 1993;388:56.)*

excess is quite problematic and refractory to suppression with physiologic cortisol replacement dosages. For this reason adrenalectomy has been proposed for specific patients. Because of this, and because in general the long-term results of replacement therapy have not been perfect, bilateral adrenalectomy has been proposed as a possible means of improving these results. Other approaches to treatment have included peripheral blockade of androgen action and estrogen production with testolactone and flutamide. It is important to emphasize that such alternatives are presently experimental and many years of follow-up will be required to judge their validity.[18]

Psychological treatment. In all patients with CAH, there is a risk of psychological problems related to having a chronic disease. In females this is complicated by a history of ambiguous genitalia and genital surgery. Adjustment is usually improved when the patient and parents understand the pathogenesis of the disorder. Appropriate glucocorticoid treatment will remediate the chronic androgen excess, and thus adherence to treatment recommendations should prevent androgen excess at puberty. There is some evidence that prenatal androgen exposure influences postnatal behavior in some females with CAH, but this is highly variable.[40]

Attenuated CAH

There is some degree of overlap between PCOS and attenuated CAH, thus some patients with CAH may have enough ovarian secretion of androgen to require addition of ovarian suppressive therapy (oral contraceptives) to reduce the virilizing symptoms.

Treatment of ACTH deficiency. As previously noted, the patients will require appropriate replacement of the deficient cortisol, as well as any other deficient hormones. When basal cortisol secretion is abnormally low, both maintenance and stress therapy are required. When basal concentrations are normal but the rapid IV ACTH test or oral metyrapone test is abnormal, only stress therapy may be required.

In patients with a deficiency of both TSH and ACTH, cortisol replacement should be initiated prior to thyroxine replacement. This is because thyroid replacement in absence of glucocorticoid may result in symptoms of acute adrenal insufficiency. On occasion, ADH deficiency is unmasked shortly after starting cortisol replacement therapy. Since cortisol is needed to excrete a water load, cortisol deficiency partially corrects the diuresis of diabetes insipidus.

Hyperadrenocorticism

The classification of adrenocortical overactivity syndromes is usually based on the clinical findings related to the specific hormone that is in excess. In some cases, there are several hormones that are over-secreted together.

In Cushing syndrome, there is cortisol excess. It is owing to a number of different etiologies (Table 5-10), including Cushing disease resulting from hypersecretion of ACTH, and other causes of cortisol excess such as primary adrenal sources and iatrogenic causes.

The so-called adrenogenital syndrome results from hypersecretion of adrenal androgens. This syndrome usually results from one of two causes, congenital adrenal hyperplasia (CAH) or masculinizing adrenal tumors. As it is now known that CAH results from a reduction of cortisol secretion, and subsequent stimulation of ACTH secretion causes overproduction of other adrenal steroids that may or may not include androgens, in this chapter CAH was covered under the section "Hypoadrenocorticism." Masculinizing tumors secrete androgen, and in many cases also secrete cortisol.

Feminizing adrenal tumors cause excess estrogen secretion of adrenal origin. These tumors rarely secrete only estrogen, and in most cases secrete both estrogen and androgen. They are termed "feminizing tumors" if the estrogen effects predominate.

Primary hyperaldosteronism or Conn syndrome is due to excessive secretion of aldosterone. Similar clinical findings may also result from dexamethasone-suppressible hypertension or apparent mineralocorticoid excess (AME).

Cushing syndrome

If one excludes iatrogenic causes, Cushing syndrome is rare in infancy childhood. In all age groups, there is a two- to threefold predominance of females. The signs and symptoms may develop over a short period of time, and after cure will regress rapidly (Figure 5-19).

Table 5-10.

Etiologies and Features of Various Types of Hypercortisolism

Disorder	Etiology	Adrenal Glands	ACTH Secretion
Cushing disease	Pituitary adenoma	Bilateral hyperplasia	+ to ++
Cushing syndrome	Adrenal adenoma	Contralateral hypoplasia	Low to absent
	Adrenal carcinoma	Contralateral hypoplasia	Low to absent
Bilateral micronodular adrenal hyperplasia	Activated ACTH receptor (eg, McCune-Albright syndrome)	Bilateral hyperplasia	Low to absent
Primary pigmented adrenal hyperplasia	Stimulating adrenal immunoglobulins (may be seen with Carney complex)	Bilateral hyperplasia with deeply pigmented nodules	Low to absent
Bilateral macronodular adrenal hyperplasia	Food-dependent Cushing syndrome	Bilateral hyperplasia	Low to absent
Ectopic ACTH (CRH)	Nonpituitary ACTH (CRH)-producing tumor	Bilateral hyperplasia	+ to +++
Pseudo-Cushing syndrome	Depression, alcoholism (increased CRH secretion)	Normal or small	+ to ++
Iatrogenic Cushing syndrome	Pharmacologic glucocorticoid therapy	Bilateral hypoplasia	Low to absent

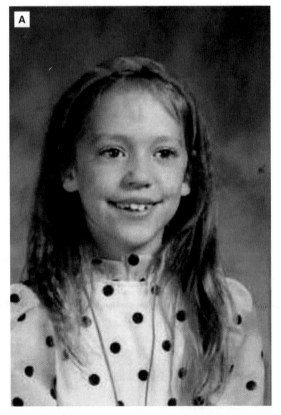
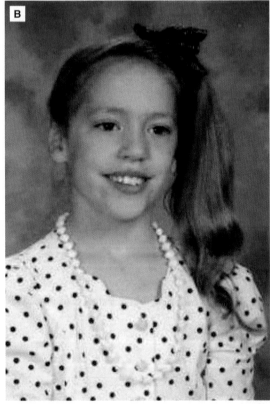

FIGURE 15-19 ■ Female child with Cushing syndrome. The photographs depict the patient at age 6 years 10 months **(A)**; 7 years 10 months **(B)**; 9 years 10 months **(C)**; 10 years 10 months, 6 weeks prior to the diagnosis of Cushing disease **(D)**; age 11 years 10 months, after surgical resection of pituitary adenoma **(E)**; and at age 16 years **(F)**.

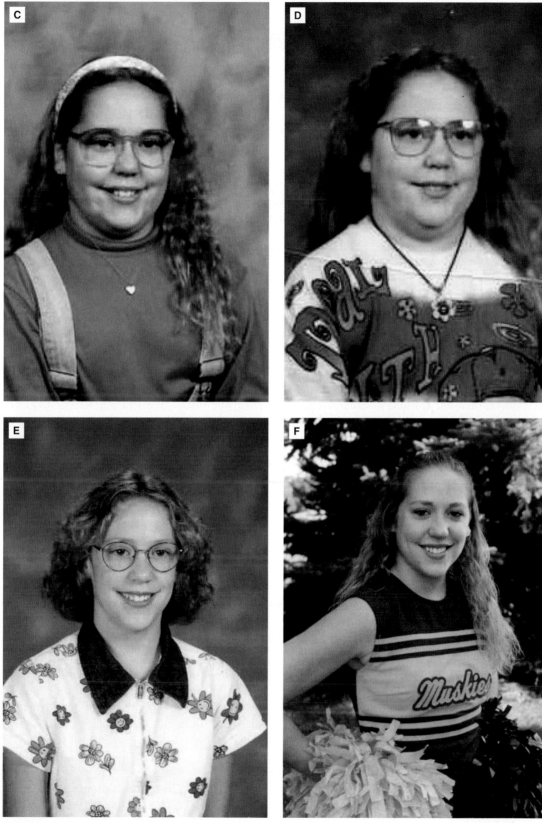

FIGURE 15-19 ■ (*Continued*)

Table 5-11.

Effects of Hypercortisolism

Tissue Effect	Laboratory Findings	Signs/Symptoms
On muscle cells		
Protein catabolism	Increased serum amino acids, negative	Muscle wasting
Decreased glucose uptake	nitrogen balance	
and glycogen storage		
On adipose tissue		
Increased lipolysis	Hyperlipidemia, hypercholesterolemia	Truncal obesity
On liver carbohydrate metabolism		
Increased gluconeogenesis	Hyperglycemia, glucosuria	Diabetes
On bones		
Increased protein matrix resorption	Possible hypocalcemia	Osteoporosis
Inhibition of vitamin D-mediated calcium		Growth retardation
absorption from gut		
On water and electrolyte balance		
Increased sodium retention and potassium loss	Hypokalemia	Muscle wasting
Water retention	Mild hypernatrmia	Hypertension

Clinical manifestations. Cushing syndrome is characterized by hypercortisolism, and its clinical features represent an exaggeration of the physiological effects of cortisol (Tables 5-1 and 5-11). The effects on skeletal muscle and fat are manifested as wasting of the extremities, truncal obesity, moon facies, and cervical fat pad ("buffalo hump"). The skeletal effects in all age groups included osteoporosis and osteomalacia. In children, there is marked inhibition of skeletal growth and maturation resulting in short stature and delayed bone age. This contrasts markedly with the growth acceleration and advanced bone age associated with common obesity in childhood. The effects on collagen result in atrophy and thinning of the skin, and violaceous striae characteristically on the abdomen and hips. Capillary fragility is another effect, and it is manifested by easy bruisability.

Hypertension is an inconsistent finding, and may result from the salt-retaining effect of cortisol or other substances. Hypokalemia, if present, may cause muscle weakness and fatigue.

In some patients, cortisol excess is accompanied by oversecretion of adrenal androgens, and the typical Cushingoid features are accompanied by generalized virilism or hirsutism. This is manifested by excess hair growth of the face, extremities, trunk, and pubic area. In some children, marked androgen effects may occur, and the time course of these changes is generally more rapid than that seen in virilizing CAH or precocious puberty.

CNS effects of excess cortisol are not well understood, but may include broad mood swings, psychosis, and idiopathic intracranial hypertension.

Stimulation of gastric acid secretion by excess cortisol may cause dyspepsia and gastric ulcers. The latter is more common in adults than in children.

Laboratory diagnosis

General. Hematological parameters show an increase in neutrophils and perhaps a high hematocrit. Electrolytes may reveal hypokalemia and/or hypochloremia. There is expansion of intravascular fluid volume, despite the stimulatory effect of cortisol on free water excretion at physiologic concentrations. Calcium concentration in the blood is usually normal despite its increased urinary excretion. Serum phosphate may be low.

Plasma amino acid concentrations are elevated because of protein catabolism. Plasma insulin levels are elevated as a result of the cortisol-related insulin resistance. Blood glucose may increase because of the combination of insulin resistance and gluconeogenesis. As a result, glucosuria may also be detected. Hyperlipidemia may result from increased lipolysis stimulated by cortisol excess, as well as the increased conversion of glucose to lipids by the high insulin concentrations.

Cortisol and ACTH concentrations. Demonstration of excess cortisol is necessary to confirm the diagnosis of Cushing syndrome, but the diagnosis often requires complex and tedious testing to confirm or rule it out. Direct measurement of cortisol concentration is helpful as a screening test, however owing to the marked increase in ACTH and cortisol during stressful situations, particularly phlebotomy in children, cortisol and

ACTH levels are often elevated in patients without Cushing syndrome. In patients with Cushing syndrome, there is not only elevation of cortisol but also loss of the normal diurnal variation, thus levels should be obtained at both 8 AM and 4 PM for comparison. A serum cortisol level at midnight has been proposed as a method of distinguishing Cushing from pseudo-Cushing syndrome. In a study of 240 patients with Cushing syndrome and 23 with pseudo-Cushing, a midnight serum cortisol concentration more than 7.5 mcg/dL had 100% specificity and 96% sensitivity for Cushing syndrome. A level of less than 1.8 mcg/dL at that time excludes the diagnosis.

ACTH should be measured simultaneously with cortisol. If ACTH concentration is quite low or undetectable (<10 pg/dL) in the face of high cortisol, then an adrenal tumor producing cortisol should be suspected. If the level of ACTH in the late afternoon is not suppressed (>20 pg/dL) in the face of high cortisol, then stress or ACTH-dependent Cushing must be considered. In some patients with suspected ACTH-dependent Cushing disease, ACTH levels measured on samples obtained from the inferior petrosal sinus can aid the localization of the ACTH secreting lesion.

Midnight salivary cortisol has been proposed as another useful test for Cushing syndrome. The sample can be collected at home, away from the stress of the health care facility or phlebotomy. In adults, cut-off values vary but values more than 0.55 mcg/dL are suggestive of Cushing syndrome, and those less than 0.35 mcg/dL rule against it.[41,42]

Urinary steroid excretion. The excretion of 17-OHCS or free cortisol is a useful assessment of the 24 hour secretion of cortisol. Urinary free cortisol is felt to be a direct reflection of unbound cortisol in blood, therefore representing the biologically active hormone. In Cushing syndrome, the increment in urinary free cortisol is proportionately greater than that in 17-OHCS. Urinary excretion of 17-OHCS is considered normal if less than 5.5 mg/m²/day. From 5.5 to 9.0 mg/m²/day is considered elevated and further evaluation for Cushing is recommended. Values more than 9.0 mg/m²/day are suspicious of Cushing syndrome. Urinary excretion of free cortisol is generally expressed as mcg/day, corrected for surface area, or corrected for creatinine excretion as mcg/mg creatinine/day. Values over 70 mcg/m²/day are considered elevated and deserving of further evaluation.

Dexamethasone suppressions tests. Suppression of ACTH secretion with dexamethasone is useful in determining the etiology of ACTH-dependent Cushing syndrome. Suppression is usually attempted with a low-dose or overnight test. An oral dose of 1.25 mg/m² (or 1.0 mg in adults) is administered at midnight, and cortisol concentration is measured at 8 AM to 9 AM the following

morning. A normal response is defined as a cortisol of less than or equal to 1.8 mcg/dL. Failure of suppression leads to the next step, with a higher dose of dexamethasone. Protocols vary, but include the Liddle 2-day test (0.5 mg every 6 hours for eight doses, starting at 9 AM). After 48 hours, cortisol is measured. A single dose high-dose test using 8 mg dexamethasone followed by tests for cortisol the following morning can also be used. In general, ACTH-dependent Cushing owing to a pituitary tumor will show suppression with the high-dose but not the low-dose test. Ectopic ACTH secreting tumors and CRH-secreting tumors are less likely to suppress with high dose dexamethasone. As an alternative to measuring the cortisol response to dexamethasone, the 24-hour urinary free cortisol or 17-OHCS can be followed. Whereas these avoid the stress of phlebotomy, they are not commonly employed because of their cumbersome and error-prone collections.

CRH stimulation test. The IV administration of ovine CRH, 100 mcg/m² (100 mcg in adults), causes an exaggerated ACTH response at 30 minutes and cortisol response at 60 minutes in patients with pituitary Cushing disease. Patients with ectopic secretion of ACTH or adrenal tumors do not show this pattern. Some investigators have demonstrated the usefulness in combining the CRH test before and after the 48 hour dexamethasone suppression test. This combination has been shown to differentiate between Cushing syndrome and Pseudo-Cushing.

Key Clinical Recommendations

Differentiating the hypercortisolism of Cushing syndrome from that of obesity—Patients with obesity have elevated cortisol secretion rates and excretion of urinary 17-OHCS. Correction of these values for body surface area normalizes them in many subjects, but not all. The low-dose dexamethasone suppression test may help in the differentiation between Cushing syndrome and common obesity. Obese subjects show suppression of urinary 17-OHCS excretion and serum cortisol concentration at 8 AM in the morning after an oral dose of dexamethasone at 11 PM of 1.25 mg/m².

Determining the etiology of hypercortisolism—In patients with clinical evidence of Cushing syndrome who have elevated blood, salivary, and urinary cortisol concentrations, it is necessary to determine the etiology in order to recommend treatment. Exogenous sources such as oral, topical, or inhaled steroids must be ruled out. In addition, one must consider the possibility of pseudo-Cushing syndrome, which is most often secondary to chronic alcoholism or depression. The latter can usually be distinguished from

Table 5-12.

Characteristics of Hormone Secretion in Various Forms of Cushing Syndrome

| | Cortisol Secretion | | | | | | |
	Baseline	Midnight Salivary	Low Dose Dex Suppression	High Dose Dex Suppression	Cortisol Response to ACTH	ACTH Response to CRH	Androgen Secretion
Pituitary adenoma	+ to ++	+ to ++	No	Yes	++	+++	+ to ++
Adrenal adenoma	+ to ++	+ to ++	No	No	–/+	–	– to normal
Adrenal carcinoma	+ to +++	++ to +++	No	No	–	–	+ to +++
Food dependent	Low to normal		No	No	–		
Micronodular hyperplasia	+ to +++		No	Variable	++		normal
Pseudo-Cushing	+	+	Yes	Yes	+	–	+
Iatrogenic	* – to ++	*– to ++	No	No	–	–	* – to +

This depends on whether the therapy is cortisol/cortisone, or synthetic glucocorticoid. The latter is not measured accurately in the cortisol assay.

Cushing syndrome based on the clinical history, along with laboratory findings (Table 5-12). Pseudo-Cushing syndrome is cured when the underlying cause is effectively treated.

An algorithm for approaching the diagnosis of Cushing syndrome in pediatric patients is shown in Figure 5-20. Over the years, myriad testing regimens have been proposed, and certain variations in the basic approach may be useful in specific patients. In general, as discussed earlier, the first screening tests include measurement of plasma cortisol and ACTH at 8 AM and 4 PM, and midnight blood or salivary cortisol. If elevated, urinary excretion of 17-OHCS and/or free cortisol are determined. If these results are elevated, the next step is a low dose or overnight dexamethasone suppression test. If suppression is adequate, Cushing syndrome is unlikely. If not, further testing with CRH stimulation, high dose dexamethasone suppression, or both, is indicated.

Radiologic studies for the determination of the etiology of hypercortisolism—Radiologic imaging studies are necessary to localize the source of excess hormone secretion. CT scans are the study of choice for the adrenal glands. Adrenal hyperplasia caused by ACTH hypersecretion is easily detected. Bilateral micronodular adrenal hyperplasia is also diagnosed by this study, as well as by biopsy. Of course,

unilateral adrenal tumors accompanied by contralateral adrenal atrophy are also visible with this test. CT scanning is also useful in the detection of ectopic ACTH secreting tumors, which are most often located in the lungs. The latter tumors are quite rare in childhood.

MRI is the study of choice for brain imaging. Unfortunately, many ACTH-secreting pituitary adenomas are quite small and avoid detection. Because surgical resection represents a cure, localization is extremely important. Therefore, some patients require bilateral inferior petrosal sinus sampling for ACTH levels to localize the tumor prior to surgical resection. The sensitivity of is study this enhanced by measuring ACTH before, and 15 and 30 minutes after administration of IV CRH.

Treatment
ACTH-dependent Cushing disease

Pituitary adenoma—The treatment of choice is resection of the pituitary tumor, which, if complete, is curative. This is most often accomplished through the transsphenoidal route. If not successful, pituitary radiation is a generally effective second-line treatment. The most common side-effect of the radiation is growth hormone deficiency, which occurs in more than 80% of patients. Most patients will have transient suppression of the normal ACTH axis after

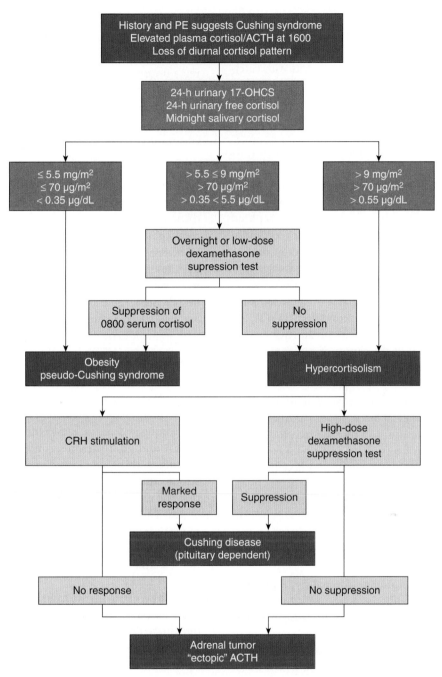

FIGURE 5-20 ■ Algorithm for the study of patients with suspected hypercortisolism versus obesity. Patients should be initially evaluated as indicated in the top panel. They can then be stratified as to low risk (left), moderate risk (middle) or higher risk (right). It should be noted that not all patients will logically follow one of these paths, and additional testing may be needed.

surgery, necessitating corticosteroid replacement therapy for several months.[43]

Ectopic ACTH-secreting tumor—As mentioned above, this is quite rare in childhood. Localization of the source, and subsequent resection are the main goals of treatment. As most of these tumors are highly malignant, treatment generally involves a combination of surgery, radiation, and chemotherapy.

CRH-secreting tumors—These are rare both in childhood and in adulthood.

Adrenocortical tumors—In very young children, 80% of Cushing syndrome is caused by a unilateral adrenal tumor. Adrenal tumors can also arise from ectopic adrenal tissue, such as in the liver. Unfortunately, these are very often malignant carcinomas demonstrating local invasion or distant metastases at the time of diagnosis.

If detected early, surgical resection can be curative. Distant metastases generally involve the lung, bone, and liver.

After surgical resection, patients with carcinomas may or may not benefit from radiation to the tumor bed. Chemotherapeutic regimens for patients with metastatic disease are generally effective. Adrenal adenomas have an excellent prognosis for complete cure after surgical resection.

After surgical resection of an adrenal tumor, there is a high risk of suppression of the CRH/ACTH/adrenal axis. The atrophied contralateral adrenal usually recovers within 6 months, thus corticosteroid therapy must be provided postoperatively, and the dosage very slowly reduced to avoid adrenal insufficiency.

Bilateral adrenal hyperplasia—The most common cause of this condition is ACTH-dependent Cushing syndrome, and treatment is the removal of the source of excess ACTH or CRH. Other more unusual causes are described later on.

Food-dependent Cushing syndrome—In these patients, bilateral macronodular adrenal hyperplasia is because of an aberrant receptor causing adrenal sensitivity to gastric inhibitory polypeptide (GIP). These patients, who have intermittent Cushing syndrome, have low ACTH levels, normal fasting cortisol concentration, and increases of plasma cortisol in response to ingestion of food or infusion of GIP. This effect can be blocked with octreotide, which is an effective medical therapy.

Bilateral micronodular adrenal hyperplasia—This rare condition is due to constitutively activated ACTH receptors on the adrenocortical cells. This activation results from mutations of the gene encoding the alpha subunit of the stimulatory G protein, Gsα. These patients, who may also have other manifestations of this mutation as seen in the McCune-Albright syndrome, require bilateral adrenalectomy to cure the hypercortisolism.

Medical treatment of Cushing syndrome. Some medications may offer palliation in patients with Cushing syndrome that cannot be cured surgically. Some choices include the steroidogenic inhibitors mitotane, metyrapone, aminoglutethimide, and ketoconazole. In terms of drugs that have a neuromodulatory effect on ACTH, the choices include bromocriptine, cyproheptadine, valproic acid, and octreotide. GR antagonism with RU-486 (mifepristone) has been used with success in a small number of patients.

Virilizing Tumors

Virilizing tumors are the most common adrenocortical tumors of childhood. In most parts of the world they remain rare, but certain clusters do occur, and suggest environmental factors or genetic contributions in isolated populations. These tumors tend to have a twofold female preponderance, and are quite unusual in the first year of life.

Clinical manifestations. In females, the tumors cause hirsutism and virilization. Usually, pubic hair appears first, followed by clitoromegaly. In older girls, the hyperandrogenism prevents normal pubertal maturation, thus breast development is delayed. In prepubertal males, there is also marked hirsutism. There is pubic hair development and growth of the phallus, without testicular enlargement. In both sexes, there is increased muscle mass, rapid skeletal growth, advanced bone age, and occasional hemihypertrophy. The tumors are rarely large enough to be detected by abdominal palpation.[44]

Hormone levels. Virilizing tumors secrete large amounts of androgen precursors without ACTH stimulation. Most patients have marked elevation of urinary 17-ketosteroids. A large fraction of the blood androgens are conjugated as sulfates, with a predominance of DHEA and androsterone. Among the unconjugated androgens, there is a marked increase in DHEA, testosterone, and androstenedione. There is good evidence that the elevated testosterone is of adrenal origin, as opposed to the peripheral conversion of androstenedione to testosterone seen in CAH.

Most patients have normal cortisol secretion, and normal electrolytes and aldosterone secretion.

Pathology. Patients with virilizing tumors that also secret excess cortisol have a poorer prognosis. It is often difficult to differentiate between an adenoma and a carcinoma. As a rule carcinomas tend to be larger and more vascular, with heterogeneous areas of cystic formation, hemorrhage, and necrosis. In advanced carcinomas, there is local invasion of the kidney or liver.

Diagnosis

Androgen secretion—The marked increase in androgen secretion can be demonstrated by elevated urinary 17-ketosteroid excretion, and elevated plasma androgens. In most cases, over 50% of the fractionated 17-KS will be DHEA.

Dexamethasone suppression test—As opposed to the hyperandrogenism of CAH, the androgen secretion from adrenal tumors is not suppressible. If dexamethasone 1.25 mg/m^2/day orally, divided every 8 hours for 5 to 7 days causes little or no change in urinary 17-ketosteroid excretion or blood androgen levels, an adreno-cortical tumor is suspected.

> **Imaging studies**—Abdominal CT is usually the preferred method of detecting these tumors, although MRI may be used as well.

Differential diagnosis. In the differential diagnosis of virilization, it must be determined if the androgens are adrenal, gonadal, or exogenous in origin. In girls, the possibilities include ovarian tumors, premature adrenarche, precocious puberty, polycystic ovary syndrome, or CAH. In boys, the possibilities include premature adrenarche, gonadotropin-dependent or independent precocious puberty, Leydig cell tumor of the testis, or ectopic hCG secretion from tumors such as a hepatoma or dysgerminoma.

Treatment. The primary treatment is surgical resection of the tumor, once localized. In most cases, if the tumor does not also produce Cushing syndrome, the lesion is fairly small and can be completely resected, resulting in a cure. In the rare metastatic tumors, the primary tumor is resected as completely as possible, as well as the metastatic tumors. When metastases are widespread and cannot be surgically resected, radiotherapy and chemotherapy are usually offered.

After surgery, the patient should be followed carefully for recurrence with serial measurements of adrenal androgens as well as for clinical signs of androgen excess.

Feminizing tumors

These tumors are quite rare in childhood, and in most patients there is a concomitant increase in androgens as well as estrogens.[45]

Clinical manifestations. In prepubertal children of both sexes, the tumor is usually small at the time of diagnosis, and is therefore not palpable on abdominal examination. There is rapid growth with skeletal age advancement.

In boys, the presenting sign is usually gynecomastia. The genitalia appear normal in size, and pubic and axillary hair are usually absent if there is no androgen hypersecretion. In prepubertal girls, there is premature breast development with estrogenization of the vaginal mucosa. There may be episodes of vaginal spotting. In the absence of hyperandrogenism, there is no development of pubic or axillary hair. In pubertal girls, the diagnosis is more difficult, and is often made later in the development of the tumor.

Diagnostic studies. The blood and urinary concentrations of estrogens are generally elevated for age, but may be in the range seen in adult women. In some patients, urinary excretion of 17-ketosteroids is elevated as a result of the concomitant secretion of adrenal androgens. This again is due mostly to the excretion of DHEA. In these patients, the blood androgen pattern may be similar to that seen in virilizing tumors. As with virilizing tumors, some patients with feminizing tumors may also manifest increased cortisol secretion and features of Cushing syndrome.

> **Dexamethasone suppression**—There will be no decrease in the estrogen secretion with dexamethasone suppression, as the secretion is not ACTH-dependent.
> **Imaging studies**—As with virilizing tumors, CT of the abdomen is the studies of choice.

Pathology. The general appearance and histology of feminizing tumors is similar to that of virilizing tumors. In many patients, it may be difficult to determine that the tumor is benign. The observation that many patients have survived many years following surgery suggests that these tumors have a low degree of malignancy.

Differential diagnosis. In patients of both sexes, an exogenous source of estrogen must be ruled out. These include oral contraceptives or premarin. Certain cosmetic and hair care products may also contain estrogens, such as those derived from placental extracts.

In boys, other causes of gynecomastia must be considered. These include benign pubertal gynecomastia, which would be accompanied by testicular enlargement, a feature generally not present in patients with feminizing tumors. Some drugs cause gynecomastia, including reserpine, digoxin, and marijuana. Klinefelter syndrome and partial androgen insensitivity are other causes of gynecomastia.

In prepubertal girls, premature thelarche and precocious puberty would need to be excluded. Elevated estrogen caused by an ovarian cyst or tumor could be diagnosed based on ultrasound examination of the ovaries. In pubertal or postpubertal girls, the diagnosis is more difficult, and as mentioned above, is often made late.

Treatment. Feminizing tumors should be resected as soon as the diagnosis is made. In general, these tumors do not produce excess cortisol, so adrenal suppression is unlikely. Most patients are cured surgically. If the bone age has been significantly advanced prior to resection of the tumor, the patient may have a risk of precocious puberty postoperatively.

Hyperaldosteronism

Syndromes of mineralocorticoid excess are rare in childhood (Table 5-13) and can be subdivided into those with elevated aldosterone levels (true aldosterone excess) and those with features of aldosterone excess but no elevation of aldosterone levels (AME). These features include hypokalemia and hypertension.

Table 5-13.
Mineralocorticoid Excess Syndromes

True aldosterone excess
   Primary hyperaldosteronism
      Bilateral adrenal hyperplasia
      Adrenocortical adenoma
   Dexamethasone-suppressible hypertension
   Hyperreninemic hyperaldosteronism
      Renal ischemia
      Juxtaglomerular cell tumors
   Bartter syndrome
Apparent mineralocorticoid excess
   11βHSD2 deficiency
   Licorice intoxication

True aldosterone excess. In the conditions of aldosterone excess, plasma levels of aldosterone are elevated, and hypokalemia is present. Patients may or may not have elevated renin levels or hypertension, depending upon the etiology of their hyperaldosteronism.

Primary hyperaldosteronism results from autonomous adrenocortical hypersecretion of aldosterone owing to bilateral nodular hyperplasia of the adrenal cortex (idiopathic hyperaldosteronism [IHA]) or an adrenocortical tumor (adenoma or carcinoma). Patients present with hypertension, hypokalemia, elevated plasma aldosterone levels, and low PRA. In IHA, the adrenal glands exhibit focal hyperplasia of normal zona glomerulosa cells, accompanied by adrenocortical nodules. Patients with IHA are treated medically with spironolactone, an inhibitor of aldosterone biosynthesis, which is usually quite effective in managing the hypertension.

Hyperaldosteronism because of an adrenocortical tumor may present with the same signs and symptoms as IHA. However, a unilateral source of aldosterone hypersecretion may be demonstrated by selective adrenal vein sampling for aldosterone levels, and a mass may be visible by radiologic imaging studies (CT or MRI scan). Adenomas are more common than carcinomas, and may also produce cortisol in a normal diurnal pattern. In adults, primary aldosteronism more often results from an adenoma than IHA. The treatment of choice is surgical resection of the tumor.[46]

Dexamethasone-suppressible hyperaldosteronism or *glucocorticoid-remediable aldosteronism (GRA)* is a rare autosomal dominant form of low-renin aldosterone excess with hypertension, hypokalemia, low PRA, elevated aldosterone levels, and lack of the normal aldosterone escape with continuous infusion of synthetic ACTH. The unique features of this syndrome are the rapid reduction of aldosterone levels into the normal range by administration of dexamethasone, and the failure of aldosterone infusion to produce hypertension in the dexamethasone-suppressed patient.[47]

The pathogenesis of GRA is a persistent and unregulated overproduction of mineralocorticoids, eventually leading to hypertension and hypokalemia. The recognition that two distinct gene products perform the terminal steps in biosynthesis of mineralocorticoid (CYP11B2) and glucocorticoid (CYP11B1) prompted the proposal that a hybrid CYP11B1/CYP11B2 gene caused the disorder. The promoter-regulatory sequences derived from CYP11B1 direct ACTH-responsive expression of the chimeric gene in the inner (fasciculata and reticularis) cortical zones. The chimeric protein, by virtue of critical amino acids encoded by CYP11B2, should perform all reactions required for aldosterone production, thus causing ACTH-dependent hyperaldosteronism. Ectopic expression of the chimeric protein in the inner cortical zones, which also express CYP17, would permit the formation of 18-hydroxy and 18-oxo-cortisol, the biochemical hallmarks of GRA. Finally, treatment with glucocorticoids, by suppressing the steroidogenesis of the zona fasciculata and reticularis, alleviates the hypertension.[48]

Determining the optimal dose of glucocorticoid can be difficult, especially in children in whom glucocorticoid requirements vary markedly at different stages of development. Alternative therapies include mineralocorticoid antagonists such as spironolactone, which competitively inhibits the mineralocorticoid receptor, and amiloride, which indirectly inhibits mineralocorticoid actions in the kidney.

In *hyperreninemic hyperaldosteronism,* the aldosterone hypersecretion is secondary to excessive renin production by the renal juxtaglomerular cells. The most common etiology of this condition is renal ischemia. In such patients, the hypertension may be responsive to medical therapy with angiotensin-converting enzyme inhibitors. Therapy directed toward correction of the underlying cause of the renal ischemia should be undertaken when possible.

Apparent mineralocorticoid excess. This is an autosomal recessive disorder caused by deficiency of the enzyme 11β-hydroxysteroid dehydrogenase (11βHSD type 2), which is necessary for the conversion of cortisol to its inactive metabolite cortisone. In 11βHSD type 2 deficiency, inappropriately high intrarenal levels of cortisol result in a clinical picture consistent with mineralocorticoid excess through its binding to the steroid type 2 or mineralocorticoid receptor. Under physiologic conditions the mineralocorticoid receptor, which has equal affinities for glucocorticoids and mineralocorticoids, is exposed essentially only to mineralocorticoids because of the efficient activity of 11βHSD type 2 in the kidney. In patients with congenital AME, the interaction of cortisol with the mineralocorticoid receptor produces volume expansion, sodium retention, hypertension, and hypokalemia. Plasma levels of renin and aldosterone are below normal. Patients with this disease have severe hypertension that is resistant to medical management. The human gene encoding 11βHSD type 2 has been cloned and mapped to chromosome 1. The molecular genetic defects in patients with AME include small intragenic deletions, missense mutations, and one intronic defect altering normal splicing. Most patients are homozygotes, suggesting a founder effect. Treatment consists of low salt diet, potassium supplementation, and spironolactone.

AME may be acquired by licorice intoxication. Patients who ingest excessive amounts of licorice may develop hypertension, hypokalemia, and fluid retention with low plasma levels of aldosterone and renin. The active components on licorice are glycyrrhizic acid and its metabolite glycyrrhetinic acid, both of which inhibit 11βHSD type 2 activity. The signs and symptoms of mineralocorticoid excess resolve within several weeks after discontinuation of licorice, however complete reversal of the renin-angiotensin system suppression may take several months.[49]

Disorders of the Adrenal Medulla

Normal hormone physiology

The adrenal medulla consists of chromaffin tissue, innervated by sympathetic nerves that originate in the splanchnic system. This sympathoadrenal system is controlled by a complex set of central neural connections that are involved in the production, storage, and secretion of catecholamines. In addition, the adrenal medulla is exposed to the relatively high concentrations of glucocorticoids found in the venous drainage of the adrenal cortex, and this exposure is required for a normal epinephrine response to stress. In patients with glucocorticoid deficiency owing to ACTH unresponsiveness, there is a marked loss of basal epinephrine secretion, as well as in the epinephrine response to upright posture, cold pressor, and exercise. These individuals have a slight compensatory increase in norepinephrine. In patients with CAH caused by CYP21 deficiency, ACTH suppression with maintenance glucocorticoid treatment reduces the adrenal medullary hormone output.

The major catecholamines in humans are dopamine, norepinephrine, and epinephrine, all of which are synthesized primarily in nerve endings. Dopamine is produced mainly in the brain, norepinephrine mainly in the sympathetic nerve endings (and to a limited extent in the adrenal medulla), and epinephrine in the adrenal medulla where it is the major product. The o'-methylated metabolites of catecholamines are excreted in the urine as fractionated metanephrines. They can also be measured as free metanephrines in the plasma.

The biosynthesis of catecholamines is illustrated in Figure 5-21. Tyrosine is hydroxylated to form DOPA, which is then converted to dopamine, a neurotransmitter within the CNS. Dopamine also acts as the precursor for synthesis

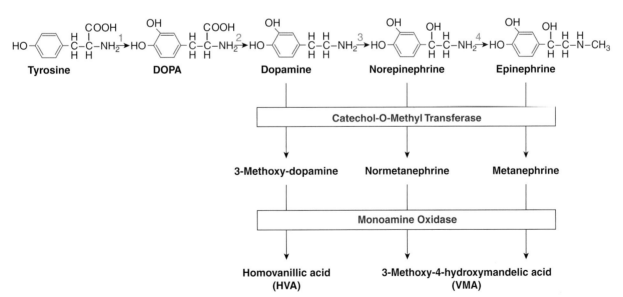

FIGURE 5-21 ■ Biosynthesis and metabolism of catecholamines. The upper part of the figure shows the biosynthetic pathway from tyrosine to epinephrine. Under the effects of two enzymes (catechol-o-methyltransferase and monoamine oxidase), dopamine and norepinephrine/epinephrine are metabolized to homovanillic acid (HVA) and 3-methoxy-4-hydroxymandelic acid (VMA), respectively. (1) Tyrosine hydroxylase; (2) aromatic L-amino acid decarboxylase; (3) dopamine β-hydroxylase; and (4) phenylethanolamine N-methyl transferase.

Table 5-14.	
Adrenergic Effects	
α	β
Vasoconstriction	Vasodilation
Sweating	Cardiac stimulation
Uterine contraction	Uterine relaxation
Pupillary dilation	Gluconeogenesis
Inhibition of insulin release	Lipolysis
Intestinal relaxation	Intestinal relaxation
Norepinephrine release	Brochodilation

of norepinephrine, the principal neurotransmitter of the sympathetic nervous system. Norepinephrine is then converted to epinephrine in an enzymatic step that is controlled by glucocorticoid. Epinephrine exerts its physiologic effects by interaction with both alpha (α1 and α2) and beta (β1 and β2) adrenergic receptors. The physiologic effects of epinephrine are widespread, and are separated into the differing alpha and beta effects (Table 5-14).

Tests of adrenal medullary function

Measurement of single random catecholamine concentrations in the blood, that is, norepinephrine and epinephrine, is rarely helpful, as patients who have excess production may have periods of low blood concentrations, and patients with normal production will have appropriately high concentrations in response to stress. In addition, there is a maturational trend in plasma epinephrine and metanephrine concentrations that is pubertal-stage and sex dependent. In normal children and adolescents, plasma epinephrine and metanephrine decrease with advancing pubertal stage, and are generally higher in boys than in girls. These hormone levels correlate inversely with blood concentrations of DHEA-S, estradiol, testosterone, leptin, and insulin.

Patients who have symptoms of catecholamine excess are better evaluated under controlled conditions by measurement of catecholamines and their metabolites normetanephrine, metanephrine, homovanillic acid (HVA), and vanillylmandelic acid (VMA) in a 24-hour urine sample. This gives an assessment of integrated catecholamine production. The metabolic pathways in the degradation of catecholamines are illustrated in Figure 5-21. Serial measurements of these compounds in blood and urine after paroxysmal attacks of catecholamine release may also be informative. Measurement of plasma catecholamine concentrations, if obtained in the fasting supine individual after 30 minutes of rest, can be as reliable

as urinary metanephrine concentrations in predicting the presence of pheochromocytoma, but the false-negative rate is fairly high.

There has been a recent trend toward the use of fractionated urinary metanephrines and plasma free metanephrines in the evaluation of patients with suspected pheochromocytoma. The combination of 24-hour urinary catecholamines and fractionated metanephrines may yield less false positives than the plasma free metanephrines, but the latter may be of more value in high-risk patients.[50]

It is important to note that some medications (radiocontrast dyes, acetaminophen, antihypertensives, monoamine oxidase inhibitors, methyldopa, quinidine, tetracyclines, and bronchodilators) may alter the results of blood or urinary catecholamine measurements. Urinary VMA concentrations may be falsely elevated with certain drugs such as aspirin, penicillin, and sulfa preparations. In addition, some dietary components (certain fruits, chocolate, vanilla, caffeine) may also affect these assays.

Several provocative tests are available to aid in the diagnosis of the etiology of elevated catecholamine concentrations, should plasma and urinary catecholamine concentrations not be diagnostic. These tests are accompanied by significant risks in some patients, including hypertensive crisis and the complications thereof. Therefore, provocative tests should only be performed in patients who have a patent IV catheter, and with phentolamine (an α-adrenergic blocking agent) available for immediate IV infusion, if needed.

The glucagon stimulation test produces a rise in blood catecholamine concentrations and often a rise in blood pressure. It is associated with less risk than histamine or tyramine stimulation tests. Glucagon (1.0-2.0 mg in adults) is given as an IV bolus, and plasma catecholamines and blood pressure are measured 1 to 3 minutes later. The test is considered positive for pheochromocytoma if there is a threefold increase in catecholamine concentrations, or an increase to a concentration greater than 2000 pg/mL.

The histamine stimulation test (0.025-0.05 mg IV) causes a normal drop in blood pressure followed by a secondary rise. The plasma and urinary catecholamine concentrations rise after histamine in patients with pheochromocytoma.

Clonidine, a centrally acting α-adrenergic agonist, has been reported to cause a decrease in plasma catecholamine concentrations (sum of epinephrine and norepinephrine concentrations) to less than 500 pg/mL in normal subjects and in patients with essential hypertension. However, patients with pheochromocytoma do not show a drop in plasma catecholamine concentrations to this degree. Hypotension is a potentially serious side effect of this test, especially in patients receiving β-adrenergic blocking agents.

Radiologic studies are invaluable in the diagnosis of adrenal medullary tumors and other causes of catecholamine excess. A CT or MRI scan may identify masses of the adrenal medulla or sympathetic chain. Selective catheterization for adrenal venous sampling may allow lateralization of a source of excess catecholamine production. Nuclear medicine studies allowing localization of catecholamine-producing tumors have become possible through the use of the isotope ^{131}I-metaiodobenzylguanidine (MIBG). MIBG is similar in structure to norepinephrine and is an analogue of guanethidine. It is concentrated in tissues that are actively synthesizing catecholamines by means of uptake into norepinephrine storage granules.

Clinical entities

Most abnormalities of the adrenal medulla are attributed to tumors, either benign or malignant, which secrete catecholamines.

Pheochromocytoma is rare in childhood, but must always be considered in a child with hypertension or other symptoms of catecholamine excess. This tumor may arise from any chromaffin tissue, but it is most often found in the adrenal medulla. Bilateral adrenal or extra-adrenal tumors are more common in children than in adults and are often associated with familial pheochromocytoma or the multiple endocrine neoplasia (MEN) syndromes, as well as the von Hippel-Lindau syndrome. The neoplasms associated with these syndromes are listed in Table 5-15. Features consistent with these associated tumors, for example, medullary carcinoma of the thyroid, should be sought in any patient with pheochromocytoma. The MEN syndromes are inherited in an autosomal dominant manner and have variable expression. Pheochromocytomas are also associated with neuroectodermal dysplasias (eg, neurofibromatosis). Pheochromocytoma is benign in greater than 90% of pediatric cases. There is a male preponderance during childhood; however, the sex ratio is reversed in adults.

Diagnosis. The signs and symptoms of pheochromocytoma are those of catecholamine excess, and include hypertension, sweating, palpitations, headache, nausea, polyuria with polydipsia, and emotional lability. These features are highly variable among different patients, and are likely to be paroxysmal in nature. However, the hypertension may be sustained, and a hypertensive crisis may occur during anesthesia necessitating adequate medical preparation for surgical procedures. The diagnosis of pheochromocytoma is based on demonstration of increased concentrations of catecholamines and their metabolites in blood and/or a 24-hour urine sample. The total urinary catecholamine excretion generally exceeds 200 to 300 mcg/24 h. Plasma catecholamine

Table 5-15.

Features of MEN Syndromes

Neoplasia	MEN1	MEN2A	MEN2B
Pheochromocytoma	–	+	+
Medullary thyroid carcinoma	–	+	+
Multiple neural tumors	–	–	+
Parathyroid tumors/ hyperplasia	+	+	–
Pancreatic tumors	+	–	–
Anterior pituitary tumors	+	–	–
Gastrinoma	+	–	–
Carcinoid	+	–	–
Other features:			
Marfanoid habitus	–	–	+
Cutaneous Lichen amyloidosis	–	+	–
Hirschsprung disease	–	+	–

concentrations above 2000 pg/mL are considered pathognomonic for pheochromocytoma. The predominant urinary catecholamine in children with pheochromocytoma is norepinephrine, whereas in adults both epinephrine and norepinephrine excretions are usually elevated. The use of fractionated urinary metanephrine excretion is also helpful. If the results are inconclusive, a pharmacologic stimulation or suppression test may be indicated. If suspected by biochemical tests, the tumor can usually be localized by radiologic imaging. Venography to demonstrate elevated concentrations of catecholamines should only be performed after adequate α-blockade to prevent a hypertensive crisis.[51]

The molecular bases of the syndromes associated with childhood pheochromocytoma are now known. The defective gene in the MEN 1 syndrome is called the MEN1 gene, which is a tumor-suppressor gene located on chromosome 11q13. Mutations of this gene do not have a strong genotype-phenotype relation in this syndrome, and the penetrance of pheochromocytomas in this syndrome is low. Somatic mutations of this gene also occur in sporadic adrenocortical tumors. MEN2 is caused by mutations in the RET-protooncogene on chromosome 10. This gene is also defective in familial medullary thyroid carcinoma. The penetrance of pheochromocytoma in MEN2 is fairly high. The von Hippel-Lindau tumor suppressor gene on chromosome 3p25 is defective in that syndrome, and in familial pheochromocytoma.[52]

Treatment. The treatment of pheochromocytoma is surgical excision. Patients should be prepared for surgery with α-adrenergic blockade, employing either oral phe-noxybenzamine or prazosin (specific α1 blocker) for 7 to 10 days prior to surgery. Patients with arrhythmias should also receive presurgical treatment with β-adrenergic blocking agents after adequate α-blockade is achieved. Intraoperative management of hypertensive crises employs IV phentolamine or sodium nitroprus-side. If bilateral adrenalectomy is necessary, treatment for primary adrenal insufficiency must be promptly instituted. Postoperative follow-up of blood pressure and catecholamine concentrations is needed to monitor for tumor recurrence. Malignant tumors are diagnosed on the basis of functional tumor in nonchromaffin tissue areas. Benign tumors may cause blood vessel or capsular invasion but do not spread beyond chromaffin tissue areas. Malignant tumors grow slowly, are resistant to radiation and chemotherapy, and the symptoms may be treated medically with α-methyl tyrosine (an inhibitor of catecholamine synthesis) with variable success.

Neuroblastoma, a malignant tumor of neural crest origin, is a common solid tumor of childhood. Neuro-blastomas may arise from the adrenal medulla as well as from other sympathetic nervous tissue. As these tumors secrete catecholamines, the diagnosis is most often made by demonstration of elevated HVA and/or VMA concen-trations in the urine. In general, urinary concentrations of epinephrine, norepinephrine, metanephrines, and VMA are lower in neuroblastoma than in pheochromo-cytoma, whereas concentrations of dopamine and HVA tend to be higher. Hypertension is less common in neu-roblastoma than in pheochromocytoma. These tumors may also secrete neuropeptides such as vasoactive intes-tinal peptide (VIP), gastrin-releasing peptide (GRP), substance P, pancreastatin, and neuropeptide Y (NPY). Pediatric reference ranges for these peptides have been developed, and this will aid in the interpretation of their levels in patients with suspected neuroblastoma.

Radiologic localization is usually achieved with CT or MRI scanning. Genetic studies of neuroblastomas reveal that many tumors contain karyotypic abnormal-ities. There is frequently a deletion of distal chromo-some 1p (1p32-1pter), which has been found in other tumor lines as well. Presence of the 1p deletion within a neuroblastoma correlates with decreased patient sur-vival. Many neuroblastoma cells also contain areas of chromatin that are composed of amplified genes, occur-ring either as extrachromosomal double minute chro-mosomes or as intrachromosomal homologously stain-ing regions. The amplified gene in these regions is the N-*myc* proto-oncogene, so termed because of its simi-larity to c-*myc*. N-*myc* is normally expressed in a variety of fetal tissues, but not normally in differentiated cells. Neuroblastoma cells contain somatostatin receptors, particularly of the subtype 2. This may eventually allow

targeting of this receptor for diagnostic and therapeutic purposes with radiolabeled somatostatin analogs.

Other tumors of adrenal medullary origin include *ganglioneuroblastoma* and *ganglioneuroma*. These tumors, as well as neuroblastoma and pheochromocytoma may present with chronic watery diarrhea caused by tumor secretion of VIP. Catecholamine-releasing nonadrenal tumors may mimic pheochromocytoma. These include paraganglioma and astrocytoma.

REFERENCES

1. Ikeda Y, Swain A, Weber T, et al. Steroidogenic factor 1 and Dax-1 colocalize in multiple cell lineages: potential links in endocrine development. *Mol Endocrinol.* 1996;10:1261-1272.

2. Omura T. Forty years of cytochrome P450. *Biochem Biophys Res Commun.* 1999;266:690-698.

3. Parker KL, Schimmer BP. Steroidogenic factor 1: a key determinant of endocrine development and function. *Endocr Rev.* 1997;18:361-377.

4. Korosi A, Baram TZ. The central corticotropin releasing factor system during development and adulthood. *Eur J Pharmacol.* 2008;583(2-3):204-214.

5. Yudt MR, Cidlowski JA. The glucocorticoid receptor: cod-ing a diversity of proteins and responses through a single gene. *Mol Endocrinol.* 2002;16(8):1719-1726.

6. Bolt RJ, van Weissenbruch MM, Popp-snijders C, Sweep FGJ, Lafeber HN, Delemarre-van de Waal HA. Maturity of the adrenal cortex in very preterm infants is related to ges-tational age. *Pediatr Res.* 2002;52:405-410.

7. Rosenfield RL. Identifying children at risk for polycystic ovary syndrome. *J Clin Endocrinol Metab.* 2007;92(3):787-796.

8. Catania A. The melanocortin system in leukocyte biology. *J Leukoc Biol.* 2007;81(2):383-392.

9. Rask E, Olsson T, Söderberg, et al. Tissue-specific dysreg-ulation of cortisol metabolism in human obesity. *J Clin Endocrinol Metab.* 2003;86:1418-1421.

10. Cooper MS, Stewart PM. Corticosteroid insufficiency in acutely ill patients. *N Engl J Med.* 2003;348(8):727-734.

11. Migeon CJ, Tyler FH, Mahoney JP, et al. The diurnal vari-ation of plasma levels and urinary excretion of 17-hydrox-ycorticosteroids in normal subjects, night workers, and blind subjects. *J Clin Endocrinol Metab.* 1956;16:622.

12. Papanicolaou DA, Mullen N, Kyrou I, Nieman LK. Nighttime salivary cortisol: a useful test for the diagnosis of Cushing's syndrome. *J Clin Endocrinol Metab.* 2002;87:4515-4521.

13. Kenny FM, Preeyasombat C, Migeon CJ. Cortisol produc-tion rate. II. Normal infants, children and adults. *Pedi-atrics.* 1966; 37:34.

14. Linder BL, Esteban NV, Yergey AL, Winterer JC, Loriaux DL, Cassorla F. Cortisol production rate in childhood and adolescence. *J Pediatr.* 1990;117:892-896.

15. Maghnie M, Uga E, Temporini F, et al. Evaluation of adrenal function in patients with growth hormone deficiency and hypothalamic-pituitary disorders: comparison between insulin-induced hypoglycemia, low-dose ACTH, standard

ACTH and CRH stimulation tests. *Eur J Endocrinol.* 2005;152(5):735-741.

16. Lin L, Acherman JC. Inherited adrenal hypoplasia: not just for kids! *Clin Endocrinol.* 2004;60:529-537.

17. Clark AJL, Weber A. Adrenocorticotropin insensitivity syndromes. *Endocr Rev.* 1998;19(828):843.

18. Joint LWPES/ESPE CAH Working Group. Consensus statement on 21-hydroxylase deficiency from the Lawson Wilkins Pediatric Endocrine Society and the European Society for Paediatric Endocrinology. *J Clin Endocrinol Metab.* 2002;87:4048-4053.

19. Pinto G, Tardy V, Trivin C, et al. Follow-Up of 68 children with congenital adrenal hyperplasia due to 21-hydroxylase heficiency: relevance of genotype for management. *J Clin Endocrinol Metab.* 2003;88(6):2624-2633.

20. Hoffman WH, Shin MY, Donohoue PA, et al. Phenotypic evolution of classic 21-hydroxylase deficiency. *Clin Endocrinol.* 1996;45:103-109.

21. Merke DP, Chrousos GP, Eisenhofer G, et al. Adrenomedullary dysplasia and hypofunction in patients with classic 21-hydroxylase deficiency. *N Engl J Med.* 2000; 343:1362-1368.

22. Fleischnick E, Awdeh ZL, Raum D, et al. Extended MHC haplotypes in 21-hydroxylase deficiency congenital adrenal hyperplasia: shared genotypes in unrelated patients. *Lancet.* 1983;1:152-156.

23. Pang S, Wallace MA, Hofman L, et al. Worldwide experience in newborn screening for classical congenital adrenal hyperplasia due to 21-hydroxylase deficiency. *Pediatrics.* 1988;81:866-874.

24. Witchel SF, Lee PA. Identification of heterozygotic carriers of 21-hydroxylase deficiency—sensitivity of ACTH stimulation tests. *Am J Med Genet.* 1998;76:337-342.

25. Mercado AB, Wilson RC, Cheng KC, New MI. Extensive personal experience: prenatal treatment and diagnosis of congenital adrenal hyperplasia owing to steroid 21-hydroxylase deficiency. *J Clin Endocrinol Metab.* 1995;80: 2014-2020.

26. Therell BL, Berenbaum SA, Manter-Kapanke V, et al. Results of screening 1.9 million Texas newborns for 21-hydroxylase-deficient congenital adrenal hyperplasia. *Pediatrics.* 1998;101:583-590.

27. White PC, Curnow KC, Pascoe L. Disorders of steroid 11b-hydroxylase isozymes. *Endocr Rev.* 1995;15: 421-438.

28. Yanase T, Simpson ER, Waterman MR. 17-hydroxylase/17,20-desmolase deficiency: from clinical investigation to molecular definition. *Endocr Rev.* 1991;12:91.

29. Simard J, Sanchez R, Durocher F, et al. Structure-function relationships and molecular genetics of the 3b-hydroxysteroid dehydrogenase gene family. *J Steroid Biochem Molec Biol.* 1995;55:489-505.

30. Carbunaru G, Prasad P, Scoccia B, et al. The hormonal phenotype of nonclassic 3 beta-hydroxysteroid dehydrogenase (HSD3B) deficiency in hyperandrogenic females is associated with insulin-resistant polycystic ovary syndrome and is not a variant of inherited HSD3B2 deficiency. *J Clin Endocrinol Metab.* 2004;89(2):783-794.

31. Bose HS, Sugawara T, Strauss III JF, Miller WL. The pathophysiology and genetics of congenital lipoid adrenal hyperplasia. *N Engl J Med.* 1998;335:1870-1878.

32. Fluck CE, Tajima T, Pandley AV, et al. Mutant P450 oxidoreductase causes disordered steroidogenesis with and without Antley-Bixler Syndrome. *Nat Genet* 2004; 36:228-230.

33. Sadeghi-Nejad A, Senior B. Adrenomyeloneuropathy presenting as Addison's disease in childhood. *N Engl J Med.* 1990;322:13-16.

34. Andersson, HC, Frentz, J, Martinez, JE, et al. Adrenal insufficiency in Smith-Lemli-Opitz syndrome. *Am J Med Genet.* 1999; 82:382.

35. Shizuta Y, Kawamoto T, Mitsuuchi Y, et al. Molecular genetic studies on the biosynthesis of aldosterone in humans. *J Steroid Biochem.* 1992;8:981-987.

36. Vogel A, Strassburg CP, Obermayer-Straub P, Brabant G, Manns MP. The genetic background of autoimmune polyendocrinopathy-candidiasis-ectodermal dystrophy and its autoimmune disease components. *J Mol Med.* 2002;80:201-211.

37. Aarskog D, Blizzard RM, Migeon CJ. Response to methopyrapone (su-4885) and pyrogen test in idiopathic hypopituitary dwarfism. *J Clin Endocrinol Metab.* 1965;25:439.

38. Riepe FG, Krone N, Morlot M, Ludwig M, Sippell WG, Partsch CJ. Identification of a novel mutation in the human mineralocorticoid receptor gene in a German family with autosomal-dominant pseudohypoaldosteronism type 1: further evidence for marked interindividual clinical heterogeneity. *J Clin Endocrinol Metab.* 2003; 88(4):1683-1686.

39. Saxena A, Hanukoglu I, Saxena D, Thompson RJ, Gardiner RM, Hanukoglu A. Novel mutations responsible for autosomal recessive multisystem pseudohypoaldosteronism and sequence variants in epithelial sodium channel-, a-, b-, and g-subunit genes. *J Clin Endocrinol Metab.* 2002;87(7):3344-3350.

40. Kino C. Glucocorticoid and mineralocorticoid resistance/hypersensitivity syndromes. *J Endocrinol.* 2001; 169(3):437-445.

41. Long DN, Wisniewski AB, Migeon CJ. Gender role across development in adult women with congenital adrenal hyperplasia due to 21-hydroxylase deficiency. *J Pediatr Endocrinol Metab.* 2004;17:1367-1373.

42. Batista DL, Riar J, Keil M, Stratakis CA. Diagnostic tests for children who are referred for the investigation of Cushing Syndrome. Pediatrics 2007; 120:e575-e586.

43. Yaneva M, Mosnier-Pudar H, Dugué M-A, Grabar S, Fulla Y, Bertagna X. Midnight salivary cortisol for the initial diagnosis of Cushing's syndrome of various causes. *J Clin Endocrinol Metab.* 2004;89:3345-3351.

44. Miller JW, Crapo L. The medical treatment of Cushing's syndrome. *Endocr Rev.* 1993;14(4):443-458.

45. Sandrini R, Ribeiro RC, DeLacerda L. Childhood adrenocortical tumors. *J Clin Endocrinol Metab.* 1997;82(7): 2027-2031.

46. Gabrilove JL, Sharma DC, Wotiz HH, et al. Feminizing adrenocortical tumors in male: a review of 52 cases including a case report. *Medicine.* 1965;44:37.

47. Ganguly A. Primary aldosteronism. *N Engl J Med.* 1998;339:1828-1834.

48. New MI, Siegal EJ, Peterson RE. Dexamethasone-suppressible hypertension. *J Clin Endocrinol Metab.* 1973; 37:93-100.

49. Pascoe L, Curnow KM, Slutsker L, et al. Glucocorticoid-suppressible hyperaldosteronism results from hybrid genes created by unequal crossovers between *CYP11B1* and *CYP11B2*. *Proc Natl Acad Sci USA*. 1992;89:8327-8331.

50. White PC, Tomoatsu M, Agarwal AK. 11b-hydroxysteroid dehydrogenase and the syndrome of apparent mineralocorticoid excess. *Endocr Rev*. 1997;18:135-156.

51. Sawka AM, Jaeschke R, Singh RJ, Young JW. A comparison of biochemical tests for pheochromocytoma: measurement of fractionated plasma metanephrines compared with the combination of 24-hour urinary metanephrines and catecholamines. *J Clin Endocrinol Metab*. 2003;88:553-558.

52. Eisenhofer G. Editorial: biochemical diagnosis of pheochromocytoma—is it time to switch to plasma-free metanephrines? *J Clin Endocrinol Metab*. 2003;88:550-552.

53. Brandi ML, Gagel RF, Angeli A, et al. Consensus: guidelines for diagnosis and therapy of MEN type 1 and type 2. *J Clin Endocrinol Metab*. 2001;86(12):5658-5671.

CHAPTER 6

Disorders of Bone and Mineral Metabolism

Andrea Kelly and Michael A. Levine

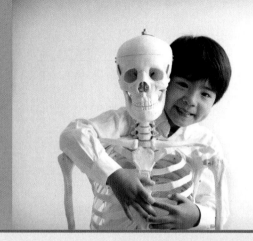

PHYSIOLOGY

Introduction

The last two decades have seen great progress in our knowledge and understanding of the genetic and biochemical control of mineral metabolism. Moreover, our understanding of vitamin D action continues to extend well beyond the conventional roles in bone and mineral metabolism and now includes functions as a transcriptional regulator of immune function.

Clinical application of these discoveries has led to significant and practical improvements in diagnosis and treatment of disorders of mineral metabolism and analysis of bone mass in children and adolescents.

Calcium/Magnesium/Phosphorus Homeostasis

Calcium

The maintenance of calcium homeostasis is a complex dynamic process involving intestinal calcium absorption and excretion, renal filtration and reabsorption, and skeletal storage and mobilization (Figure 6-1).

Circulating calcium. Only 1% of the total body calcium is within extracellular fluids and soft tissues. Approximately 50% of total serum calcium is in the ionized form (Ca^{2+}) at normal serum protein concentrations and represents the biologically active component of the total serum calcium concentration. Another 8% to 10% is complexed to organic and inorganic acids (eg, citrate, sulfate, and phosphate); together, the ionized and complexed calcium fractions represent the diffusible portion of circulating calcium. Approximately 40% of serum calcium is protein-bound, primarily to albumin (80%) but also to globulins (20%). The protein-bound calcium is not biologically active but provides a readily available reserve of calcium should the need for increased ionized calcium arise acutely.

Sudden changes in the distribution of calcium between ionized and bound Ca^{2+} may cause symptoms of hypocalcemia. Increases in the extracellular fluid concentration of anions, such as phosphate, citrate, bicarbonate, or edetic acid, will chelate calcium and decrease ionized calcium. Alkalosis increases the affinity of albumin for calcium, and thereby decreases the concentration of Ca^{2+}. By contrast, acidosis decreases the binding of calcium to albumin and increases Ca^{2+} concentrations.

Physiologically relevant information is best obtained by determination of the Ca^{2+} concentration, particularly when evaluating patients who have abnormal circulating proteins or acid-base and electrolyte disorders[1] (eg, total serum calcium will be low in a child with decreased serum albumin while the concentration of Ca^{2+} will typically be normal). One widely used algorithm estimates that total serum calcium declines by approximately 0.8 mg/dL for each 1 g/dL decrease in albumin concentration.

The cytoplasmic concentration of Ca^{2+} affects many intracellular enzymes including adenylate cyclase, guanylate cyclase, troponin C, calmodulin, and protein kinase C. The normal intracellular calcium concentration is about 0.1 mmol/L, or about ten-thousandth the concentration in plasma. Therefore, only minute amounts of calcium, either released from endoplasmic reticulum or from stimulated influx through calcium channels, are needed to raise the concentration by the factor of 10 that is ordinarily necessary to activate an

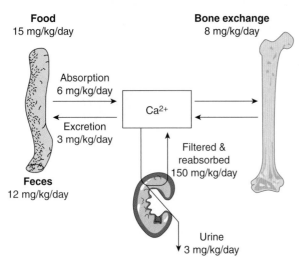

Food
15 mg/kg/day

Bone exchange
8 mg/kg/day

Absorption
6 mg/kg/day

Ca²⁺

Excretion
3 mg/kg/day

Filtered &
reabsorbed
150 mg/kg/day

Feces
12 mg/kg/day

Urine
3 mg/kg/day

FIGURE 6-1 ■ The dynamics of calcium homeostasis in a normal adult. In growing children intestinal calcium absorption and skeletal deposition are increased.

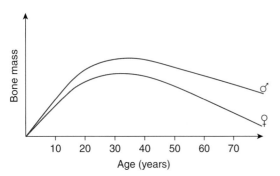

FIGURE 6-2 ■ Relationship between bone mass, sex, and age.

enzyme. The activity of cell membrane calcium channels and ion pores in the endoplasmic reticulum is regulated by potential membrane as well as by interactions with membrane receptors and phospholipids.[2]

Calcium intake. Calcium intake and requirements vary considerably for different age groups. The primary demand for dietary calcium is to enhance bone mineral deposition. Skeletal calcium accumulates at a rate of 80 to 150 mg/day between birth and 10 years of age; this rate increases to a maximum of 200 mg/day in girls and 270 mg/day in boys during the adolescent growth spurt and gradually falls to zero with cessation of growth. Approximately 90% of the total bone mass is formed by the age of 20. The remaining 10%, which determines the maximum attainable bone mass, is accumulated during the second and third decade. Subsequently, bone mass decreases continually (Figure 6-2).

While calcium requirements may change across the lifespan, both dietary constituents and genetic variability highly influence the net calcium intake. Thus, the interactions of these factors complicate

Table 6-1.

Regulation of Bone Metabolism

	Bone Formation	Bone Resorption
Calcium Regulating hormones		
PTH	(+)	+ (−)
Calcitriol	(+)	+ (−)
Calcitonin		−
Other Systemic hormones		
Glucocorticoid	−	
Thyroid	+	+
Insulin	+	
Growth hormone	+	
Estrogen	+	−
Androgens	+	−
Growth factors		
IGF-1	+	
Epidermal growth factor	+	+
FGF		+

(+) signifies the effect increases; (−) signifies the effect decreases

determination of a universal calcium "requirement" for all children.[3] In response, dietary guidelines recommend calcium intake levels that are predicted to benefit most children (Table 6-1).

Intestinal regulation. Calcium absorption from the intestine is a regulated process, controlled by calcium intake and requirements.[4] The efficiency of calcium absorption is much greater from the duodenum/jejunum than from the ileum. The intestinal calcium absorption occurs by two processes, a saturable, active transfer in the upper and mid section of the small intestine and a nonsaturable, vitamin D-independent diffusional transfer along the entire small intestine. Impaired calcium absorption can result from chronic diarrhea, particularly in disorders in which there is fat malabsorption with precipitation of calcium in the intestinal lumen as insoluble calcium salts of fatty acids, so called calcium soaps. Excessive intake of fats, phosphates, phytates, and oxalates also decreases the intestinal absorption of calcium by their combining with calcium to form insoluble salts.[4]

Renal regulation. Renal tubular calcium reabsorption is an important determinant of extracellular fluid (ECF) calcium concentration. Normally, about 99% of filtered calcium is reabsorbed by the tubules, but the fractional excretion of calcium can be modified by active transport mechanisms that are controlled by local and systemic factors (eg, parathyroid hormone [PTH] and calcitriol). PTH and calcitriol appear to increase the activity and/or expression of multiple calcium transport proteins (eg, TRPV5).[5] Besides this hormonal control, it has been recognized recently that ECF calcium is able to regulate its own reabsorption by the mammalian tubule. Consistent with its polarized localization on the basolateral membrane in the thick ascending limb of the distal nephron, the calcium-sensing receptor (CaSR) is involved in the control of active reabsorption of calcium and magnesium in this region of the tubule. Indeed, a large body of evidence supports the view that ECF calcium exerts this action in almost an "auto-regulatory" mechanism via activation of the CaSR. First, increasing ECF calcium concentration elicits a marked increase in urinary calcium (and magnesium) excretion and this occurs independently of any change in the calcium-regulating hormones. Second, the inhibitory effect of ECF calcium on its own reabsorption is shared by other CaSR agonists, for example, magnesium (Figure 6-3).

Both calcium and magnesium are passively reabsorbed in the cortical portion of the thick ascending limb (cTAL) along an electrical gradient through the paracellular pathway. The electrical gradient is related to transcellular NaCl reabsorption. In addition, potassium recycling hyperpolarizes the apical membrane. Chloride exits the cell across the basolateral membrane, which depolarizes the basolateral membrane, and the overall consequence is a lumen-positive transepithelial voltage that drives calcium, magnesium and also sodium through the paracellular pathway. The pathway permeability for calcium and magnesium requires the presence of a specific protein, paracellin-1 (also known as claudin-16), which is co-expressed with occluding in the tight junctions of TAL. Inactivating mutations of the paracellin-1 gene cause a specific decrease in cTAL calcium and magnesium reabsorption and renal loss of both cations without renal sodium loss, which is the landmark of an inherited disease referred to as hypercalciuric hypomagnesaemia with nephrocalcinosis

The diuretics that specifically inhibit urinary sodium resorption (eg, furosemide) also inhibit calcium reabsorption resulting in calciuria. These diuretics, therefore, can be useful in the emergency treatment of hypercalcemia along with aggressive fluid therapy with saline. Urinary calcium excretion is also increased by systemic acidosis and by high protein intake, and this may be exaggerated in stone formers.

Bone. At all ages approximately 99% of total body calcium is in the skeleton, where in combination with 89% of the total body phosphorus, it constitutes the major inorganic matrix of bone. Skeletal regulation of calcium will be described separately later in the text.

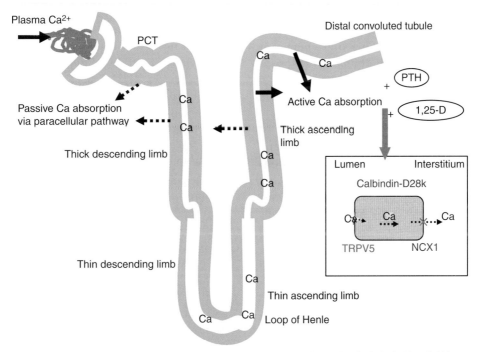

FIGURE 6-3 ■ Regulation of renal calcium. Passive calcium absorption occurs in the proximal convoluted tubules (PCT) and thick ascending limb. Active calcium absorption occurs primarily in the distal convoluted tubule and collecting duct. Active absorption occurs through the permeable transient receptor potential V5 channel (TRPV5), located on the luminal membrane of the renal tubular cell. Intracellular transport occurs via calbindin-D28k and calbindin D9k. Intracellular calcium exchange with sodium to the interstitium occurs through the plasma membrane Ca^{2+} ATPase (PMCA) and the Na^+/Ca^{2+} exchanger (NCX1), located on the basolateral membrane. Active absorption is stimulated by PTH and 1,25-$(OH)_2$-D (1,25-D) via increased expresson of these calcium transport proteins.

Magnesium

Magnesium and calcium are closely interrelated, and any disturbance in homeostasis of one of these ions is commonly associated with disturbance in the other. Total body magnesium amounts to about 260 mg/kg in the infant and increases to about 330 mg/kg in adults. Sixty percent of the body's magnesium is in bone, and most of the remaining 40% is intracellular. Only 20% to 30% of the intracellular magnesium is exchangeable, the rest being bound to proteins. The plasma concentration of magnesium is similar in infants, children, and adults, and ranges from 1.6 to 2.4 mg/dL (0.70-1.00 mmol/L), and seems to be maintained largely independently of calciotropic hormone influence. Of the total serum magnesium, approximately 30% is protein bound, chiefly to albumin, 55% is ionized, and 15% is complexed. The ionized and complexed fractions of magnesium constitute the ultrafiltrable magnesium. Like calcium, the concentration of ionized magnesium is influenced by serum pH, with a rise in pH leading to an increase in the proportion of magnesium that is protein-bound.

Magnesium intake/intestinal/renal regulation.

The intake of magnesium in children ranges from 120 to 300 mg/day depending upon age. Magnesium is principally absorbed in the small intestine by passive and active mechanisms that have yet to be fully delineated. About 50% to 75% of ingested magnesium is absorbed. In contrast to calcium balance, the maintenance of magnesium balance depends primarily on urinary excretion. Normally, less than 5% of the filtered magnesium is excreted. The major sites of reabsorption are the proximal tubule and the TAL. Both magnesium and calcium have the capacity to diminish the resorption of the other.

Phosphorus/phosphate

Phosphorus plays a critical role in skeletal development, mineral metabolism, and diverse cellular functions involving intermediary metabolism and energy-transfer mechanisms. It is a vital component of bone mineral, membrane phospholipids, nucleotides that provide energy and serve as components of DNA and RNA, and phosphorylated intermediates in cellular signaling. Plasma phosphorus exists in an inorganic form and an organic form. Approximately 20% of the plasma inorganic phosphorus is protein bound, and the remainder circulates as free phosphate ions HPO_4^{2-} or $H_2PO_4^{-}$. Phosphorus in the form of phosphate ions is filtered at the glomerulus. However, measurement of plasma and urine phosphate content is expressed in terms of elemental phosphorus. Since organic phosphorus is in the form of phosphate, the latter term is used in this chapter.

Eighty to ninety percent of body phosphate is present in bone mineral as a major component of hydroxyapatite. The rest is in soft tissue, blood cells, and in the extracellular fluid. In cells, phosphate is bound to sugars, lipids, proteins, nucleic acids, and various nucleotides. In plasma, two-thirds of total phosphate is present as phospholipids. These compounds are insoluble in acid and are not measured in routine plasma phosphate determinations. The concentration of phosphate in plasma is not set at a steady level like that of calcium, but varies in relation to age and growth.[6] The average plasma concentration in premature infants is 7.9 mg/dL (2.6 mmol/L), in full-term infants 6.1 mg/dL (2.0 mmol/L), in children and adolescents 4.6 mg/dL (1.5 mmol/L), and in adults 3.5 mg/dL (1.15 mmol/L).

Phosphate intake.

The principal sources of dietary phosphate are milk, dairy products, and meat. Recommended daily intake is 880 mg/day for children 1 to 10 years of age and 1200 mg/day for older children. Serum concentrations of phosphate also exhibit a diurnal rhythm, with levels lowest in the morning and increasing during the day. Monitoring of plasma phosphate concentrations in patients on oral phosphate supplementation is therefore best done in the fasting state and at a consistent time of day

Renal regulation.

The principal organ that regulates phosphate homeostasis is the kidney (Figure 6-4). Serum inorganic phosphorus (Pi) is filtered by the glomerulus, and 80% of the filtered load is reabsorbed predominantly along the proximal nephron. Regulation of proximal renal tubular reabsorption of phosphate is achieved through changes in the activity, number, and intracellular location of type 2 sodium-phosphate cotransporters (Npt2a and Npt2c). Phosphate reabsorption is a saturable process and is dependent on both glomerular filtration rate (GFR) and plasma phosphate concentration. The tubular maximum rate of phosphate reabsorption (TmP) is not an absolute constant, since it can be set at different levels according to physiological or pathological conditions. The TmP in relation to GFR (TmP/GFR) is the most reliable quantitative estimate of the overall tubular phosphate transport capacity. The TmP/GFR is 4.0 to 5.9 mg/dL in normal children between 6 and 14 years of age and declines to adult values of 2.5 to 4.2 mg/dL by the age of 20 years. PTH inhibits phosphate reabsorption by lowering the TmP/GFR via cAMP-dependent inhibition of Npt2a and Npt2c expression, resulting in phosphaturia. PTH is the best-characterized physiological regulator of phosphate reabsorption, but its principal function is to maintain calcium homeostasis. By contrast, both acute and chronic Pi deprivation initiates an adaptive increase in brush border membrane sodium phosphate transport through microtubule-dependent recruitment of Npt2 proteins to the apical membrane surface.

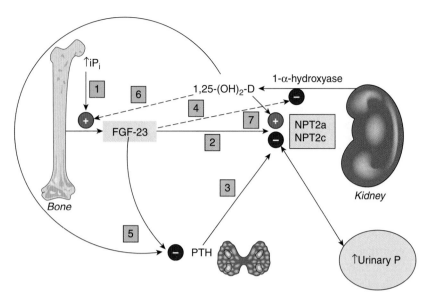

FIGURE 6-4 ■ Renal regulation of phosphate. (1) Increased plasma inorganic phosphate (Pi) increases FGF-23 secretion. (2) FGF-23 decreases expression of renal tubule sodium-phosphate cotransporters Npt2a and Npt2c, leading to decreased Pi reabsorption. (3) PTH also decreases expression of renal Npt2a and Npt2c. (4) FGF-23 decreases expression of renal 25-hydroxycalciferol 1-α-hydroxylase thereby indirectly decreasing intestinal Pi absorption. The net effect is lowering of plasma Pi. (5) FGF-23, like 1,25-(OH)$_2$D, inhibits PTH secretion. (6) In contrast, 1,25-(OH)$_2$D increases FGF-23 secretion, presumably offsetting 1,25-(OH)$_2$D-mediated increases in intestinal Pi absorption, and (7) likely increases Npt2a and Npt2c expression.

An additional hormone, fibroblast growth factor 23 (FGF23), has also emerged as an important regulator of phosphate homeostasis. FGF23 reduces expression of the renal tubular sodium phosphate co-transporters Npt2a and Npt2c, thus impairing phosphate reabsorption in the proximal renal tubule. In addition, FGF23 suppresses activity of the renal 1-α-hydroxylase (CYP27B1) while inducing activity of the renal 24-hydroxylase (CYP24).

Many other hormones and cytokines influence phosphate reabsorption in the proximal renal tubule. GH, IGF-I, insulin, epidermal growth factor, thyroid hormone, and dietary phosphate depletion stimulate renal Pi reabsorption. In contrast, renal phosphate reabsorption is inhibited by parathyroid hormone-related protein (PTHrP), calcitonin, atrial natriuretic factor, TGF-α and TGF-β, and glucocorticoids.

Intestinal absorption. Up to two-thirds of the dietary phosphate is absorbed from the intestine, primarily in the jejunum. The percentage of inorganic phosphate absorbed increases as inorganic phosphate intake decreases, but the absolute absorption of inorganic phosphate increases proportionally with increasing intake. Active absorption of phosphate is mediated by the type 2b sodium-phosphate cotransport (Npt2b) which is located in the brush border of enterocytes.

Dietary phosphate restriction and hypophosphatemia stimulate calcitriol synthesis via enhanced activity of the 25(OH)D-1β-hydroxylase (CYP27B1) in the kidney, leading to increased calcium and phosphorus absorption in the intestine and enhanced mobilization

of calcium and phosphorus from bone. It appears that this effect reflects inhibition of FGF23 secretion by hypophosphatemia. The resultant increased serum levels of calcium and calcitriol inhibit PTH secretion, which leads to increased urinary calcium excretion and increased tubular reabsorption of phosphate. Thus, normal serum calcium levels are maintained and serum phosphorus levels are normalized (Figure 6-4).

Bone Metabolism

Bone mass is determined both by modeling and remodeling. Bone begins to form (modeling) during early fetal life, and the skeleton continues to enlarge by replacement and expansion of existing bone (remodeling) well into the early third decade of life (early 20s) soon after statural growth has ceased. There then appears a period of relatively stable bone mass (balanced remodeling), followed by a decline in women, influenced by changes of the menopause, and in both genders, as a function of advancing age (enhanced remodeling, followed by unbalanced remodeling). "Peak bone mass" accumulation appears to be under strong genetic influence, and, based on studies in mono- and di-zygotic twins, genetic variation may account for up to 80% of achieved peak bone mass. A substantial influence, perhaps 20% or more, of environmental factors such as nutrition, exercise, or the introduction of disease, on acquisition of peak mass is also at play. Pubertal gain in bone mass represents the largest percentage increase after that seen in the first year of life.

Bone cells

The structural and metabolic functions of the skeleton require the coordinated interaction of osteoblasts and osteoclasts and a great many systemic and local factors (Table 6-1). Osteoblasts are bone-forming cells, and are derived from pluripotent mesenchymal stem cells that can also differentiate into muscle, adipocytes, cartilage, or fibrous tissue. Populations of partially differentiated precursor cells appear committed to differentiating only into osteoblasts.

Bone formation. In the process of bone formation, preosteoblasts and osteoblasts synthesize collagen and alkaline phosphatase followed by osteocalcin, an osteoblast-specific protein that contains γ-carboxylated glutamic acid. Osteocalcin, or bone GLA protein, is a vitamin K-dependent, noncollagenous bone protein that is secreted by osteoblasts and is involved in the mineralization process. Osteocalcin is found predominantly in bone matrix, but decarboxylated osteocalcin is released into the circulation where it appears to function as hormone that participates in the regulation of glucose metabolism and fat mass. Cell-based studies show that decarboxylated osteocalcin can increase insulin secretion and proliferation of pancreatic beta cells, and can also enhance adiponectin secretion from fat cells. These actions suggest that osteocalcin can regulate glucose metabolism and affect insulin sensitivity and fat mass and provide further evidence of metabolic interaction between the skeleton and fat tissue.[7] Osteoblastic activity is associated with serum osteocalcin, and measurement of plasma osteocalcin concentration is therefore considered a useful clinical marker of bone formation, and indirectly, of bone remodeling or turnover. However, levels of osteocalcin correspond better with the rate of bone mineralization rather than osteoblastic activity *per se*, and osteocalcin concentrations are typically not elevated in children with active rickets despite greatly increased levels of bone alkaline phosphatase.[8,9] The kidneys excrete osteocalcin, and serum values are increased in renal failure. In normal individuals osteocalcin and other markers of bone formation follow the same pattern as the markers of bone resorption, because the two processes are coupled during bone remodeling. Concentrations of osteocalcin are greatest during infancy and at puberty, with levels varying in parallel to the normal pattern of growth and puberty. After adolescence bone remodeling slows, and the concentrations of these markers declines.[10] Although the variations in the plasma concentration of osteocalcin are similar to the changes observed in the concentration of calcitriol, no sustained correlation has been found between plasma osteocalcin and calcitriol.

Fully differentiated osteoblasts are spatially arranged on the bone surface so that the deposition of collagen and noncollagen proteins occurs in a manner that is favorable for mineralization. Mineralization is delayed for several days, during which time the collagen fibrils are cross-linked to enhance strength.

As osteoblast production of collagen and noncollagen protein is completed, a few of the osteoblasts are buried in the matrix and become osteocytes. Many cell processes that lie in canaliculi within the bone connect the osteoblasts and osteocytes to each other. This syncytium of interconnected cells is probably critical for sensing mechanical forces.

Osteoblasts have receptors for factors that influence bone remodeling, and they produce many regulators of bone growth. These receptors include those for PTH, calcitriol, glucocorticoids, sex hormones, growth hormone, (GH) and thyroid hormone. Receptors for interleukin (IL)-1, tumor necrosis factor-alpha (TNF-α), prostaglandins insulin-like growth factors (IGFs), transforming growth factor (TGF)-β, bone morphogenetic proteins, fibroblast growth factors, and platelet-derived growth factor are also present. Factors produced by osteoblasts that probably act locally include prostaglandins, IL-6, IGFs and their binding proteins (IGF-BPs), TGF-β, bone morphogenetic proteins, fibroblast growth factors, platelet-derived growth factor, and vascular-endothelial growth factor.

Bone is resorbed by osteoclasts, large, multinucleated cells that can dissolve mineral and degrade matrix. Osteoclasts are related to monocyte/macrophage cells and are derived from granulocyte/macrophage-forming colony units (CFU-GM).[11,12] Osteoclast progenitors are present in the marrow, spleen, and in small numbers in the circulation. During development, osteoclast precursors probably migrate to the bone from extramedullary sites of hematopoiesis. The lifespan of an osteoclast may be as long as 3 to 4 weeks.

Actively resorbing osteoclasts are firmly attached to bone by a zone of membrane that is relatively devoid of subcellular particles (the "sealing" zone). The sealing zone surrounds an area of highly convoluted membrane, the "ruffled border," where resorption occurs.

Osteoclast formation requires an interaction with cells of the osteoblastic lineage, which may depend upon cell-cell contact and specific cytokines of the receptor activator of NF-kappa B (RANK) system described in the section "Resorption." Osteoblasts may also be the source of the M-CSF that is required for osteoclastogenesis (Figure 6-5). Excessive osteoclastic resorption occurs in osteoporosis, Paget disease, hyperparathyroidism, and inflammatory bone loss. On the other hand, osteoclastic resorption is deficient in osteopetrosis.

Bone modeling

Modeling produces growth of the skeleton and changes in bone shape. Linear growth during childhood and adolescence occurs by growth of cartilage at the end plates of long bones, followed by endochondral bone formation. The width of the bones increases by periosteal apposition. During childhood, this is accompanied by

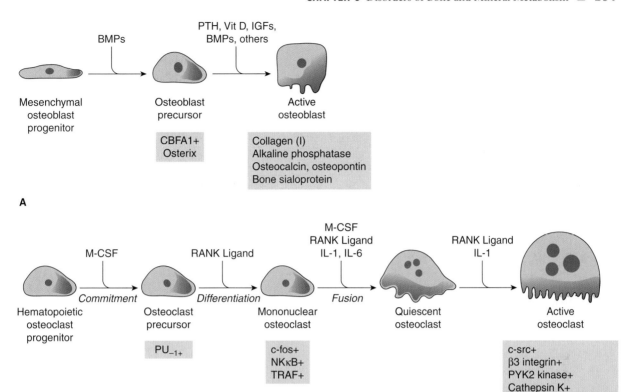

FIGURE 6-5 ■ Regulation of osteoblast **(A)** and osteoclast **(B)** development. Hormones, cytokines, and growth factors regulating cell proliferation and differentiation are shown above the arrows. Transcription factors regulating cell proliferation and differentiation are shown below the arrows. BMPs, bone morphogenic proteins; PTH, parathyroid hormone; Vit D, vitamin D; IGFs, insulin-like growth factors; CBFA1, core binding factor A1; M-CSF, macrophage colony-stimulating factor; PU-1, a monocyte- and B lymphocyte-specific ets family transcription factor; NFkB, nuclear factor kB; TRAF, tumor necrosis factor receptor-associated factors; RANK ligand, receptor activator of NFkB ligand; IL-1, interleukin 1; IL-6, interleukin. *(From Jameson JL. Principles of Endocrinology. In: Jameson JL, ed. Harrison's Endocrinology. New York, NY: McGraw-Hill; 2006, Figure 23-1, p. 412.)*

endosteal resorption. The endosteal (or inner) surface is in contact with the marrow; thus, endosteal resorption results in a concomitant enlargement of the marrow cavity. In general, the first bone formed from mesenchyme in early development as well as bone formed during rapid repair has a relatively disorganized pattern of collagen fibers and is termed "woven" bone. Subsequent bone is laid down in an orderly fashion with successive layers of well-organized collagen, and is termed "lamellar bone."

During puberty and early adult life, endosteal apposition and trabecular thickening provide maximum skeletal mass and strength (peak bone mass). Locally and systemically produced factors and mechanical forces influence these processes. The adult skeleton continues to undergo remodeling throughout life; approximately 15% of the mature skeleton is replaced each year to maintain mineral homeostasis, to repair damaged bone, and to respond to changes in skeletal stress.[13]

Bone remodeling

Bone remodeling occurs most often in skeletal sites rich in cancellous (trabecular) bone. Trabecular bone is found inside the long bones, in the inner portions of the pelvis and other large flat bones, and throughout the bodies of the vertebrae, where it provides important mechanical support to the spine. Trabecular or cancellous bone constitutes only 20% of the skeleton, but it has an enormous surface area and is particularly active metabolically.

A second form of bone, termed cortical bone, is less metabolically active but provides great strength and integrity to the skeleton. Cortical bone comprises 80% of the skeleton, and constitutes the outer part of all skeletal structures. Cortical bone is dense and compact, and the lamellae may be extensive (circumferential) or tightly packed in concentric circles in osteons. Cortical bone primarily provides mechanical strength and protection, but with severe or prolonged mineral deficits it can participate in metabolic responses.

The remodeling cycle. Bone remodeling is a process that takes place in a cyclic fashion at specific sites or skeletal lacunae. Each remodeling cycle lasts about 90 to 120 days. Bone turnover begins with activation of surface osteoblasts and ostecytes. The signals for initiation of remodeling include changes in the serum concentration of a number of systemic factors, such as PTH, thyroxine, growth hormone, and estrogen. Cytokines and growth factors (eg, IL-1, IL-6, IL-11, insulin-like growth factor I, and TGF-β) trigger the bone-synthesizing activity of osteoblasts.[13]

> **Resorption**—Once cells of the osteoblast lineage are activated, these cells undergo shape changes and secrete collagenase and other enzymes that lyse proteins on the bone surface; they also express a factor that is termed osteoclast differentiating factor or RANK ligand (RANKL). RANKL interacts with a receptor on osteoclast precursors that is identical to the receptor involved in interaction of T-cells and dendritic cells called RANK. RANKL stimulates activation, migration, differentiation, and fusion of hematopoietic cells of the osteoclast lineage to begin the process of resorption.[14,15]

Osteoclasts secrete protons and proteases that dissolve the mineral matrix. Osteoclasts also have acid phosphatase anchored to their cell membranes. Multinucleated osteoclasts remove mineral and matrix to a limited depth on the trabecular surface or within cortical bone. What stops this process is not clear, but high local concentrations of calcium or substances released from the matrix may be involved.

> **Reversal**—After osteoclastic resorption is completed, a reversal phase occurs, in which mononuclear cells, possibly of monocyte/macrophage lineage, appear on the bone surface. These cells prepare the surface for new osteoblasts to begin bone formation. A layer of glycoprotein-rich material is laid down on the resorbed surface, the so-called "cement line," to which the new osteoblasts can adhere.

> **Formation**—The formation phase follows, with successive waves of osteoblasts laying down bone until the resorbed bone is completely replaced and a new bone structural unit is fully formed. When this phase is complete, the surface is covered with flattened lining cells and a prolonged resting period with little cellular activity on the bone surface ensues until a new remodeling cycle begins. The major structural protein in bone matrix is type 1 collagen, which is synthesized by the osteoblasts. Type 1 collagen is the most abundant protein in bone, and is assembled as a complex structure containing two α-1 chains and one α-2 chains. The α-1 and α-2 chains are the products of distinct genes, and after synthesis many of the proline and lysine residues in the collagen chains are

hydroxylated to hydroxyproline and hydroxylysine, respectively. Then, one α-2 and two α-1 chains intertwine to form a helical structure known as procollagen, followed by cleavage of their amino-terminal and carboxy-terminal peptides to form tropocollagen.[16,17]

Hormonal regulation of bone metabolism

PTH normally increases the number and the activity of osteoclasts, through at least two mechanisms: upregulation of RANKL production and inhibition of osteoprotogerin (OPG) production. Both PTH and calcitriol act in concert to increase bone resorption and elevate plasma calcium concentration. However, both hormones also have long-term effects that cause inhibition of bone resorption and/or stimulation of bone formation, resulting in a net increase in bone mass. Calcitonin has a direct and acute inhibitory effect on osteoclastic bone resorption and may also decrease the formation of osteoclasts. Calcitonin has no major effect on bone formation.

Glucocorticoids have complex and multiple effects on bone and calcium homeostasis. When used in pharmacologic doses glucocorticoids inhibit both bone formation and resorption. The inhibition of bone formation is probably the major mechanism responsible for the osteopenia associated with glucocorticoid excess.[18] Glucocorticoids also stimulate expression of RANKL and M-CSF, which, in conjunction with the steroid's antiapoptotic effects on mature osteoclasts, would predict increased rather than decreased degradative activity. However, accelerated bone resorption does not appear to contribute to the osteoporosis that occurs with prolonged glucocorticoid therapy. Glucocorticoids also reduce osteoblast number by decreasing osteoblast formation from precursors, inhibit osteoblast activity, and stimulate apoptosis of mature osteoblasts. Thyroid hormones cause a marked increase in bone turnover, and osteopenia is common in patients with hyperthyroidism, particularly those over the age of 50 years. This effect is likely as a result of a direct stimulatory effect on osteoclastic bone resorption. Insulin has direct and indirect effects on both cartilage and bone formation. Some patients with longstanding type 1 diabetes mellitus may develop osteopenia. The effect of insulin is thought to be mediated through increased production of insulin-like growth factor 1 (IGF-1) and calcitriol. IGF-1 stimulates protein synthesis and sulfation in cartilage, and both insulin and IGF-1 stimulate bone collagen synthesis. The effects of insulin and IGF-1 on bone are closely related and not additive, suggesting a similar mechanism of action. Growth hormone also stimulates both cartilage and bone formation. This effect is probably mediated through increased production of IGF-1.

Sex steroids accelerate skeletal growth and bone maturation, and contribute to bone accumulation and are antiresorptive. These effects may be direct or conferred through interaction with the GH system or mechanical loading. Estrogens alone and estrogens in combination with testosterone increase bone mineral density to a greater extent than testosterone alone, suggesting that least some of androgen action is mediated through estrogens.[19] The estrogen receptor-α is responsible for at least some of these effects as highlighted by the abnormal bone histology described in a male with genetic mutations that led to a loss of estrogen receptor- α loss function.[20] Androgens, either directly or through accrual of lean mass, also target periosteal bone apposition. The androgen receptor is important for the action of androgens. The osteoclast is the target of antiresorptive effects of estrogen; the androgen site is not yet defined.[21]

Hormonal Regulation of Calcium and Phosphate Homeostasis

Parathyroid hormone

PTH synthesis and secretion. PTH is synthesized and secreted by chief cells, the major cells of the parathyroid glands. PTH is produced by a two-step

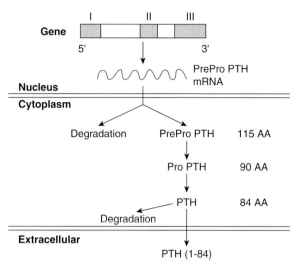

FIGURE 6-6 ■ PTH synthesis from gene transcript to secretion.

proteolytic conversion of the primary gene product, prepro PTH, yielding first proPTH and then native hormone (Figure 6-6), a single chain polypeptide comprised of 84 amino acids with a molecular weight of 9500 daltons (9.5 kDa) (Figure 6-7). Biological activity, as defined by hypercalcemic potency, resides within the

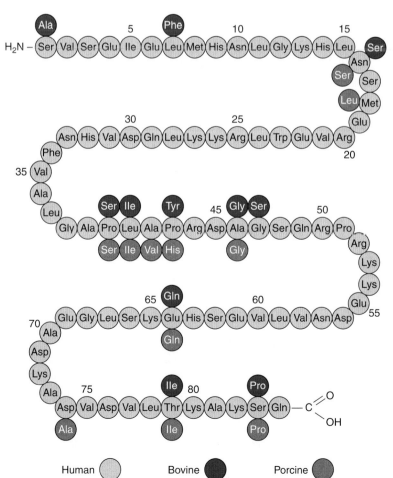

FIGURE 6-7 ■ Complete amino acid sequence of human, bovine, and porcine PTH.

34 amino acids at the amino terminus, which shows the greatest degree of sequence homology among different species and with the related molecule, PTHrP. The first two amino acids are essential for activation of the receptor, and region 3 to 34 contains the structural determinants necessary for receptor binding.

PTH synthesis and secretion from the parathyroid glands occurs at a rate that is inversely proportional to the serum ionized calcium concentration. PTH release is pulsatile and temporally coupled with the plasma concentrations of calcium and phosphate. In addition, a circadian periodicity in plasma PTH concentrations exists with a characteristic nocturnal increase. PTH secretion is also regulated by calcitriol, which reduces hormone secretion, and by extracellular phosphate, which stimulates PTH secretion.[22,23]

Extracellular calcium, and to a lesser extent other divalent cations, strictly regulate PTH synthesis and secretion through interaction with specific calcium-sensing receptors (CaSRs) that are expressed on the surface of parathyroid cells. These receptors are also present on several other cell types, including the calcitonin-secreting C-cells of the thyroid and renal tubular cells. The CaSR consist of a single polypeptide chain that is spans the plasma membrane seven times (ie, heptahelical), forming three extracellular and three or four intracellular loops and a cytoplasmic carboxyl-terminal tail. The heptahelical receptors are coupled by heterotrimeric ($\alpha\beta\gamma$) G proteins[24] to signal effector molecules (eg, adenylyl cyclase, phospholipase C, potassium channels) that are localized to the inner surface of the plasma membrane (see references 25 and 26 for reviews).

Binding of extracellular calcium to the CaSR activates the receptor and facilitates its interaction and activation of G proteins that stimulate phospholipase C activity (G_q and G_{11}) and inhibit adenylyl cyclase (G_i).[27] Activation of phospholipase C leads to the generation of the second messengers inositol 1,4,5-trisphosphate and diacylglycerol, which increase levels of cytosolic calcium via release from intracellular stores and stimulate protein kinase C activity, respectively. These second messenger systems mediate the parathyroid cell's responses to elevated concentrations of extracellular calcium, which include inhibition of PTH release, suppression of *PTH* gene expression, and accelerated degradation of intracellular PTH.

A decrease in extracellular calcium rapidly increases the secretion of PTH from a pool of stored intracellular hormone that is sufficient to sustain PTH secretion for only 60 to 90 minutes. Under conditions of protracted hypocalcemia the parathyroid cell relies upon two mechanisms to increase PTH availability: First, inhibition of intracellular hormone degradation and second, increased levels of PTH mRNA (with hyperplasia if needed). A basal, nonsuppressible PTH secretion that is independent of extracellular calcium also exists and is proportional to the mass of chief cells. As a result, basal PTH secretion is markedly increased by parathyroid gland hyperplasia.

The extracellular magnesium concentration also seems to have a role in the regulation of PTH secretion. Severe magnesium deficiency results in decreased secretion of PTH as well as refractoriness to PTH action in target cells and can cause hypocalcemia.[28] Conversely, elevated serum levels of magnesium can directly inhibit PTH secretion via interaction of the divalent cation with CaSRs.[29,30]

Metabolism. Once secreted into the circulation, PTH has a short half-life, probably of the order of less than 5 minutes. It is taken up by hepatic Kupffer cells where cathepsin enzymes cleave the region between amino acids 33 and 43, thereby generating amino- and carboxyterminal fragments. Carboxyl region fragments are released back into circulation, whereas the amino region portions are probably further degraded so that they are not released as bioactive entities. The kidney is also known to have PTH cleaving enzymes, but apparently neither carboxyl nor amino region fragments are released back into the circulation from the kidney.

Actions. The primary function of PTH is to increase the extracellular fluid calcium (1) directly, by stimulating the rates of renal calcium reabsorption and bone resorption and (2) indirectly, by increasing the rate of intestinal calcium absorption via increased renal formation of calcitriol. These PTH effects are mediated by specialized target cells present in bone and kidney that express specific plasma membrane G protein–coupled receptors. The classical PTH receptor is an approximately 75-kD glycoprotein that is often referred to as the PTH/PTHrP or type 1 PTH receptor (type 1 PTH-r). The type 1 receptor expressed on bone and kidney cells is identical. The type 1 PTH-r binds both PTH and PTHrP, a factor made by diverse tumors that cause humorally mediated hypercalcemia, with equivalent affinity. The type 1 PTH-r is most abundantly expressed in the physiological target tissues for PTH action (ie, kidney and bone), but it is also found in a wide variety of fetal and adult tissues where it appears to mediate the paracrine/autocrine signaling pathways of PTHrP rather than the endocrine actions of PTH. By contrast, a second PTH receptor, termed the type 2 receptor protein, interacts with PTH but not PTHrP,[31,32] and has a very restricted tissue distribution that does not include classical PTH target tissues (ie, bone and kidney). It is more likely that the hypothalamic peptide termed TIP39 is the physiological ligand for the type 2 PTH receptor,[32-34] but the biological functions mediated by this receptor remain largely unknown.

The type 1 PTH receptor couples to G proteins[35] that stimulate adenylyl cyclase (Gs) (Figure 6-8) and

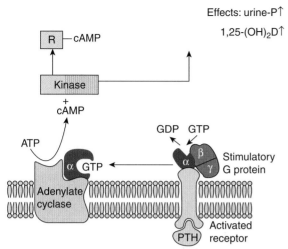

Effects: urine-P↑
1,25-(OH)₂D↑

FIGURE 6-8 ▪ Mechanism of action of PTH in the kidney. The activation of adenylate cyclase is mediated by the G$_s$-protein which consists of α, β, and γ-subunits. The α-subunit contains the guanine nucleotide-binding site that, in the nonactivated state, is occupied by GDP. Binding of PTH to the receptor induces a change in the conformation of the α-subunit leading to an exchange of bound GDP for GTP. The α-GTP complex then dissociates from the rest of the G$_s$-protein and activates adenylate cyclase. Cyclic AMP is produced and binds to the regulatory subunit (R) of cAMP-dependent protein kinase, liberating the catalytic subunit of the enzyme which subsequently phosphorylates and activates enzymes involved in tubular phosphate transport and 1-α-hydroxylation of 25-(OH)D.

phospholipase C (Gq/11) which activate protein kinase A and protein kinase C signaling pathways, respectively. Thus, receptor activation leads to rapid generation of the second messengers cAMP,[36,37] inositol 1,4,5-trisphosphate and diacylglycerol,[38,39] and cytosolic calcium.[40-43]

Action on the kidney. The renal handling of phosphate appears to be the main determinant of plasma phosphate concentration. PTH inhibits phosphate reabsorption by resetting the TmP/GFR to a lower level resulting in phosphaturia and, in turn, reduced plasma phosphate concentration. PTH mediates this effect by controlling the concentration of Npt2a and Npt2c cotransporters on the brush border membrane located at the apical surface of proximal tubular cells. In hypoparathyroid states TmP/GFR is set at a higher level resulting in increased phosphate resorption and increased plasma phosphate concentration.

PTH-enhanced reabsorption of calcium in distal tubules is mediated directly (and indirectly via calcitriol) by increased expression or activity of the transient receptor potential cation channel 5 (TRPV5) (Figure 6-3). In hyperparathyroidism the opposing forces of increased filtered load because of hypercalcemia and increased tubular reabsorption due directly to PTH determine the urinary excretion of calcium. PTH also has a minor effect on tubular transport of bicarbonate and amino acids so that aminoaciduria and a rise in pH

and bicarbonate content of the urine can be present in hyperparathyroid states. PTH stimulates the rate-limiting enzyme in vitamin D activation, 1-α-hydroxylase in the kidney, (see section "Vitamin D" stated later on). Thus, PTH indirectly increases intestinal calcium and phosphate absorption by stimulating calcitriol production in the proximal tubule.

Action on bone. Osteoblasts possess PTH receptors, whereas osteocytes and mature osteoclasts do not appear to bind PTH. The available data indicate that PTH acts primarily on mature osteoblasts to enhance their function, their lifespan, or both, and it may also enhance the differentiation of cells in the osteoblastic lineage. These findings indicate that the PTH stimulation of osteoclastic bone resorption is mediated through osteoblasts. One of the most important consequences of PTH action is mediated via increased expression of RANK ligand (RANKL) on the cell surface (described in section "Action on the Kidney" stated earlier). PTH also decreases production of osteoprotegerin (OPG), a soluble decoy receptor that can bind RANKL and block its interaction with RANK.[44,45] By increasing production of RANKL and decreasing production of the natural antagonist OPG, PTH increases osteolastic bone resorption. PTH and calcitriol act in concert to elevate the plasma calcium by stimulating bone resorption.

PTH also increases bone formation in a manner that appears to require IGF-1.[46,47] PTH stimulates osteoblasts to synthesize and secrete IGF-1 into the local microenvironment, where it behaves as an autocrine or paracrine factor to stimulate osteoblasts and osteoblast precursors.[47-49]

Measurement of PTH in plasma. Immunometric "sandwich" assays have replaced conventional radioimmunoassay for PTH. The first-generation immunometric PTH assay not only detects the intact hormone, but also additional PTH fragments that are truncated at the amino terminus and consist principally of PTH (7-84). A second-generation immunometric PTH assay uses a detection antibody that recognizes antigenic determinants at the extreme amino-terminal (1-4) end of the PTH molecule, making the assay specific for biologically active "whole" PTH-(1-84) and possibly PTH fragments that are truncated at the carboxyl-terminus. This assay will not measure PTH-(7-84) fragments, which are directly released from the parathyroid gland in humans and appear to exert a hypocalcemic effect by inhibiting the calcemic effect of PTH-(1-84) and its stimulatory effect on bone turnover.[50]

Measures of biologically active PTH provide the most accurate index of parathyroid activity. Hence, the successful development of "third" generation whole PTH 1-84 immunoassays has provided superior diagnostic sensitivity over older assays in patients with primary hyperparathyroidism and has allowed more meaningful interpretation of PTH trends.[51] Since the half-life of 1-84 PTH is much shorter than that for the 7-84 PTH fragment, the development of this assay for intraoperative monitoring has advanced the surgical management of hyperparathyroidism.

Parathyroid hormone-related protein

PTHrP was originally discovered as the cause of humorally mediated hypercalcemia of malignancy. PTHrP interacts with shared PTH/PTHrP (type 1 PTH) receptors in the kidney and bone through its amino terminus, which is homologous with the amino terminus of PTH.[52,53] The PTH and PTHrP genes have presumably evolved from a common ancestor through an ancient gene duplication event. Overall, PTH and PTHrP share significant amino acid homology only at the amino terminus, where 8 of the first 13 amino acids are identical. Remarkably, even in the primary receptor binding domain (amino acids 18-34), PTH and PTHrP do not have recognizable primary sequence homologies. PTH and PTHrP bind to the type 1 PTH receptor with equivalent affinity, which no doubt explains why biological actions that are mediated via the amino terminus of the two molecules appear to be very close in both range of biological activities and potency.

Compared to PTH, PTHrP is considerably longer, with variants containing either 139, 141, or 173 amino acids. PTHrP plays a significant role in regulating skeletal development and fetal calcium homeostasis, and is widely expressed in adult tissues including cartilage, bone, smooth muscle, placenta, central nervous system (CNS), and epithelial tissues such as breast, hair follicle, intestine, and tooth enamel.

Vitamin D

The observation by Palm in 1890 that rickets could be treated by exposure to sunlight marked the beginning of a scientific quest that led to the discovery of vitamin D by Windaus and coworkers in 1932.[6] The appreciation of calcitriol as the principal and most potent form of vitamin D, along with the elucidation of a molecular mechanism of action analogous to that of classic steroid hormones, led to the recognition of vitamin D as a precursor of a potent steroid hormone rather than a vitamin in the context of an essential nutritional substance. The distribution of vitamin D receptors in many tissues in addition to the intestine, the skeletal system, and the kidney implies that the hormone has biological functions besides its classical role in mineral homeostasis.

Sources and transport. The D vitamins constitute a family of fat-soluble biologically active secosteroids (Figure 6-9). The term vitamin D refers to both vitamin

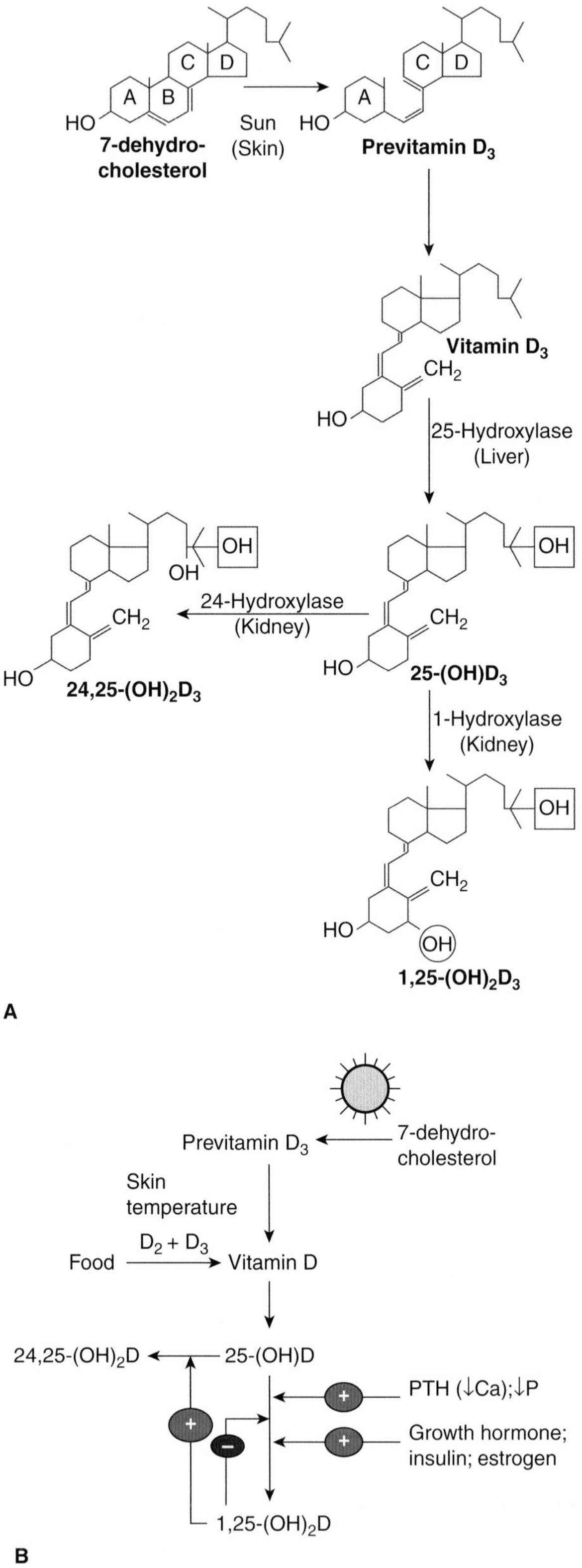

FIGURE 6-9 ■ (A) Pathway of vitamin D metabolism. The rate-limiting step in the activation of vitamin D is the 1-α-hydroxylation of 25-(OH)D$_3$ to calcitriol and is directly stimulated by PTH and low serum phosphate concentration. **(B)** Regulation of vitamin D metabolism. PTH is the main stimulator of calcitriol synthesis. The effect of ionized calcium is indirect and mediated by PTH. Calcitriol inhibits its own synthesis and stimulates the production of 24,25-(OH)$_2$D$_3$, an inactive vitamin D metabolite.

D_2 (ergocalciferol) that originates in plants and to vitamin D_3 (cholecalciferol) produced in the body. Both vitamin D_2 and vitamin D_3 are used to fortify foods. Vitamin D_2 and vitamin D_3 have generally been considered to be of near equal potency in humans,[54] but some studies suggest that vitamin D_3 may be slightly (two- to threefold) more potent than vitamin D_2 in humans in maintaining serum levels of 25-(OH)D[55-57] as it and its 25-hydroxylated metabolite may bind vitamin D–binding protein (DBP) with greater affinity than vitamin D_2 (see below).[57]

Vitamin D_3 is produced in the skin via opening of the B-ring of 7-dehydrocholesterol. During exposure to sunlight, 7-dehydrocholesterol absorbs solar radiation with energies between 290 and 320 nm (UVB ultraviolet light), and is transformed into previtamin D_3. Over the next several hours previtamin D_3 isomerizes to vitamin D_3 by a temperature dependent process. This process permits the skin to continue the synthesis of vitamin D_3 for up to 3 days after a single exposure to sunlight. Once vitamin D_3 is formed, the DBP in plasma translocates it preferentially into the circulation, and this ensures the efficient conversion of previtamin-D_3 to vitamin D_3 by shifting the equilibrium toward vitamin D_3.

For most individuals, daily requirements for vitamin D can be satisfied by exposure of hands, face, and arms to sunlight for 20 to 30 minutes three times per week. Many factors can influence the efficiency of cutaneous production of vitamin D. Sunscreens, even those with a sunlight protection factor rating as low as 8 (SPF 8), can markedly reduce, by as much as 97%, the cutaneous production of vitamin D. Moreover, chronic use can result in vitamin D deficiency.[58-61] The melanin in skin pigment absorbs UVB photons and can thereby behave as a natural sunscreen, such that dark-skinned people will require greater exposure (five- to tenfold) than light skinned people to synthesize equivalent amounts of vitamin D.[58-60] Similarly, street clothing can decrease the amount of cutaneous vitamin D synthesized in response to UVB radiation.[62,63] Latitude, time of day, and season can also affect the efficiency of solar irradiation on cutaneous synthesis of vitamin D. Very little cutaneous vitamin D is formed during the winter months (October through March in the northern latitudes and April through September in the southern latitudes) owing to increased clothing worn, decreased time spent outdoors during winter, and decreased ultraviolet radiation reaching the earth.[64-66] During sunlit hours, vitamin D_3 production is maximal at midday and small quantities are still being formed between 8:00 and 9:00, and between 16:00 and 17:00 during the summer. For most individuals, the cutaneous production of vitamin D during the spring, summer, and fall is in excess of daily requirements, and fat-stored cholecalciferol (3000-5000 IU/day) is used to provide more than 80% of daily needs

during the winter months.[67] Finally, aging also reduces the ability of skin to synthesize vitamin D.[58,62,68] Excessive sunlight exposure is unlikely to cause vitamin D intoxication, as previtamin D can be degraded by further UVB radiation to the inert photoproducts lumisterol and tachysterol and vitamin D_3 can be photoisomerized to suprasterol and other biologically inactive products.

Humans obtain calciferols either endogenously through metabolism of precursors in the skin, or exogenously as a dietary component or dietary supplement. For practical purposes, the metabolism and actions of vitamin D_3 and vitamin D_2 are similar in humans, although slight distinctions in the processing of these two steroids have been recently noted. In the temperate zones the vitamin D status is mainly determined by exposure to solar irradiation and reflects season, global latitude and average hours of sunlight exposure.

Metabolism. Vitamin D must undergo two hydroxylation steps before it becomes biologically active (Figure 6-9). Once vitamin D_2 or vitamin D_3 enters the circulation it is transported by the DBP to the liver to form 25-hydroxyvitamin D (25(OH)D). The principal cytochrome P450 enzyme 25-hydroxylase (CYP2R1) is present in the microsomal fractions of the liver cells.[69] At normal circulating concentrations 25(OH)D is essentially inert, but as it is the major circulating form of vitamin D the measurement of its plasma concentration is used in the assessment of the vitamin D status of an individual. Available evidence suggests that this hydroxylation step is not tightly regulated, even though a mild degree of product feedback inhibition may occur.

Although 25(OH)D is two to five times more potent than the parent vitamin, it is not biologically active at physiologic concentrations. To achieve full potency, 25(OH)D must be transported to the kidney where it is further hydroxylated at the C1 position to the hormonal form, calcitriol. The 1-α-hydroxylase enzyme system is located in the mitochondria of the proximal convoluted and straight tubules of the nephron and appears to be a classical mixed-function cytochrome P-450 steroid hydroxylase (CYP27B1).[70] The activity of the renal 1-α-hydroxylase is tightly regulated and thus the production of calcitriol remains relatively steady over a wide range of substrate concentrations. PTH activates enzyme activity through a cAMP mediated pathway. Enzyme activity is also stimulated directly by calcitonin and indirectly by growth hormone and prolactin. Calcitriol, phosphate, FGF-23, and calcium inhibit 1-α-hydroxylation. In humans, the circulating concentration of calcitriol is approximately one thousandth that of 25(OH)D.

In the past the kidney was considered the sole organ of calcitriol production. However, following the finding of elevated plasma concentrations of calcitriol in an anephric patient with sarcoidosis, this concept was no longer tenable.[71] Subsequently, synthesis of calcitriol was demonstrated in alveolar macrophages and in lymph node homogenates from patients with sarcoidosis. Elevated plasma levels of calcitriol have also been observed in hypercalcemic patients with other granulomatous disorders such as candidiasis, tuberculosis, subcutaneous fat necrosis of the newborn, and in silicon-induced granulomas. In addition, *in vitro* studies have disclosed that tissues such as placenta, colon, breast, as well as osteoblasts, activated macrophages, and keratinocytes are capable of converting 25(OH)D to calcitriol. Local production of calcitriol may serve an autocrine role in regulating cell growth and/or other activities as these tissues and cells also express vitamin D receptors. In fact, the role of PTH-independent metabolism of vitamin D in immune regulation has received much attention with respect to cancer, infections, and immune disorders.

Both calcitriol and 25(OH)D are catabolized by CYP24 (also known as 24-hydroxylase) in the kidney, which is followed by sequential metabolism, yielding the terminal product calcitroic acid. Calcitriol also undergoes CYP3A4-dependent 23- and 24-hydroxylations in the liver and small intestine (Figure 6-9). The balance between bioactivation and degradation of calcitriol ensures appropriate biological effects and is tightly controlled *in vivo*. In normal prepubertal and pubertal children the plasma concentration of (relatively inactive) $24,25\text{-}(OH)_2D$ is approximately 50 to 100 times that of calcitriol and 3% to 6% that of 25(OH)D. Another nuclear receptor, the steroid and xenobiotic receptor (SXR; also known as pregnane X receptor [PXR], PAR, and NR1I2) is expressed at high levels in the liver and small intestine, where it acts as a xenobiotic sensor that regulates the expression of CYP3A4 and other enzymes that regulate xenobiotic clearance. A variety of drugs (eg, rifampin, phenobarbital, etc) that bind to SXR can induce expression of CYP3A4 and thereby accelerate the degradation of calcitriol and 25(OH)D.[72]

Over 99% of vitamin D metabolites circulate bound to plasma proteins. The DBP is the principal carrier protein, but albumin also contributes to the transport. DBP is an α-globulin of 58,000 D[73] and is synthesized in the liver. It is a major component of plasma (normal concentration 10^{-5} M) and has multiple isoforms,[74] many of which were extensively studied for their genetic diversity long before a function in calciferol transport was recognized.

The major vitamin D metabolites are bound to a single high-affinity binding site with preferential affinity for the 25-hydroxylated forms. Normally, less than 5% of the binding sites are occupied. The affinity constants of both DBP and albumin are 10- to 20-fold higher for 25(OH)D than for calcitriol. Under normal circumstances approximately 85% of the total calcitriol is bound to DBP, about 15% to albumin, and about 0.03% is free. Only the free fraction of circulating calcitriol is thought to be available to exert metabolic effects in target cells. The plasma concentrations of DBP and total calcitriol are increased during pregnancy and after intake of oral contraceptives and estrogen, whereas the level of the free and presumably physiologically active fraction remains essentially unchanged.[75] Polymorphisms in DBP may partly explain differences in measured 25(OH)D.[76] Data to support a role for DBP in the vitamin D endocrine system apart from that of a transport protein are currently scant.

Actions. The biological actions of calcitriol are mediated through the vitamin D receptor (VDR), a 50-kDa intracellular nuclear receptor that functions in a manner similar to that described for classical steroid hormones such as glucocorticoids and estrogens.[77] The VDR is found in small intestine, kidney and bone, the major classical vitamin D target tissues, and also in other tissues including testis, ovary, pituitary, parathyroid, skin, breast, muscle, lymphocytes, and some tumor cell lines.[78] The VDR, similar to other steroid hormone receptors, contains discrete functional domains, including a hormone-binding domain at the carboxy terminus and a DNA-binding domain at the amino terminus characterized by two fingers anchored via Zn^{2+} atoms to cysteine residues (Chapter 1). The binding affinity of different vitamin D metabolites is correlated with their biologic potencies. Calcitriol is the most potent natural calciferol metabolite, with a binding affinity that is approximately 1000-fold greater than that of 25(OH)D in most test systems. Calcitriol binds to the hormone-binding domain of the VDR, and the VDR must complex with the retinoic acid X receptor (RXR) to form a heterodimeric complex.[79-81] The DNA-binding domain of the VDR is then able to bind to a vitamin D response element (VDRE) in target genes, thereby regulating gene transcription to increase or decrease the synthesis of specialized proteins mediating the biological effect of the hormone[81] (Figure 6-10). Some of the target genes are known (*e.g.,* intestinal calcium binding protein, osteocalcin, osteopontin, and calmodulin [77] (Table 6-2.). Calcitriol also has some cellular effects that are not mediated by a genomic pathway.[82-85]

Action on intestine. The most important physiologic action of calcitriol is stimulation of active calcium transport across the duodenum from lumen to bloodstream.[86] Vitamin D compounds are believed to increase transcellular calcium absorption by inducing expression of the Ca^{2+}-selective channels TRPV5 and TRPV6 on the luminal membrane, cytosolic calcium-binding proteins (eg, calbindin D9k), and the calcium

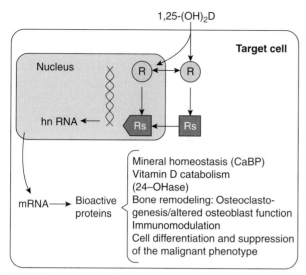

FIGURE 6-10 ■ Mode of action of calcitriol. For detailed explanation see text (hn RNA, Heterogenous Nuclear RNA).

Table 6-2.	
Receptor-Mediated Effects of Calcitriol	
Calbindin (CaBP)	+
Osteocalcin	+
Alkaline phosphatase	+
Fibronectin	+
Type 1 collagen	+
Vitamin D receptor (VDR)	+
1-α-hydroxylase (CYP27B1)	−
24-α-hydroxylase (CYP24)	+

transporters PMCA1b and NCX1 on the basolateral membrane of enterocytes in the duodenum and upper jejunum. The intestinal absorption of phosphate occurs principally in the jejunum and ileum, and is less dependent on calcitriol than is the case for calcium. Thus in vitamin D deficiency the reduction of phosphate absorption is proportionally much less than the reduction of calcium absorption. Specifically, adults who are vitamin D replete can absorb approximately 30% of dietary calcium and 70% to 80% of dietary phosphate, whereas adults who are vitamin D deficient can absorb no more than 10% to 15% of dietary calcium and 60% of dietary phosphate.

Action on bone. Calcitriol is essential for normal bone growth and mineralization. The effect on bone mineralization is probably indirect by providing minerals for incorporation into bone matrix through increased intestinal absorption of calcium. Calcitriol inhibits proliferation and collagen synthesis in fetal bone and in fetal osteoblasts, whereas in osteoblast-like cells from adult humans calcitriol stimulates collagen synthesis. Differing effects on alkaline phosphatase have been reported in several systems; however, there is general agreement that in rapidly growing osteoblast-like cells alkaline phosphatase levels are low and that they rise in response to calcitriol (Table 6-2).

Although vitamin D is essential for bone mineralization, calcitriol also has a bone-resorbing effect. *In vivo* and in organ culture, calcitriol is a potent activator of osteoclasts. Calcitriol induces monocyte stem cells in the bone marrow to differentiate to osteoclasts. Once osteoclasts have matured they no longer respond directly to

calcitriol and do not contain VDR's. Osteoclastic activity is stimulated indirectly by calcitriol through its action on osteoblasts and osteocytes, which produce a variety of cytokines, including RANKL (see in section "Action on the Kidney" stated earlier).

Action on kidney. Probably the most important effect of calcitriol on the kidney is the inhibition of its own synthesis through suppression of CYP27B1 and the concomitant enhancement of its degradation through induction of CYP24. These actions are both direct, through genomic effects, and indirect via induction of FGF23 (see in section "Regulation" stated later).[87] Calcium absorption in the distal tubule is also regulated by calcitriol though its ability to induce expression of the TRPV5 calcium channel, calbindin-D28k, and calbindin-D9k, and the basolateral membrane calcium transporters NCX1 and PMCA1b.

Regulation. The conversion of 25(OH)D to the active hormonal form calcitriol is highly regulated. The factors include PTH, calcium, phosphate, calcitriol itself, FGF-23, and various other hormones (Figure 6-11). PTH is the main trophic hormone for 1-α-hydroxylation, and elevated calcitriol levels are found in both primary and secondary hyperparathyroidism. Additionally, calcitriol inhibits its own synthesis in the kidney, whereas the production in alveolar macrophages is largely independent of both calcitriol and PTH.[88] The regulatory effects of calcium and phosphate are both likely indirect and mediated by PTH and FGF-23, respectively. According to this concept, hypocalcemia stimulates PTH secretion, which, in turn, stimulates calcitriol production, leading to (1) increased circulating calcium, which, inhibits PTH secretion and (2) increased phosphate absorption, thereby offsetting the PTH-mediated phosphaturia.

Dietary phosphorus seems to have more of a long-term regulatory effect. Phosphate restriction and hypophosphatemia produce an increase in calcitriol

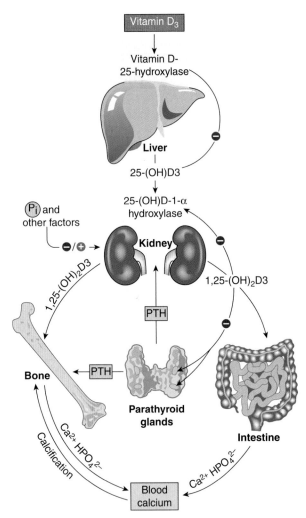

FIGURE 6-11 ■ Regulation of vitamin D metabolism. PTH is the main stimulator of calcitriol synthesis. The effect of Ca++ is indirect and mediated by PTH. Calcitriol inhibits its own synthesis and stimulates 24,25-(OH)$_2$D production.

plasma concentration within several days, whereas a high intake of phosphate decreases the level of calcitriol. FGF-23 appears to mediate these effects.

Several other endocrine factors (GH, IGF-1) have direct or indirect effect on renal 1-α-hydroxylase activity, although the exact relationships and their clinical significance remain to be clarified (Figure 6-11). Growth hormone and IGF-1 may also be involved in mediating the increase in serum calcitriol concentration induced by restriction of dietary phosphorus. Newly diagnosed children with insulin dependent diabetes have moderately reduced plasma concentrations of calcitriol which increase to normal within 3 weeks of insulin treatment. Decreased circulating levels of calcitriol have been described in hyperthyroidism, and, in contrast, elevated levels in hypothyroidism. Estrogen treatment in relatively high doses leads to a modest increase in the serum

concentration of calcitriol. This effect is attributed to a concomitant rise in DBP, resulting in a selective increase of the protein-bound fraction, and essentially unchanged level of biologically active free calcitriol fraction.[89] Pubertal girls with anorexia nervosa have low serum concentrations of calcitriol in face of normal concentrations of DBP resulting in low levels of the unbound free fraction.

The renal 24-hydroxylase CYP24 responds to many of the same modulators as the 1-α-hydroxylase, but in the opposite direction (Figure 6-11). Thus, calcitriol inhibits the renal production of calcitriol and enhances the formation of 24,25-(OH)$_2$D. This induction of the 24-hydroxylase by calcitriol has been found in virtually all other tissues that have calcitriol receptors. An assessment of the 24,25-(OH)$_2$D synthesizing capacity has therefore been extensively used to indicate receptor-mediated responsiveness of a given tissue to calcitriol.

Other effects. During the last few years a series of discoveries has suggested that calcitriol may influence the proliferation and differentiation of both normal and malignant tissues, and that the hormone also may have immunoregulatory properties.[90,91] Most cells in the body express the VDR, although the exact physiological function of calcitriol in many non-classical target tissues remains obscure (Table 6-3).

Measurements and normal values. Although cholecalciferol and 1,25-(OH)$_2$D can be measured in the circulation, the best estimates of vitamin D status are provided by measurement of 25-(OH)D. This is owing to its long serum half-life (~3 weeks) and because the 25-hydroxylation step is unregulated, thus reflecting substrate availability. In contrast, cholecalciferol has a short half-life (~24 hours) so that serum levels depend on recent sunlight exposure and vitamin D ingestion.

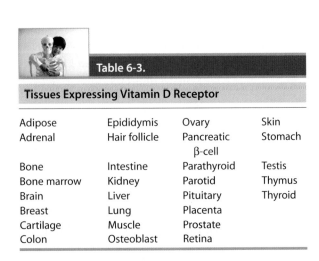

Table 6-3.

Tissues Expressing Vitamin D Receptor

Adipose	Epididymis	Ovary	Skin
Adrenal	Hair follicle	Pancreatic β-cell	Stomach
Bone	Intestine	Parathyroid	Testis
Bone marrow	Kidney	Parotid	Thymus
Brain	Liver	Pituitary	Thyroid
Breast	Lung	Placenta	
Cartilage	Muscle	Prostate	
Colon	Osteoblast	Retina	

The assay is difficult owing to the lipophilic nature of the molecule and no commercial versions are available.

Because most 25-(OH)D in the circulation is protein-bound, chromatographic separation requires an extraction step to release 25-(OH)D from its binding proteins, which can be subject to variable coprecipitation. On the other hand, nonextracted immunoassay methods may be susceptible to matrix effects, particularly owing to the lipophilic nature of 25-(OH)D. In the context of the low (nanomolar) levels of vitamin D metabolites in serum, these factors have made the routine measurement of 25-(OH)D an analytical challenge.

Although immunoassays remain the most commonly used assay, not all currently available commercial immunoassays will detect 25-(OH)D$_2$ with adequate sensitivity, thus laboratory assessment of vitamin D status in patients receiving ergocalciferol can be problematic. To improve the assay for 25-(OH)D, a number of laboratories have developed HPLC methods for vitamin D determination, and today analysis of 25-(OH)D by HPLC with UV detection is considered by many to be the gold standard method. Regardless of the methodology used to measure 25-(OH)D, standardization of results between methods and laboratories remains a significant problem. This may be owing to variability with temperature of antigen-antibody or protein-binding protein interactions as well as to differences in recognition of the 25-(OH)D$_2$ and 25-(OH)D$_3$ forms. The Diasorin RIA shows good correlation with HPLC in experienced hands but may not perform well in a laboratory that has not validated the method.

The plasma concentration of 25-(OH)D reflects the vitamin D status of an individual, and is primarily determined by sunlight exposure and the dietary supply of parent vitamin D. Seasonal variation must to be taken into account, with the highest concentrations observed in late summer and lowest in late winter. Recent studies now highlight problems and controversies with defining normal levels of 25-(OH)D. Traditionally, serum 25-(OH)D levels below 5 to 10 ng/mL were recognized to lead to rickets or osteomalacia and serum levels above 10 to 12 ng/mL were considered normal or adequate. However, observational and experimental studies have shown that serum PTH levels are suppressed and intestinal calcium absorption is optimized when serum 25-(OH)D levels are greater than 31 ng/mL (78 nm/L).[92,93] Thus, a new classification of vitamin D status has been proposed that defines serum 25-(OH)D levels that are more than 32 ng/mL (>80 nmol/L) as "desirable," serum levels between 10 and 30 ng/mL (25 and 75 nmol/L) as vitamin D insufficiency, and 25-(OH)-D levels below 10 ng/mL (25 nmol/L) as deficient. This new classification contrasts with previous attempts to define a normal range for serum 25-(OH)D concentrations that were based on statistical analyses (ie, mean ±2 SDs) of values obtained in populations that undoubtedly included many individuals who were vitamin D insufficient or deficient.[94,95]

In normal children the plasma concentration of calcitriol ranges between 25 and 85 pg/mL (60-120 pmol/L), with the higher values seen in infancy and adolescence.[96,97] These probably reflect increased intestinal mineral absorption needed during periods of rapid growth. The plasma concentration of calcitriol is not affected by sunlight exposure. The other two dihydroxylated metabolites 24,25-(OH)$_2$D and 25,26-(OH)$_2$D show seasonal variation and their plasma concentrations are positively correlated to 25-(OH)D. In normal children the plasma concentration of 24,25-(OH)$_2$D ranges between 3% and 6% of the 25-(OH)D level, whereas the concentration of 25,26-(OH)$_2$D is about 1% of the 25-(OH)D level.[96]

Phosphatonins

Until recently, regulation of phosphate metabolism has been relegated a subordinate role to calcium homeostasis. The identification of specific disorders arising from congenital and acquired defects in phosphate regulation has established the importance of phosphatonins. Thus far, the best characterized phosphatonin is FGF-23. FGF-23 is the largest member of the FGF family, contains 251 amino acids, including a 24 amino acid hydrophobic amino terminus that is a signal sequence.[98] The receptor for FGF23 is composed of the widely expressed FGFR3 plus the coreceptor Klotho, a protein with a more restricted distribution in bone, kidney, and parathyroid. Klotho has homology to β-glucosidase, and exists as both a secreted or membrane-bound protein.

Calcitriol increases FGF-23 while FGF-23 inhibits 1α-hydroxylase activity. In mouse models, both overexpression and exogenous administration of FGF-23 decreased renal expression of Npt2a (and Npt2c), decreased renal phosphate reabsorption, decreased calcitriol production, and lower serum phosphate have all been observed. Klotho-deficient mice have similar abnormalities.[99] It appears that FGF-23 is an important modulator of phosphate homeostasis in normal individuals, as there is a positive relationship between changes in dietary phosphate and circulating levels of FGF23.[100-103] Autosomal dominant hypophosphatemic rickets arises from FGF-23 gene mutations which prevent its proteolytic inactivation.

Other factors that appear important in tumor-induced osteomalacia include secreted frizzled related protein 4 (sFRP-4) and MEPE [104].

Calcitonin

Synthesis and secretion. Calcitonin is a 32 amino acid peptide synthesized and secreted by the parafollicular, or C cells, of the thyroid gland. The gene for calcitonin is composed of six exons and five introns, and the gene transcript can undergo alternative tissue-specific RNA processing to produce two different peptides (Figure 6-12). In the thyroid, the major product of the calcitonin gene is calcitonin, whereas in the brain, it is the calcitonin gene-related peptide (CGRP).

In all species, calcitonin is composed of 32 amino acids with a 1-7 amino terminal disulfide bridge and a carboxy-terminal prolinamide residue. The whole peptide is necessary for biological activity. Nonmammalian forms of calcitonin have greater potency than mammalian forms, even when tested in mammalians. Calcitonin is synthesized as a large precursor with a N-proCTpeptide flanking the amino terminal end and a C-proCTpeptide flanking the carboxy terminus (Figure 6-12). Proteolytic processing of procalcitonin cleaves off these flanking peptides. C-proCT is cosecreted with calcitonin in equimolar amounts, and radioimmunological measurement of the peptide may have clinical value in monitoring patients with medullary thyroid carcinoma.

Metabolism and regulation.

Human calcitonin has a plasma half-life of 5 to 10 minutes. The kidney represents the predominant site of metabolism and subsequent clearance of the circulating hormone. The concentration of calcitonin in plasma may therefore be elevated in patients with renal failure.

The secretion of calcitonin is directly regulated by the plasma concentration of calcium.[97] When blood calcium rises acutely, plasma calcitonin increases proportionally. Conversely, an acute decrease in plasma calcium produces a corresponding decrease in plasma calcitonin. However, the effects of chronic hypercalcemia and hypocalcemia are more complex; for example, normal, elevated, and decreased levels of calcitonin have been reported in hyperparathyroidism. Chronic hypocalcemia may result in increased storage of calcitonin in C-cells, but does not appear to have any consistent effect on calcitonin secretion. C calcitonin is also released in response to the gastrointestinal factors gastrin, pentagastrin, cholecystokinin and secretin and to neuroendocrine factors such as the α-agonist isoproterenol and the α-antagonist phentolamine.[97] However, the physiological significance of these factors in regulation of calcitonin secretion remains unclear. Notably, most studies in humans fail to demonstrate an increase in plasma calcitonin after calcium-rich meals unless plasma calcium increases.

Actions.

As for many other peptide hormones, calcitonin mediates its effects via activation of adenylyl cyclase to increase in intracellular cAMP generation. The major biological effect of calcitonin is to decrease bone resorption by inhibiting the activity of osteoclasts.[105] In addition, calcitonin may reduce the formation and maturation of osteoclasts. However, athyroid patients and patients with tumors that secrete calcitonin (eg, medullary thyroid carcinoma) have no obvious abnormalities in either bone histomorphometry or calcium homeostasis. The diminished inhibition of calcium resorption from skeletal tissue in long-term *in vitro* experiments is probably owing to desensitization of the calcitonin receptor.

Measurement.

Calcitonin circulates in several forms, including monomeric, dimeric, and larger forms of the hormone. The plasma concentration of monomeric calcitonin is very low in healthy children and adults (~10 pg/mL). So far, the clinical use of calcitonin measurements in plasma has mainly been to detect increased secretion in patients with medullary thyroid carcinoma.

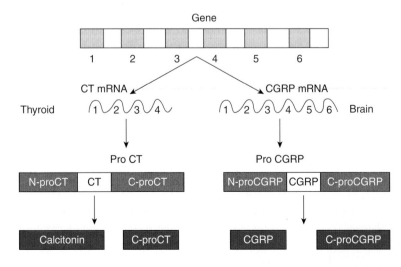

FIGURE 6-12 ■ Calcitonin gene expression. Calcitonin is preferentially expressed in the thyroid and calcitonin gene related peptide (CGRP) in the brain. Both prohormones are flanked by amino- and carboxy-terminal peptides.

CLINICAL PRESENTATION AND MANAGEMENT OF HYPOCALCEMIA

Neonatal Hypocalcemia

Definitions

Neonatal hypocalcemia is the most prevalent type of hypocalcemia encountered by the pediatrician and is relatively common in the neonatal intensive care unit. A fall of total calcium below 7.5 mg/dL (1.75 mmol/L), or 2.5 mg/dL (0.63 mmol/L) in the ionized calcium concentration usually defines neonatal hypocalcemia. In infants up to 3 months of age, hypocalcemia is defined as a total serum calcium less than 8.8 mg/dL or ionized calcium less than 4.9 mg/dL (1.22-1.4 mM). The relationship of the total calcium concentration to the ionized calcium concentration is atypical in preterm infants, and measurement of the ionized calcium concentration is required for accurate assessment of these infants.

Pathogenesis

In order to meet the high demand for minerals required by the developing skeleton, the fetus maintains higher blood calcium and phosphorus levels than the ambient maternal level. This high demand is accomplished through active transport of calcium across the placenta by a calcium pump in the basal membrane that maintains a 1:1.4 maternal to fetal calcium gradient. A midregion fragment of PTHrP produced by the parathyroids and many other tissues is largely responsible for regulating the calcium gradient, but intact parathyroids and PTH are also required for maintenance of normal fetal levels of calcium (as well as magnesium and phosphate), and lack of parathyroids and PTH cause a greater fall in fetal serum calcium concentration than lack of PTHrP. The role of calcitriol in fetal physiology is not completely understood, but it appears to play a role in skeletal development.

Fetal circulating calcium levels, as reflected in the cord blood total serum calcium concentration, increase with advancing gestational age, and at term the fetus is hypercalcemic relative to maternal concentrations of serum calcium. With birth the infant is abruptly disconnected from the placenta and the maternal calcium supply, and thus becomes entirely dependent upon intestinal absorption of dietary calcium and upon skeletal calcium reserves to maintain serum calcium levels. During this transition the response of the parathyroid gland to falling levels of ionized calcium is somewhat deficient, resulting in a physiologic nadir in neonatal serum calcium levels within the first 2 days of life. The ability of the parathyroid glands to respond to the relative hypocalcemic challenge of birth depends upon gestational age. Term infants typically achieve normal levels of serum calcium during the second week of life. Circulating

concentrations of ionized calcium tend to be higher in neonates (range 1.0-1.5 mmol/L) than in older children or adults (range 1.12-1.32 mmol/L)

The newborn has an especially high degree of adaptability for absorption of calcium depending upon the amount of calcium present in the diet. Mature human milk contains 34 mg of calcium per 100 mL, and standard commercial formulas contain approximately 50 mg/100 mL. Thus, infants fed low calcium human milk have 86% absorption of calcium compared to infants fed high calcium cow's milk, who have an absorption of only 44%. Human milk fed and formula fed infants supplemented with vitamin D exhibit significantly greater absorption of calcium compared with their unsupplemented counterparts. The term infant appears to be able to absorb and retain more calcium than preterm infants. Nonetheless, in preterm infants, as calcium intake increases, so does the intestinal absorption of calcium. For preterm infants, though, the calcium contents of human milk and standard formulas are low when compared to the amount needed to match intrauterine calcium accretion rates of 100 to 150 mg/kg/day, and low calcium intake is thought to be a factor in the decreased bone mineralization of preterm infants. Fortunately, intestinal maturation with regard to vitamin D responsiveness is accelerated by preterm delivery, indicating that absorption of calcium is not a limiting issue for the preterm infant. Of note, lactose increases calcium absorption, possibly by reduction of the intestinal pH, or formation of calcium-lactose chelates that prevent the precipitation of unabsorbable calcium phosphate salts.

Clinical presentation

Infants with low calcium levels may lack specific symptoms or signs, and hypocalcemia may only be detected by routine blood chemistry studies. Common features include neuromuscular irritability in the form of myoclonic jerks, "twitching," exaggerated startle responses, and seizures. Apnea, cyanosis, tachypnea, tachycardia, vomiting, laryngospasm, or heart failure may also be seen. Markedly reduced ionized calcium concentrations may be associated with prolongation of the Q_o-Tc interval on the electrocardiogram and decreased cardiac contractility.

Differential diagnosis/classification

Early neonatal hypocalcemia. Early neonatal hypocalcemia occurs within the first 3 days of birth and may be regarded as an accentuation of the physiologic fall in the plasma calcium concentration that takes place in all newborn infants the first 2 to 3 days of life (Figure 6-13). Early neonatal hypocalcemia apparently results from insufficient release of PTH by immature parathyroid glands or inadequate responsiveness of the renal tubule cells to PTH. An exaggerated rise in calcitonin secretion in premature infants may play a contributory

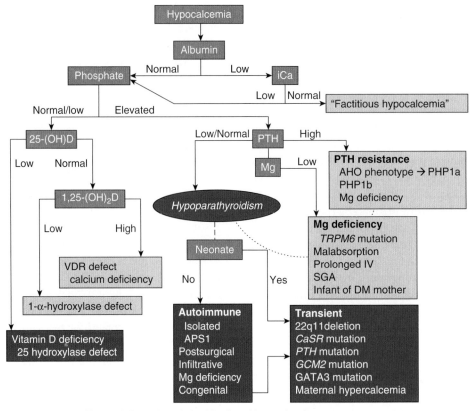

FIGURE 6-13 ■ Differential diagnosis and classification of hypocalcemia.

role. Prematurity, low birth weight, hypoglycemia, maternal diabetes mellitus, difficult delivery, and respiratory distress syndrome are common associated findings. Hypomagnesemia has especially been observed in newborn infants of diabetic mothers, but it is usually mild, transient, and unlikely to play a prominent role in the pathophysiology of neonatal hypocalcemia in these infants. A more severe form of transient neonatal hypoparathyroidism and tetany occurs in infants who were exposed to maternal hypercalcemia in utero. Intrauterine hypercalcemia suppresses parathyroid activity in the developing fetus and apparently leads to impaired responsiveness of the parathyroid glands to hypocalcemia after birth

Late neonatal hypocalcemia. Classically, infantile tetany occurs after the first week of life in both full term and prematurely born infants fed a cow's milk formula. The high phosphate content of cow's milk and some modified cow's milk formulas results in hyperphosphatemia and, in turn, depression of the plasma concentration of calcium. Since human milk is low in phosphate, breast-fed infants rarely, if ever, develop late hypocalcemia. Hyperphosphatemia, and consequent hypocalcemia, may also arise from phosphate enemas.

Transient hypoparathyroidism might contribute to the hypocalcemia in some of these infants since the normal compensatory increase in PTH secretion to increase the urinary excretion of phosphate and elevate the plasma concentration of calcium is often lacking. In other infants normal PTH secretion but relative resistance of the immature kidney to PTH occurs, causing renal retention of phosphorus and hypocalcemia. These biochemical features strongly resemble those of pseudohypoparathyroidism (PHP), but in contrast to genetic forms of PHP that are associated with defects in the *GNAS* gene, infants with this transient form of PTH resistance show normal nephrogenous cyclic AMP responses to administered PTH. Rarely, late onset hypocalcemia may occur as a manifestation of maternal hypercalcemia

The plasma concentration of magnesium may be moderately decreased, whereas the calcitriol concentration remains normal or slightly elevated. In most infants, restoration of normal calcium homeostasis occurs within 1 to 2 weeks, but the hypocalcemia may persist for 4 weeks. If hypocalcemia and hyperphosphatemia persist beyond 4 weeks, other causes of parathyroid dysfunction such as congenital hypoparathyroidism or specific magnesium deficiency disorders should be suspected (see the section "Hypocalcemia in children and adolescents").

Treatment

Symptomatic hypocalcemia should be treated with intravenous 10% calcium gluconate in a dosage of 1 to 2 mL/kg given as a slow infusion over 10 minutes. If intravenous catheters are used, they should not be placed near the heart because of the danger of cardiac arrest from inadvertent rapid calcium infusion. Avoiding extravasation is important, since 10% calcium gluconate is injurious to the soft tissue and causes severe necrosis with precipitation of calcium in the injured tissue. Some infants will require protracted treatment with intravenous calcium, which can be administered as a continuous infusion (1-3 mg/kg/h of elemental calcium) when fluid volume is not a concern. In those infants who cannot tolerate excess intravenous fluids, calcium may be administered by bolus infusion every 4 to 6 hours. In infants with accompanying hypomagnesemia, the plasma magnesium concentration usually increases spontaneously as the plasma concentration of calcium returns to normal. Termination of intravenous therapy should be guided by repeated plasma calcium determinations, and, ideally, done gradually by halving the intravenous dosage successively for 2 days before discontinuation.

To sustain normal plasma calcium concentrations, calcium lactate or gluconate in a dosage of 75 mg of elemental calcium/kg/day in neonates and 50 mg/kg/day in older infants should be added to the milk feeding. Calcium levels of symptomatic infants can be increased within 1 to 2 days by supplementing artificial formulas with sufficient calcium to achieve a high (3:1 to 4:1) calcium/phosphorus ratio. Calcium lactate powder is 13% calcium by weight whereas calcium gluconate is 9% calcium. In late neonatal hypocalcemia a formula containing low amounts of phosphate or breast milk should be used. One useful approach has been to supplement a low phosphorus formula such as Similac PM 60/40 (11.2 mg calcium and 5.5 mg phosphorus per oz). For example, 5 oz of Similac PM 60/40 contains 1.4 mmol (56 mg) of calcium and 0.90 mmol (28 mg) of phosphorus, which corresponds to a Ca:P ratio of 1.4:0.90. In order to achieve a desired 4:1 Ca:P ratio, one needs 2.2 mmol of calcium (88 mg), which could be achieved by addition of 220 mg of calcium carbonate to 5 oz of formula. As treatment decreases the plasma phosphate concentration, the plasma calcium returns to normal. At this point, the calcium supplement is reduced in steps, not stopped abruptly, since the phosphate level may rise precipitously leading to a fall in the calcium concentration to tetanic levels (Box 6-1).

Hypocalcemia in Children and Adolescents

Clinical presentation

The clinical presentation of hypocalcemia can vary from an asymptomatic biochemical finding to a life-threatening

---

> **Box 6-1. When to Refer**
>
> Hypocalcemia
>
> Appropriate referral to the endocrinologist or other specialist should be made for hypocalcemia that is not attributable to a significant intercurrent illness or intervention or that is persistent. Such disorders include:
>
> - Severe vitamin D deficiency
> - 25-α-hydroxylase deficiency
> - 1-α-hydroxylase deficiency
> - Vitamin D receptor defects
> - Hypoparathyroidism
> - Pseudohypoparathyroidism
> - Gain of function mutations in calcium-sensing receptor

---

condition. The manifestations of hypocalcemia are due primarily to enhanced neuromuscular excitability (tetany) of the central and peripheral nervous system, and in general reflect the level of ionized calcium, rather than total calcium, as well as the rate of decline. In addition, the signs and symptoms of hypocalcemic tetany can be potentiated by other electrolyte abnormalities, particularly hypomagnesemia. The total plasma calcium concentration varies with the degree of PTH deficiency and may range from about 5 mg/dL (1.25 mmol/L) to low-normal values. At normal plasma protein levels, symptoms referable to hypocalcemia might be seen at calcium concentrations of about 7 to 7.5 mg/dL (1.75-1.87 mmol/L). Patients with chronic hypocalcemia sometimes have few, if any, symptoms of neuromuscular irritability despite markedly depressed serum calcium concentrations. By contrast, patients with acute hypocalcemia frequently manifest many symptoms of tetany. Most patients with hypocalcemia will have some mild features of tetany, including circumoral numbness, paresthesias of the distal extremities, or muscle cramps. Symptoms of fatigue, hyperirritability, anxiety, and depression are also common.

Latent or manifest tetany is the hallmark of hypocalcemia in children. Muscular pain, stiffness, and cramps are early manifestations. A typical attack of tetany begins with tingling sensations in the fingertips, and sometimes in the feet. The muscles then feel tense and go into spasm. The hands are most commonly involved producing the classic carpal spasm, that is, adduction of the thumb and extension of the fingers. Spasm in the feet is less common with plantar flexion of the toes, arching of the feet, and contraction of the calf muscle. The muscle spasm causes pain, which may be severe. Tetany attacks may be provoked by prolonged muscular exercise, emotional stress, or febrile illness. Spasm, including laryngospasm, can also be precipitated by hyperventilation leading to alkalosis and reduction of ionic calcium concentration.

The Chvostek, Trousseau, and Erb signs are indicative of hyperirritability and may be useful in the clinical diagnosis of latent tetany. Chvostek sign is elicited by tapping the facial nerve 1 to 2 cm anterior to the earlobe with a fingertip. The muscle twitching in response to the stimulus can be graded as follows: twitching of upper lip at the corner of mouth only (grade 1), progress of twitching to include alae nasi (grade 2), and to include contraction of orbicularis oculi (grade 3). A grade 1 response may occur in somewhat more than 25% of normal children and in 10% to 30% of adults with normal serum calcium levels.[106] Trousseau sign is evoked by inflating a blood pressure cuff on the upper arm above systolic pressure for up to 3 minutes to produce carpal spasm. Trousseau sign is present if carpal spasm occurs after compression of the nerves in the upper arm. In the presence of hypocalcemia, the neuro-ischemia caused by application of pressure to the upper arm induces sufficient irritability to yield a positive response: flexion of the wrist and metacarpophalangeal joints, extension of the interphalangeal joints, and adduction of the digits. The Erb peroneal sign is the flexion and eversion of the foot when the peroneal nerve is tapped just behind the head of the fibula. All of these signs can be absent even in patients with definite hypocalcemia.

Seizures resembling epilepsy may occur. Measurement of plasma calcium concentration should therefore be done routinely in the clinical workup of patients with seizures. Longstanding untreated hypocalcemia in children may result in mental retardation and poor school performance. In patients with hypoparathyroidism, and especially PHP, untreated for many years, small irregular calcifications may be seen in basal ganglia on skull radiographs. These lesions, as well as diffuse calcification at the grey-white matter interface of the cerebrum, are particularly evident on CT scans. These lesions are irreversible but most often do not affect the function of the nervous system.

Papilledema may be found in longstanding hypoparathyroidism and cause suspicion of an intracranial tumor (pseudotumor cerebri). The papilledema is moderate in degree and is not accompanied by hemorrhage or impaired vision. Following treatment the papilledema usually begins to subside within a few days of normocalcemia, but it may take several weeks to disappear. Lenticular cataracts are a common complication of chronic hypocalcemia. They first appear as discrete punctate or lamellar opacities in the cortex, separated by a clear zone from the capsule. These ocular manifestations are irreversible but normalization of the plasma calcium arrests further progression.

Hypocalcemia delays ventricular depolarization and prolongs the Q-T and ST intervals on the electrocardiogram. A 2:1 heart block and, rarely, congestive cardiac failure may develop. Dry and scaly skin and brittle and fissured nails are ectodermal manifestations of chronic hypocalcemia. In addition, the hair may be coarse, dry, fractured, and easily shed. Eruption of teeth may be delayed and the formation of enamel may be irregular and hypoplastic.

Pathogenesis

Hypocalcemia is typically a manifestation of defective vitamin D homeostasis or inadequate PTH secretion or action (Figure 6-13). In general, serum levels of intact PTH are elevated and serum concentrations of phosphate are depressed in patients with defects in vitamin D homeostasis. Bone remodeling is increased but mineralization is impaired. By contrast, in states of functional hypoparathyroidism, in which PTH secretion or action is deficient, the normal effects of PTH on bone and kidney are absent. Bone resorption, and release of calcium from skeletal stores, is diminished. Renal tubular reabsorption of calcium is decreased, but because of hypocalcemia and low filtered load, urinary calcium excretion is low. In the absence of PTH action, urinary clearance of phosphate is decreased, and hyperphosphatemia ensues. The plasma phosphate concentrations range from 7 to 12 mg/dL (2.24-3.84 mmol/L). The deficiency of PTH action and the hyperphosphatemia together impair renal synthesis of calcitriol, and absorption of calcium from the intestine is markedly impaired. Calcitriol is also a potent stimulator of bone resorption, and its absence also decreases the availability of calcium from bone (Figure 6-14).

Differential diagnosis/classification

Hypoparathyroidism. Functional hypoparathyroidism (HP) may be owing to impaired PTH synthesis, impaired PTH secretion, or target organ resistance to the effects of PTH (ie, PHP) (Figure 6-13). Severe hypomagnesemia might cause both deficient PTH secretion as well as diminished target-cell response. In clinical practice an etiological classification based on sporadic or familial occurrence, age at onset of symptoms, and presence or absence of associated disorders or malformations can be useful (Table 6-4).

Hypoparathyroidism as part of a complex developmental syndrome. Congenital defects in parathyroid gland development may be isolated or, more commonly, occur with other developmental defects. Depending on the severity of the glandular defect, symptoms of hypoparathyroidism might develop neonatally or later in childhood. Late manifestation may arise from failure of a hypoplastic gland to adapt to increased demand for PTH during growth or intercurrent illness.

22q Deletion syndrome (DiGeorge sequence)— The DiGeorge anomaly or sequence (DGS) is an etiologically heterogeneous developmental field defect in which cardiovascular malformations, hypocalcemia, thymic hypoplasia, and

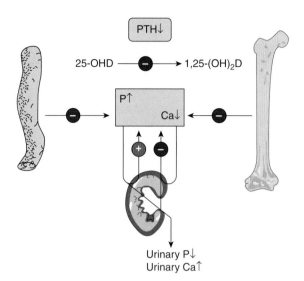

FIGURE 6-14 ■ Pathophysiology of hypoparathyroidism. Hypocalcemia and hyperphosphatemia are the biochemical hallmarks of deficient PTH action. Hypocalcemia results directly from decreased mobilization of calcium from the skeleton and its reabsorption from the renal tubules and, indirectly, from decreased calcium absorption from the intestine because of decreased PTH-dependent synthesis of calcitriol. Hyperphosphatemia results mainly from increased tubular reabsorption of phosphate in the absence of the phosphaturic effect of PTH.

characteristic dysmorphisms are major clinical features. The triad of congenital absence of the thymus, congenital hypoparathyroidism, and cardiac anomalies, commonly of the outflow tract or aortic arch (ie, conotruncal defects), was originally described by DiGeorge in 1965. The 22q11.2 deletion is the most common single etiology of DGS, although a number of other chromosomal abnormalities and teratogens, including maternal diabetes, have been implicated as well. The 22q11 deletion syndrome is considered one of the most frequent genomic disorders, and the most common human contiguous gene deletion syndrome, with an incidence of 1 out of 2000 to 4000 births.[107] It arises from variable sized deletions at 22q11, 85% of which include a "typically deleted region." The high mutation rate is thought to arise from significant DNA duplication that predisposes to recombination in this region. Depending upon the series, 6% to 25% of deletions are inherited. The clinical spectrum induced by this genomic disorder is expansive and includes cardiac, thymic, parathyroid, neurologic, behavioral, psychiatric, and craniofacial defects.

The basic embryological defect is inadequate development of the facial neural crest tissues that results in maldevelopment of branchial pouch derivatives. The facial features that have been described in association with 22q11 deletion syndrome include hypertelorism or telecanthus, short or hypoplastic philtrum, micrognathia, and low-set, posteriorly rotated ears (Case 6-1). These features can be seen in various other syndromes and are therefore not specific for 22q11 deletion syndrome. Cardiac defects occur in approximately 70% of children with 22q11 deletion syndrome[108] but this of course may reflect ascertainment bias. Common cardiac outflow abnormalities in 22q11 deletion syndrome include type B interrupted aortic arch, truncus arteriosus, tetrology of Fallot, and perimembranous ventricular septal defects,[109] and children with these disorders should be evaluated for 22q11 deletion syndrome.

The degrees of thymic hypoplasia and immune dysfunction are also variable. While failure of thymic hypoplasia and decreased circulating T lymphocytes are common, severe thymic aplasia is rare. Thymic transplant,[110] hematopoietic cell transplant,[111] and donor lymphocyte infusions have all been used successfully in severe immune deficiency.

Lastly, the degree of parathyroid hypoplasia and ensuing hypoparathyroidism is variable, and in some patients parathyroid dysfunction may evolve over time.[112] Other patients may experience a spontaneous resolution of hypoparathyroidism as they mature.[113] However, latent hypoparathyroidism is presumably present in these patients, and under conditions of stress hypocalcemia may ensue.[114]

Many commercial laboratories now offer genetic testing services that can identify these microdeletions in 22q11 by fluorescent *in situ* hybridization (FISH) or comparative genomic hybridization microarray.

Haploinsufficiency of transcription factor *TBX1* has emerged as the likely explanation for the developmental defects of the heart, ears, and parathyroids. Studies of TBX1 regulation during embryogenesis have yielded unexpected insights into the pathogenesis of the DiGeorge phenotype. For example, the observation that retinoic acid represses expression of TBX1 now provides a likely explanation for the development of the DiGeorge phenotype in children who were exposed *in utero* to maternal use of retinoic acid products.[115]

Other syndromes—Other complex genetic syndromes are associated with hypoparathyroidism, while exposure to retinoic acid and poorly controlled diabetes are been associated with a DiGeorge sequence phenotype (Table 6-4).

Table 6-4.

Classification of Hypoparathyroidism

Clinical Context	Example	Parathyroid Defect	Age of Onset*	Associated Features
Transient	Transient neonatal	Physiologic suppression	2-10 d	Maternal hypercalcemia
Complex genetic syndromes	DiGeorge sequence	Parathyroid dysgenesis	0-1 mo, childhood and older reported	Del22q11; *TBX1* mutation. Cardiac and thymic (immune) deficits
	HDR syndrome (Barakat syndrome)	Parathyroid dysgenesis	Childhood and older	Renal dysplasia and deafness; *GATA3* mutation
	Kenny-Caffey/Sanjad-Sakati syndrome	Parathyroid dysgenesis	Childhood and older	Short stature, osteosclerosis, growth retardation; *TBCE* mutation
	Mitochondrial syndromes	Parathyroid agenesis	Childhood and older	Kearns-Sayre; MELAS, Pearson-Marrow-Pancreas syndromes; LCHAD deficiency
Autoimmune	Type 1 polyglandular autoimmune syndrome	Autoimmune destruction or activating antibodies	3+ y	Mutation of *AIRE* gene. Mucocutaneous candidiasis, adrenal failure.
Nonsyndromic hypoparathyroidism	Autosomal dominant hypocalcemia	Reduced: "set point" for Ca^{2+}	Infancy and childhood	Activating mutation of *CaSR* gene; positive family history; hypercalciuria
	Isolated hypoparathyroidism	Parathyroid aplasia	Infancy and childhood	Loss of function mutation of *GCM2*; autosomal recessive or dominant inhibitor mutations
	PTH deficiency	Decreased synthesis of PTH	Infancy and childhood	Loss of function mutations in the *PTH* gene
	X-linked	Parathyroid agenesis	Infancy	?SOX3 mutations
Parathyroid destruction	Thalassemia/iron overload	Iron deposition	Adolescence and beyond	Cardiac, liver, and endocrine dysfunction
	Postsurgical	Removal or damage	Any	Following thyroidectomy
PTH resistance	Pseudohypoparathyroidism	Resistance to PTH	Infancy to 10 y	
	Hypomagnesemia	Reduced PTH production and/or resistance to PTH	Any	Specific intestinal defect or generalized malabsorption

*Most typical ages given. Individual cases may vary widely.
PTH, parathyroid hormone.

Isolated hypoparathyroidism. Nonsyndromic, isolated hypoparathyroidism, in which PTH deficiency is not associated with other endocrine disorders or developmental defects, is usually sporadic but may occur on a familial basis (Table 6-4). Hypoparathyroidism can be inherited by autosomal dominant, autosomal recessive, and X-linked modes of transmission. Genetic defects that impair PTH synthesis (ie, *PTH* gene defects) or secretion (ie, *CASR* gene defects) as well as parathyroid gland development (ie, *GCMB* gene defects) are now recognized. The age at onset covers a broad range (1 month to 30 years), but the hypoparathyroidism is most commonly diagnosed during childhood.

PTH gene mutations—Defects in the *PTH* gene are an uncommon cause of hypoparathyroidism, and mutations have been identified in only three families, one with autosomal dominant and two with autosomal recessive forms of isolated hypoparathyroidism.[116-119]

Calcium-sensing receptor—Autosomal dominant gain-of-function mutations in the *CASR* gene encoding the CaSR have been identified in many subjects with a mild variant of hypoparathyroidism, associated with low or low-normal levels of serum PTH and relative hypercalciuria. Molecular defects in this gene may be the most common cause of mild isolated hypoparathyroidism.

GCMB gene mutations—Mutations in the *GCMB* (also *GCM2*) gene located at 6p23-24 are associated with parathyroid aplasia and congenital hypoparathyroidism in both humans[120] and mice.[121] Homozygous loss of function mutations or heterozygous dominant inhibitor mutations of *GCMB* cause autosomal recessive or autosomal dominant isolated hypoparathyroidism, respectively.[122] These observations implicate GCM2 as the master regulator of parathyroid development during embryogenesis.

X-linked hypoparathyroidism—Isolated hypoparathyroidism can also be inherited as an X-linked recessive trait (MIM307700). Affected males present with infantile hypocalcemic seizures while hemizygous females are unaffected. Autopsy of an affected individual revealed complete agenesis of the parathyroid glands as the cause of hypoparathyroidism. Linkage analysis has localized the underlying mutation to a 1.5 Mb region on Xq26-q27,[123] and recent molecular studies have identified a deletion-insertion involving chromosomes Xq27 and 2p25 as the basis for the defect.

Autoimmune. Autoimmune hypoparathyroidism may occur alone or in the context of an autoimmune polyglandular syndrome. Patients with isolated hypoparathyroidism have a high incidence of parathyroid antibodies. These cases may represent isolated autoimmune hypoparathyroidism or may actually be incomplete expression of the autoimmune polyglandular syndrome (APS-1). Some patients may possess antibodies that inhibit the secretion of PTH[124] rather than cause parathyroid gland destruction. The major features of APS-1 include mucocutaneous candidiasis, hypoparathyroidism, and adrenal insufficiency. APS-1 may be sporadic or familial with an autosomal recessive inheritance pattern. Many affected patients have additional autoimmune features. The syndrome is generally first recognized in early childhood, although a few individuals have developed the condition after the first decade of life. The clinical onset of the three principal components of the syndrome typically follows a predictable pattern, in which mucocutaneous candidiasis first appears at a mean age of 5 years, followed by hypoparathyroidism at a mean age of 9 years and adrenal insufficiency at a mean age of 14 years. Patients may not manifest all three components of the clinical triad. In about two-third of the patients, hypoparathyroidism is the first manifestation of endocrinopathy followed later by the insidious development of adrenal insufficiency. Less than a year to decades may elapse between the diagnosis of one disease and the second in the same individual. The development of hypercalcemia in a hypoparathyroid patient who has been normocalcemic over a long period on a stable dose of vitamin D might herald the insidious development of adrenal insufficiency.

Alopecia occurs in about one-third of patients with the highest incidence at ages 5 to 9 years. It appears as hairless patches, and may proceed to complete baldness and lack of eye and body hair (Case 6-2). Some patients will develop additional features, such as keratoconjunctivitis, malabsorption and steatorrhea, gonadal failure, pernicious anemia, chronic active hepatitis, thyroid disease, and insulin-requiring diabetes mellitus. Enamel hypoplasia of teeth is also common, and appears to be unrelated to hypoparathyroidism. The presence of these additional defects in patients with APS-1 has led to the suggestion that a more inclusive term be used to describe the syndrome: "autoimmune polyendocrinopathy-candidiasis-ectodermal dystrophy" (APECED). In those cases that have been examined pathologically, complete parathyroid atrophy or destruction has been demonstrated. In some patients, treatment of hypoparathyroidism has been complicated by apparent vitamin D *resistance,* possibly related to coexistent hepatic disease or steatorrhea, or both.

The autoimmune basis for the disorder is suggested by the findings of circulating autoantibodies directed against the parathyroid, thyroid, and adrenal glands in many patients[125] and a T-cell abnormality has been described.[126] Recent studies indicate that patients with APS-1 and hypoparathyroidism have circulating antibodies that react with the NALP5 protein and damage or destroy the parathyroid glands.[127] An alternative pathophysiology implicates the presence of circulating antibodies that bind and activate the CaSR, thereby reducing PTH secretion from parathyroid cells (and increasing calcium excretion from the kidney).[128]

The molecular defect in patients with APS-1 has been identified, thus facilitating genetic diagnosis of the syndrome. Based on linkage analyses, APS-1 candidate gene was first assigned to 21q22.3.[129] Subsequent studies used positional cloning to identify the APS-1 gene, termed *AIRE* for autoimmune regulator, and sequence analysis of genomic DNA from affected subjects has disclosed common *AIRE* mutations in different geo-ethnic patient groups. The *AIRE* gene encodes a predicted 57.7 kDa protein that is expressed in thymus, lymph nodes and fetal liver, and which contains motifs, including two PHD zinc fingers, that are suggestive of a role as a transcriptional regulator. Mutations in the *AIRE* gene are predicted to lead to truncated forms of the protein that lack at least one of the PHD zinc fingers, and which fail to localize to the cell nucleus.[130]

Other forms of hypoparathyroidism. The most common cause of hypoparathyroidism in adults is surgical excision of or damage to the parathyroid glands as a result of total thyroidectomy for thyroid cancer, radical neck dissection for other cancers, or repeated operations for primary (or tertiary) hyperparathyroidism. Prolonged hypocalcemia, which may develop immediately or weeks to years after neck surgery, suggests permanent hypoparathyroidism. Postoperative hypoparathyroidism occurs in approximately 1% of thyroid and parathyroid procedures. Rarely, hypoparathyroidism occurs in patients who receive extensive radiation to the neck and mediastinum. It is also reported in metal overload diseases such as hemochromatosis and Wilson disease, and in neoplastic or granulomatous infiltration of the parathyroid glands. Hypoparathyroidism may be present in as many as 14% of patients with thalassemia who develop iron overload owing to frequent blood transfusion. Hypoparathyroidism has also been observed in association with HIV disease.

Several syndromes owing to deletions in mitochondrial DNA have been associated with hypoparathyroidism. These include the Kearns-Sayre syndrome (encephalomyopathy, ophthalmoplegia, retinitis pigmentosa, heart block), the Pearson Marrow-Pancreas syndrome (sideroblastic anemia, neutropenia, thrombocytopenia, pancreatic dysfunction), and the maternally inherited diabetes and deafness syndrome. Hypoparathyroidism has also been described in the MELAS (**M**itochondrial myopathy, **E**ncephalopathy, **L**actic **A**cidosis, and **S**troke-like episodes) syndrome, owing to point mutations in mitochondrial tRNA. In addition, mutations in the mitochondrial trifunctional protein (MTP) that result in either isolated long-chain 3-hydroxy-acyl-coenzyme A dehydrogenase (LCHAD) deficiency or loss of all three MTP enzymatic activities have been associated with hypoparathyroidism in a few unrelated patients. This condition manifests as hypoketotic hypoglycemia, cardiomyopathy, hepatic dysfunction, and developmental delay and is associated with maternal fatty liver of pregnancy.

PTH resistance states

Pseudohypoparathyroidism. The term pseudohypoparathyroidism (PHP) describes a group of disorders characterized by biochemical hypoparathyroidism (ie, hypocalcemia and hyperphosphatemia), increased secretion of PTH, and target tissue (bone, kidney) unresponsiveness to the biological actions of PTH. A classification is provided in Table 6-5. Thus the pathophysiology of PHP differs fundamentally from true hypoparathyroidism, in which PTH secretion rather than PTH responsiveness is defective.

Type 1 pseudohypoparathyroidism. Cyclic AMP mediates many of the actions of PTH on kidney and bone, and that administration of biologically active PTH to normal subjects leads to a significant increase in the urinary excretion of nephrogenous cAMP and phosphate. The blunted nephrogenous cAMP response to exogenous PTH in subjects with PHP type 1 indicates that PTH resistance is caused by a defect in the hormone-sensitive signal transduction pathway that activates adenylyl cyclase in renal proximal tubule cells.

Current evidence now clearly links the pathophysiology of PHP type 1 to defective expression of *GNAS*, the gene that encodes the alpha chain of Gs (Gα_s), the signaling protein that couples PTH/PTHrP receptors to stimulation of adenylyl cyclase.[131] Subjects with PHP type 1a have defects in *GNAS* that reduce expression or function of Gα_s in a variety of cell types. Consistent with a generalized defect in Gα_s expression, patients with PHP type 1a have resistance not only to PTH, but also to additional hormones, including TSH, gonadotropins, glucagon, calcitonin, and growth hormone releasing hormone, whose receptors interact with Gs to stimulate adenylyl cyclase.[132]

Table 6-5.

Classification of PTH Resistance/Pseudohypoparathyroidism

Type	AHO Phenotype	Response to PTH	Hormone Resistance	Molecular Defect	Transmission
PHP 1a	+	↓ cAMP ↓ Phos	Multiple (PTH, TSH, GHRH, LH, FSH)	*GNAS*	Maternal
PPHP	!	Normal*	None	*GNAS*	Paternal
POH	Ectopic ossification only	Normal	None	*GNAS*	Paternal
PHP 1b	Some w/ mild brachydactyly	↓ cAMP ↓ Phos	PTH; possible mild TSH resistance	Epigenetic defects in *GNAS*	Maternal
PHP 1c (probably 1a variant)	+	↓ cAMP ↓ Phos	Multiple (PTH, TSH, GHRH, LH, FSH)	*GNAS*	Maternal
PHP 2	−	Normal cAMP ↓ Phos	PTH only	Likely vitamin D deficiency	None known

*Normal: 10- to 20-fold increase in urinary cAMP

Although patients sometimes present with mild congenital hypothyroidism, often detected during neonatal screening, or with late onset neonatal hypocalcemia, most patients are identified after the age of 3 years with hypocalcemia and hyperphosphatemia. Calcification of the basal ganglia has been observed in most patients at the time of diagnosis, and indicates that hypocalcemia and hyperphosphatemia have been present for several years. Similar ectopic calcifications of the basal ganglia are sometimes seen in HP, but they are much more frequent in patients with PHP. Convulsions seem to be more prevalent than in HP and may occur in about two-thirds of cases. The plasma concentration of PTH is elevated in all patients with hypocalcemia, and is often mildly increased in patients with normal serum calcium levels.

In addition to hormone resistance, patients with PHP type 1a (OMIM 30080, #103580) also manifest a peculiar constellation of developmental and somatic defects that are collectively termed Albright hereditary osteodystrophy (AHO).[133,134] The AHO phenotype consists of short stature, round faces, brachydactyly, and subcutaneous ossifications (Case 6-3), but dental defects and sensory-neural abnormalities may also be present. In the past obesity had been considered a general feature of AHO, but recent studies indicate that obesity is limited to PHP type 1a, and reflects a defect in metabolic regulation of energy homeostasis.[135] Brachydactyly usually includes shortening of the distal phalanges of the thumbs and the third and fourth metacarpals and metatarsals. The shortening of the metacarpals results in the appearance of dimples rather than knuckles over these digits when the hand is clenched (ie, Archibald sign). Mild or moderate mental retardation is frequent.

The subsequent identification of individuals with AHO who lacked apparent hormone resistance led Albright to propose the rather awkward term *pseudopseudohypoparathyroidism* (pseudoPHP) to describe this normocalcemic variant of PHP.[136] Subjects with pseudoPHP have a normal urinary cAMP response to PTH, which distinguishes them from occasional patients with PHP type 1a who maintain normal serum calcium levels without treatment. PseudoPHP is genetically related to PHP type 1a. Within a given kindred, some affected members will have only AHO (ie, pseudoPHP) while others will have hormone resistance as well (ie, PHP type 1a), despite equivalent functional deficiency of $G\alpha_s$ in tissues that have been analyzed.[137]

Osteoma cutis and progressive osseous heteroplasia (POH) represent alternative manifestations of AHO in which only heterotopic ossification occurs. In osteoma cutis ectopic ossification is limited to the superficial skin, whereas in POH heterotopic ossification involves the skin, subcutaneous tissue, muscles, tendons, and ligaments. POH can be disabling as extensive dermal ossification occurs during childhood, followed by widespread ossification of skeletal muscle and deep connective tissue. Nodules and lace-like webs of heterotopic bone extend from the skin into the subcutaneous fat and deep connective tissues, and may cross joints, thus leading to stiffness, joint locking, and permanent immobility.

$G\alpha_s$ deficiency in patients with PHP type 1a and pseudoPHP results from heterozygous inactivating mutations in the *GNAS* gene, a complex gene that maps to 20q13.3.[138] Molecular studies of DNA from subjects with AHO have disclosed a variety of *GNAS* gene mutations that account for autosomal dominant inheritance of the disorder. The striking variability in the biochemical and clinical phenotypes of patients with PHP type 1a and pseudoPHP is consistent with a model in which tissue-specific expression of *GNAS* is controlled by genomic imprinting,[132] a process whereby the expression level of the alleles of a gene depends upon their parental origin. At least three unique, alternative first exons, and their respective promoters, are located upstream of the *GNAS* exon 1, and each has a differentially methylated region (DMR) that correlates with parent-of-origin specific allelic transcription. Despite the reciprocal imprinting in both the paternal and maternal directions of the *GNAS* gene, expression of $G\alpha_s$ appears to be biallelic in most tissues that have been examined. However, predominant monoallelic expression from the maternally derived allele has been documented in tissues that are associated with hormone resistance in patients with PHP type 1a. Accordingly, patients who inherit the defective *GNAS* gene maternally express that allele preferentially in imprinted tissues, such as the PTH-sensitive renal proximal tubule, resulting in a near absence of functional $G\alpha_s$ protein. In contrast, patients with pseudoPHP, osteoma cutis, and progressive osseous heteroplasia have inherited a defective paternal *GNAS* allele. Because the maternal allele is preferentially expressed in imprinted tissues, a paternal defect does not result in reduced $G\alpha_s$ expression in maternally imprinted tissues. Patients with PHP type 1a and pseudoPHP (and osteoma cutis and progressive osseous heteroplasia) have an approximately 50% reduction in $G\alpha_s$ expression in nonimprinted tissues, which express both *GNAS* alleles, and which may account for more variable and moderate hormone resistance in these sites.

Pseudohypoparathyroidism type 1b. The characteristics of PHP type 1a contrast sharply with those of PHP type 1b (OMIM #603233), a less common and clinically distinct variant of PHP type 1. Although most cases of PHP type 1b appear to be sporadic, familial cases have been described with autosomal dominant transmission of the disorder. Subjects with PHP type 1b lack typical features of AHO but may have mild brachydactyly. The primary feature is decreased responsiveness to PTH, but resistance to TSH has also been described.[139] Despite renal resistance to PTH, subjects with PHP type 1b who have elevated levels of PTH often manifest skeletal lesions similar to those that occur in patients with hyperparathyroidism. PHP type 1b arises from an epigenetic imprinting defect: loss of normal methylation of the exon1a DMR on the maternal allele leads to a paternal-specific imprinting pattern of the exon 1A region on both alleles.[140] Causative mutations have been identified in most cases of familial but not sporadic PHP type 1b.

PHP type 2. In subjects with PHP type 2, PTH resistance is characterized by a reduced phosphaturic response to administration of PTH, despite a normal increase in urinary cAMP excretion.[141,142] These observations suggest that the PTH receptor-adenylyl cyclase complex functions normally to increase nephrogenous cAMP in response to PTH, but that intracellular cAMP is unable to act upon downstream targets such as the sodium phosphate transporter. PHP type 2 lacks a clear genetic or familial basis, and a similar clinical and biochemical picture occurs in patients with severe deficiency of vitamin D. Taken together, it is likely that[143] most, if not all, cases of PHP type 2 are actually examples of unsuspected vitamin D deficiency.[143-145]

Diagnosis. Recombinant human PTH(1-34) peptide is now available for use in the differential diagnosis of hypoparathyroidism. In response to 200 to 300 units (25-40 μg) of rhPTH(1-34), normal subjects and patients with hormonopenic hypoparathyroidism usually display a 10- to 20-fold increase in urinary cAMP excretion, whereas patients with pseudoPHP, regardless of their serum calcium concentration, will show a markedly blunted response. Thus, this test can distinguish patients with so-called "normocalcemic" PHP (ie, patients with PTH resistance who are able to maintain normal serum calcium levels without treatment) from subjects with pseudoPHP who will have a normal urinary cAMP response to PTH.[137,146] The urinary cAMP and phosphate responses to PTH are dependent upon the endogenous serum PTH and calcium levels,[147] and treatment with vitamin D to normalize serum calcium levels may normalize the phosphaturic response to PTH in patients with PHP type 1. Measurement of plasma cAMP or plasma 1,25-dihydroxyvitamin D after intravenous (or subcutaneous) administration of rhPTH(1-34) may also differentiate PHP type 1 from other causes of hypoparathyroidism.

Treatment of hypoparathyroidism and pseudohypoparathyroidism

The treatment of hypocalcemia in patients with PHP does not differ significantly from that of patients with hypoparathyroidism. In both disorders the aim of treatment is to maintain the plasma calcium concentration in the lower normal range, that is, about 8.5 to 9.5 mg/dL (2.12-2.37 mmol/L) to avoid episodic hypercalcemia and hypercalciuria. The plasma phosphate concentration also decreases with treatment, but this decrease lags behind the rise of plasma calcium and often some degree of hyperphosphatemia may persist.

Patients with tetany or cardiovascular manifestations of hypocalcemia should be treated with slow intravenous injection of 10% calcium gluconate in a dose of 1 to 2 mL/kg up to 10 mL. Care should be taken to avoid subcutaneous leakage owing to dangers of local necrosis. If tetany persists, the dose could be repeated at 6 to 8 hour intervals or provided as a continuous infusion of elemental calcium at 1 to 3 mg/kg/h. Calcium salts should be administered orally as soon as possible, preferably with meals, to reduce serum phosphorus concentrations as well as maintain normal levels of serum calcium. For the first 1 to 2 days a total of 4 to 6 g of elemental calcium daily may be given in 1 g doses.

Long-term treatment requires administration of a 1-α-hydroxylated form of vitamin D; the addition of supplemental oral calcium with meals ensures a consistent intake of calcium and also serves to control serum phosphorus levels. A reasonable starting dosage is 25 to 50 ng/kg/day of calcitriol or 1-α-OHD. Patients with PHP require lower doses of vitamin D and vitamin D metabolites and have less risk of treatment-related hypercalciuria than patients with hypoparathyroidism. Plasma calcium should initially be monitored at short intervals to tailor the minimal dosage required to sustain the ideal plasma level of calcium. During long-term treatment, the plasma calcium concentration needs to be monitored every 2 to 3 months to avoid hypercalcemia. The urinary excretion of calcium should also be monitored regularly.

Preliminary studies of PTH replacement in both adults and children with hypoparathyroidism are promising. Recombinant human PTH(1-34) can be administered by subcutaneous injection, and less significant calcium fluctuation appears to occur with twice daily dosing compared to once daily dosing.[148] Urinary calcium excretion also improves on this therapy, suggesting that rhPTH(1-34) may be a reasonable option in individuals in whom nephrocalcinosis is a concern. Control of hyperphosphatemia is not improved, however.

Treatment of any associated endocrinopathies does not differ from the standard approach. The development of chronic active hepatitis might create a particularly serious problem. The therapy of mucocutaneous candidiasis has improved by the introduction of the orally active antifungal drug, ketoconazole.

Magnesium Deficiency

Pathogenesis

Magnesium homeostasis is tightly regulated and depends on the balance between intestinal absorption and renal excretion. As described earlier, hypomagnesemia can lead to either impaired secretion of PTH or resistance to PTH, leading to functional hypoparathyroidism.

Differential diagnosis

Transient hypomagnesemia. Hypomagnesemia has been observed in newborn infants of diabetic mothers, in SGA infants, in infants with early or late tetany, and in infants with malabsorption syndromes, following shortening of the small intestine by surgical removal and after prolonged intravenous fluid therapy with magnesium-free fluids (Table 6-6).

Congenital hypomagnesemia. The combination of hypomagnesemia and secondary hypocalciuria can occur in patients with rare magnesium malabsorption or more commonly owing to renal tubular transport disorders: Gitelman syndrome and autosomal dominant isolated renal magnesium wasting. Distinct genetic defects for these two renal disorders have been elucidated, and the defective proteins have been localized within the distal convoluted tubule (DCT), a segment of the nephron known to play an important role in active magnesium reabsorption. In isolated renal magnesium wasting (OMIM 154020), a dominant-negative mutation has been reported in *FXYD2* that results in a trafficking defect of the γ-subunit of the

Na^+/K^+-ATPase.[149,150] The majority of patients with Gitelman syndrome carry inactivating mutations in the *SLC12A3* gene encoding the sodium-chloride cotransporter located in the distal convoluted tubule.[151] This defect results not only in hypomagnesemia but also metabolic alkalosis, hypokalemia, and hypocalciuria. By contrast, hypomagnesemia is not a constant finding in Bartter syndrome, and urinary calcium excretion is normal or high.[152] Bartter syndrome, owing to mutations in the chloride channel gene *CLCNKB*,[153] is often diagnosed neonatally and associated with subsequent growth retardation and nephrocalcinosis. Other congential disorders of hypomagnesemia include familial hypomagnesemia with hypercalciuria and nephrocalcinosis, which results from mutations in paracellin-1, a tight-junction protein that appears to be important in conducting or regulating paracellular cation transport in the thick ascending limb of Henle loop. Impaired function of paracellin-1 leads specifically to urinary losses of magnesium and calcium, but because transcellular transport is intact these patients do not have hypokalemia or salt wasting.

Renal injury. More commonly magnesium-wasting is owing to renal tubule injury following treatment with aminoglycoside antibiotics such as gentamicin. In most cases the nephrotoxicity has been reported in patients treated with a combination of gentamicin and cephalosporin.

Table 6-6.

Classification of Hypomagnesemia

	Etiology		Additional Features
Transient			
	Infant of diabetic mother		
	SGA		
	Malabsorption		
	Prolonged intravenous therapy		
	Short gut		
	Neonatal hypocaclemia		
Congenital			
	Gitelman syndrome	Autosomal recessive *SLC12A3* mutations	Renal magnesium wasting w/metabolic alkalosis, hypokalemia, hypocalcemia
	Isolated renal magnesium wasting	Dominant-negative *FXYD2* mutation	Hypocalciuria
	Dent disease	X-linked *CLCN5* or *OCRL* mutations	Hypercalciuria, nephrocalcinosis, renal failure
	Familial hypomagnesemia with hypercalciuria and nephrocalcinosis	Autosomal recessive *CLDN16* mutations	Renal failure
Acquired			
	Renal injury	Aminoglycosides	

Treatment

When associated with early neonatal tetany the hypomagnesemia tends to be mild and transient and may not require treatment with magnesium. In late neonatal tetany, however, the infants may fail to respond to calcium treatment until magnesium levels have been returned to normal. Severe hypomagnesemia is initially treated with intramuscular injection of magnesium sulfate, 0.2 mL/kg of 25% solution repeated at 6-hour intervals. Long-term treatment requires oral magnesium supplementation with Mg-chloride, citrate, or lactate in a dose of 24 to 48 mg/kg/day in four divided doses up to a maximum of 1 g magnesium per day. If these doses of magnesium salts aggravate the diarrhea in patients with resection or disease of the small intestine, it may be necessary to resort to intramuscular injection of magnesium sulfate (Table 6-7).

Table 6-7.

Treatments for Calcium/Magnesium/Phosphate Disorders

		Formulation	Trade Names	Approach to Specific Disorders
Vitamin D				

D_2	Ergocalciferol	8000 IU/mL solution
		50,000 IU gelcaps
		25,000 IU tablet
		50,000 IU tablet
			Calciferol
			Drisdol
				Vitamin D deficiency rickets:
				Dietary deficiency: 2000-4000 IU/d
				  until evidence of resolution
				Malabsorption syndromes:
				  4000-10,000 IU/d

D_3	Cholecalciferol	400 IU/drop
		1,000 IU tablets
		50,000 IU tablets
			D-Drops
			Delta-D
			Vitamin D_3 OTC
				Vitamin D deficiency rickets:
				Dietary deficiency: 2000-4000 IU/d
				  until evidence of resolution
				Malabsorption syndromes:
				  4000-10,000 IU/d
				Mild VDD2: 2,00,000-2,000,000 IU/d
				Hypophosphatemic rickets:
				Initial: 15-20 ng/kg/d
				Maintenance: 30-60 ng/kg/d

1,25-$(OH)_2D3$	Calcitriol	0.25 mcg softgel 0.5 mcg softgel 1 mcg/mL oral solution 1 mcg/mL injection solution	Rocaltrol Calcijex	Hypoparathyroidism: 25-50 ng/kg/d VDD1 with active rickets: 1-4 mcg/d VDD1 with healed rickets: 0.5-2 mcg/d Intermediate VDD2: 5-60 mcg/d
Calcium				

	Gluconate	9 mg elemental/mL,
		  10% solution
			Kalcinate	Symptomatic hypocalcemia:
				  1-2 mL/kg IV over 10 min followed by
				  1-3 mg elemental/kg/h

	Chloride	27.2 mg elemental /mL, solution	Cal Plus	**Hypocalcemia (after stabilization)** Neonate:75 mg elemental/kg/d

	Carbonate	500 mg elemental/mL
		  solution
		400 mg elemental/g
		  tab
			Tums
			Caltrate
				Infant: 50 mg elemental/kg/d
				Child: 4-6 g daily for 1-2 d, then
				  1-3 g daily for 1-2 wk depending
				  upon calcium

	Glubionate	115 mg elemental/5 mL	Calcionate	
Magnesium				
	Magnesium sulfate Magnesium chloride Magnesium citrate Magnesium lactate			0.2 mL 25% magnesium sulfate IM q6 h 24-48 mg/kg/d (max 1 g)/4 doses
Phosphorus	Potassium-phosphate	250 mg tab 250 mg	K-Phos Neutral Neutra-Phos powder	Hypophosphatemia Neonate: 30-40 mg/kg/d Hypophosphatemic rickets: 1-3 mg elemental/kg/d/q4-6

Disorders of Vitamin D Supply, Activation, or Action

Definitions

Rickets is a term applied to an abnormality of growing bones related to a failure of normal mineralization. The essential bone lesion is an accumulation of excess osteoid tissue owing to lag in the mineralization of the cartilaginous epiphyseal plate. Osteomalacia is simply rickets occurring after cessation of linear growth of the skeleton, since remodeling of bone continues with resorption of bone and new formation of unmineralized osteoid. Worldwide, rickets is most commonly owing to vitamin D deficiency, but dietary deficiency of calcium as well as genetic defects in vitamin D action or phosphate metabolism can also cause rickets.

Rickets and osteomalacia were widespread problems until the discovery of the calciferols, after which they were used for prevention and treatment. However, some cases did not respond to the usual doses of calciferols, and multiple genetic and other causes were subsequently recognized. Most hereditary cases showed biochemical features different from those of calciferol

nutritional deficiency, and are now classified as phosphate diabetes or X-linked hypophosphatemia.

Pathogenesis

Regardless of etiology, low serum phosphate, rather than reduced vitamin D action or hypocalcemia per se, likely accounts for the defect in mineralization and rickets. Evidence for this notion derives from analysis of bone in patients with hypoparathyroidism: despite hypocalcemia and low circulating concentrations of calcitriol, mineralization defects do not occur, presumably because of the normal or elevated levels of serum phosphate.

Classification

Rickets and osteomalacia may conveniently be classified according to cause into three main categories, as listed in Table 6-8. The most frequent cause is vitamin D deficiency, which may arise from poor diet, lack of sunlight, malabsorption of fat-soluble nutrients, or less commonly from ineffective conversion of 25-(OH)D to calcitriol. Rickets caused by dietary calcium deficiency is unusual under normal conditions, but has been described in infants fed with a low calcium soy-based formula as the main source

Table 6-8.

Classification of Rickets

Type of rickets		P	Ca	HCO$_3$	25-(OH)D	1,25-(OH)$_2$D	PTH	Ca
		Serum Concentration					**Urine**	
Nutritional	Vitamin D deficiency	L to H	L	N	L	L to H	H	L
	Calcium deficiency	L	L	N	N	H	H	L
	Prematurity*	L	N	N	N	H	N	H
Hypophosphatemic	X-linked (PHEX)	L	N	N	N	N	N to H[†]	N to H[†]
	Autosomal dominant (FGF23)/autosomal recessive (DMP1)	L	N	N	N	N	N	N
	Hereditary hypophosphatemic rickets with hypercalciuria (SLC34A3)	L	N	N	N	H	L	H
	Fanconi syndrome	L	N	L	N	N to L	N to H	N to H
Vitamin D–dependent rickets	Type 1 (1-α-hydroxylase deficiency; CYP27B)	L to N	L	N	N	L	H	L
	Type 2 (Calcitriol resistance, VDR)	L to N	L	N	N	H	H	L
Uremic	Osteodystrophy	H	L to H	L	N	L	H	L to H

*Most commonly owing to relative phosphorus deprivation.
†Elevated PTH and urine Ca seen as consequences of treatment.
Notes: Alkaline phosphatase and other markers of bone turnover are increased in all forms.
PTH, parathyroid hormone; L, low; N, normal; H, high.

of nutrition as well as in children with low dietary calcium intakes both in the developing world and more recently in the United States. The resulting calcipenia leads to secondary hyperparathyroidism, increased urinary phosphate excretion, and subsequent hypophosphatemia.

In the second category, the primary cause is end-organ resistance to calcitriol owing to defective expression or activity of the nuclear receptor for vitamin D (VDR). In these rare conditions, secondary hyperparathyroidism results in very high plasma

In the third category rickets is caused by phosphate deficiency, most commonly owing to impairment of renal tubular reabsorption of phosphate. Secondary hyperparathyroidism usually does not occur in this type of rickets.

Environmental vitamin D deficiency

Epidemiology. Rickets has been present since ancient times, but the incidence increased dramatically during the industrial revolution in children of the crowded alleys of the air polluted industrial cities of Northern Europe and North America. Following the introduction of prophylactic vitamin D administration in the 1930s and early 1940s in most industrialized nations, vitamin D deficiency rickets was almost completely eradicated. In the Muslim countries and also among non-Muslim populations of India and China, rickets is still quite prevalent. Typically, affects infants who have received prolonged breast-feeding and have had minimal sunlight exposure. The mothers who wear the traditional veil are vitamin D deficient owing to lack of sunlight exposure and often have frank osteomalacia. In pregnant women with severe osteomalacia the fetus might develop severe rickets in utero and present with hypocalcemic tetany at birth (congenital rickets). More recently, vitamin D deficiency and rickets have been recognized as significant health problems among infants in North America who have been breast-fed for more than 6 months without receiving either vitamin D supplements or other foods that are fortified with vitamin D.[154]

In today's Northern Europe and North America the children at risk of developing vitamin D deficiency rickets are mainly dark-skinned individuals and children on strict vegetarian, cult, or other fad diets. In most developed nations, commercially produced cow's milk is fortified with vitamin D, but many other dairy products (eg, yogurts and cheeses) do not contain supplemental vitamin D. In addition, some soy-based milk substitutes do not contain vitamin D and can place infants at unsuspected risk. By contrast, many juices, cereals, and other foods are now vitamin D-fortified. Rickets typically occurs toward the end of the first and during the second year of life. Later in childhood, manifest vitamin D deficiency is rare, and has mainly been reported in adolescent Asian immigrants in Britain. The precise

cause of adolescent rickets in Asian immigrants remains to some extent obscure. However, the increased need of vitamin D associated with the adolescent growth spurt is clearly the trigger superimposed on cultural food habits and insufficient sunlight exposure.

Clinical presentation. The early manifestations of rickets are biochemical rather than clinically recognizable or radiographic signs. The important finding at this stage is slight hypocalcemia with some or only moderate elevation of alkaline phosphatase activity (Table 6-8). The fall in plasma calcium leads to increased PTH secretion which, in turn, normalizes plasma calcium. However, if the rickets proceed to a moderate stage the compensatory secondary hyperparathyroidism leads to increased urinary excretion of cAMP, aminoaciduria, phosphaturia with subsequent fall in plasma phosphate, and rise of alkaline phosphatase. In the florid forms of rickets, increased PTH secretion and calcium mobilization from bone can no longer compensate for the deficient calcium absorption from the intestine, and the plasma calcium concentration may drop sufficiently to induce symptoms of tetany (Table 6-8, Figure 6-15).

Infants with florid rickets typically present during the late winter or early spring at the age of 6 to 12 months, often with tetany or frank convulsions owing to hypocalcemia. Latent tetany may be revealed by observing a positive Chvostek, Trousseau, or Erb sign (see section "Hypocalcemia in Children and Adolescents" discussed earlier). The plasma calcium concentration is usually below less than 6 mg/dL (1.5 mmol/L). Muscle tone and strength are decreased, and motor development is usually delayed.

The osseous manifestations depend on the age of onset and the relative growth rate of different bones. In the first year of life the skull, upper limbs, and ribs are the fastest growing bones and thus most prone to be affected. Accordingly, in the youngest infants craniotabes, frontal bossing, thickening of the wrist, and visible enlargement or palpable swelling of the costochondral junction (rachitic rosary) are the characteristic skeletal manifestations. Late ambulation and delayed tooth eruption are additional clinical findings. Owing to softening of the ribs a depression corresponding to the costal insertion of the diaphragm (Harrison sulci) might also be visible. Craniotabes is owing to thinning of the skull and is particularly found in prematurely born infants. By pressing firmly over the occiput or posterior parietal bones a ping-pong ball sensation will be felt.

In the second year of life the legs grow more quickly, and the effect of weight-bearing results in bowing of the legs, or genu varum. On rare occasions this bowing may be confused with exaggerated physiological bowing or Blount disease. The angulation is especially pronounced at the junction of the lower third and upper

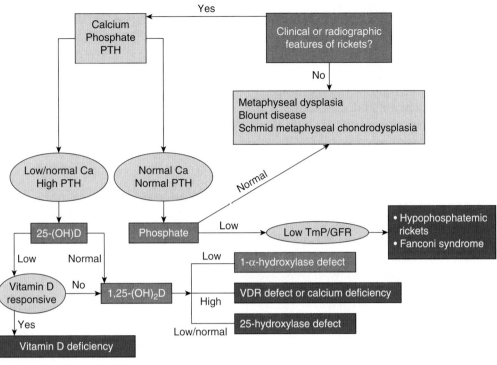

FIGURE 6-15 ▪ Classification of bone deformities suggestive of rickets.

two-thirds of the leg. The most prominent osseous manifestation of adolescent rickets is the occurrence of "knock knee", or genu valgum. Toddlers may have walking problems and adolescents may exhibit a waddling gait.

Diagnosis. The plasma concentration of 25(OH)D is a sensitive index of vitamin D nutritional status, and is typically found at the lower limit (<10 ng/mL). Previously published normal ranges for plasma 25(OH)D were not correct, and a normal lower limit for plasma 25(OH)D is likely closer to 30 ng/mL rather than 10 ng/mL. No apparent relationship between the 25(OH)D concentration and the severity of the rickets has been appreciated. Even more perplexing perhaps, the plasma concentration of calcitriol can be low, normal, or elevated in nutritional vitamin D deficiency, and thus can be more confusing than illuminating. Indeed, most untreated patients have normal or even elevated plasma concentration of calcitriol owing to the secondary hyperparathyroidism and increased activity of the renal 1-α-hydroxylase (Table 6-8). Following treatment with vitamin D this increased enzyme activity results in a prompt rise of calcitriol to levels well above the upper limit of the normal range, often with transient hypercalcemia.

Radiological examination of the distal ends of radius and ulna, perhaps in conjunction with measurement of the serum level of 25(OH)D, appears to be the most useful screen for the early diagnosis of rickets. The earliest radiological finding is a slight widening of the growth plate owing to proliferation of uncalcified cartilage and osteoid. In severe rickets the metaphyses appear widened, splayed, cupped, and frayed, in contrast to the normally sharply demarcated and slightly convex ends (Case 6-4 A-D).

Treatment. Rickets can be prevented by sufficient exposure to ultraviolet light and/or by oral supplementation of vitamin D. For most children and adolescents of the world, exposure to sunlight is the principal source of vitamin D. The capacity of the human skin to produce vitamin D is quite large, but is not sufficient during the winter months in the temperate zones. Few foods contain vitamin D naturally, and several countries therefore practice the fortification of some foods. Traditionally, an adequate intake of vitamin D in most countries has been defined as 200 to 400 IU, or 5 to 10 μg daily. In temperate zones, oral substitution with 400 IU daily during the winter months (eg, from September through April in the northern hemisphere) is currently recommended but may not be sufficient to protect children with a normal outdoor lifestyle from rickets. In fact, in 1997 the Institute of Medicine could only propose an adequate intake rather than a recommended daily allowance because of the dearth of investigation into dietary vitamin D. With the recent recognition that (1) many children are vitamin D deficient, (2) higher serum vitamin D levels than previously thought are necessary for bone health, and

(3) 400 IU of dietary vitamin D are not adequate to attain optimal vitamin D levels at least in adults in whom it has been better studied, the recommendations for vitamin D dosing are likely to change. Because human milk contains inadequate amounts of vitamin D, all infants who are exclusively breast-fed should receive 400 IU of vitamin D daily within days of birth.[155] An alternative approach has been suggested: high dose replacement in breastfeeding mothers. Cholecalciferol doses of 6400 IU daily to breastfeeding mother's safely lead to serum 25(OH)D levels in their breastfed infants that are comparable to those of breastfed infants supplements with 400 IU vitamin D.[156]

Vitamin D deficiency rickets can be safely and effectively healed by daily doses of 50 to 100 μg or 2000 to 4000 IU vitamin D. Radiological signs of healing will usually be evident within 2 to 4 weeks. More protracted therapy for 6 to 8 weeks with daily doses of 2000 IU vitamin D may be beneficial in longstanding rickets to replenish vitamin D fat stores. In some cases, administration of a large dose of vitamin D (150,000-300,000 IU) at one time, so called "stoss" therapy, may be more practical. However, the incidence of hypercalcemia after large dose vitamin D treatment is significant, and this form of treatment should be reserved for those children who have failed more usual treatment regimens because of poor compliance. If no healing occurs, the rickets is probably resistant to vitamin D.

Severe or symptomatic tetany should be treated with slow, intravenous injection of 10% calcium gluconate in a dose of 1 to 2 mL/kg up to 10 mL (93 mg of elemental calcium). Care should be taken to avoid subcutaneous leakage owing to dangers of local necrosis. To sustain the plasma calcium concentration above the tetany level, calcium supplements should be provided. For example, calcium chloride in 1% to 2% solution can be added to the milk or fruit juice. For the first 1 to 2 days, a total of 4 to 6 g of elemental calcium daily may be given in 1 g doses, with a doubling of the initial dose. The treatment should then be continued with smaller doses of calcium (eg, 50 mg/kg/day of elemental calcium) for 1 to 2 weeks. Calcium chloride in more concentrated solutions should be avoided because of danger of gastric ulceration, and larger doses may cause acidosis. Other salts of calcium (eg, calcium carbonate, calcium citrate, calcium lactate, calcium glucobionate) are also suitable, and may be more convenient to use, but contain less elemental calcium (Box 6-2).

Hepatic and intestinal disorders (vitamin D malabsorption)

Pathogenesis. Under conditions in which the major source of vitamin D is the diet rather than exposure to sunlight, deficient absorption of the vitamin in conjunction with hepatic and intestinal disorders can result

---

Box 6-2. When to Refer

Rickets

Appropriate referral to the endocrinologist or other specialist should be made for rickets unresponsive to pharmacologic doses of vitamin D or if other forms of rickets are suspected such as:

- 25-α-hydroxylase deficiency
- 1-α-hydroxylase deficiency
- Vitamin D receptor defects
- Disorders of fat malabsorption
- Use of pharmacologic agents disrupting vitamin D metabolism
- Hypophosphatemic rickets
- If osteogenesis imperfecta is suspected

---

in rickets. Reduced levels of 25(OH)D have been reported following small-intestinal resection, and in patients with malabsorption because of cystic fibrosis and celiac disease. However, the occurrence of rickets is rare, and may be owing to a combination of deficient resorption of both vitamin D and calcium and a probable defect in the entero-hepatic circulation of vitamin D and its metabolites. Additional risk factors for metabolic bone disease in patients with inflammatory bowel disease include overall poor nutrition, decreased weight-bearing, and elevated circulating levels of proinflammatory cytokines (eg, interleukin (IL) 1, IL-6, and TNF-α) that are known to enhance bone resorption. Metabolic bone disease and osteomalacia have also been reported in patients who receive long-term parenteral nutrition. The discovery that bone resorption is stimulated by the interaction of RANKL with the receptor to activated NF-kappa B (RANK) expressed by osteoclasts now provides a potential association between mucosal or systemic inflammation and bone remodeling, as RANK-RANKL are also involved in lymphopoiesis and T-cell apoptosis.

A variety of cholestatic diseases and syndromes, and particularly biliary atresia, might cause rickets and osteomalacia. The vitamin D deficiency probably results from complex causes involving reduced exposure to sunlight, reduced dietary intake of vitamin D, and malabsorption in patients with steatorrhoea. In most types of chronic liver disease, mean plasma levels of 25(OH)D are usually insufficient by current standards, and in patients with rickets and osteomalacia they are usually deficient. Reduced production of DBP in the liver may contribute to the reduction of 25(OH)D, and also the plasma concentration of calcitriol without reducing the biologically active free fraction. The finding of subnormal plasma concentrations of 25(OH)D and calcitriol in these patients should therefore be interpreted with caution.

Treatment. Adequate exposure to sunlight is sufficient to protect the majority of patients with gastrointestinal or liver disease from the clinical manifestations of vitamin D deficiency. Since rickets is mainly related to vitamin D malabsorption in these children, treatment would require somewhat higher oral doses of vitamin D than those necessary to heal ordinary nutritional rickets. Thus, 4000-10,000 IU of vitamin D (100-250 μg) should be given daily, along with oral calcium supplementation as described above. If the desired vitamin D level is not obtained with high dose vitamin D replacement, UV light therapy is a valuable alternative.

Anticonvulsant therapy

Epidemiology. Long-term treatment with anticonvulsant drugs that induce hepatic P450 enzymes such as CYP3A4 has been associated with rickets and osteomalacia as well as osteopenia and osteoporosis. Defective mineralization is rather uncommon, but has been especially found in institutionalized epileptic children treated with polytherapy, which produces a greater risk of a disturbance in bone metabolism than monotherapy.

Pathogenesis. The combination of phenobarbital and phenytoin appears to be most deleterious to bone and mineral metabolism, as phenobarbital, phenytoin, primidone, and carbamazepine increase activity of the hepatic cytochrome CYP3A4 enzyme system, which accelerates the catabolism of 25-(OH)D and calcitriol into more polar, inactive products leading to a reduction in vitamin reserves and increasing daily needs. Exposure to adequate sunlight reduces the risk of anticonvulsant-induced vitamin D insufficiency, as subjects residing in latitudes near the equator rarely develop this complication.

Diagnosis. In overt rickets and osteomalacia, the plasma concentrations of calcium, 25(OH)D and 24,25-(OH)$_2$D are reduced, whereas the calcitriol concentration usually is within the normal range. Other mechanisms such as lack of exposure to sunlight, low dietary intake of vitamin D and calcium, together with drug-induced inhibition of calcium absorption may also contribute.

Treatment. Upon initiation of anticonvulsant therapy, all children should receive year round vitamin D supplementation. Children at greater risk, such as institutional epileptic patients, may require prevention with prophylactic vitamin D supplementation at doses up to 2000 IU/day. A calcium intake of 600 to 1000 mg/day should also be ensured. If an osteopenic/osteoporotic disorder exists, treatment with 2000 to 4000 IU/day vitamin D is appropriate. Overt rickets and osteomalacia in these children are treated similarly to vitamin D deficiency rickets.

Vitamin D dependency type 1 (1-α-hydroxylase deficiency)

Definitions and Epidemiology. Vitamin D-dependent rickets type 1 (VDD1) is a rare autosomal disorder also known as Pseudovitamin D deficiency rickets. The plasma concentration of calcitriol is low in patients with pseudodeficiency rickets and does not increase in response to PTH administration. This disorder represents a defect in the renal 1-α-hydroxylase (CYP27B1) that converts 25(OH)D to calcitriol. A continuing requirement for high doses of vitamin D to sustain the remission indicates a state of vitamin D dependency. Thus, this condition is also known as "selective and simple deficiency of calcitriol," "hereditary vitamin D-pseudodeficiency type 1," and "hereditary 25D, 1-α-hydroxylase deficiency rickets." VDD1 is a rare cause of rickets, but the disorder occurs with unusual frequency in the French-Canadian population.

Clinical presentation. The clinical findings of this condition are similar to those of ordinary vitamin D deficiency rickets, but rickets develops despite a history of adequate vitamin D intake. The most distinctive clinical feature is the failure of the rickets to heal in response to normal therapeutic doses of vitamin D, whereas complete healing and restoration of plasma concentrations of calcium and phosphate are achieved after treatment with doses approximately 100 times the normal daily requirement.

Pathogenesis. Defects in the 1-α-hydroxylase gene have been identified in patients with VDD1. A wide variety of mutations have now been identified that explain deficient expression or activity of the 1-α-hydroxylase. Despite the high prevalence of VDD1 within the relatively isolated French-Canadian population of Quebec, the allelic diversity suggests that more than one genetic founder must account for the disorder in these patients.[157]

Treatment. The drugs of choice in treatment are calcitriol or its synthetic analogue, 1-α(OH)D. Both compounds have much shorter biological half-life than the parent vitamin D, which is an advantage in the event of inadvertent overtreatment. The biological activity of 1-α(OH)D is about one-half to two-third that of calcitriol. The recommended doses in treatment of active rickets are 2 to 8 μg/day of 1-α(OH)D, or 1 to 4 μg/day of calcitriol. Following radiologically evident healing of the rickets, the lifelong substitution therapy will require 1 to 3 μg/day of 1-α(OH)D or 0.5 to 2 μg/day of calcitriol (Table 6-7). To avoid overtreatment, the plasma concentration of calcium and phosphate, as well as urinary calcium excretion, should be measured periodically.

Vitamin D dependency type 2 (end-organ resistance)

Definitions. Vitamin D-dependent rickets 2 (VDD2) is a rare hereditary disease because of target organ resistance to calcitriol. The hallmarks of the disorder include early onset rickets, hypocalcemia, secondary hyperparathyroidism, and very high plasma concentrations of calcitriol (Table 6-8).

Clinical presentation. The clinical features are almost identical to those that occur in patients with VDD1, but in VDD2, alopecia (head and body) is found in about half of the patients. Patients with VDD2 appear normal at birth and develop features of calciferol deficiency over the first 2 to 8 months of life. Alopecia generally develops at 2 to 12 months but may be present at birth. It may be partial or complete. Sometimes a selective sparing of the eyelashes occurs. Alopecia seems to be a marker of the more severe forms of the disease, as judged by earlier onset of hypocalcemia, more marked clinical presentation, and poor response to therapy. Other ectodermal defects have been reported in small numbers of cases and have an uncertain relation to the syndrome; these include oligodontia, epidermal cysts, and multiple milia.

In some cases neonatal development is normal and dysfunction is not evident until late in childhood or even in adulthood. These patients do not have alopecia and respond to high doses of calciferols, indicating a mild variant of the syndrome.

Pathogenesis. The disorder is inherited by autosomal recessive transmission. Studies of cultured skin fibroblasts from affected individuals and family members indicate that the disorder encompasses a heterogenous group of molecular defects of the vitamin D receptor which contain discrete functional domains involved in hormone-binding and DNA-binding (see Chapter 1).

Treatment. Patients with VDD2 are usually responsive to high doses of calcitriol, or 1-α(OH)D, with or without calcium supplementation. Such treatment can often heal the rickets and normalize calcium homeostasis, but alopecia never improves. Cases with mild-to-moderate resistance respond to very high doses of vitamin D, which should then be in the order of 0.5 to 5 mg/day, that is, 2,00,000 to 2 million IU/day (Table 6-7). By increasing substrate in this way, these patients can sustain very high plasma levels of calcitriol in part because of deficient receptor-mediated feedback inhibition.

In cases with intermediate severity VDD2, endogenous production of calcitriol cannot be sufficiently increased with vitamin D therapy, and extremely high doses of calcitriol or 1-α(OH)D (in the order of 5-60 μg/day) are required. A supplementation dose of about 2 g calcium per day is an important adjunct to avoid fluctuations of the plasma concentration of calcium owing to variable dietary calcium content.

In the most severely affected patient complete refractoriness to the action of calcitriol on intestinal calcium absorption is present. Even to calcitriol doses achieving sustained plasma concentrations in the order of 2000 pg/mL, that is, 300 to 400 times above normal, are inadequate. In such cases the only effective therapy is high doses of oral or intravenous calcium. Such a therapeutic regimen presents a considerable practical problem for long-term use.

As is true for therapy of vitamin D-deficiency rickets and VDD1, a catch-up mineralization of accumulated osteoid tissue in the early stage of treatment occurs. This "catch up" requires higher doses of both calcitriol and calcium supplementation than needed for long-term maintenance therapy.

CLINICAL PRESENTATION AND MANAGEMENT OF HYPERCALCEMIA

Definitions

Interpretation of a serum calcium level in a child with possible hypercalcemia requires that the child's age and the serum albumin concentration be considered (Figure 6-16). The laboratory evaluation of hypercalcemia must include determination of the serum phosphorus concentration, a step that is often overlooked now that phosphorus measurement is no longer included as a standard component of the comprehensive metabolic panels (eg, SMAC or SMA12) that are processed using multichannel autoanalyzers. Hypophosphatemia can cause hypercalcemia, particularly in the case of the premature or very-low-birth weight infant who receives inadequate dietary phosphorus.

Clinical Presentation

The clinical manifestations of hypercalcemia will be dependent upon both the age of the child and the degree of hypercalcemia. Infants with mild increases in serum calcium (11-13 mg/dL or 2.75-3.25 mmol/L) often lack specific symptoms of hypercalcemia. Nonspecific signs and symptoms such as anorexia, vomiting, abdominal pain, and constipation (rarely diarrhea) may occur with moderate to severe hypercalcemia. Neurologic symptoms can range from drowsiness or irritability to confusion; in the extreme cases, stupor and coma can ensue. Failure to thrive may be the only sign of chronic hypercalcemia. The nonspecific or absence of symptoms of hypercalcemia in young children is problematic as unrecognized hypercalcemia in newborns or infants can cause significant morbidity or death. Polyuria caused by

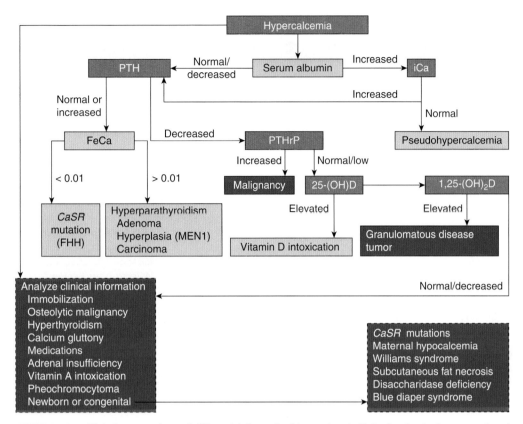

FIGURE 6-16 ■ Clinical presentation and differential diagnosis of hypercalcemia (FeCa, fractional urinary excretion of calcium; iCa, ionized calcium).

renal resistance to vasopressin can lead rapidly to severe dehydration in infants. Elevated serum concentrations of calcium can cause hypertension and affect cardiac conduction with shortening of the ST segment and heart block. Severe hypercalcemia can affect the nervous system and cause lethargy and seizures. Renal complications such as nephrocalcinosis, nephrolithiasis, or hematuria may be the earliest clinical manifestation of hypercalcemia and hypercalciuria. Thus, timely recognition and treatment of hypercalcemia in infants and children is critical in determining the prognosis.

Differential Diagnosis

Primary hyperparathyroidism

Neonatal transient primary hyperparathyroidism. Hypercalcemia is far less common than hypocalcemia in the neonatal period and early infancy. In many cases a thorough investigation of the infant's mother will disclose previously recognized but poorly treated hypoparathyroidism or clinically unsuspected hypocalcemia, which during pregnancy had induced severe secondary hyperparathyroidism in the developing fetus, (Figure 6-16 and Table 6-9). In general, hyperparathyroidism and hypocalcemia are transient in the affected infant.

The birth weights are frequently less than 2500 g, but otherwise these infants usually appear normal at birth. The pathogenetic mechanism probably involves fetal hyperparathyroidism secondary to decreased calcium transport from the hypocalcemic mother to the fetus leading to fetal hypocalcemia. The secondary increased secretion of fetal PTH mobilizes calcium from the fetal skeleton causing generalized skeletal demineralization and subperiosteal resorption. The hyperfunction of the parathyroid glands may persist after birth, resulting in moderate transient hypercalcemia, although most neonates have been normocalcemic and have had somewhat elevated rather than depressed plasma phosphate concentrations. Following birth, the skeleton avidly takes up calcium, and the bone lesions heal spontaneously within 4 to 6 months. Careful management of the plasma calcium concentration in hypoparathyroid women during pregnancy will prevent the development of secondary hyperparathyroidism in the fetus.

Familial benign hypocalciuric hypercalcemia and neonatal severe hyperparathyroidism. Patients with familial (benign) hypocalciuric hypercalcemia (FBHH) are asymptomatic despite mild to moderate hypercalcemia, and the disorder usually comes to light by the incidental finding of hypercalcemia in a patient

Table 6-9.

Causes of Hypercalcemia in Childhood

Type	Serum					Notes
	Pi	25(OH)D	Calcitriol	PTH	UCa	
Williams syndrome	N	N	N/H	L	H	Contiguous deletion at 7q11.23. Cognitive impairment Elfin facies, aortic stenosis
Childhood hyperparathyroidism	L	N	H	H	H	Often genetic (multiple endocrine neoplasia)
Severe neonatal hyperparathyroidism	L	N	H	H	L/N	*CASR* loss-of-function mutation, generally homozygous
Familial hypocalciuric hypercalcemia	N	N	N	N	L	*CASR* loss-of-function mutation, generally heterozygous; benign
Immobilization	N	N	L	L	H	
Malignancy (metastatic)	N	N	L	L	H	
Malignancy (nonmetastatic)	L	N	L	L ↑ PTHrP	H	Unregulated and excessive secretion of bone resorbing substances; notably PTHrP, less frequently 1,25(OH)$_2$D

Pi, phosphate; PTH, parathyroid hormone; PTHrP, parathyroid hormone–related peptide; UCa, urinary calcium; CaSR, calcium-sensing receptor gene.

investigated for an unrelated condition, or during the evaluation of relatives of a patient with hypercalcemia. FBHH is an autosomal dominant disorder with high penetrance of hypercalcemia at all ages. The hypercalcemia may be present at birth, and the diagnosis is frequently made during infancy and childhood, which is an important distinguishing feature from other forms of familial or sporadic PHPT. Despite hypercalcemia, nearly all patients have relative hypocalciuria, but an occasional patient may have hypercalciuria. A relatively benign course is a distinctive feature.

The circulating concentrations of PTH are normal or high-normal (Table 6-9). However, in the presence of hypercalcemia such concentrations are inappropriately high and indicate that the set-point of the parathyroid calciostat regulating PTH secretion functions at a higher than normal level (as discussed earlier). The hypercalcemia and hypophosphatemia are similar in magnitude to those found in mild cases of primary hyperparathyroidism. Most patients display no symptoms attributable to the hypercalcemia, although some may experience mild muscle weakness and easy fatiguability.

Neonatal severe hyperparathyroidism (NSHPT) is genetically related to FBHH. In contrast to the benign nature of FBHH, however, NSHPT is a severe and often life-threatening disorder. NSHPT may have its onset in fetal life and usually manifests symptoms in the first week of life. The fetal onset is suggested by the occasional finding of skeletal lesions in the neonate characteristic of hyperparathyroidism, that is, generalized

demineralization and osteopenia as well as localized erosions at the ends of the long bones and subperiosteal resorption along the shafts of the tubular bones. The parathyroid glands are enlarged with chief cell hyperplasia. Affected infants often have severe hypercalcemia with markedly elevated PTH levels, normal to low serum phosphate, normal to high serum magnesium, elevated alkaline phosphatase, and inappropriately normal or low urinary calcium excretion.[158]

Pathogenesis. Both FBHH and NSHPT have been attributed to mutations in the *CASR* gene at 3q13.3-21 that inactivate the CaSR,[159] (Figure 6-17). In many families, NSHPT and FBHH are the respective homozygous and heterozygous manifestations of the same genetic defect. NSHPT can also occur in heterozygous infants born to affected fathers but unaffected normocalcemic mothers, or in neonates with an apparent *de novo* heterozygous mutation in the *CASR* gene. Mutations that inactivate the CaSR have been found scattered throughout the *CASR* gene, and most families have private mutations. Reduced expression or function of parathyroid CaSRs decreases the sensitivity of the parathyroid cells to extracellular Ca^{2+}, which increases the set point for calcium-dependent inhibition of PTH release and leads to mild parathyroid hyperplasia and elevated circulating levels of PTH. Decreased receptor activity in the kidney is thought to account for relative hypocalciuria, the hallmark of the disorder.[160] Children who survive NSHPT but who remain hypercalcemic can have

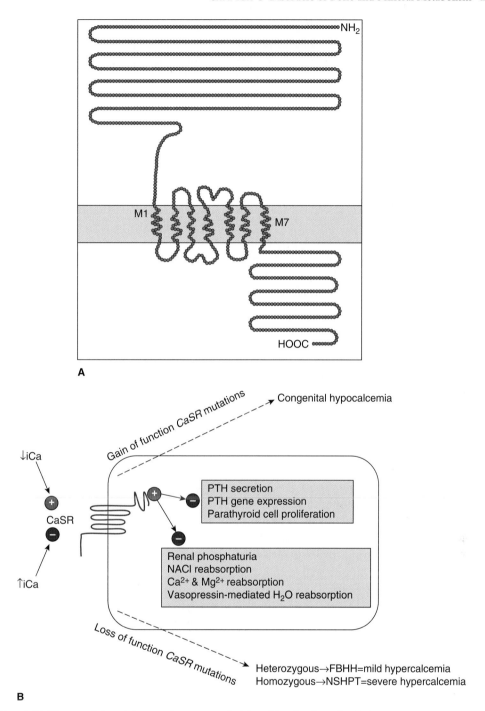

FIGURE 16-17 ■ (**A**) and (**B**) Diagram of the calcium-sensing receptor (CaSR) and its disorders. The shaded area depicts the cell membrane, with the extracellular space at the top of the figure. The CaSR is a protein of 1078 amino acids (the circles represent its secondary structure). Three structural regions are present: a large amino-terminal extracellular domain involved in Ca^{2+} binding; seven transmembrane helices characteristic of the G protein-coupled receptor superfamily (see Chapter 1); and a cytoplasmic carboxy-terminal domain. Activation of the CaSR on the parathyroid cells and renal tubules suppresses PTH release and increases urinary calcium excretion, whereas inactivation of the receptor facilitates PTH release and reduces urinary calcium excretion.

poor feeding with failure to thrive, hypotonia, and developmental delay, and may be at risk of subsequent neurodevelopmental deficits.

Diagnosis. The diagnosis of NSHPT is based on the presence of inappropriately normal or elevated PTH levels along with relative hypocalciuria in an infant with hypercalcemia. A family history of FHH or NSHPT in a sibling can provide strong confirmation of the diagnosis. Care must be taken to distinguish these disorders from the transient neonatal hyperparathyroidism associated with maternal hypocalcemia, as seen in mothers with pseudohypoparathyroidism or renal tubular acidosis. Genetic testing for FBHH and NSHPT is available commercially. Although FHH and NSHPT have been associated with mutations in the *CASR* gene at 3q13.3-21 in nearly all affected subjects, in some families the disorder has been linked to unknown genes present on the long or short arms of chromosome 19, suggesting genetic heterogeneity.

Patients have a tendency to elevated plasma levels of magnesium and hypocalciuria, but neither of these features can differentiate FBHH from other forms of primary hyperparathyroidism with absolute certainty. The fractional clearance of calcium (ratio of calcium clearance to creatinine clearance, FeCa) is usually less than 0.01 in FBHH, whereas a FeCa above 0.01 is a typical finding in other forms of primary hyperparathyroidism. The plasma level of calcitriol in FBHH is usually in the midnormal range in contrast to a tendency to elevated levels in primary hyperparathyroidism.

Primary hyperparathyroidism in children and adolescents

Epidemiology. Primary hyperparathyroidism (PHPT) is uncommon in both children and adolescents, and generally constitutes less than 5% of all cases of PHPT. In a review of 35 cases the ages at diagnosis ranged from 3 to 15 years with a mean of 12.8 years. The clinical and biochemical features of PHPT in children and adolescents who are younger than 20 years at time of diagnosis differ significantly[161] from the typical form of PHPT that occurs in older adults. Firstly, an equal distribution between males and females is found instead of the female predominance that is typical of adult onset PHPT. Secondly, symptomatic disease is much more common (81%-83%) with renal involvement as the most common presenting symptom and evidence of bone disease in over 50% of patients.

Diagnosis. In contrast to the differences in disease presentation and epidemiology, many important similarities between PHPT in children and adults are found. For example, levels of intact PTH are consistently elevated or inappropriately normal. Circulating levels of intact PTH in children have been shown to be either lower (eg, <36 pg/mL) or similar to those levels in adults. Sestimibi SPECT scintigraphy appears as useful in children as in adults for preoperative localization of enlarged parathyroid glands,[161] which makes possible the use of minimally invasive parathyroid surgery techniques in young patients.

Pathogenesis. The normal parathyroid cell has a mechanism sensing the extracellular calcium concentration which, in turn, regulates the PTH secretion in a negative feedback fashion. In PHPT, a poorly defined defect in the regulation of this feedback mechanism occurs. Parathyroid adenomas display decreased expression of cell surface CaSRs, with a resultant loss of

sensitivity to extracellular calcium that leads to excessive and inappropriate secretion of PTH. In PHPT caused by hyperplasia, the set-point for PTH release in response to plasma calcium is normal, but the mass of cells is so great that the total amount of PTH secreted is increased. In some cases even normal parathyroid cells cannot be completely suppressed. Thus, when the mass of secretory tissue is increased, this basal nonsuppressible PTH may be sufficient to cause the clinical manifestations of hyperparathyroidism (Figure 6-18). Nearly all parathyroid tumors are clonal, suggesting a defect in a gene (or genes) that regulates growth of the parathyroid cell. External neck irradiation in childhood, recognized as an underlying factor in some patients with PHPT, may induce defects in one or more of these genes.

PHPT may be sporadic or inherited as an autosomal dominant condition (Table 6-10). The majority of children and adolescents with PHPT have a single benign parathyroid tumor (adenoma), whereas multiple hypercellular glands are present in about 30% to 40% (primary hyperplasia or "double adenomas") of patients. Parathyroid carcinoma is rare. Parathyroid adenomas usually occur spontaneously as monoclonal neoplasms. A monoclonal tumor may result from a set of somatic mutations or other "hits" in one parent cell, whereas a polyclonal expansion is to be expected when multiple original cells respond to an exogenous or endogenous stimulus. The development of monoclonal adenomas as a result of somatic mutation supports the suggestion that parathyroid

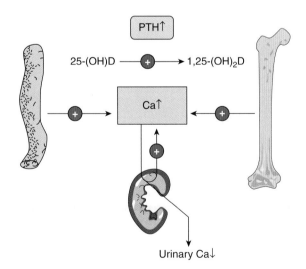

FIGURE 6-18 ■ Pathophysiology of hyperparathyroidism. Hypercalcemia is the biochemical hallmark of increased PTH action, and results from increased mobilization of calcium from the skeleton and, indirectly, from increased calcium absorption from the intestine because of increased PTH-dependent synthesis of calcitriol. The urinary output of calcium is determined by the opposite forces of increased filtered load of calcium and increased tubular reabsorption.

Table 6-10.

Genetic Syndromes Associated with Primary Hyperparathyroidism and Parathyroid Hyperplasia

	FBHH/NSHPT	MEN 1	MEN2a	Hyperparathyroidism-Jaw Tumor Syndrome (HPT- JT)	MEN 4	Familial Hyperparathyroidism
Tissues affected	Parathyroid Kidney	Parathyroid Pituitary	MTC Adrenal (pheochromocytoma)	Parathyroid Jaw	Parathyroid Pituitary	Parathyroid
		Pancreas Skin	Parathyroid	Kidney		
Presentation	Hypercalcemia	Hypercalcemia	Medullary thyroid carcinoma	Hypercalcemia; parathyroid carcinoma; jaw and renal tumors	Hypercalcemia	Hypercalcemia
Gene defect	CaSR	*MEN1* gene 11q13	*RET*	*CDC73* gene encoding parafibromin 1q25	*CDKN1B*, cyclin-dependent kinase inhibitor 1B (p27,^{Kip}1)	Some *MEN1* or *CASR*, rarely *CDC73*; most unknown

adenomas may be induced by neck irradiation. The cyclin D1/PRAD1 gene was identified as a clonally activated oncogene in parathyroid adenomas and, with cyclin D1 being a key regulator of the cell cycle, has subsequently been implicated in the pathogenesis of 20% to 40% of sporadic parathyroid adenomas. In sporadic parathyroid tumors, not associated with familial MEN1, biallelic somatic mutations inactivating *MEN1* occur in 12% to 17%, or about half the tumors with allelic losses on 11q.[162] Somatic mutation of another tumor suppressor gene, *HRPT2*, which causes the rare autosomal dominant hyperparathyroidism-jaw tumor (HPT-JT) syndrome, also occurs in some benign parathyroid adenomas and in most parathyroid carcinomas. Finally, other mutations affecting the CaSR, which when partially or markedly deficient because of germline mutation can cause familial hypocalciuric hypercalcemia or neonatal severe hyperparathyroidism, must still be considered as having a potentially important secondary role in the manifestations of sporadic parathyroid tumors.

Inherited PHPT with multiple gland enlargement can occur as a manifestation of several autsomal dominant syndromes. The most common owing to mutation of the *MEN1* gene, and is associated with multiple enlarged parathyroid glands (90%), pancreatic islet cell (>50%) and pituitary (25%-40%) adenomas, and dermal lesions (70%-90%) such as angiofibromas and collagenomas. PHPT occurs with lesser frequency in patients with MEN2a, owing to germline *RET* gene mutations, in which medullary thyroid carcinoma and pheochromocytoma are common. PHPT is very unusual in the MEN2b

variant, in which medullary carcinoma of the thyroid and pheochromocytoma are associated with ganglioneuromas of the gastrointestinal tract and a marfanoid habitus. Finally, mutations that inactivate p27^{kip1}, a multifunctional cyclin-dependent kinase inhibitor, cause a fourth form of MEN (so called MEN type 4) that is associated with benign tumors of the parathyroids and pituitary.

Treatment of primary hyperparathyroidism. The treatment of life-threatening hypercalcemia requires urgent medical intervention. The natural history of NSHPT suggests that hyperparathyroidism and severe hypercalcemia may improve with time in many infants, and that appropriate medical treatment can preclude the need for surgical intervention in selected cases. The first principle in medical emergency treatment of neonatal hypercalcemia is to increase the urinary excretion of sodium since sodium clearance and calcium clearance are very closely linked during water or osmotic diuresis. Infants with NSHPT are often dehydrated, and two-thirds to full strength saline containing 30 mEq of potassium chloride per liter should be infused to correct dehydration and maximize glomerular filtration rate. Furosemide has traditionally been used to enhance calciuresis once hydration has been optimized as this agent can inhibit tubular reabsorption of calcium as well as sodium and water, but evidence demonstrating efficacy in the treatment of hypercalcemia is lacking.[163] Additional concerns that powerful loop diuretics may induce dehydration and thereby worsen hypercalcemia further reduce enthusiasm for the routine use of these agents.

Because hypercalcemia is caused by excessive release of calcium (and phosphorus) from the skeleton Figure 6-18, treatment will require an agent that can directly reduce osteoclastic bone resorption. Calcitonin (4 U/kg every 6-12 hours) given by subcutaneous injection may reduce serum calcium levels modestly for a short period of time, but resistance to the hormone occurs quite rapidly. More reliable and durable inhibition of bone resorption can be achieved with bisphosphonates. These agents are analogues of inorganic pyrophosphate, which adsorb to the hydroxyapatite matrix of bone and inhibit osteoclast-mediated bone resorption. Nitrogen-containing bisphosphonates, including alendronate, ibandronate, pamidronate disodium, risedronate, and zoledronic acid, are potent inhibitors of osteoclast-mediated bone resorption. Zoledronic acid is a new-generation, heterocyclic nitrogen-containing bisphosphonate and the most potent inhibitor of bone resorption identified to date. The more powerful parenteral bisphosphonates (eg, pamidronate disodium and zoledronic acid) can acutely lower serum and urinary calcium in patients with PHPT. Glucocorticoids are relatively ineffective in the treatment of hypercalcemia associated with PHPT.

Parathyroid surgery is recommended for symptomatic patients and patients who are under the age of 50 years. Other criteria that favor parathyroidectomy in patients with mild or asymptomatic disease include:

1. Serum calcium ≥ 1 mg/dL above normal
2. Kidney stone or extreme hypercalciuria (24 hour urine calcium > 400 mg/day)
3. Creatinine clearance reduced by 30% compared to age-matched normal individuals
4. Reduced bone density compared to peak bone mass (T score < −2.5) at hip, lumbar spine or distal radius
5. Patients for whom medical surveillance is neither desirable nor possible (eg, patients for whom serial monitoring is impractical or unacceptable)

Based on the age criteria described above, surgical management of PHPT for all children and adolescents is reasonable, unless extenuating circumstances indicate otherwise. Patients with FBHH, regardless of age, represent an important exception to this management guideline. As noted above, patients with FBHH are typically asymptomatic and do not develop the long-term complications that are common in other forms of PHPT. Thus, they will not benefit from parathyroidectomy. Moreover, patients with FBHH have multigland hyperplasia, and removal of all parathyroid tissue has been necessary when a surgical approach to management of hypercalcemia has been undertaken. Practically, this results in the infliction of surgical hypoparathyroidism

Box 6-3. When to Refer

Hypercalcemia
Appropriate referral to the endocrinologist or other specialist should be made for hypercalcemia that is not attributable to a significant intercurrent illness or intervention that is persistent. Such disorders include:

■ Loss of function mutations in calcium-sensing receptor
■ Vitamin D intoxication
■ Vitamin A intoxication
■ Hyperparathyroidism
■ Williams syndrome
■ Granulomatous disease
■ Neoplastic or paraneoplastic disorder
■ Immobilization

as a treatment for asymptomatic hyperparathyroidism. Thus, diagnosing FBHH and screening first-degree relatives, in order to avoid performing unnecessary parathyroid surgery in these patients, are critically important. No effective medical therapy for long-term management of PHPT is currently available or recommended for children. Calcimimetics, such as cinacalcet, increase the sensitivity of the CaSR to calcium and can lower serum calcium levels, but only limited information regarding their usefulness and safety in children and adolescents with PHPT is available[164] (Box 6-3).

Idiopathic infantile hypercalcemia and Williams syndrome

In 1961, Williams and coworkers first called attention to the association of peculiar facies and supravalvular aortic stenosis in children with growth retardation. The association of so-called elfin facies and infantile hypercalcemia is now termed Williams syndrome.

Clinical presentation. The craniofacial features which comprise the elfin facies include dolichocephaly, asymmetry, bitemporal depression, flat nasal bridge, full cheeks, periorbital fullness, epicanthal folds, stellate or lacy iris patterns, full nasal tip with anteverted nostrils, long philtrum, full lips, and wide mouth. The facial features tend to be more pronounced with age (Case 6-5). Musculoskeletal manifestations of Williams syndrome include hallux valgus, fifth finger clinodactyly, hypoplastic, deep-set nails, pectus excavatum, joint limitations, kyphosis, scoliosis, and awkward gait. About 80% of the patients have a cardiac murmur, which may either disappear or become less marked with time. Supravalvular aortic stenosis is the most frequent cardiovascular anomaly and occurs in about 30% of cases. Intracardiac defects include valvular aortic stenosis, pulmonary stenosis, ventricular and atrial septal defect. Additional extracardiac anomalies include mesenteric, celiac, and renal artery stenosis. Hypertension has been noted in about 50% of adult patients.

A unique constellation of neurocognitive characteristics have been described in children with Williams syndrome, and constitute a characteristic behavioral phenotype. These factors begin in infancy with development of salient attachment behaviors. Patients with Williams syndrome have a generalized developmental delay, and IQ ranges from 50 to 90. In general, patients with the more severe form of Williams syndrome tend to have only mild to moderate mental retardation. Interestingly, despite delayed acquisition of speech, they are quite sociable ("cocktail personality") and have remarkable linguistic abilities. Many patients with Williams syndrome also appear to be musically gifted. Their personality is often described as friendly and loquacious. Their growth pattern is characterized by moderate prenatal growth deficiency, a delay during the first 4 years of life, catch-up growth in childhood, and low ultimate adult height. Special growth charts for children with Williams syndrome are now available.[165]

Williams syndrome is associated with hypercalcemia in approximately 15% of cases, although hypercalciuria may be more frequent. The hypercalcemia typically occurs during infancy and usually resolves between 2 and 4 years of age. PTH is suppressed or inappropriately normal, and hypercalciuria is common even in children who do not have hypercalcemia. Nephrocalcinosis and soft-tissue calcifications may also be found. Because hypercalcemia resolves during infancy or early childhood, most patients with Williams syndrome are normocalcemic at the time of diagnosis, but the presence of nephrocalcinosis and other soft tissues calcifications suggests the previous presence of hypercalcemia. Osteosclerosis, especially of the base of the skull and, to lesser extent of the long bones and vertebral column, is found occasionally by radiological examination during infancy (Case 6-6).

Pathogenesis. Williams syndrome has been associated with microdeletions at 7 q11.13, and likely represents a contiguous gene deletion that typically includes the genes for elastin (*ELN*) LIM kinase 1, RFC2, CYLN2, GTF2IRD, and GTF2. Hemizygosity of the *ELN* gene likely accounts for the associated cardiac defects, but cannot explain the hypercalcemia or other phenotypic features and developmental abnormalities. Williams syndrome has also been associated with other chromosomal abnormalities including an interstitial deletion of chromosome 6(q22.2q23), a terminal deletion of chromosome 4[46,XX,del(4)(q33)], as well as chromosomal translocations. However, the definitive basis remains unknown. In most cases, fluorescent *in situ* hybridization (FISH) using a probe for *ELN* is diagnostic.

Patients with Williams syndrome typically show exaggerated responses to pharmacological doses of vitamin D_2 and blunted calcitonin responses to calcium loading. Elevated plasma concentrations of calcitriol have been reported in some patients despite circulating levels of PTH that are low or normal. However, studies have failed to show any consistent abnormality in the metabolism of vitamin D that might explain these features. However, the discovery that the Williams syndrome transcription factor (WSTF) is part of a multiprotein regulatory complex that facilitates VDR genomic action, including transrepression of the 1-α-hydroxyase gene,[166] suggests aberrant activity of the vitamin D pathway may be responsible.

Some children with hypercalcemia show similar disturbances in vitamin D sensitivity but lack other phenotypic features of Williams syndrome and do not have a 7q11.13 deletion. This condition, which may be familial, has been termed "idiopathic infantile hypercalcemia" (IIH). The hypercalcemia in IIH usually resolves within the first few years of life, but persistent hypercalciuria is common. Clinical evaluation and genetic testing provide the ability to differentiate between Williams syndrome and IIH in more than 95% of cases.

Treatment. The most important aspect of the treatment of hypercalcemia is a low calcium diet with elimination of vitamin D. The daily calcium intake should be kept below 100 mg and preferably as low as 25 to 35 mg. Both elimination of vitamin D intake and protection from excessive exposure to direct sunlight are helpful. Maintenance of the low calcium, low vitamin D diet for at least 9 months after the serum calcium has become normal is recommended. Corticosteroids may be a useful adjunct in the acute stage to induce rapid lowering of the plasma calcium level. Steroid therapy can usually be discontinued after a few days when the diet has produced its effects.

Hypervitaminosis D
Pathogenesis. Hypercalcemia resulting from hypervitaminosis D is usually seen as a complication of vitamin D overtreatment of hypoparathyroidism, pseudohypoparathyroidism, hypophosphatemic rickets, or renal osteodystrophy. Neonates whose mothers ingest excessive amounts of vitamin D and/or its derivatives during pregnancy can develop hypercalcemia. This excessive intake usually occurs during treatment of the mother for a hypocalcemic disorder, but can occur by self-medication. Rarely, excessive vitamin supplements over a long period of time lead to hypervitaminosis D in infants. Approximately 2000 units/kg body weight per day as vitamin D_2 or vitamin D_3 over a period of many months will cause hypercalcemia and hypercalciuria in most patients, and 20,000 to 40,000 units per day can

lead to fatal hypercalcemia in infants. Intermittent high-dosage vitamin D prophylaxis, or so-called "Stosstherapie," which has been used for the prevention of rickets in some central European countries, is another cause of hypervitaminosis D, and may lead to transient hypercalcemia, hypercalciuria, and nephrocalcinosis. A typical "Stosstherapie" scheme that provides an oral dosage of 6,00,000 IU, or 15 mg vitamin D, every 3 to 5 months for the first 18 months of life, is clearly excessive, and must be considered unsafe. Excessive fortification of milk with vitamin D is an unusual cause of vitamin D intoxication and hypercalcemia. Hypervitaminosis D produces hypercalcemia by increasing the intestinal absorption of calcium and enhancing bone resorption.

Clinical presentation. The symptoms are those of hypercalcemia and include anorexia, constipation, nausea, vomiting, polydipsia, polyuria, and failure to thrive, but the earliest evidence of vitamin D intoxication may be the development of renal complications such as polyuria, hematuria, or nephrocalcinosis. In infants and young children, roentgenographic examination may show a characteristic intense line of mineralization of the provisional zone of calcification at the metaphyseal end of the long bones. The line is not only denser, but also usually wider than the line of calcified cartilage seen in normal growing bone. The skull may also show increased density of mineralization of the base and the orbits. More prolonged hypercalcemia may lead to soft-tissue calcifications, nephrocalcinosis, and renal insufficiency.

Diagnosis. The plasma phosphate concentration is normal or high depending on the state of the renal function. Alkaline phosphatase activity is usually low. The plasma concentrations of 25(OH)D and 24,25-(OH)$_2$D are markedly elevated while plasma calcitriol usually remains within the normal range. Because vitamin D is stored in adipose tissue, elevated plasma concentrations of 25(OH)D may persist for months after withdrawal of vitamin D medication.

Treatment. If the hypercalcemia is only moderate, discontinuation of vitamin D treatment is usually sufficient. For patients requiring continued vitamin D intervention for an underlying disorder, vitamin D therapy can be reinstituted with a 20% to 50% lower dose when normocalcemia has been reestablished. With more severe hypercalcemia some of the measures discussed earlier in the emergency treatment of hypercalcemia may be instituted. Glucocorticoids (eg, prednisone at a dose of 1-2 mg/kg/day) can be of benefit.

Vitamin D has a prolonged and cumulative action but with a relatively wide therapeutic-toxic range. Therefore, vitamin D is no longer recommended as the drug of choice for high-dose replacement therapy, since

calcitriol and its analog 1-α-(OH)D$_3$ have the advantage of much shorter biological half-life in the event of inadvertent overdosage.

Hypervitaminosis A
Pathogenesis. Vitamin A is essential for normal bone growth and maturation. Deficiency of vitamin A may cause growth impairment, and excess vitamin A increases bone fragility and may be a rare cause of hypercalcemia. Excessive vitamin A intake nowadays is usually found among food faddists taking megavitamin preparations. In children excessive vitamin A intake has arisen from use of candy-like chewable vitamin supplements. Excessive vitamin A intake has also been described in the setting of supplementation in the context of cystic fibrosis. Neonates and children who have impaired renal function appear to be at particular risk of vitamin A-induced hypercalcemia. More recently, severe hypercalcemia has been associated with the administration of the vitamin D analog all-trans-retinoic acid (ATRA) during therapy for acute promyelocytic leukemia. Historically, acute vitamin A intoxication occurred in the Arctic explorers and hunters who ate the liver of seals and polar bears, which are rich in vitamin A. The pathophysiology of the hypercalcemia involves vitamin A stimulation of osteoclastic bone resorption.

Clinical Presentation. Chronic hypervitaminosis A appears after ingestion of excessive doses for several weeks or months. The child develops anorexia, pruritus, yellow-orange skin pigmentation (with white sclerae), pseudotumor cerebri, irritability, bone pain, and tender swellings of bone. Roentgenograms might show osteopenia, signs of increased osteoclastic bone resorption, hyperostosis of the shafts of the long bones, periosteal calcifications particularly in the hands, and osteophyte formation, particularly in the thoracic spine.

Treatment. Spontaneous recovery with alleviation of hypercalcemia follows discontinuation of vitamin A intake. In cases of severe hypercalcemia, patients can be treated using the same approach as for hypervitaminosis D.

Subcutaneous fat necrosis
Clinical presentation. Subcutaneous fat necrosis is common in neonates with a complicated delivery and may lead to hypercalcemia within days or weeks of birth. The subcutaneous fat necrosis usually develops within 1 to 2 weeks after birth and presents as reddish or purple subcutaneous nodules at sites of pressure such as the back, buttocks, and thighs or in areas of direct trauma that occur during a difficult birth process, such as with forceps or vacuum extraction. Failure-to-thrive

is the most common clinical sign associated with subcutaneous fat necrosis, which is associated with a surprisingly high 15% mortality. Affected infants often have a history of birth asphyxia. X-ray examination might show calcifications in the kidney and increased mineralization at the metaphyses of the long bones.

Pathogenesis. The histopathological findings are subcutaneous fat necrosis with mononuclear and giant-cell infiltration. Hypercalcemia results from excess circulating 1,25-(OH)$_2$D that is produced by macrophages present within the granulomatous reaction to the necrotic fat. The hypercalcemia is also compounded by calcium release from fat tissues and increased prostaglandin E activity. The macrophages express ectopic 25-(OH)D$_3$-1-α-hydroxylase activity that is not regulated by PTH, calcium, phosphorus, or 1,25-(OH)$_2$D but which is responsive to glucocorticoids.

Treatment. Severe hypercalcemia may require emergency medical treatment according to the principles described under the section on neonatal primary hyperparathyroidism stated earlier. Glucocorticoids (eg, prednisone at a dose of 1-2 mg/kg/day) may be effective both in lowering plasma calcium concentration and dampening the inflammation of the fat necrosis. Calcitonin and even bisphosphonates can be beneficial for long-term management of mild but symptomatic hypercalcemia. The hypercalcemia may persist for weeks, and the infant should be given a low calcium, reduced vitamin D diet until the plasma and/or urinary calcium concentration normalizes.

Phosphate depletion

Pathogenesis. Hypercalcemia in association with phosphate depletion is most commonly seen in low-birth-weight infants who are fed human milk, which has relatively low phosphate content. The laboratory evaluation of hypercalcemia must include determination of the serum phosphorus concentration, a step that is often overlooked now that phosphorus measurement is no longer included as a standard component of the comprehensive metabolic panels (eg, SMAC or SMA12) that are processed using multichannel autoanalyzers. Hypophosphatemia stimulates renal synthesis of calcitriol, which activates intestinal absorption and skeletal resorption of calcium (and phosphorus). In the presence of hypophosphatemia, only limited amounts of calcium can be deposited in the rapidly growing bones, and hypercalcemia and hypercalciuria result. The plasma concentration of 25(OH)D is normal.

Hypophosphatemia not uncommonly leads to the development of rickets, which of course does not respond to standard therapy with vitamin D.

Treatment. Both the hypercalcemia and rickets respond to phosphate repletion, which can be achieved by supplementing human milk with 30 to 40 mg/kg/day of phosphorus as disodium phosphate, or by switching from human milk to a proprietary formula with higher phosphate content.

Malignancy associated hypercalcemia

Hypercalcemia occurs in less than 1% of children with cancer. Hypercalcemia has been associated with many kinds of cancer in children including leukemia, lymphoma, myeloma, neuroblastoma, hepatocellular carcinoma, hepatoblastoma, rhabdomyosarcoma, brain, and ovarian tumors. Two mechanisms account for the development of hypercalcemia with nonparathyroid tumors: (1) direct invasion of the skeleton by tumor cells and (2) tumor secretion of humoral factors. The most commonly identified humoral factor to cause hypercalcemia of malignancy is PTH-related peptide (PTHrP), which acts not only as a paracrine and intracrine factor, but under conditions of neoplastic derepression tumors can secrete sufficient PTHrP to yield circulating levels that are high enough to induce hypercalcemia via interaction with the type 1 PTH receptor.[167-169] The specific tumors that characteristically produce humoral hypercalcemia of malignancy via secretion of PTHrP include squamous cell carcinoma of the lung, head, and neck, renal cell carcinoma, breast carcinoma, adult T-cell leukemias, and multiple myeloma. Acute lymphoblastic leukemia is another important cause in children. Other tumor factors that play a role in producing hypercalcemia include prostaglandins, IL-1 and IL-6, transforming growth factor-β, tumor necrosis factor, and calcitriol. Specific treatment of hypercalcemia will often be necessary in conjunction with aggressive therapy of the underlying malignancy. Vigorous hydration and intravenous bisphosphonates constitute the primary approach to management of malignancy-associated hypercalcemia, but glucocorticoids will be effective when calcitriol is the tumor-derived mediator of hypercalcemia.

Immobilization

Epidemiology. During the poliomyelitis epidemic of the 1950s, prolonged immobilization of children and young adults was commonly associated with hypercalcemia and/or hypercalciuria. In recent years, immobilization hypercalciuria and hypercalcemia have most frequently been encountered in adolescents and young adults immobilized by spinal-cord injuries or by multiple skeletal fractures requiring extensive plaster casts. However, hypercalcemia can occur in growing children and adolescents after single-limb fractures. In fact, the most typical scenario is the active adolescent boy who has experienced a femur fracture. The sudden transition from an active physical life to complete immobilization, especially if both extremities are immobilized, can cause severe hypercalcemia. Infants and children who have any disorder causing limited mobility, especially those who are wheelchair-bound or bedridden, are at high risk for developing immobilization hypercalcemia.

Pathogenesis. Hypercalcemia associated with immobilization arises from increased bone resorption relative to bone formation. Immobilization of a rapidly growing child will lead to a marked decrease in osteoblastic bone formation and a dramatic increase in osteoclastic bone resorption. This imbalance in bone remodeling causes increased movement of calcium (and phosphorus) out of the skeleton with a consequent net loss of bone mass that is termed disuse osteoporosis. Hypercalciuria can develop within a few days of immobilization, and hypercalcemia may follow within 1 to 3 weeks. In most cases the hypercalcemia is moderate, but the plasma calcium concentration may rise as high as 18 mg/dL (4.5 mmol/L).

The immobilization-induced hypercalcemia and/or hypercalciuria arise from a primary bone resorbing process in which the PTH-calcitriol axis is suppressed. The diminished PTH-induced calcium reabsorption in the distal nephron and the reduction of calcitriol synthesis, and thereby reduced intestinal calcium absorption, presumably serve as protective mechanisms minimizing the possibility that increased skeletal calcium resorption will lead to hypercalcemia.

Clinical presentation. Hypercalciuria may lead to calcium oxalate nephrolithiasis and can cause abdominal pain mimicking an acute surgical crisis. Evidence of impaired renal function with reduced creatinine clearance is a common finding. Plasma phosphate values and the renal phosphate threshold (TmP/GFR) are elevated or high normal. Hypercalcemia is often overlooked in an immobilized child. The child's anorexia, nausea, weight loss, lethargy, and depression might be attributed to hospitalization and immobilization rather than hypercalcemia.

Treatment. Restriction of calcium in the diet of immobilized patients has no effect on urinary calcium excretion. Dietary calcium restriction, with its concomitant limitations in protein intake and selection of foods, therefore have no place in the management of immobilization hypercalcemia and hypercalciuria. The treatment should be aimed at prevention by mobilizing the patient as much as possible. Patients with mild hypercalcemia should be maintained on a high sodium and water intake to increase urinary calcium excretion and prevent hypercalcemic crisis. If plasma calcium exceeds 14 mg/dL (3.5 mmol/L), saline infusion should be started as outlined above. The recent demonstration that bisphosphonates can rapidly reverse the hypercalcemia and hypercalciuria of immobilization provides additional justification to monitor young patients for the development of these complications.[170-172]

Miscellaneous conditions associated with hypercalcemia

Many inborn disorders of metabolism are associated with hypercalcemia (Table 6-11). *Blue diaper syndrome* is caused by a defect in tryptophan metabolism. The block in tryptophan metabolism leads to urinary excretion of excessive amounts of indole derivatives, including a derivative called "indican" that gives the urine-soaked diaper a blue tint. The mechanism of hypercalcemia in this disorder is unknown.

Congenital lactase deficiency can cause hypercalcemia and medullary nephrocalcinosis during the first few months of life. The hypercalcemia resolves after initiation of a lactose-free diet, but later in childhood (ages 2-10 years) patients may still have hypercalciuria and/or nephrocalcinosis. The etiology of the hypercalcemia

Table 6-11.

Inborn Errors of Metabolism Associated with Hypercalcemia

	Clinical Manifestations	Etiology of Hypercalcemia	
Blue diaper syndrome	Indicanuria Nephrocalcinosis	Unknown	Defect in tryptophan metabolism
Congenital lactase deficiency	Watery diarrhea	?metabolic acidosis ?increased intestinal calcium absorption owing to increased gut lactose	Recessive *LCT* mutations
Infantile hypophosphatasia	Premature loss of deciduous teeth, failure to thrive, hypotonia	Imbalance between intestinal calcium absorption and reduced skeletal deposition	Recessive *TNSALP* mutations ↑ urinary phosphoethanolamine

is unclear, but is thought to be related to metabolic acidosis and/or an increase in intestinal calcium absorption secondary to increased gut lactose.[173] A similar pathophysiology occurs in patients with disaccharide intolerance.

Several cases of hypercalcemia, hypercalciuria, and nephrocalcinosis have been reported in infants and toddlers with *Down syndrome*. The etiology of the hypercalcemia was initially thought to be secondary to overingestion of cow's milk. However, this has not been found in all cases. The hypercalcemia is now thought to be specifically associated with the genetic defect(s) of Down syndrome, although the mechanism remains unclear.

Hypophosphatasia is a rare inborn error of metabolism characterized by defective bone mineralization due to deficiency of tissue nonspecific alkaline phosphatase (TNSALP).[174,175] Five clinical forms of hypophosphatasia have been described: perinatal (lethal), infantile, childhood, adult, and odontohypophosphatasia. The most severe forms of the disease (perinatal and infantile) are transmitted as an autosomal recessive trait, while clinically milder forms, including childhood and adult hypophosphatasia and odontohypophosphatasia, demonstrate both autosomal recessive and autosomal dominant transmission. Premature loss of deciduous teeth in children less than 5 years of age is a significant clue to the diagnosis, and is the result of hypoplasia or aplasia of the dental cementum. Hypercalcemia is a feature of infantile hypophosphatasia, which presents before 6 months of age when failure to thrive and hypotonia become apparent. Hypercalcemia and hypercalciuria reflect an imbalance between intestinal calcium absorption and reduced skeletal deposition. Serum concentrations of calcitriol and PTH are low or suppressed in hypercalcemic patients.

The characteristic radiological findings are severe demineralization of the skeleton but less pronounced than in the perinatal form. The fontanels appear widely open due to hypomineralized areas of calvarium, but in fact functional craniosynostosis can occur with raised intracranial pressure.[176] Rachitic skeletal deformities, including flail chest, predispose to pneumonia and more than 50% of patients die during the first year of life (Case 6-7). Those children who survive beyond infancy seem to show some improvement.

TNSALP hydrolyzes inorganic pyrophosphate in a reaction that removes inorganic pyrophosphate (PPi), a potent inhibitor of hydroxyapatite crystal nucleation and growth, while providing inorganic monophosphate ions (Pi) that perhaps further condition mineralization. In hypophosphatasia excess extracellular inorganic pyrophosphate hinders hydroxyapatite crystal growth and proliferation and thereby impairs mineralization. Low plasma ALP, or hypophosphatasia, is the biochemical hallmark of hypophosphatasia, although some cases of cleidocranial dysplasia can also have low serum alkaline phosphatase. Increased urinary excretion of phosphoethanolamine

support the diagnosis, and this biochemical marker of the disorder is readily measured in most clinical laboratories as part of the quantitative amino acid profile. In addition to phosphoethanolamine, inorganic pyrophosphate is also elevated in plasma and in the urine. Serum pyridoxal-phosphate (PLP) concentrations are also markedly elevated, and in the absence of vitamin B_6 supplementation, an elevated serum PLP level is the most sensitive and specific marker for hypophosphatasia.

Traditional treatment for the rickets should be avoided because it exaggerates the hypercalcemia. Reduction of dietary calcium and glucocorticoid therapy may reduce the plasma concentration of calcium, but lead to further demineralization of the skeleton. Bone marrow transplantation and transplantation of bone fragments and cultured osteoblasts, and recombinant human alkaline phosphatase hold some promise as future therapies.

CLINICAL PRESENTATION AND MANAGEMENT OF HYPOPHOSPHATEMIA

Definitions and Classification

Hypophosphatemia is common in the various forms of vitamin D deficiency and dependency rickets and osteomalacia of moderate or severe degree. The hypophosphatemia predominantly reflects the decrease in TmP/GFR induced by secondary hyperparathyroidism in these conditions (see "Parathyroid hormone; Action on Kidney"). However, several other disorders leading to rickets or osteomalacia, are recognized in which hypophosphatemia occurs in the absence of vitamin D deficiency, and with minimal, if any, hyperparathyroidism and without significant net changes in serum concentrations of PTH or calcium (Table 6-12). These diseases, which are characterized by hypophosphatemia, hyperphosphaturia, and defective bone mineralization include X-linked and autosomal forms of hypophosphatemia and tumor induced osteomalacia (TIO). The observation that patients with these diseases generally have low or normal serum calcitriol concentrations, despite hypophosphatemia, had historically been unexpected given that low phosphate should stimulate 1-α-hydroxylase activity. The discovery of circulating humoral factors that alter phosphate regulation has provided significant insight into these syndromes. In these forms of phosphopenic, vitamin D-resistant rickets, the hypophosphatemia is caused by decreased renal tubular reabsorption of phosphate. The tubular phosphate transport may be affected alone, or in association with defective transport of glucose or glycine, or as part of a multiple renal tubular defect as seen in Fanconi syndrome.

Table 6-12.

Classification of Hypophosphatemic States

Inadequate intestinal absorption of phosphate
Poor nutrition
Chelation by phosphate-binders
Total parental nutrition

Renal loss of phosphate
Genetic forms of hypophosphatemic rickets
Tumor-associated hypophosphatemic rickets
Hypophosphatemic rickets with hypercalciuria
Fanconi syndrome
Nephropathic cystinosis
Tyrosinosis, type 1
Lowe syndrome
Hereditary fructose intolerance
Wilson disease
Renal tubular acidosis

Other causes
Intracellular shift

Differential Diagnosis

Genetic forms of hypophosphatemic rickets

Familial X-linked hypophosphatemic rickets (XLH) (also termed hypophosphatemic vitamin D-resistant rickets, MIM 307800) is the most common form of inherited hypophosphatemia, but autosomal dominant and autosomal recessive hypophosphatemic rickets share many features in common. In each condition, reabsorption of phosphate in the proximal renal tubule is reduced and metabolism of vitamin D is impaired. Serum levels of phosphate are reduced, and serum calcitriol levels are inappropriately normal while serum calcium and PTH levels are normal (Table 6-8). Aberrant regulation of the 25-(OH)-D-1-α-hydroxylase accounts for the paradoxical occurrence of inappropriately normal or reduced calcitriol levels in the presence of hypophosphatemia. In children with active rickets, a variable degree of reduced intestinal absorption of both phosphate and calcium also occurs.

X-linked hypophosphatemic rickets

Epidemiology. Despite occasional sporadic cases, as well as families with autosomal dominant inheritance, most cases of familial hypophosphatemic rickets are transmitted as an X-linked dominant trait with no evidence of a gene dosage effect, imprinting, or genetic anticipation, and little, if any, difference in the severity or extent of the disorder in affected males and females has been found. XLH has a prevalence of approximately 1 in 20,000 and accounts for 80% of cases of familial phosphate wasting.

Pathogenesis. XLH is caused by mutations in the *PHEX* gene (phosphate regulating gene with homologies to endopeptidases on the X chromosome). *PHEX*, located on Xp22.1, is composed of 22 exons and encodes a 749-amino acid protein. At present, the native substrate for the *PHEX* enzyme has not yet been identified. *PHEX* is expressed in a restricted fashion and is found in osteoblasts, odontoblasts, ovary, lung, parathyroids, brain, and muscle. Notably, *PHEX* is not expressed in kidney.

A wide range of *PHEX* defects have been identified in patients with XLH, and include deletions, insertions, duplications, as well as missense and nonsense mutations and splice site mutations (see http://www.phexdb.mcgill.ca/ for Phexdatabase). These defects are scattered throughout the gene and invariably result in loss of function. Commercial laboratories now provide clinical testing for mutations in the *PHEX* gene, and defects can be identified in approximately 80% of patients with suspected XLH. However, the presence of the trait may be readily ascertained in most patients by 6 months of age by determination of plasma phosphate concentration. Extensive analysis of phenotype/genotype relationships has failed to show a correlation between severity of disease and type or location of *PHEX* mutation. Because *PHEX* is located on the X chromosome, random X chromosome inactivation in females is predicted to result in a less severe phenotype compared with males who are completely *PHEX* deficient. However, males and females seem to be affected equally with similar biochemical indices and skeletal manifestations. X chromosome inactivation analysis of the *PHEX* gene has demonstrated that the *PHEX* gene is randomly inactivated. Thus, preferential inactivation of the normal *PHEX* allele is excluded as a potential basis for the similar phenotype observed between males and females with XLH.

Animal studies confirm the presence of a circulating factor that inhibits renal phosphate reabsorption through down regulation of the sodium-dependent phosphate cotransporter, NPT2a/Npt2a, which is expressed in the renal tubule cell. A similar pathogenetic mechanism was shown to be operative in XLH after transplantation of an unaffected sister's kidney into a brother with XLH led to renal phosphate wasting by the normal kidney.[177]

In addition to hypophosphatemia, an intrinsic osteoblast defect also contributes to the bone disease in XLH. Even after adequate treatment with phosphorus and calcitriol, XLH patients continue to have hypomineralized periosteocytic lesions in bone. The dual defect in the osteoblast and evidence for a humoral factor has led to the hypothesis that the intrinsic bone defect leads to release of humoral factors that effect bone mineralization, calcitriol synthesis, and proximal tubular Pi absorption.

Finally, abnormalities in the metabolism of vitamin D are also characteristic of individuals with XLH, and levels of serum calcitriol are inappropriately normal for the degree of hypophosphatemia. Stimulators of calcitriol synthesis such as PTH or low phosphate diets fail to increase calcitriol synthesis in patients with XLH. The pathogenesis of the renal phosphate wasting is dissociable from the vitamin D synthetic defect. This suggests that the circulating phosphaturic factor implicated in XLH and other hypophosphatemic syndromes has two independent effects—one inhibits renal phosphate conservation and the other impairs renal calcitriol synthesis.

Clinical presentation. The primary clinical manifestations of hypophosphatemic rickets are skeletal pain and deformity, bone fractures, slipped epiphyses, and abnormalities of growth. Classic skeletal features of rickets, such as frontal bossing, may appear as early as 6 months of age in untreated infants. Boys with XLH have early severe deformities viz., shortness of stature and skeletal disproportions, which become apparent during childhood with the legs short relative to the trunk. The deformities include bilateral coxa vara, anterior and lateral femoral bowing, genu valgum or varum, and medial deviation and torsion of the lower one-third of the tibia (Case 6-8). Unlike the findings in infants with vitamin D deficiency rickets, craniotabes and rachitic rosary are not seen. Proximal myopathy is absent in contrast to the findings in hypophosphatemia that occurs in patients with tumor induced osteomalacia or antacid-induced hypophosphatemia. Thus, the waddling gait seen in boys and severely affected girls is probably owing to coxa vara. Poor dental development and spontaneous tooth abscesses may occur. Considerable variation in the severity of the disease particularly is seen among girls and between families. Although the genetic defect is highly penetrant, the severity of disease and specific clinical manifestations are variable, even among members of the same family.

The roentgenological manifestations are evident by 1 to 2 years of age and include widening, splaying and cupping of the metaphyses, and coarse trabeculation of the whole skeleton. These findings are most pronounced in the lower extremities. The characteristic wedge-shaped defect of the medial surface of proximal tibia in patients with genu varum deformity is probably the result of the increased weight on the medial side of the knee (Case 6-4).

Diagnosis. The renal reabsorption of phosphate is the main determinant of plasma phosphate concentration, and the TmP/GFR is the most reliable estimate of the overall tubular phosphate transport capacity. TmP/GFR in patients with hypophosphatemic rickets is depressed to less than 2 mg/dL compared with 4.0 to 5.9 mg/dL in normal children from 6 to 14 years of age. Because of placental phosphate transport, the plasma phosphate concentration is normal at birth even when the mother has XLH. During the course of the next few months of life the plasma phosphate decreases, but diagnostic hypophosphatemia, that is, plasma phosphate below 4 mg/dL (1.3 mmol/L), may not be found until 6 months of age. The growth of the affected infant is also within normal range for the first 6 to 9 months of life, but as plasma phosphate decreases, the growth rate diminishes and stunted growth becomes manifest during early childhood.

Elevation of the plasma alkaline phosphatase activity is an early and useful indicator of rickets even before the hypophosphatemia becomes manifest. The plasma calcium concentration is normal or low normal, and the PTH concentration is usually normal. The plasma concentration of calcitriol in untreated patients is also within normal limits, but may be considered inappropriately low in view of the hypophosphatemia. Urinary cAMP excretion is normal, and aminoaciduria is not a feature of XLH.

Treatment. Optimal management includes combined treatment with oral phosphate and calcitriol or 1-α-OHD. Patients respond extremely well to a regimen of adequate phosphate and calcitriol, but healing of rickets and osteomalacia are not universal outcomes. Combined therapy often improves growth velocity, and if treatment starts before 5 years of age a catch-up growth and spontaneous correction of lower limb deformities can be obtained. However, refractoriness to growth-promoting effects of treatment is not uncommon, and some patients may benefit from treatment with recombinant growth hormone. Use of growth hormone alone, however, may aggravate skeletal deformities in this population despite improving phosphate and vitamin D status.[178] In treated girls with XLH, the pubertal growth is nearly normal despite suboptimal metabolic control, and the major height loss occurs prior to puberty and is not recovered during the pubertal growth spurt.

The recommended therapy consists of 1 to 3 g of elemental phosphorus daily in four to six divided doses to achieve a maintenance serum phosphate concentration of at least 1 mmol/L (3.1 mg/dL). To avoid gastrointestinal intolerance of phosphate, the initial dose should be small and increased slowly over several months. The initial dose of calcitriol is 15 to 20 ng/kg/day, and is increased over several months to a maintenance dose of 30 to 60 ng/ kg/day. During long-term treatment, the plasma concentrations of calcium, phosphate, and PTH and the alkaline phosphatase activity as well as urine calcium/ creatinine ratios should be monitored by regular checkups at 1 to 3 month intervals. A urinary calcium/creatinine (both in mg/dL) ratio above 0.25 is indicative of hypercalciuria and that the calcitriol dosage should be decreased. In patients in whom the calcitriol dose is inadequate obligating high dose oral phosphate therapy, a secondary hyperparathyroidism, which can exaggerate the renal tubular loss of phosphate, can occur. If not managed properly, secondary hyperparathyroidism can progress to autonomous (so-called "tertiary") hyperparathyroidism.

Radiologic evaluation of the hands, wrists, ankles, and knees as well as renal ultrasound examinations should be carried out at 12-month intervals to assess healing of rickets and provide early detection of nephrocalcinosis. Using a sensitive ultrasonographic grading score to detect early changes, nephrocalcinosis has been detected in about 75% of patients on combined phosphate/calcitriol therapy, with a significant association between the severity of nephrocalcinosis and the dose of phosphate. Progression of nephrocalcinosis may be prevented by use of thiazide diuretics. Regular renal imaging and frequent assessment of renal function are therefore essential in the long-term care of the patients. Additional complications of combined therapy include cardiovascular abnormalities such as hypertension and ventricular hypertrophy.

If skeletal deformities are severe enough that joint damage might ensue, corrective osteotomies can be considered during the growing period. Because of the short half-life of calcitriol and 1-α-(OH)D, interrupting these treatments prior to surgery is not necessary, and the combined phosphate/calcitriol regimen can be maintained throughout the hospitalization period. However, monitoring the urinary calcium excretion is mandatory. If the urinary calcium to creatinine ratio becomes greater than 0.25, calcitriol should be stopped for a few days.

Autosomal dominant hypophosphatemic rickets
Clinical Presentation. Autosomal dominant hypophosphatemic rickets (ADHR; OMIM 193100) is characterized by low serum phosphorus concentration, phosphaturia, inappropriately low or normal calcitriol levels, and bone mineralization defects that result in rickets, osteomalacia with bone pain, lower extremity deformities, and muscle weakness. By contrast to XLH, greater variability in the age of onset and expression of the biochemical and clinical features of ADHR is apparent. Those with childhood onset look phenotypically like XLH, but some patients present with an apparent adult onset form of the disorder, with osteomalacia, bone pain, weakness, and fractures, but no skeletal deformity. Thus, ADHR is a phenotypically variable disorder with incomplete penetrance, delayed onset, and, in several kindreds, postpubertal reversal of renal phosphate wasting.

Dental abscesses are a prominent feature of the syndrome. The pattern of inheritance with evidence of male-to-male transmission and the phenotypic variability distinguish this disorder from XLH.

Pathogenesis. Specific mutations in fibroblast growth factor (FGF)-23 were identified in several kindreds with ADHR.[179]

Treatment. Treatment of ADHR is similar to the treatment of XLH described earlier.

Autosomal recessive hypophosphatemic rickets.
Recently, individuals from two separate families were described as having recessive hypophosphatemic rickets. In one family, rickets was evident in infancy while in the other mild genu valgum was noted later in childhood. The affected individuals had biochemical data consistent with other forms of hypophosphatemic rickets: decreased serum phosphate, decreased TmP/GFR, increased alkaline phosphatase, inappropriately normal calcitriol, increased FGF-23, and eucalciuria. Based upon the hypophosphatemic rickets observed in mice null for the DMP gene which encodes dentin matrix protein 1 (DMP1) expressed in osteocytes, mutations in *DMP* were sought and subsequently found in these individuals.[180,181] As DMP1 inhibits secretion of FGF-23 from osteocytes, it seems reasonable to assume that loss of DMP1 action accounts for the increase in circulating FGF-23 that occurs in these patients. Rickets is treated with calcitriol and phosphate.

Hypophosphatemic rickets with hypercalciuria.
Hypophosphatemic rickets with hypercalciuria is a distinct form of hypophosphatemic rickets that arises from mutations in the *SLC34A3* gene encoding the Npt2c sodium-phosphate cotransporter.[182,183] This condition is termed hereditary hypophosphatemic rickets with hypercalciuria (HHRH).

Pathogenesis. Patients with HHRH have hypophosphatemia and appropriately elevated serum levels of calcitriol. Such high levels of calcitriol may lead to a higher than usual efficiency of calcium absorption from the gastrointestinal tract, enhanced bone resorption, and reduced synthesis and secretion of PTH. Together, these changes in calcium homeostasis favor hypercalciuria and promote kidney stone formation.

Treatment. Treatment with phosphate salts alone has resulted in improvement of clinical and roentgenological abnormalities, decreases urinary calcium excretion and plasma concentration of calcitriol, and reverses hypophosphatemia.[184,185] Vitamin D treatment is contraindicated in this condition because it may further increase intestinal absorption of calcium and increase the risk of nephrolithiasis.

Tumor-associated hypophosphatemia

Definitions and epidemiology. Hypophosphatemic rickets associated with neoplasia, so called tumor-induced osteomalacia (TIO), is uncommon, and fewer than 20% of affected patients are younger than 20 years at presentation. The cardinal feature of the condition is the remission of the rickets or osteomalacia after the resection of the coexisting tumor. The tumors are of most commonly of a primitive, mixed connective tissue or mesenchymal origin and typically behave in a benign manner. The tumors may be located either within the bone or in extraskeletal connective tissue. They have included histiocytoma, hemangiopericytoma, fibroangioma, and ossifying mesenchymal tumors as well as malignancies such as breast, lung, and prostate carcinoma and chronic lymphocytic leukemia. Similar features also occur in patients with widespread fibrous dysplasia of bone, the linear sebaceous nevus syndrome, and neurofibromatous.

Clinical presentation. Patients with TIO have severe hypophosphataemia, which results in osteomalacia, bone fractures, and generalized muscle weakness, most pronounced in the proximal muscle groups of the lower extremities. The biochemical findings include normocalcemia, elevated alkaline phosphatase activity, hypophosphatemia, and markedly diminished TmP/GFR, indicative of renal phosphate wasting. In addition, the plasma concentration of calcitriol is markedly decreased despite hypophosphatemia.

Pathogenesis. The pathophysiological basis for tumor-associated rickets and osteomalacia is the excessive production of phosphatonin(s) by the tumor or abnormal tissue. Several lines of evidence implicate FGF-23 as a leading candidate for the tumor-associated phosphatonin.

Treatment. Conventional treatment with oral phosphate and calcitriol is often inadequate and frequently leads to complications. By contrast, surgical resection of tumors results in prompt resolution of biochemical defects and remineralization of bone.[186] Thus, the preferred, and only curative, treatment of TIO is surgical removal of the tumor, which of course is predicated on successful localization of the tumor.

If no tumor can be found and removed after careful search, the patients should be given combined treatment with calcitriol and oral phosphate as outlined above for the treatment of XLH, and they should be monitored carefully.

Renal disorders associated with hypophosphatemia

Tables 6-13 and 6-14 summarize renal disorders associated with hypophosphatemia .

Metabolic bone disease of prematurity

Definitions and epidemiology. Bone disease, or rickets of prematurity occurs mainly in small premature infants with birth weights less than 1500 g who are fed with breast milk or regular commercial infant formulas, or in ill newborns on total parenteral nutrition. Even when the vitamin D intake is adequate, these infants may develop osteopenia and rickets because of an insufficient supply of calcium and phosphate to meet the needs of bone mineral accretion after birth.

Pathogenesis. Mineral accretion rates for both calcium and phosphate increase through pregnancy to

Table 6-13.

Inborn Errors of Metabolism Associated with Fanconi Syndrome

Disorder	Additional Clinical Features	Disease-Specific Treatment	Genetic Mutation
Nephropathic cystinosis	Growth failure, hypothyroidism, blond hair, fair complexion (melanin synthesis defect), photophobia (owing to conjunctival cystine crystals)	Cysteamine	AR *CTNS* mutations
Tyrosinosis type 1	FTT, progressive cirrhosis	NTBC	AR *FAH* mutations
Lowe syndrome	Buphthalmos, glaucoma, cataract, blindness, severe muscle hypotonia, mental retardation		XR *OCRL* mutations
Hereditary fructose intolerance	Fructose-induced liver injury	Fructose avoidance	AR *ALDOB* mutations

AR, autosomal recessive; XR, X-linked recessive.

Table 6-14.

A General Classification of Childhood Osteoporosis

Category	Diagnosis	Comment
Genetic disorders of connective tissue or osteoblast	Osteogenesis imperfecta Ehlers-Danlos syndrome Marfan syndrome (some) Homocystinuria Lysinuric protein intolerance Osteoporosis-pseudoglioma syndrome	
Locally mediated bone resorption	Malignancy Sickle cell anemia Thalassemia Other causes of bone marrow expansion or proliferation	Skeletal pain may be severe May be exacerbated by chelating agents used to manage iron overload
Cytokine-mediated catabolic states affecting connective tissue matrix	Inflammatory bowel disease Inflammatory arthritis	May be worsened by corticosteroid use
Endocrine and metabolic	Hyperparathyroidism Hypercortisolism Thyrotoxicosis Pubertal disorders Hypogonadism Anorexia nervosa	Includes Klinefelter and Turner syndromes, congenital adrenal hyperplasia, aromatase deficiency, and estrogen receptor defects
Disuse and underuse	Paraplegia Muscular dystrophy Cerebral palsy	
Unclassified	Idiopathic juvenile osteoporosis	Usually remits at puberty; heritable disorders of collagen identified in some cases

reach a maximum during the third trimester of about 150 mg/kg/day for calcium and about 70 mg/kg/day for phosphate. Human milk fed at 200 mL/kg/day will provide only one-fifth of the intrauterine supply of calcium and only about one-third of the requirement for phosphate. During the 48 hours after birth, PTH secretion increases two- to fivefold, and in response, the kidney reabsorbs calcium and actively excretes phosphate. Phosphate depletion is therefore more likely to develop more rapidly because of initial urinary loss, and because the protoplasmic metabolic requirements for phosphate are greater than for calcium. Preterm infants fed human milk are therefore at particular risk of phosphopenia. The resulting hypophosphatemia stimulates the renal production of calcitriol. By the third day of life, the plasma concentration of calcitriol is markedly increased, which in turn increases the intestinal absorption of both calcium and phosphate and inhibits PTH secretion.

These pathophysiological events are reflected by a fall in the plasma phosphate from 6.2 mg/dL to 3.1-4.6 mg/dL (2 mmol/L to 1.0-1.5 mmol/L) over the first week. The plasma phosphate concentrations often reach a nadir during the second week after birth. In infants depleted of phosphate as a result of poor intake and urinary loss, a further reduction to less than 3.1 mg/dL (1 mmol/L) may occur, and this has been reported to be associated with the later development of biochemical and radiological evidence of bone disease. As already alluded to, the urinary phosphate excretion initially may be increased but by day 5 is usually negligible. By contrast, because of increased calcitriol stimulated intestinal absorption and diminished PTH-dependent renal reabsorption, urinary calcium losses increase and persist during the period that tissue phosphate stores remain depleted. For practical purposes, a prolonged absence of phosphate from urine with persisting calciuria would imply continued phosphate depletion and the need for further mineral supplementation.

The natural history of plasma alkaline phosphatase activity is to rise over the first 3 weeks, reaching a plateau by the age of 5 to 6 weeks. Rises that occur after this are seen principally in infants with persistently low plasma phosphate concentrations receiving low phosphate diets. Peak concentrations of greater than 5 to 7.5 times the maximum adult normal value for the particular alkaline phosphatase assay used have been associated with reduced linear growth velocity and growth potential. Roentgenological changes of bone disease are usually not seen until the age of 6 weeks, with reduced bone density and cupping, splaying and fraying of metaphyses, and, in severe cases, fractures of ribs and long bones.

Treatment. The management of bone disease of prematurity should essentially follow the dictum "Prevention is better than cure." Vitamin D should be given routinely to all preterm infants in a daily dose of 400 to 600 IU (10-15 μg). In clinical practice, the infants likely to require mineral supplementation are those with a birth weight less than 1500 g. A reasonable prophylactic measure would be to add 30 to 40 mg/kg/day of inorganic phosphorus and 50 to 60 mg/kg/day of elemental calcium to the expressed breast milk or a regular formula. Addition of the phosphorus salt, usually disodium phosphate, first is important so that it can enter the fat micelles. Calcium is usually given as gluconate or gluceptate, and an appreciable risk of precipitation exists if calcium is added before phosphorus. Supplementation should be given as soon as enteral feeds are started and continue until the infant has achieved a weight of 2000 g. A urinary calcium to phosphate ratio of more than 1.0 at the age of 3 weeks is an indication for further supplementation.

CLINICAL PRESENTATION AND MANAGEMENT OF OSTEOPOROSIS

Definition

In osteoporosis bone mass is reduced but mineralization is generally normal. The bones are thus rendered brittle and susceptible to fracture. Mild degrees of osteoporosis, insufficient to cause symptoms, are often referred to as osteopenia. The clinical definition of osteoporosis, as developed for the adult population, is a bone disorder associated with low bone mass relative to peak bone density and a propensity for fragility fractures. This definition cannot be applied to children, who have not yet achieved peak bone mass. Presently, no one clinical definition of osteoporosis in children is generally accepted, but a diagnosis of osteoporosis is reasonable in a child with low bone mass for age, gender, and race who has sustained a fragility fracture or skeletal deformity. A summary of some causes of osteoporosis in childhood is given in Table 6-14.

Assessment of Bone Mass

Assessment of bone mass in children has special challenges. Techniques to measure bone density in adults have assumed that bone mass is reflective of the extent and breadth of bone remodeling rates at specific sites,

such as the spine, and portions of the hip. In children, the growing skeleton undergoes both (1) modeling, with the processes of endosteal resorption and periosteal new bone formation occurring on distinct bone surfaces, and (2) remodeling, in which osteoclastic-mediated bone resorption is followed by osteoblast-directed bone formation on the same bone surface. Bone modeling occurs at many sites not measured by conventional bone densitometers, and alterations in modeling may account for much more of the lack of bone mass accretion than changes in remodeling. As a result, assessment of distinct trabecular and cortical bone compartments is more critical for understanding the bone mass dynamics in children than in adults.

Dual energy x-ray absorptiometry (DXA) is the preferred technique to assess bone mineral density (BMD). DXA can provide highly accurate measurements of BMD in adults, but this technique has significant deficiencies when used to assess BMD in growing children. For example, because DXA provides an analysis of areal bone mineral density (aBMD), rather than a true determination of volumetric bone mineral density (vBMD), the size (ie, area) of the bone assessed will have a disproportionate impact on the derived measurements for BMD (Figure 6-19). Because the size of bones is related to the height of a child, databases must be developed that account for height-adjusted age. Other variables that affect the reliability of DXA in children include pubertal status and body composition. Overall, the application of DXA to measurement of BMD in young patients is limited by the lack of appropriate reference databases that allow for adjustments, if any, for bone size or height,

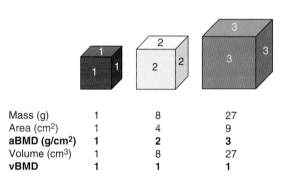

Mass (g)	1	8	27
Area (cm²)	1	4	9
aBMD (g/cm²)	**1**	**2**	**3**
Volume (cm³)	1	8	27
vBMD	**1**	**1**	**1**

FIGURE 6-19 ■ Technical limitation of dual x-ray absorptiometry. Total bone mineral density describes the amount of bone mineral (bone mass) divided by the bone volume, the volume enclosed by the periosteal bone surface. Because DXA is a two-dimensional projection technique, it cannot measure volume directly. Instead, bone volume is approximated through geometric algorithms, and an areal bone mineral density (aBMD) rather than a volumetric BMD (vBMD) is derived. As a result, BMD may be underestimated in smaller bones. As shown above, the true density (mass/volume) of all cubes is 1 g/cm³, but the aBMD varies with bone size when the aBMD (mass/area) is derived.

weight, maturity, pubertal status, and other clinical variables. Not surprisingly, given these unique characteristics of growing children, interpretation of their DXA results is often incorrect or inadequate.

By contrast, quantitative computed tomography (qCT) can accurately determine vBMD in children, with separation of cortical and trabecular compartments. However, qCT is not satisfactory for repeated testing because of the relatively high radiation dose delivered. A more promising application of qCT in children and adolescents is based on application of the technology to assess bone density in peripheral bone sites (pQCT). The lower radiation exposure of pQCT allows for repeated studies, which may encourage wider use of this technology in the future.

Ultrasound technology has been applied to both measurement of bone mass and assessment of bone strength in adults and children, and is an attractive option with great promise for future clinical use in children.

A general limitation of bone densitometry in children derives from uncertainty regarding the clinical implications of low BMD. In children, upper extremity fractures, particularly forearm fractures, appear to be associated with reduced BMD. However, BMD alone likely does not explain fracture risk in children (or adults), and bone quality, bone turnover, and the nature of trauma are also likely to be important contributors to the risk of fractures. Thus, BMD criteria for "fracture threshold" in children have not been established. By contrast, the proven association between low BMD and fractures in older adults led the World Health Organization (WHO) to propose quantitative criteria for "osteopenia" and "osteoporosis" that are based solely on BMD T scores, which reflect the number of standard deviation's above or below peak bone mass. Expressing BMD in children using T scores is inappropriate, as children and adolescents have not yet achieved peak bone mass, and they will normally have negative T scores. The use of T scores, rather than age-adjusted Z scores, to express BMD in children and adolescents is a leading cause of misinterpretation of bone densitometry, and often leads to an inappropriate diagnosis of osteoporosis. Taken in context, bone densitometry can be a valuable *adjunct* in the diagnosis of osteoporosis in children and adolescents, but by itself should not be relied upon to provide a clinical diagnosis.

Differential Diagnosis

The sensitivity of the developing skeleton to nutrition and exercise is still unknown, but deprivation of protein, vitamin D, and minerals can reduce bone mass and or quality. Similarly, the absence of weight-bearing exercise, such as with immobilization, leads to increased bone resorption and a consequent reduction in bone mass.

In severely affected children, low impact (fragility) fractures begin in childhood, and skeletal pain and bone deformities may occur. Table 6-14 provides a general classification of osteoporosis in children and adolescents.

In children, osteopenia is often a consequence of disuse atrophy of the skeleton (eg, after immobilization for severe trauma), neuromuscular disease (eg, Duchenne muscular dystrophy), or a consequence of glucocorticoid therapy. Osteoporosis is also seen in association with malignancy (eg, leukemia or neuroblastoma) and in cancer survivors, and after bone marrow and solid organ transplantation. Low bone density is also present in many children with celiac disease as well as many chronic inflammatory diseases (eg, inflammatory bowel disease and juvenile idiopathic arthritis). In addition, low bone mass is a characteristic of Klinefelter, Ehlers-Danlos, and Turner syndromes, where osteoporosis may be present in more than 50% of untreated patients older than 18 years. Reduced bone density is also common in children with delayed puberty, hypogonadism, anorexia nervosa, and the female athlete triad (amenorrhea, disordered eating, and osteoporosis), and may occur in some patients with Marfan syndrome. Osteoporosis occurs in approximately 40% of children with idiopathic hypercalciuria. Osteoporosis is also a feature of many rare inherited disorders such as homocystinuria, galactosemia, lysinuric protein intolerance, as well as osteoporosis pseudoglioma syndrome. During the pubertal growth spurt, a lag in mineralization of rapidly growing bone may lead to a transient reduction in BMD that is accompanied by temporary bone fragility that promotes fractures.

Idiopathic juvenile osteoporosis

Idiopathic juvenile osteoporosis (IJO) is a rare condition that follows a rather predictable clinical pattern. IJO occurs in previously apparently healthy children of either sex in the years immediately preceding puberty. Patients present with osteoporotic collapse of one or more (usually lumbar) spinal vertebrae or with fractures of long bones, mostly at metaphyseal sites, on minor trauma. Radiological evidence of osteoporotic new bone is characteristic. A waddling gait is common. Bone histology sometimes shows an excess of osteocytes associated with woven bone and normal mineralization. No extraskeletal biochemical abnormalities are present.

Although disability and deformity can be severe during the active phase of the disease, IJO tends to remit spontaneously soon after the onset of puberty, although skeletal deformity may persist. The recovery presumably occurs under the influence of gonadal steroid secretion. The cause of the disease is unknown, and no satisfactory methods of therapy have been described. In severe cases, orthopedic maneuvers (splinting, casting) might be needed, but it should be remembered that the consequent local immobilization can make the degree of bone loss even worse.

Osteogenesis imperfecta

Osteogenesis imperfecta (OI) is characterized primarily by low bone mass and an increased incidence of bone fractures in connection with minimal trauma. There are at least eight forms of OI, of which type 1 is the most common. The distinguishing characteristic of type 1 is a persistent blueness of the sclerae (blue sclerae are normal in infancy) and in most cases normal stature. Bone mineral density can be normal at birth, but fails to increase appropriately. OI occurs with an incidence at birth of approximately 1 out of 10,000 with a population prevalence

of about 1 out of 20,000. Frequency seems to be similar in all ethnic and racial groups. Most forms of OI are caused by mutations that affect the nature or synthetic rate of the peptide chains that constitute type 1 collagen, the major collagen of the skeleton. Although some nonosseous connective tissues are also affected in OI, the principal impact of defects in production or assembly of type 1 collagen is on the skeleton.

OI is divided into subtypes that are genetically, pathologically, and clinically distinct from one another (described in Table 6-15).

Table 6-15.

Expanded Classification of Osteogenesis Imperfecta (After Sillance)

Type	Fragility	Sclerae	Teeth	Inheritance	Typically Associated Mutations	OMIM	Comments
IA	Present	Blue	Abnormal	Autosomal dominant	Premature stop codon in *COL1A1*	166240	Relatively common; normal height or mild short stature
IB	Present	Blue	Normal	Autosomal dominant	Premature stop codon in *COL1A1*	166200	Variable severity
IIa	Extreme	Blue*	—	? dominant (germ cell)	Glycine substitutions in *COL1A1* or *COL1A2*	166210	Perinatal lethal; multiple rib and long bone fractures at birth; low density of skull bones
IIb	Extreme	Blue	—	Autosomal recessive	*CRTAP*		As above
III	Severe	Greyish	Abnormal	? dominant (germ cell)	Glycine substitutions in *COL1A1* or *COL1A2*	259420	Severe deformity; very short with triangular face
IVA	Present	Normal	Abnormal	Autosomal dominant	Glycine substitutions in *COL1A1* or *COL1A2*	166220	Uncommon
IVB	Present	Normal	Normal	Autosomal dominant	Glycine substitutions in *COL1A1* or *COL1A2*		Variable severity; moderately short, mild to moderate scoliosis
V	Present	Normal	Normal	Autosomal dominant	?	610967	Moderately deforming; mild to moderate short stature; dislocation of radial head; mineralized interosseous membrane; hyperplastic callus; mesh-like bone lamellation
VI	Present	Faintly blue	Normal	Autosomal recessive	?	610968	Moderately short; excess osteoid and fish-scale pattern of bone lamellation
VII	Present	Normal	Normal	Autosomal recessive	*CRTAP*	610682	Mild short stature; short humeri and femora; coxa vara
VIII	Present	Normal	Normal	Autosomal recessive	*LEPRE1*	610915	Similar to VII

*Sclerae are often blue in normal infants.

Treatment

As a first principle, it seems reasonable to recommend that all children with osteoporosis maintain an adequate calcium intake and receive sufficient supplemental vitamin D to sustain normal serum levels of 25(OH)D (ie, greater than 32 ng/mL).

When possible, weight-bearing activity should be maximized, which in healthy children and adolescents has been shown to increase bone mineral accrual and bone size. In ambulant and nonambulant children with spastic cerebral palsy, weight-bearing activity has been shown to significantly improve femoral neck bone mineral content and volumetric BMD compared to controls. In nonambulant children with cerebral palsy, a standing frame to facilitate an upright position has been shown to improve BMD, with the gains in BMD being proportional to the duration of standing. Recent pilot studies in nonambulant children have demonstrated that high frequency low-magnitude strain, applied through a vibration platform, increases volumetric BMD in several skeletal sites.

Bisphosphonates can increase bone density and reduce fractures in children and adults with osteoporosis, but these agents must still be considered experimental in children.[187] Bisphosphonates are potent antiresorptive agents that disrupt osteoclastic activity by interfering with the mevalonate pathway of cholesterol biosynthesis. In OI, histomorphometric studies have shown that pamidronate, a powerful nitrogen-containing bisphosphonate, increases cortical thickness and trabecular number. Pamidronate suppresses bone turnover in children with OI to well below that of normal age-matched controls. This can interfere with bone modeling and result in undertubularization of long bones. In the growing skeleton, a reduction in bone remodeling results in the accumulation of mineralized cartilage within the bone. The mineralized cartilage has a high density, which contributes to the increase in bone density seen with pamidronate treatment. Persistence of calcified cartilage accounts for the characteristic sclerotic metaphyseal lines seen on long bone radiographs of children receiving cyclic pamidronate therapy. Suppressed bone remodeling can also interfere with the repair of microdamage and may account for the delay in osteotomy and possibly fracture repair seen in children with OI who receive pamidronate. Oral bisphosphonates such as alendronate have also been used with limited success in patients with OI. Oral bisphosphonates may result in chemical esophagitis.

Many studies, most of which have been uncontrolled, have shown that administration of bisphosphonates, particularly cyclical intravenous pamidronate (mean dose 6.8 mg/kg IV every 4-6 months) to children with severe OI can alleviate bone pain, reduce the incidence of fractures, enhance growth, and improve the overall quality of life. Optimal responsiveness to pamidronate therapy occurs in children who are first treated in infancy. Reduction in radiologically confirmed fractures and improved ambulation are seen, but treatment does not affect fracture healing, the growth rate, or the appearance of growth plates. Children report substantial relief of chronic pain and fatigue. An "acute-phase reaction" is common during the first infusion cycle, which can be controlled with acetaminophen and does not usually recur during subsequent treatment cycles.

Both intravenous and oral bisphosphonates have been used successfully in children and adolescents with other forms of osteoporosis. Intravenous pamidronate also appears to be a useful therapeutic option in childhood osteoporosis. Treated children have reported rapid pain relief following the first treatment, followed by large increments in lumbar spine bone density over 1 year (eg, increments of 26%-54% as compared to the expected increases owing to growth of 3%-15%).

Bisphosphonates are contraindicated during pregnancy and all females of reproductive age should have a negative pregnancy test before each treatment cycle or before commencing oral bisphosphonates. Because bisphosphonates persist in mineralized bone for many years, the theoretical concern exists that bisphosphonates administered before conception could be released from the maternal skeleton during the pregnancy and affect the fetus.

REFERENCES

1. Berry EM, Gupta MM, Turner SJ, Burns RR. Variation in plasma calcium with induced changes in plasma specific gravity, total protein, and albumin. *Br Med J.* 1973;4(5893):640-643.
2. Carafoli E, Penniston JT. The calcium signal. *Sci Am.* 1985;253(5):70-78.
3. Food and Nutrition Board. Institute of Medicine. Dietary Reference Intakes for Calcium, Phosphorus, Magnesium, Vitamin D, and Fluoride. 1997. Tertiary Food and Nutrition Board. Institute of Medicine. Dietary Reference Intakes for Calcium, Phosphorus, Magnesium, Vitamin D, and Fluoride.
4. Harrison HE. Vitamin D, the parathyroid and the kidney. *Johns Hopkins Med J.* 1979;144(6):180-191.
5. van Abel M, Hoenderop JG, Bindels RJ. The epithelial calcium channels TRPV5 and TRPV6: regulation and implications for disease. *Naunyn Schmiedebergs Arch Pharmacol.* 2005;371(4):295-306.
6. Harrison HE, Harrison HC. *Disorders of Calcium and Phosphate Metabolism in Childhood and Adolescence: Major Problems in Pediatrics.*. Philadelphia, PA: Saunders; 1979.
7. Ferron M, Hinoi E, Karsenty G, Ducy P. Osteocalcin differentially regulates beta cell and adipocyte gene expression

and affects the development of metabolic diseases in wild-type mice. *Proc Natl Acad Sci U S A.* 2008;105(13): 5266-5270.

8. Kruse K, Kracht U. Evaluation of serum osteocalcin as an index of altered bone metabolism. *Eur J Pediatr.* 1986;145:27-33.

9. Daniels ED, Pettifor JM, Moodley GP. Serum osteocalcin has limited usefulness as a diagnostic marker for rickets. *Eur J Pediatr.* 2000;159(10):730-733.

10. Robins SP. Biochemical markers for assessing skeletal growth. *Eur J Clin Nutr.* 1994;48(1):S199-209.

11. Ash P, Loutit JF, Townsend KM. Osteoclasts derived from haematopoietic stem cells. *Nature.* 1980;283(5748): 669-670.

12. Massey HM, Flanagan AM. Human osteoclasts derive from CD14-positive monocytes. *Br J Haematol.* 1999; 106(1):167-170.

13. Manolagas SC, Jilka RL. Bone marrow, cytokines, and bone remodeling. Emerging insights into the pathophysiology of osteoporosis. *N Engl J Med.* 1995;332(5):305-311.

14. Fuller K, Wong B, Fox S, Choi Y, Chambers TJ. TRANCE is necessary and sufficient for osteoblast-mediated activation of bone resorption in osteoclasts. *J Exp Med.* 1998;188(5):997-1001.

15. Lean JM, Matsuo K, Fox SW, et al. Osteoclast lineage commitment of bone marrow precursors through expression of membrane-bound TRANCE. *Bone.* 2000;27(1):29-40.

16. Myllyharju J, Kivirikko KI. Collagens and collagen-related diseases. *Ann Med.* 2001;33(1):7-21.

17. Prockop DJ, Kivirikko KI. Collagens: molecular biology, diseases, and potentials for therapy. *Annu Rev Biochem.* 1995; 64:403-434.

18. Kim HJ, Zhao H, Kitaura H, et al. Glucocorticoids suppress bone formation via the osteoclast. *J Clin Invest.* 2006;116(8):2152-2160.

19. Rochira V, Zirilli L, Madeo B, et al. Skeletal effects of long-term estrogen and testosterone replacement treatment in a man with congenital aromatase deficiency: evidences of a priming effect of estrogen for sex steroids action on bone. *Bone.* 2007;40(6):1662-1668.

20. Smith EP, Specker B, Bachrach BE, et al. Impact on bone of an estrogen receptor-alpha gene loss of function mutation. *J Clin Endocrinol Metab.* 2008;93(8):3088-3096.

21. Vanderschueren D, Gaytant J, Boonen S, Venken K. Androgens and bone. *Curr Opin Endocrinol Diabetes Obes.* 2008;15(3):250-254.

22. Rodriguez M, Almaden Y, Hernandez A, Torres A. Effect of phosphate on the parathyroid gland: direct and indirect? *Curr Opin Nephrol Hypertens.* 1996;5(4):321-328.

23. Almaden Y, Hernandez A, Torregrosa V, et al. High phosphate level directly stimulates parathyroid hormone secretion and synthesis by human parathyroid tissue in vitro. *J Am Soc Nephrol.* 1998;9(10):1845-1852.

24. Neer EJ. Heterotrimeric G proteins: organizers of transmembrane signals. *Cell.* 1995;80:249-257.

25. Gudermann T, Nurnberg B, Schultz G. Receptors and G proteins as primary components of transmembrane signal transduction. Part 1. G-protein-coupled receptors: structure and function. *J Mol Med.* 1995;73(2):51-63.

26. Nurnberg B, Gudermann T, Schultz G. Receptors and G proteins as primary components of transmembrane

27. Yamaguchi T, Chattopadhyay N, Brown EM. G protein-coupled extracellular Ca^{2+} (Ca^{2+}o)-sensing receptor (CaR): roles in cell signaling and control of diverse cellular functions. *Adv Pharmacol.* 2000;47:209-253.

28. Matsumoto T. Magnesium deficiency and parathyroid function [editorial; comment]. *Intern Med.* 1995;34(7): 603-604.

29. Mayan H, Hourvitz A, Schiff E, Farfel Z. Symptomatic hypocalcaemia in hypermagnesaemia-induced hypoparathyroidism, during magnesium tocolytic therapy—possible involvement of the calcium-sensing receptor. *Nephrol Dial Transplant.* 1999;14(7):1764-1766.

30. Cholst IN, Steinberg SF, Tropper PJ, Fox HE, Segre GV, Bilezikian JP. The influence of hypermagnesemia on serum calcium and parathyroid hormone levels in human subjects. *N Engl J Med.* 1984;310(19):1221-1225.

31. Behar V, Pines M, Nakamoto C, et al. The human PTH2 receptor: binding and signal transduction properties of the stably expressed recombinant receptor. *Endocrinology.* 1996;137(7):2748-2757.

32. Usdin TB, Gruber C, Bonner TI. Identification and functional expression of a receptor selectively recognizing parathyroid hormone, the PTH2. *J Biol Chem.* 1995;270:15455-15458.

33. Usdin TB. Evidence for a parathyroid hormone-2 receptor selective ligand in the hypothalamus. *Endocrinology.* 1997;138(2):831-834.

34. Hoare SR, Clark JA, Usdin TB. Molecular determinants of tuberoinfundibular peptide of 39 residues (TIP39) selectivity for the parathyroid hormone-2 (PTH2) receptor. N-terminal truncation of TIP39 reverses PTH2 receptor/PTH1 receptor binding selectivity. *J Biol Chem.* 2000;275(35):27274-27283.

35. Schwindinger WF, Fredericks J, Watkins L, et al. Coupling of the PTH/PTHrP receptor to multiple G-proteins. Direct demonstration of receptor activation of Gs, Gq/11, and Gi(1) by [alpha-32P]GTP-gamma-azidoanilide photoaffinity labeling. *Endocrine.* 1998;8(2):201-209.

36. Melson GL, Chase LR, Aurbach GD. Parathyroid hormone-sensitive adenyl cyclase in isolated renal tubules. *Endocrinology.* 1970;86:511-518.

37. Chase LR, Fedak SA, Aurbach GD. Activation of skeletal adenyl cyclase by parathyroid hormone in vitro. *Endocrinology.* 1969;84:761-768.

38. Civitelli R, Reid IR, Westbrook S, Avioli LV, Hruska KA. PTH elevates inositol polyphosphates and diacylglycerol in a rat osteoblast-like cell line. *Am J Physiol.* 1988;255:E660-E667.

39. Dunlay R, Hruska K. PTH receptor coupling to phospholipase C is an alternate pathway of signal transduction in bone and kidney. *Am J Physiol.* 1990;258:F223-F231.

40. Gupta A, Martin KJ, Miyauchi A, Hruska KA. Regulation of cytosolic calcium by parathyroid hormone and oscillations of cytosolic calcium in fibroblasts from normal and pseudohypoparathyroid patients. *Endocrinology.* 1991;128:2825-2836.

41. Civitelli R, Martin TJ, Fausto A, Gunsten SL, Hruska KA, Avioli LV. Parathyroid hormone-related peptide transiently increases cytosolic calcium in osteoblast-like cells: comparison with parathyroid hormone. *Endocrinology.* 1989;125:1204-1210.

42. Reid IR, Civitelli R, Halstead LR, Avioli LV, Hruska KA. Parathyroid hormone acutely elevates intracellular calcium in osteoblastlike cells. *Am J Physiol.* 1987;253:E45-E51.

43. Yamaguchi DT, Hahn TJ, Iida-Klein A, Kleeman CR, Muallem S. Parathyroid hormone-activated calcium channels in an osteoblast-like clonal osteosarcoma cell line. *J Biol Chem.* 1987;262:7711-7718.

44. Hofbauer LC, Heufelder AE. Role of receptor activator of nuclear factor-kappaB ligand and osteoprotegerin in bone cell biology. *J Mol Med.* 2001;79(5-6):243-253.

45. Hofbauer LC, Khosla S, Dunstan CR, Lacey DL, Boyle WJ, Riggs BL. The roles of osteoprotegerin and osteoprotegerin ligand in the paracrine regulation of bone resorption. *J Bone Miner Res.* 2000;15(1):2-12.

46. Bagi C, van der MM, Brommage R, Rosen D, Sommer A. The effect of systemically administered rhIGF-I/IGFBP-3 complex on cortical bone strength and structure in ovariectomized rats. *Bone.* 1995;16(5):559-565.

47. Bikle DD, Sakata T, Leary C, et al. Insulin-like growth factor I is required for the anabolic actions of parathyroid hormone on mouse bone. *J Bone Miner Res.* 2002;17(9):1570-1578.

48. Billiard J, Grewal SS, Lukaesko L, Stork PJ, Rotwein P. Hormonal control of insulin-like growth factor I gene transcription in human osteoblasts: dual actions of cAMP-dependent protein kinase on CCAAT/enhancer-binding protein delta. *J Biol Chem.* 2001;276(33):31238-31246.

49. Watson P, Lazowski D, Han V, Fraher L, Steer B, Hodsman A. Parathyroid hormone restores bone mass and enhances osteoblast insulin-like growth factor I gene expression in ovariectomized rats. *Bone.* 1995;16(3):357-365.

50. Yamashita H, Gao P, Cantor T, et al. Large carboxy-terminal parathyroid hormone (PTH) fragment with a relatively longer half-life than 1-84 PTH is secreted directly from the parathyroid gland in humans. *Eur J Endocrinol.* 2003;149(4):301-306.

51. Silverberg SJ, Gao P, Brown I, LoGerfo P, Cantor TL, Bilezikian JP. Clinical utility of an immunoradiometric assay for parathyroid hormone (1-84) in primary hyperparathyroidism. *J Clin Endocrinol Metab.* 2003;88(10):4725-4730.

52. Karaplis AC. PTHrP: novel roles in skeletal biology. *Curr Pharm Des.* 2001;7(8):655-670.

53. Jans DA, Thomas RJ, Gillespie MT. Parathyroid hormone-related protein (PTHrP): a nucleocytoplasmic shuttling protein with distinct paracrine and intracrine roles. *Vitam Horm.* 2003; 66:345-384.

54. Holick MF, Biancuzzo RM, Chen TC, et al. Vitamin D2 is as effective as vitamin D3 in maintaining circulating concentrations of 25-hydroxyvitamin D. *J Clin Endocrinol Metab.* 2008;93(3):677-681.

55. Tjellesen L, Hummer L, Christiansen C, Rodbro P. Different metabolism of vitamin D2/D3 in epileptic patients treated with phenobarbitone/phenytoin. *Bone.* 1986;7(5):337-342.

56. Trang HM, Cole DE, Rubin LA, Pierratos A, Siu S, Vieth R. Evidence that vitamin D3 increases serum 25-hydroxyvitamin D more efficiently than does vitamin D2. *Am J Clin Nutr.* 1998;68(4):854-858.

57. Armas LA, Hollis BW, Heaney RP. Vitamin D2 is much less effective than vitamin D3 in humans. *J Clin Endocrinol Metab.* 2004;89(11):5387-5391.

58. Holick MF. Vitamin D—new horizons for the 21st century. *Am J Clin Nutr.* 1994;60(4):619-630.

59. Matsuoka LY, Wortsman J, Hanifan N, Holick MF. Chronic sunscreen use decreases circulating concentrations of 25-hydroxyvitamin D. A preliminary study. *Arch Dermatol.* 1988;124(12):1802-1804.

60. Matsuoka LY, Ide L, Wortsman J, MacLaughlin JA, Holick MF. Sunscreens suppress cutaneous vitamin D3 synthesis. *J Clin Endocrinol Metab.* 1987;64(6):1165-1168.

61. Holick MF, Matsuoka LY, Wortsman J. Regular use of sunscreen on vitamin D levels. *Arch Dermatol.* 1995;131(11):1337-1339.

62. Matsuoka LY, Wortsman J, Dannenberg MJ, Hollis BW, Lu Z, Holick MF. Clothing prevents ultraviolet-B radiation-dependent photosynthesis of vitamin D3. *J Clin Endocrinol Metab.* 1992;75(4):1099-1103.

63. Menter JM, Hatch KL. Clothing as solar radiation protection. *Curr Probl Dermatol.* 2003;31:50-63.

64. Pettifor JM, Moodley GP, Hough FS, et al. The effect of season and latitude on in vitro vitamin D formation by sunlight in South Africa. *S Afr Med J.* 1996;86(10):1270-1272.

65. Holick MF. Environmental factors that influence the cutaneous production of vitamin D. *Am J Clin Nutr.* 1995;61(3):638S-645S.

66. Webb AR, Kline L, Holick MF. Influence of season and latitude on the cutaneous synthesis of vitamin D3: exposure to winter sunlight in Boston and Edmonton will not promote vitamin D3 synthesis in human skin. *J Clin Endocrinol Metab.* 1988;67(2):373-378.

67. Heaney RP, Davies KM, Chen TC, Holick MF, Barger-Lux MJ. Human serum 25-hydroxycholecalciferol response to extended oral dosing with cholecalciferol. *Am J Clin Nutr.* 2003;77(1):204-210.

68. Holick MF, Matsuoka LY, Wortsman J. Age, vitamin D, and solar ultraviolet. *Lancet.* 1989;2(8671):1104-1105.

69. Cheng JB, Levine MA, Bell NH, Mangelsdorf DJ, Russell DW. Genetic evidence that the human CYP2R1 enzyme is a key vitamin D 25-hydroxylase. *Proc Natl Acad Sci U S A.* 2004;101(20):7711-7715.

70. Holick MF. McCollum Award Lecture, 1994: vitamin D—new horizons for the 21st century. *Am J Clin Nutr.* 1994;60(4):619-630.

71. Barbour GL, Coburn JW, Slatopolsky E, Norman AW, Horst RL. Hypercalcemia in an anephric patient with sarcoidosis: evidence for extrarenal generation of 1,25-dihydroxyvitamin D. *N Engl J Med.* 1981;305(8):440-443.

72. Zhou C, Assem M, Tay JC, et al. Steroid and xenobiotic receptor and vitamin D receptor crosstalk mediates CYP24 expression and drug-induced osteomalacia. *J Clin Invest.* 2006;116(6):1703-1712.

73. Haddad JG, Kowalski MA, Sanger JW. Actin affinity chromatography in the purification of human, avian and other mammalian plasma proteins binding vitamin D and its metabolites (Gc globulins). *Biochem J.* 1984;218(3):805-810.

74. Coppenhaver DH, Sollenne NP, Bowman BH. Post-translational heterogeneity of the human vitamin D-binding

protein (group-specific component). *Arch Biochem Biophys.* 1983;226(1):218-223.

75. Cooke NE, Haddad JG. Vitamin D binding protein (Gc-globulin). *Endocr Rev.* 1989;10(3):294-307.

76. Engelman CD, Fingerlin TE, Langefeld CD, et al. Genetic and environmental determinants of 25-hydroxyvitamin D and 1,25-dihydroxyvitamin D levels in Hispanic and African Americans. *J Clin Endocrinol Metab.* 2008;93(9):3381-3338.

77. Jurutka PW, Bartik L, Whitfield GK, et al. Vitamin D receptor: key roles in bone mineral pathophysiology, molecular mechanism of action, and novel nutritional ligands. *J Bone Miner Res.* 2007;22(2):V2-10.

78. Haussler MR, Haussler CA, Jurutka PW, et al. The vitamin D hormone and its nuclear receptor: molecular actions and disease states. *J Endocrinol.* 1997;154:S57-73.

79. Pathrose P, Barmina O, Chang CY, McDonnell DP, Shevde NK, Pike JW. Inhibition of 1,25-dihydroxyvitamin D3-dependent transcription by synthetic LXXLL peptide antagonists that target the activation domains of the vitamin D and retinoid X receptors. *J Bone Miner Res.* 2002;17(12):2196-2205.

80. Jin CH, Kerner SA, Hong MH, Pike JW. Transcriptional activation and dimerization functions in the human vitamin D receptor. *Mol Endocrinol.* 1996;10(8):945-957.

81. Sone T, Kerner S, Pike JW. Vitamin D receptor interaction with specific DNA. Association as a 1,25-dihydroxyvitamin D3-modulated heterodimer. *J Biol Chem.* 1991;266(34):23296-23305.

82. Baran DT. Nongenomic actions of the steroid hormone 1 alpha,25-dihydroxyvitamin D3. *J Cell Biochem.* 1994;56(3):303-306.

83. Baran DT, Quail JM, Ray R, Leszyk J, Honeyman T. Annexin II is the membrane receptor that mediates the rapid actions of 1alpha,25-dihydroxyvitamin D(3). *J Cell Biochem.* 2000;78(1):34-46.

84. Barsony J, Marx SJ. Rapid accumulation of cyclic GMP near activated vitamin D receptors. *Proc Natl Acad Sci U S A.* 1991;88(4):1436-1440.

85. Boland R, de Boland AR, Buitrago C, et al. Non-genomic stimulation of tyrosine phosphorylation cascades by 1,25(OH)(2)D(3) by VDR-dependent and -independent mechanisms in muscle cells. *Steroids.* 2002;67(6):477-482.

86. Christakos S, Barletta F, Huening M, et al. Vitamin D target proteins: function and regulation. *J Cell Biochem.* 2003;88(2):238-244.

87. Barthel TK, Mathern DR, Whitfield GK, et al. 1,25-Dihydroxyvitamin D3/VDR-mediated induction of FGF23 as well as transcriptional control of other bone anabolic and catabolic genes that orchestrate the regulation of phosphate and calcium mineral metabolism. *J Steroid Biochem Mol Biol.* 2007;103(3-5):381-388.

88. Reichel H, Koeffler HP, Norman AW. The role of the vitamin D endocrine system in health and disease. *N Engl J Med.* 1989;320(15):980-991.

89. Aarskog D, Aksnes L, Markestad T, Rodland O. Effect of estrogen on vitamin D metabolism in tall girls. *J Clin Endocrinol Metab.* 1983;57(6):1155-1158.

90. Holick MF. Evolution and function of vitamin D. *Recent Results Cancer Res.* 2003;164:3-28.

91. Holick MF. Vitamin D and bone health. *J Nutr.* 1996;126(4):1159S-1164S.

92. Heaney RP, Dowell MS, Hale CA, Bendich A. Calcium absorption varies within the reference range for serum 25-hydroxyvitamin D. *J Am Coll Nutr.* 2003;22(2):142-146.

93. Heaney RP. Vitamin D, nutritional deficiency, and the medical paradigm. *J Clin Endocrinol Metab.* 2003;88(11):5107-5108.

94. Holick MF. The parathyroid hormone D-lema. *J Clin Endocrinol Metab.* 2003;88(8):3499-3500.

95. Gomez AC, Naves DM, Rodriguez GM, Fernandez Martin JL, Cannata Andia JB. Review of the concept of vitamin D "sufficiency and insufficiency." *Nefrologia.* 2003;23(2):73-77.

96. Aksnes L, Aarskog D. Plasma concentrations of vitamin D metabolites in puberty: effect of sexual maturation and implications for growth. *J Clin Endocrinol Metab.* 1982;55(1):94-101.

97. Lichtenstein P, Specker BL, Tsang RC, Mimouni F, Gormley C. Calcium regulating hormones and minerals from birth to 18 months of age: a cross-sectional study. I. Effects of sex, race, age, season and diet on vitamin D status. *Pediatrics.* 1986;77:1138-1144.

98. Yamashita T, Yoshioka M, Itoh N. Identification of a novel fibroblast growth factor, FGF-23, preferentially expressed in the ventrolateral thalamic nucleus of the brain. *Biochem Biophys Res Commun.* 2000;277(2):494-498.

99. Kuro-o M, Matsumura Y, Aizawa H, et al. Mutation of the mouse klotho gene leads to a syndrome resembling ageing. *Nature.* 1997;390(6655):45-51.

100. Ferrari SL, Bonjour JP, Rizzoli R. Fibroblast growth factor-23 relationship to dietary phosphate and renal phosphate handling in healthy young men. *J Clin Endocrinol Metab.* 2005;90(3):1519-1524.

101. Antoniucci DM, Yamashita T, Portale AA. Dietary phosphorus regulates serum fibroblast growth factor-23 concentrations in healthy men. *J Clin Endocrinol Metab.* 2006;91(8):3144-3149.

102. Saito H, Maeda A, Ohtomo S, et al. Circulating FGF-23 is regulated by 1alpha,25-dihydroxyvitamin D3 and phosphorus in vivo. *J Biol Chem.* 2005;280(4):2543-2549.

103. Burnett SM, Gunawardene SC, Bringhurst FR, Juppner H, Lee H, Finkelstein JS. Regulation of C-terminal and intact FGF-23 by dietary phosphate in men and women. *J Bone Miner Res.* 2006;21(8):1187-1196.

104. Shaikh A, Berndt T, Kumar R. Regulation of phosphate homeostasis by the phosphatonins and other novel mediators. *Pediatr Nephrol.* 2008;23(8):1203-1210.

105. Zaidi M, Inzerillo AM, Moonga BS, Bevis PJ, Huang CL. Forty years of calcitonin—where are we now? A tribute to the work of Iain Macintyre, FRS. *Bone.* 2002;30(5):655-663.

106. Hoffman E. The Chvostek sign: a clinical study. *Am J Surg.* 1958;96:33.

107. Shprintzen RJ. Velo-cardio-facial syndrome: 30 Years of study. *Dev Disabil Res Rev.* 2008;14(1):3-10.

108. Goldmuntz E, Clark BJ, Mitchell LE, et al. Frequency of 22q11 deletions in patients with conotruncal defects. *J Am Coll Cardiol.* 1998;32(2):492-498.

109. Goldmuntz E. DiGeorge syndrome: new insights. *Clin Perinatol.* 2005;32(4):963-978, ix.

110. Markert ML, Boeck A, Hale LP, et al. Transplantation of thymus tissue in complete DiGeorge syndrome. *N Engl J Med.* 1999;341(16):1180-1189.

111. Land MH, Garcia-Lloret MI, Borzy MS, et al. Long-term results of bone marrow transplantation in complete DiGeorge syndrome. *J Allergy Clin Immunol.* 2007; 120(4):908-915.

112. Cuneo BF, Driscoll DA, Gidding SS, Langman CB. Evolution of latent hypoparathyroidism in familial 22q11 deletion syndrome. *Am J Med Genet.* 1997;69(1):50-55.

113. Wilson DI, Burn J, Scambler P, Goodship J. DiGeorge syndrome: part of CATCH 22. *J Med Genet.* 1993;30(10): 852-856.

114. Hasegawa T, Hasegawa Y, Aso T, et al. The transition from latent to overt hypoparathyroidism in a child with CATCH 22 who showed subnormal parathyroid hormone response to ethylenediaminetetraacetic acid infusion. *Eur J Pediatr.* 1996;155(3):255.

115. Zhang L, Zhong T, Wang Y, Jiang Q, Song H, Gui Y. TBX1, a DiGeorge syndrome candidate gene, is inhibited by retinoic acid. *Int J Dev Biol.* 2006;50(1):55-61.

116. Ahn TG, Antonarakis SE, Kronenberg HM, Igarashi T, Levine MA. Familial isolated hypoparathyroidism: a molecular genetic analysis of 8 families with 23 affected persons. *Medicine.* 1986;65:73-81.

117. Thakker RV. The molecular genetics of hypoparathyroidism. In: Bilezikian JP, Marcus R, Levine MA, eds. *The Parathyroids: Basic and Clinical Concepts.* 2nd ed. San Diego, CA: Academic Press; 2001:779-790.

118. Sunthornthepvarakul T, Churesigaew S, Ngowngarmratana S. A novel mutation of the signal peptide of the preproparathyroid hormone gene associated with autosomal recessive familial isolated hypoparathyroidism. *J Clin Endocrinol Metab.* 1999;84(10):3792-3796.

119. Parkinson DB, Thakker RV. A donor splice site mutation in the parathyroid hormone gene is associated with autosomal recessive hypoparathyroidism. *Nat Genet.* 1992;1(2):149-152.

120. Ding C, Buckingham B, Levine MA. Familial isolated hypoparathyroidism caused by a mutation in the gene for the transcription factor *GCMB. J Clin Invest.* 2001;108(8):1215-1220.

121. Gunther T, Chen ZF, Kim J, et al. Genetic ablation of parathyroid glands reveals another source of parathyroid hormone. *Nature.* 2000;406(6792):199-203.

122. Maret A, Ding C, Kornfield SL, Levine MA. Analysis of the GCM2 gene in isolated hypoparathyroidism: a molecular and biochemical study. *J Clin Endocrinol Metab.* 2008;93(4):1426-1432.

123. Thakker RV, Davies KE, Read AP, et al. Linkage analysis of two cloned DNA sequences, DXS197 and DXS207, in hypophosphatemic rickets families. *Genomics.* 1990;8: 189-193.

124. Posillico JT, Wortsman J, Srikanta S, Eisenbarth GS, Mallette LE, Brown EM. Parathyroid cell surface autoantibodies that inhibit parathyroid hormone secretion from dispersed human parathyroid cells. *J Bone Miner Res.* 1986;1(5):475-483.

125. Blizzard RM, Chee D, Davis W. The incidence of parathyroid and other antibodies in the sera of patients with idiopathic hypoparathyroidism. *Clin Exp Immunol.* 1966;1(2):119-128.

126. Verghese MW, Ward FE, Eisenbarth GS. Lymphocyte suppressor activity in patients with polyglandular failure. *Hum Immunol.* 1981;3(2):173-179.

127. Alimohammadi M, Bjorklund P, Hallgren A, et al. Autoimmune polyendocrine syndrome type 1 and NALP5, a parathyroid autoantigen. *N Engl J Med.* 2008;358(10):1018-1028.

128. Kifor O, McElduff A, LeBoff MS, et al. Activating antibodies to the calcium-sensing receptor in two patients with autoimmune hypoparathyroidism. *J Clin Endocrinol Metab.* 2004;89(2):548-556.

129. Chen QY, Lan MS, She JX, Maclaren NK. The gene responsible for autoimmune polyglandular syndrome type 1 maps to chromosome 21q22.3 in US patients. *J Autoimmun.* 1998;11(2):177-183.

130. Peterson P, Peltonen L. Autoimmune polyendocrinopathy syndrome type 1 (APS1) and AIRE gene: new views on molecular basis of autoimmunity. *J Autoimmun.* 2005;25:49-55.

131. Levine MA, Germain-Lee E, Jan de Beur SM. Genetic basis for resistance to parathyroid hormone. *Horm Res.* 2003;60(3):87-95.

132. Bastepe M. The GNAS locus and pseudohypoparathyroidism. *Adv Exp Med Biol.* 2008;626:27-40.

133. Albright F, Burnett CH, Smith PH. Pseudohypoparathyroidism: an example of "Seabright-Bantam syndrome." *Endocrinology.* 1942;30:922-932.

134. Mann JB, Alterman S, Hills AG. Albright's hereditary osteodystrophy comprising pseudohypoparathyroidism and pseudo-pseudohypoparathyroidism with a report of two cases representing the complete syndrome occuring in successive generations. *Ann Intern Med.* 1962;56:315-342.

135. Long DN, McGuire S, Levine MA, Weinstein LS, Germain-Lee EL. Body mass index differences in pseudohypoparathyroidism type 1a versus pseudopseudohypoparathyroidism may implicate paternal imprinting of Galpha(s) in the development of human obesity. *J Clin Endocrinol Metab.* 2007;92(3):1073-1079.

136. Albright F, Forbes AP, Henneman PH. Pseudopseudohypoparathyroidism. *Trans Assoc Am Physicians.* 1952;65: 337-350.

137. Levine MA, Jap TS, Mauseth RS, Downs RW, Spiegel AM. Activity of the stimulatory guanine nucleotide-binding protein is reduced in erythrocytes from patients with pseudohypoparathyroidism and pseudopseudohypoparathyroidism: biochemical, endocrine, and genetic analysis of Albright's hereditary osteodystrophy in six kindreds. *J Clin Endocrinol Metab.* 1986;62:497-502.

138. Levine MA, Modi WS, O'Brien SJ. Mapping of the gene encoding the alpha subunit of the stimulatory G protein of adenylyl cyclase (GNAS1) to 20q13.2—q13.3 in human by in situ hybridization. *Genomics.* 1991;11:478-479.

139. Mantovani G, Bondioni S, Linglart A, et al. Genetic analysis and evaluation of resistance to TSH and GHRH in Pseudohypoparathyroidism type Ib. *J Clin Endocrinol Metab.* 2007;92(9):3738-3742.

140. Liu J, Nealon JG, Weinstein LS. Distinct patterns of abnormal GNAS imprinting in familial and sporadic pseudohypoparathyroidism type IB. *Hum Mol Genet.* 2005;14(1):95-102.

141. Juppner H, Linglart A, Frohlich LF, Bastepe M. Autosomal-dominant pseudohypoparathyroidism type Ib is caused by different microdeletions within or upstream of the GNAS locus. *Ann N Y Acad Sci.* 2006;1068: 250-255.

142. Drezner MK, Neelon FA, Lebovitz HE. Pseudohypoparathyroidism type II: a possible defect in the reception of the cyclic AMP signal. *N Engl J Med.* 1973;280:1056-1060.

143. Rao DS, Parfitt AM, Kleerekoper M, Pumo BS, Frame B. Dissociation between the effects of endogenous parathyroid hormone on adenosine 3',5'-monophosphate generation and phosphate reabsorption in hypocalcemia due to vitamin D depletion: An acquired disorder resembling pseudohypoparathyroidism type II. *J Clin Endocrinol Metab.* 1985;61:285-290.

144. Shriraam M, Bhansali A, Velayutham P. Vitamin D deficiency masquerading as pseudohypoparathyroidism type 2. *J Assoc Physicians India.* 2003;51:619-620.

145. Srivastava T, Alon US. Stage I vitamin D-deficiency rickets mimicking pseudohypoparathyroidism type II. *Clin Pediatr (Phila).* 2002;41(4):263-268.

146. Chase LR, Melson GL, Aurbach GD. Pseudohypoparathyroidism: defective excretion of 3',5'-AMP in response to parathyroid hormone. *J Clin Invest.* 1969;48:1832-1844.

147. Stone MD, Hosking DJ, Garcia-Himmelstine C, White DA, Rosenblum D, Worth HG. The renal response to exogenous parathyroid hormone in treated pseudohypoparathyroidism. *Bone.* 1993;14:727-735.

148. Winer KK, Sinaii N, Peterson D, Sainz B Jr, Cutler GB Jr. Effects of once versus twice-daily parathyroid hormone1-34 therapy in children with hypoparathyroidism. *J Clin Endocrinol Metab.* 2008;93(9):3389-3395.

149. Meij IC, Koenderink JB, de Jong JC, et al. Dominant isolated renal magnesium loss is caused by misrouting of the Na+,K+-ATPase gamma-subunit. *Ann N Y Acad Sci.* 2003;986:437-443.

150. Kantorovich V, Adams JS, Gaines JE, et al. Genetic heterogeneity in familial renal magnesium wasting. *J Clin Endocrinol Metab.* 2002;87(2):612-617.

151. Simon DB, Nelson-Williams C, Bia MJ, et al. Gitelman's variant of Bartter's syndrome, inherited hypokalaemic alkalosis, is caused by mutations in the thiazide-sensitive Na-Cl cotransporter. *Nat Genet.* 1996;12(1):24-30.

152. Shaer AJ. Inherited primary renal tubular hypokalemic alkalosis: a review of Gitelman and Bartter syndromes. *Am J Med Sci.* 2001;322(6):316-332.

153. Konrad M, Vollmer M, Lemmink HH, et al. Mutations in the chloride channel gene CLCNKB as a cause of classic Bartter syndrome. *J Am Soc Nephrol.* 2000;11(8):1449-1459.

154. Greer FR. 25-Hydroxyvitamin D: functional outcomes in infants and young children. *Am J Clin Nutr.* 2008;88(2):529S-533S.

155. Misra M, Pacaud D, Petryk A, Collett-Solberg PF, Kappy M. Vitamin D deficiency in children and its management: review of current knowledge and recommendations. *Pediatrics.* 2008;122(2):398-417.

156. Wagner CL, Hulsey TC, Fanning D, Ebeling M, Hollis BW. High-dose vitamin D3 supplementation in a cohort of breastfeeding mothers and their infants: a 6-month follow-up pilot study. *Breastfeed Med.* 2006;1(2):59-70.

157. Kim CJ, Kaplan LE, Perwad F, et al. Vitamin D 1α-hydroxylase gene mutations in patients with 1α-hydroxylase deficiency. *J Clin Endocrinol Metab.* 2007;92(8):3177-3182.

158. Pidasheva S, D'Souza-Li L, Canaff L, Cole DE, Hendy GN. CASRdb: calcium-sensing receptor locus-specific database for mutations causing familial (benign) hypocalciuric hypercalcemia, neonatal severe hyperparathyroidism, and autosomal dominant hypocalcemia. *Hum Mutat.* 2004;24(2):107-111.

159. Pollak MR, Brown EM, Chou YW, et al. Mutations in the human Ca^{2+}-sensing receptor gene cause familial hypocalciuric hypercalcemia and neonatal severe hyperparathyroidism. *Cell.* 1993;75:1297-1303.

160. Attie MF, Gill JR Jr, Stock JL, et al. Urinary calcium excretion in familial hypocalciuric hypercalcemia. Persistence of relative hypocalciuria after induction of hypoparathyroidism. *J Clin Invest.* 1983;72:667-676.

161. Mallet E. Primary hyperparathyroidism in neonates and childhood. The French experience (1984-2004). *Horm Res.* 2008;69(3):180-188.

162. Heppner C, Kester MB, Agarwal SK, et al. Somatic mutation of the MEN1 gene in parathyroid tumours. *Nat Genet.* 1997;16(4):375-378.

163. LeGrand SB, Leskuski D, Zama I. Narrative review: furosemide for hypercalcemia: an unproven yet common practice. *Ann Intern Med.* 2008;149(4):259-263.

164. Henrich LM, Rogol AD, D'Amour P, Levine MA, Hanks JB, Bruns DE. Persistent hypercalcemia after parathyroidectomy in an adolescent and effect of treatment with cinacalcet HCl. *Clin Chem.* 2006;52(12):2286-2293.

165. Pober BR, Morris CA. Diagnosis and management of medical problems in adults with Williams-Beuren syndrome. *Am J Med Genet C Semin Med Genet.* 2007;145C(3):280-290.

166. Kato S, Fujiki R, Kim MS, Kitagawa H. Ligand-induced transrepressive function of VDR requires a chromatin remodeling complex, WINAC. *J Steroid Biochem Mol Biol.* 2007;103(3-5):372-380.

167. Massfelder T, Helwig JJ. The parathyroid hormone-related protein system: more data but more unsolved questions. *Curr Opin Nephrol Hypertens.* 2003;12(1):35-42.

168. Fiaschi-Taesch NM, Stewart AF. Minireview: parathyroid hormone-related protein as an intracrine factor—trafficking mechanisms and functional consequences. *Endocrinology.* 2003;144(2):407-411.

169. DeLellis RA, Xia L. Paraneoplastic endocrine syndromes: a review. *Endocr Pathol.* 2003;14(4):303-317.

170. McIntyre HD, Cameron DP, Urquhart SM, Davies WE. Immobilization hypercalcaemia responding to intravenous pamidronate sodium therapy. *Postgrad Med J.* 1989;65(762):244-246.

171. Massagli TL, Cardenas DD. Immobilization hypercalcemia treatment with pamidronate disodium after spinal cord injury. *Arch Phys Med Rehabil.* 1999;80(9):998-1000.

172. Kedlaya D, Brandstater ME, Lee JK. Immobilization hypercalcemia in incomplete paraplegia: successful treatment with pamidronate. *Arch Phys Med Rehabil.* 1998;79(2):222-225.

173. Saarela T, Simila S, Koivisto M. Hypercalcemia and nephrocalcinosis in patients with congenital lactase deficiency. *J Pediatr.* 1995;127(6):920-923.

174. Caswell AM, Whyte MP, Russell RG. Hypophosphatasia and the extracellular metabolism of inorganic pyrophosphate:

clinical and laboratory aspects. *Crit Rev Clin Lab Sci.* 1991;28(3):175-232.

175. Whyte MP. Hypophosphatasia. In: Scriver CR, Beaudet AL, Sly WS, Valle D, Childs B, eds. *The Metabolic and Molecular Bases of Inherited Disease.* 8th ed. New York, NY: McGraw-Hill; 2001:5313-5329.

176. Glass RB, Fernbach SK, Norton KI, Choi PS, Naidich TP. The infant skull: a vault of information. *Radiographics.* 2004;24(2):507-522.

177. Morgan JM, Hawley WL, Chenoweth AI, Retan WJ, Diethelm AG. Renal transplantation in hypophosphatemia with vitamin D-resistant rickets. *Arch Intern Med.* 1974;134(3):549-552.

178. Makitie O, Toiviainen-Salo S, Marttinen E, Kaitila I, Sochett E, Sipila I. Metabolic control and growth during exclusive growth hormone treatment in X-linked hypophosphatemic rickets. *Horm Res.* 2008;69(4):212-220.

179. The ADHR Consortium. Autosomal dominant hypophosphataemic rickets is associated with mutations in FGF23. *Nat Genet.* 2000;26(3):345-348.

180. Feng JQ, Ward LM, Liu S, et al. Loss of DMP1 causes rickets and osteomalacia and identifies a role for osteocytes in mineral metabolism. *Nat Genet.* 2006;38(11):1310-1315.

181. Lorenz-Depiereux B, Bastepe M, Benet-Pages A, et al. DMP1 mutations in autosomal recessive hypophosphatemia implicate a bone matrix protein in the regulation of phosphate homeostasis. *Nat Genet.* 2006;38(11):1248-1250.

182. Bergwitz C, Roslin NM, Tieder M et al. SLC34A3 mutations in patients with hereditary hypophosphatemic rickets with hypercalciuria predict a key role for the sodium-phosphate cotransporter NaPi-IIc in maintaining phosphate homeostasis. *Am J Hum Genet.* 2006;78(2):179-192.

183. Lorenz-Depiereux B, Benet-Pages A, Eckstein G, et al. Hereditary Hypophosphatemic Rickets with Hypercalciuria Is Caused by Mutations in the Sodium-Phosphate Cotransporter Gene SLC34A3. *Am J Hum Genet.* 2006;78(2):193-201.

184. Chen C, Carpenter T, Steg N, Baron R, Anast C. Hypercalciuric hypophosphatemic rickets, mineral balance, bone histomorphometry, and therapeutic implications of hypercalciuria. *Pediatrics.* 1989;84(2):276-280.

185. Tieder M, Arie R, Bab I, Maor J, Liberman UA. A new kindred with hereditary hypophosphatemic rickets with hypercalciuria: implications for correct diagnosis and treatment. *Nephron.* 1992;(2):176-181.

186. Ward LM, Rauch F, White KE, et al. Resolution of severe, adolescent-onset hypophosphatemic rickets following resection of an FGF-23-producing tumour of the distal ulna. *Bone.* 2004;34(5):905-911.

187. Bachrach LK, Ward LM. Clinical review. Bisphosphonate use in childhood osteoporosis. *J Clin Endocrinol Metab.* 2008;2009;94(2):400-409.

ATLAS

Case 1

DiGeorge anomaly in a 3-month-old boy with congenital hypoparathyroidism and dysplastic thymus. Note short philtrum, receding chin, and posteriorly inclined, malformed ears.

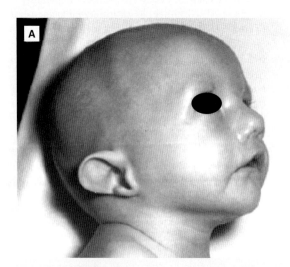 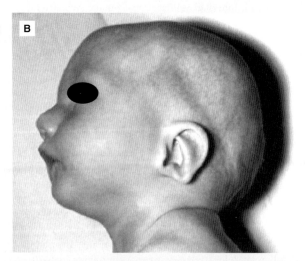

(Reproduced from Aarskog D, Harrison H. Disorders of Calcium, Phosphate, PTH and Vitamin D. In: Kappy MS, Blizzard RM, Migeon CJ, eds. The Diagnosis and Treatment of Endocrine Disorders in Childhood and Adolescence, 4th ed. Springfield: Thomas;1994:1027-1092. 1994; with permission.)

Case 2

Autoimmune hypoparathyroidism. Same boy photographed at 8 **(A)** and 14 **(B)** years of age. He developed adrenal insufficiency at 5 years hypoparathyroidism 15 months later. Note alopecia which started with hairless patches and proceeded to complete baldness and lack of eye and body hair.

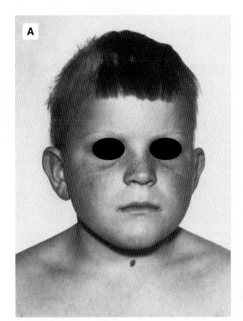
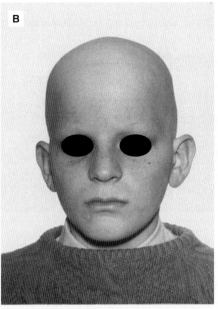

(Reproduced from Aarskog D, Harrison H. Disorders of Calcium, Phosphate, PTH and Vitamin D. In: Kappy MS, Blizzard RM, Migeon CJ, eds. The Diagnosis and Treatment of Endocrine Disorders in Childhood and Adolescence, 4th ed. Springfield: Thomas;1994:1027-1092; with permission.)

Case 3

Pseudohypoparathyroidism, type 1 in a 13-year-old boy. Note round facies and stocky, obese body. Height at 10th percentile.

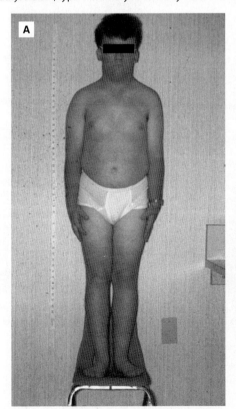
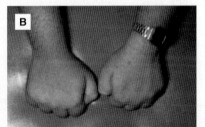
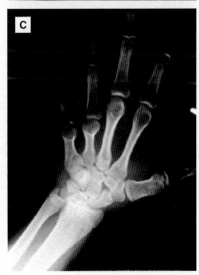

Case 4

Radiographs of a 15-month-old infant with vitamin D deficiency rickets.

A. Characteristic radiological finding of untreated rickets with splayed, cupped, and frayed metaphyses at the knee.
B. Similar radiological findings of untreated rickets at the wrist.
C. Radiographs of the knee of the same child after 4 months of treatment with pharmacologic doses of vitamin D. Radiologic signs of healing are evident.
D. Similarly, radiologic signs of healing are evident at the wrist after treatment with vitamin D.

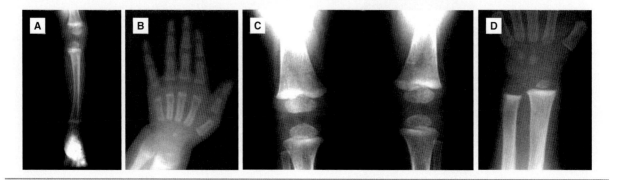

Case 5

Williams syndrome. Same boy photographed at 17 months (**A**) and at 8 years (**B**) of age. The characteristic facial features have become more pronounced.

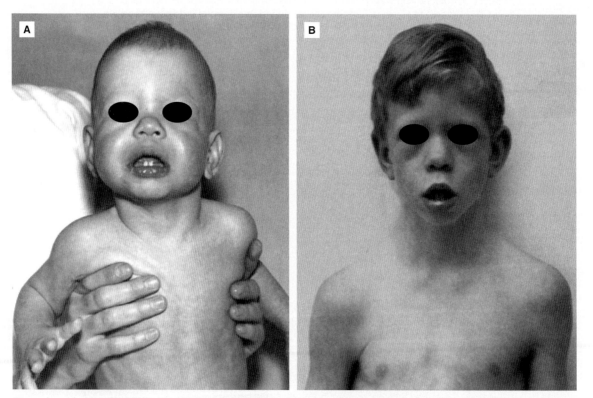

(Reproduced from Aarskog D, Harrison H. Disorders of Calcium, Phosphate, PTH and Vitamin D. In: Kappy MS, Blizzard RM, Migeon CJ, eds. The Diagnosis and Treatment of Endocrine Disorders in Childhood and Adolescence, 4th ed. Springfield: Thomas; 1994:1027-1092; with permission.)

Case 6

Osteosclerosis in a 15-month-old boy with Williams syndrome and hypercalcemia.

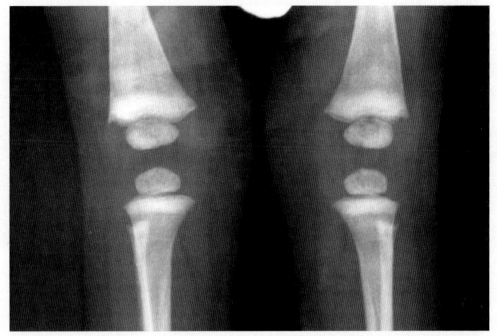

(Reproduced from Aarskog D, Harrison H. Disorders of Calcium, Phosphate, PTH and Vitamin D. In: Kappy MS, Blizzard RM, Migeon CJ, eds. The Diagnosis and Treatment of Endocrine Disorders in Childhood and Adolescence, *4th ed. Springfield: Thomas;1994:1027-1092; with permission.)*

Case 7

Chest of a 2-year-old boy with nephropathic cystinosis causing Fanconi syndrome with rickets. Note swelling of the costochondral junctions (rachitic rosary) and depression of the costal diaphragmatic insertion (Harrison groove).

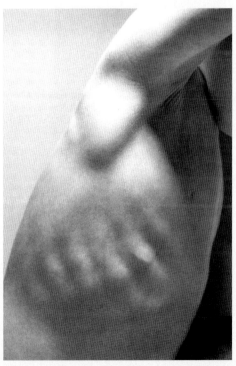

(Reproduced from Aarskog D, Harrison H. Disorders of Calcium, Phosphate, PTH and Vitamin D. In: Kappy MS, Blizzard RM, Migeon CJ, eds. The Diagnosis and Treatment of Endocrine Disorders in Childhood and Adolescence, *4th ed. Springfield: Thomas;1994:1027-1092; with permission.)*

Case 8

Five-year-old and two-year-old sisters with X-linked hypophosphatemic rickets.

A and B. Showing frontal bossing.
C. Showing marked genu varum.
D. Radiograph of the 5-year-old girl shows the extent of her genu varum as well as metaphyseal flaring at the knee.

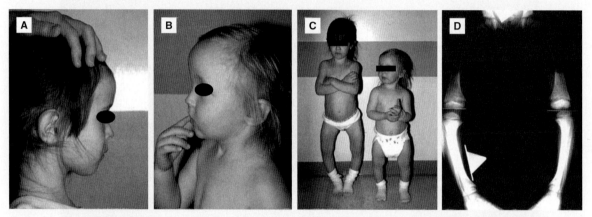

(Reproduced from Aarskog D, Harrison H. Disorders of Calcium, Phosphate, PTH and Vitamin D. In: Kappy MS, Blizzard RM, Migeon CJ, eds. The Diagnosis and Treatment of Endocrine Disorders in Childhood and Adolescence, 4th ed. Springfield: Thomas; 1994:1027-1092; with permission.)

CHAPTER 7

Puberty

Jon M. Nakamoto,
Sherry L. Franklin, and
Mitchell E. Geffner

GENERAL INTRODUCTORY COMMENTS

Puberty is the transitional process leading to reproductive maturity. Proper diagnosis and management of pubertal disorders requires understanding of: (1) basic endocrinology of the hypothalamic-pituitary-gonadal axis; (2) developmental changes that occur at different points throughout childhood; and (3) the wide variability in timing of physical changes of puberty seen in normal children.

BASIC ENDOCRINOLOGY OF PUBERTY

The three anatomic sites most pertinent to pubertal development are the hypothalamus, the anterior pituitary gland, and the gonads (ovaries or testes), known collectively as the hypothalamic-pituitary-gonadal (HPG) axis (Figure 7-1). Also shown in this figure are the critical hormones and feedback loops of the HPG axis.

Kisspeptins are peptides secreted by neurons in the arcuate and anteroventral periventricular nucleus of the hypothalamus.[1] These peptides bind to a G protein-coupled receptor called *GPR54* on hypothalamic neurons that secrete *gonadotropin-releasing hormone (GnRH)*. The resulting pulses of GnRH in turn induce pulsatile secretion of the *gonadotropins, luteinizing hormone (LH), and follicle-stimulating hormone (FSH)*. LH and FSH working in concert lead to germ cell (spermatozoa or ova) maturation and also stimulation of *sex steroid (androgen or estrogen)* secretion by the gonads, along with gonadal peptides such as *inhibins*. The sex steroids exert a negative feedback effect at both hypothalamic and pituitary levels, reducing the secretion of kisspeptin, GnRH, and LH, while inhibins control FSH secretion via a separate negative feedback loop at the pituitary level. Later in life, once menstrual cycles begin, women also develop a positive feedback cycle whereby estrogens stimulate gonadotropin release during phases of the cycle critical for ovulation.

These basic hormonal pathways are modulated by many different central nervous system (CNS) inputs, including stimulatory effects of glutaminergic neural systems, inhibitory effects of gamma-aminobutyric acid (GABA)-ergic systems, and direct interactions between glial cells and hypothalamic neurons. The CNS in turn integrates the effects of many external factors such as nutrient availability, exercise, stress, social/psychological factors, and indirect effects of chronic disease.

DEVELOPMENTAL CHANGES RELEVANT TO PUBERTY

Fetal Period

Four critical developmental steps during fetal life establish the required anatomy for the HPG axis and normal pubertal development. First, GnRH-producing neurons must migrate from the olfactory region to proper positions in the hypothalamus, with dependence on products of the *KAL-1 (Kallmann syndrome 1)* and FGFR1 *(fibroblast growth factor receptor-1)* genes for normal anatomic development. Second, the mechanism for pulsatile GnRH secretion and responsiveness must be established, with dependence upon genes such as *KISS-1* (producing kisspeptin) and *GnRHR* (GnRH receptor). Third, normal development of the hypothalamus and

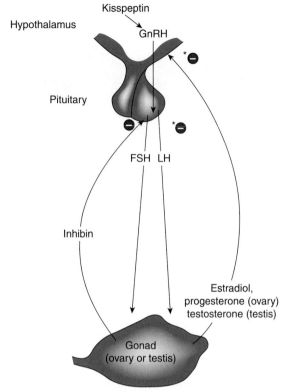

FIGURE 7-1 ■ Schematic diagram of the hypothalamic-pituitary-gonadal axis.

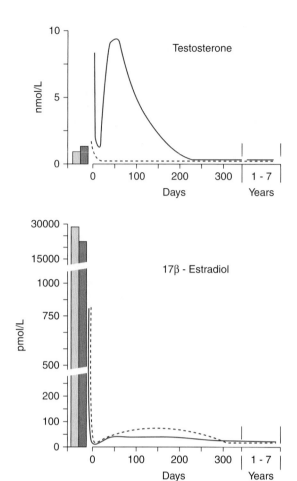

FIGURE 7-2 ■ Patterns of sex steroid secretion during the first year of life. The yellow (female) and green (male) bars represent the mean values of the measured hormones as found in cord blood.

gonadotropin-secreting cells of the pituitary depends upon genes such as *NR5A1 (SF-1), NROB1 (DAX-1), PROP1, HESX1, LHX, LH-β, LHR (LH receptor), FSH-β,* and *FSHR (FSH receptor)* among others.[2] Fourth, the gonads must form properly, with differentiation of Leydig and Sertoli cells in the testis, and granulosa and theca cells in the ovary.

Neonatal Period, Infancy, and Childhood

Providing that the above developmental steps occur properly, the pubertal mechanism is already active for brief periods during fetal, neonatal, and early infant life ("mini-puberty of infancy"). Knowing when infants normally have elevated LH, FSH, and sex steroids (Figure 7-2) allows efficient laboratory assessment whenever the integrity of the HPG axis is in question, as with congenital or acquired CNS, pituitary, or gonadal abnormalities. After the first year of life, the pubertal mechanisms are quiescent, reflecting an active suppression of GnRH pulsatile secretion that remains in place until the child approaches the time of adolescence. During this period of pubertal latency, it is difficult to distinguish the child who has *hypogonadotropic hypogonadism*

(pathological inability to produce sex steroids owing to hypothalamic-pituitary abnormalities) from the normal subject whose GnRH secretion is still under active restraint. In addition, the knowledge that the underlying pubertal mechanism is dormant only because of active CNS restraint helps explain why CNS abnormalities are often associated with precocious puberty.

Preadolescence and Adolescence

The harbinger of puberty is the increase in pulsatile release of GnRH, which occurs first at night, well over a year before any physical signs of puberty appear. While measurement of GnRH in peripheral blood in humans is of little clinical value for assessment of puberty, LH serves as a good proxy for the return of GnRH pulsatility, providing that an ultrasensitive LH assay (with analytical sensitivity down to 0.1 IU/L) is used. For most of these ultrasensitive assays, an LH level above 0.3 to 0.55 IU/L is suggestive of early central activation of puberty.

In boys, the rise in testosterone matches the increase in LH levels. The binding protein for both testosterone and estradiol, sex hormone binding globulin (SHBG) declines as testosterone increases, leading to a rapid rise in the free (active) fraction of testosterone. Estrogen levels also increase somewhat in boys during puberty mostly from peripheral conversion (aromatization) of testosterone to estradiol. The peak of this estradiol rise is typically seen around the age of 13, corresponding to mid-puberty, the period during which adolescent male breast enlargement (gynecomastia) is most often seen.

In girls, estradiol secretion during early puberty is episodic, making random measurement of estradiol an insensitive marker for pubertal onset, especially compared to ultrasensitive assays for LH. Although rising levels of estradiol should theoretically increase SHBG levels in girls as they progress through puberty, what is actually observed is a mild downward trend in SHBG, likely caused by other factors known to decrease SHBG, such as rising insulin-like growth factor-1 (IGF-1), increase in average insulin levels during adolescence, and increased secretion of androgens by the adrenals and the ovaries.

Gonadal peptides

Inhibins are dimeric gonadal proteins that inhibit FSH secretion by the pituitary gland. The two major forms of inhibin are inhibin A and inhibin B. Inhibin A is a product of ovarian follicles and is only measurable in females. Inhibin B is the product of granulosa cells in girls and of Sertoli cells in boys, and may be useful for evaluation of testicular abnormalities, including cryptorchidism.

Activins are dimeric gonadal proteins that stimulate FSH secretion, although there appears to be less clinically relevant information gleaned from measuring activins than there is from measuring inhibins.

Adrenarche

Although often used as a synonym for *pubarche*, the first appearance of pubic hair, the term *adrenarche* is better defined biochemically as a detectable increase in the secretion of adrenal androgens, including androstenedione and dehydroepiandrosterone (DHEA), or its longer-lived sulfated metabolite, DHEAS. These biochemical changes represent a gradual process that may start well before the age of 6, several years before pubic hair appears or puberty actually begins.

Pubertal changes of the growth hormone (GH)—IGF-1 axis

GH pulses increase in amplitude during puberty, with a resulting increase in circulating IGF-1 levels. These changes may explain the transient insulin resistance seen during early and mid-puberty, a phenomenon which is independent of any insulin resistance arising from increased body mass index (BMI) or total adipose tissue.

TIMING OF PHYSICAL CHANGES OF PUBERTY

The end result of the developmental and endocrinological changes described above is the appearance of the physical changes that characterize the final phase of puberty. In girls, the most obvious changes involve breast development (thelarche), the presence of pubic hair (pubarche), and the onset of menstrual periods (menarche). For boys, the focus is on genital and pubic hair development as well as increase in muscle strength, deepening of the voice, and appearance of facial hair. Any delay in pubertal onset also delays the expected acceleration of growth, so that the very common referrals of adolescents for short stature and delayed growth also requires assessment of pubertal status.

All guidelines for pubertal norms should be viewed with circumspection, as studies of puberty in children are fraught with major methodological (issues with design or measurement) and statistical difficulties.[3,4] Therefore, while a study may demonstrate convincingly that breast development in a 7-year-old girl can be normal, such a study cannot be used to predict that breast development in a specific 7-year-old patient is normal. More information from medical history and physical examination, and perhaps biochemical evaluation is required.

Factors Affecting the Timing of Puberty[5]

Genetic factors

Family studies, particularly twin studies, suggest that genetic factors contribute to at least half to three-quarters of the variability in timing of puberty.[2] Ethnicity is a known factor, with black girls showing earlier onset of breast development as compared to white girls. Table 7-1 lists many of the genes associated with normal puberty or with pubertal disorders.

BMI and fat mass

A girl's nutritional status, as assessed by BMI and/or measurement of body fat mass, is strongly associated with alterations in pubertal timing.[6] Girls who are significantly underweight or who have extremely low body fat are more likely to have delayed menarche and/or secondary amenorrhea. Higher BMI/obesity in girls is associated with earlier appearance of breasts, pubic hair, and onset of menstrual periods, with evidence pointing to *leptin*, a product of adipose tissue, as a signal that must reach a minimum threshold for the initiation of puberty.[7] Based on these findings and arguments from evolutionary biology, the current hypothesis is that increased body fat is a cause of earlier puberty in girls, although alternate hypotheses (eg, increased fat is the

Table 7-1.

Genes Playing a Role in Pubertal Development

Gene	Gene Product	Pubertal Disorder Associated with Gene Defect
FGFR1	Fibroblast growth factor receptor 1	Kallmann syndrome
FSH-β	FSH-β subunit	Idiopathic hypogonadotropic hypogonadism
FSHR	FSH receptor	Idiopathic hypogonadotropic hypogonadism
GNAS	$G_s\alpha$ protein	Precocious puberty (activating mutation) in McCune-Albright syndrome
GNRHR	GnRH receptor	Idiopathic hypogonadotropic hypogonadism
GPR54	Kisspeptin receptor	Idiopathic hypogonadotropic hypogonadism
HESX-1	"Homeobox gene expressed in ES cells" HESX1 protein	Abnormal hypothalamic-pituitary development
KAL1	Anosmin-1	Kallmann syndrome
KISS-1	Kisspeptin	
LEP	Leptin	Idiopathic hypogonadotropic hypogonadism and obesity
LEPR	Leptin receptor	Idiopathic hypogonadotropic hypogonadism and obesity
LH-β	LH-β subunit	Idiopathic hypogonadotropic hypogonadism
LHR	LH receptor	Idiopathic hypogonadotropic hypogonadism (inactivating mutation); "testotoxicosis" (activating mutation)
LHX3	"LIM family of homeobox transcription factors"	Abnormal hypothalamic-pituitary development
NELF	Nasal embryonic luteinizing hormone-releasing hormone factor	Kallmann syndrome
NR5A1 (SF-1)	Nuclear receptor, subfamily 5, group A, member 1 (Steroidogenic factor-1)	Abnormal hypothalamic-pituitary development, adrenal hypoplasia
NR0B1 (DAX-1)	Nuclear receptor, subfamily 0, group B, member 1 (dosage-sensitive sex reversal—Adrenal hypoplasia congenital critical region on the X chromosome)	Abnormal hypothalamic-pituitary development, adrenal hypoplasia
PC1	Prohormone convertase-1	Idiopathic hypogonadotropic hypogonadism and hypoglycemia
PROK2	Prokineticin-2	Kallmann syndrome
PROKR2	Prokineticin receptor 2	Kallmann syndrome
PROP1	"Prophet of Pit-1"	Abnormal hypothalamic-pituitary development

result, rather than the cause of, an accelerated pubertal process) may still be possible.

The link between higher body fat and altered timing of puberty is less obvious in boys, which may either reflect different evolutionary pressures or simply the greater methodological difficulty of scoring male genital development (as opposed to noting onset of menarche in girls) for studies of puberty in boys. The trend appears to be that higher BMI in boys is associated with later, rather than earlier, onset of puberty.

Environmental chemicals

The effect of environmental chemical exposures on the timing of puberty is a topic under great debate and active research.[8] A wide variety of endocrine-disrupting chemicals have been identified that have the ability to mimic (agonists) or block (antagonists) the effects of sex steroids, or have toxic effects on critical components of the reproductive axis. Examples include pollutants such as polychlorinated or polybrominated biphenyls, dioxins, pesticide or fungicide residues, phthalates and other compounds from plastics, toxins such as lead, or even naturally occurring food components such as soy isoflavones. Further complicating the story is that endocrine-disrupting chemicals may exert their effects during the prenatal or prepubertal years as well as in the immediate peripubertal period, making epidemiological study of these compounds an extremely ambitious task. While awaiting results of further studies, the clinician can provide some reassurance to anxious parents that these compounds are generally two or more orders of magnitude weaker than primary sex steroids like estradiol.

Chronic illness

Typically, significant chronic disease in childhood is associated with a later onset of puberty. Exceptions include diseases involving the CNS, where there may be disturbances of the normal mechanisms which restrain puberty during the childhood years. In some cases the effects are mixed, as with cerebral palsy, where onset of breast development may occur earlier, despite later onset of menstrual periods.

Physical Changes in Girls: Thelarche

Thelarche is the onset of breast enlargement in girls. Asymmetrical breast development, with one breast developing before the other, or a mild difference in size between the two breasts, is not uncommon. Criteria for Tanner staging of breast development are shown in Figure 7-3. A common difficulty in staging of breast development is encountered with overweight girls, where even a physician may not be able to distinguish by observation alone between fatty tissue in the breast area *versus* actual glandular tissue. Palpation of breast tissue is a more accurate method for determining if Tanner stage B2 has truly been attained. Other issues include the lack of an absolute objective boundary between stage B2 and B3, as well as determining the difference between a large breast at stage B3 and a small breast at stage B5. In the latter case, a more developed papilla (the pigmented projection of the nipple) close to 1 cm in diameter suggests stage B5.

A number of recent studies suggest that the mean age at thelarche is somewhere between 10 and 11 years in white girls, 9 and 10 years in black girls, and somewhere in between for Hispanic girls.[9] Mean age, however, is not particularly helpful when faced with patients referred for evaluation of precocious or delayed puberty. The lower age threshold for breast development in healthy girls remains

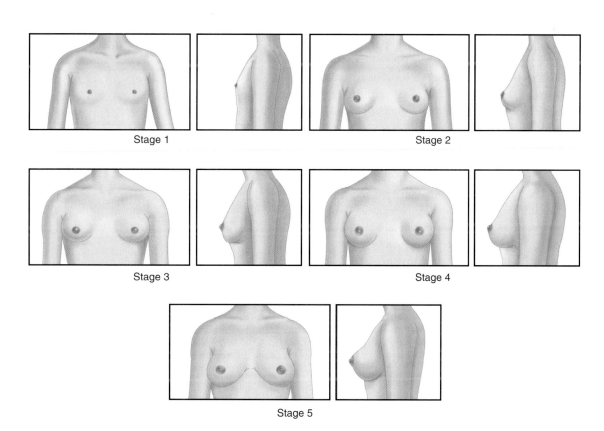

Stage 1

Stage 2

Stage 3

Stage 4

Stage 5

Stage 1   Preadolescent: juvenile breast with elevated papilla and small flat areola.

Stage 2   The breast bud forms under the influence of hormonal stimulation. The papilla and areola elevate as a small mound, and the areolar diameter increases.

Stage 3   Continued enlargement of the breast bud further elevates the papilla. The areola continues to enlarge; no separation of breast contours is noted.

Stage 4   The areola and papilla separate from the contour of the breast to form a secondary mound.

Stage 5   Mature: areolar mound recedes into the general contour of the breast; papilla continues to project.

FIGURE 7-3 ■ Tanner staging of breast development. (*From Greydanus DE, Pratt HD. Adolescent growth and development, and sport participation. In: Patel DR, Greydanus DE, Baker RJ, eds.* Pediatric Practice: Sports Medicine. *New York, NY: McGraw-Hill; 2009:18.*)

somewhat controversial, with some pediatric endocrinologists in the United States subscribing to an age threshold of 7 years in white girls and 6 years in black girls.[10] In contrast, other pediatric endocrinologists, particularly in Europe, retain the age threshold of 8 years in white girls and 7 years in black girls.[4,11] At the upper end, the +2 standard deviation (SD) age threshold for breast development is just under 13 years of age. Regardless of which cut-offs are used, statistically derived age thresholds should never be used as absolute indicators of health or disease without additional clinical and biochemical information.

Physical Changes in Girls: Pubarche

Pubarche is the first appearance of pubic or axillary hair, although typically axillary hair appears 1 to 2 years after pubic hair in white girls (this time gap may be shorter in black girls). Because pubarche is so dependent upon adrenal androgen secretion, the terms pubarche and adrenarche are frequently used interchangeably, although, as noted above, the onset of increased adrenal androgen secretion may actually precede pubarche by a few years. Although pubarche typically occurs around the same time as gonadarche (activation of the hypothalamic-pituitary-gonadal axis), each is actually the result of different regulatory pathways (adrenal *versus* gonadal) and may, on occasion, follow significantly different timing patterns. Therefore, the appearance of pubic hair should not be considered a sign of true pubertal onset.

Criteria for Tanner staging of pubic hair development are shown in Figure 7-4. In some ethnic groups, the amount of pubic hair is less for any given Tanner stage. There is no Tanner staging scale for axillary hair, which is rated on a simple three-point scale, where stage 1 signifies no hair, stage 3 signifies axillary hair adult in quantity and quality, and stage 2 is somewhere in between.

From available studies, the median age of pubarche is 10.5 to 10.9 years in white girls, 8.8 to 9.4 years in black girls, and around 10.4 years in Mexican-American girls. Estimates of the lower age limit for pubarche vary widely among different studies, ranging from 8 to 9 years in white girls.[3] Black girls have a significantly earlier pubarche, with at least one study noting that 5.2% of 4-year-old healthy black girls already had some pubic hair.

Timing of menarche

Menarche is the onset of menstruation in girls. The mean age of menarche is about 12.6 years in white girls, 12.1 years in black girls, and 12.2 years in Mexican-American girls. The lower (~ −2 SD) age threshold is about 10.5 years in white girls and 10 years in black girls. The upper (+2 SD) cut-off is between 14.5 and 15 years for white girls and about 14 and 14.5 years in black girls.

Of note, girls who have earlier thelarche may have a slightly longer period of time before menarche. Thus, a

Female

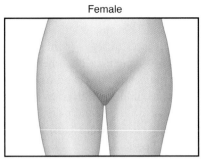

Stage 2

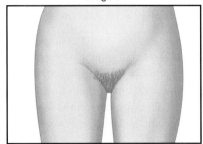

Stage 3

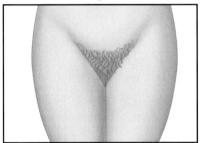

Stage 4

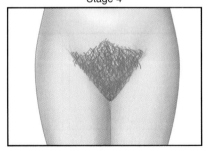

Stage 5

FEMALE

Stage 1	Preadolescent; no pubic hair present; a fine vellus hair covers the genital area.
Stage 2	A sparse distribution of long, slightly pigmented straight hair appears bilaterally along medial border of the labia majora.
Stage 3	The pubic hair pigmentation increases; the hairs begin to curl and to spread sparsely over the mons pubis.
Stage 4	The pubic hairs continue to curl and become coarse in texture. The number of hairs continues to increase.
Stage 5	Mature: pubic hair attains an adult feminine triangular pattern, with spread to the surface of the medial thigh.

FIGURE 7-4 ■ Tanner staging of pubic hair development in females. (*From Greydanus DE, Pratt HD. Adolescent growth and development, and sport participation. In: Patel DR, Greydanus DE, Baker RJ, eds. Pediatric Practice: Sports Medicine. New York, NY: McGraw-Hill; 2009:19.*)

girl with thelarche at the age of 9 years may have 2.8 years before menarche, while another girl with thelarche at the age of 11 years may only have 1.8 years until menarche. There are also girls who have early thelarche, but whose tempo of pubertal progression is slow, with a normal final outcome; thus, the tempo of puberty should be part of the assessment of pubertal development.

Physical Changes in Boys: Testicular Enlargement

Although there exists a system for Tanner staging of male genital development during puberty (Figure 7-5), in practice, the differences among the intermediate stages are too subjective for consistency from observer

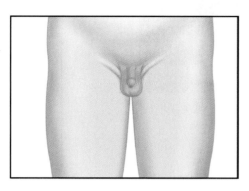

Stage 1

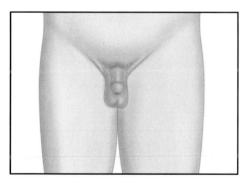

Stage 2

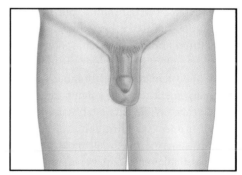

Stage 3

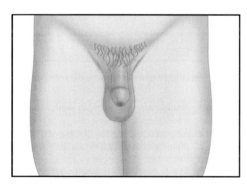

Stage 4

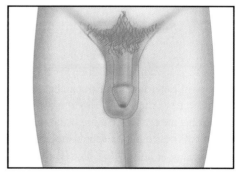

Stage 5

Stage 1   Preadolescent: testes, scrotum, and penis identical to early childhood.

Stage 2   Enlargement of testes as result of canalization of seminiferous tubules. The scrotum enlarges, developing a reddish hue and altering its skin texture. The penis enlarges slightly.

Stage 3   The testes and scrotum continue to grow. The length of the penis increases.

Stage 4   The testes and scrotum continue to grow; the scrotal skin darkens. The penis grows in width, and the glans penis develops.

Stage 5   Mature: adult size and shape of testes, scrotum, and penis.

FIGURE 7-5 ■ Tanner staging of male genital development. (*From: Greydanus DE, Pratt HD. Adolescent growth and development, and sport participation. In: Patel DR, Greydanus DE, Baker RJ, eds.* Pediatric Practice: Sports Medicine. *New York, NY: McGraw-Hill; 2009:20.*)

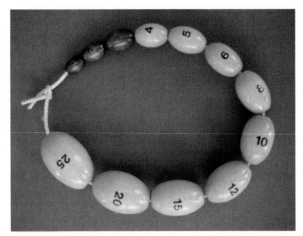

FIGURE 7-6 ■ Prader orchidometer for determination of testicular volume.

to observer. Much more accurate is the measurement of testicular size using a model such as the Prader orchidometer, shown in Figure 7-6. A volume of 3 to 4 mL is considered to be an indicator of pubertal onset, as the seminiferous tubular volume increases under gonadotropin stimulation. If an orchidometer is not available, a testis length of 2.5 cm along the longest axis corresponds to approximately 4 mL volume. Mean age at testicular enlargement to 3 mL volume ranges from about 11 to 12 years.[3] While data establishing the normal lower and upper age thresholds of testicular enlargement are sparse, in general, most physicians would consider testicular enlargement before the age of 8 to 9 years to be early, and lack of testicular enlargement by the age of 14 years to be significantly delayed.

Physical Changes in Boys: Pubarche

Tanner staging criteria for pubic hair in boys are shown in Figure 7-7. As with girls, androgen secretion from the adrenals is an important determinant of pubarche. However, androgen secretion from the testis is also a major factor in pubarche, increasing the chances that precocious pubic hair development in boys may signify true precocious puberty.

The average age of pubarche in boys is around 12 to 12.5 years in white and Hispanic boys, with black boys starting about 1 year earlier. Pubarche before the age of 10 years is commonly considered worthy of further observation and clinical workup, while lack of pubic hair development after the age of 14.5 years in white and Hispanic males (after 14 years in blacks) can be considered delayed. Axillary hair typically appears about 1 to 2 years after pubic hair.

Physical Changes in Boys: Other

Spermarche, the ability to produce and ejaculate sperm, typically occurs around the age of 13.5 years. Voice

Male

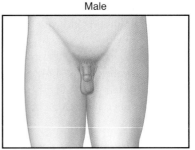

Stage 2

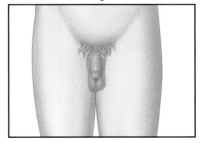

Stage 3

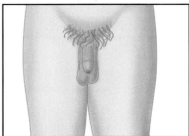

Stage 4

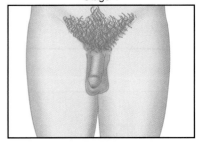

Stage 5

MALE

Stage 1   Preadolescent; no pubic hair present; a fine vellus hair covers the genital area.

Stage 2   A sparse distribution of long, slightly pigmented hair appears at the base of the penis.

Stage 3   The pubic hair pigmentation increases; the hairs begin to curl and to spread laterally in a scanty distribution.

Stage 4   The pubic hairs continue to curl and become coarse in texture. An adult type of distribution is attained, but the number of hairs remains fewer.

Stage 5   Mature: the pubic hair attains an adult distribution with spread to the surface of the medial thigh. Pubic hair will grow along linea alba in 80% of males.

FIGURE 7-7 ■ Tanner staging of pubic hair development in males. (*From Greydanus DE, Pratt HD. Adolescent growth and development, and sport participation. In: Patel DR, Greydanus DE, Baker RJ, eds.* Pediatric Practice: Sports Medicine. *New York, NY: McGraw-Hill; 2009:19.*)

break, the transition to the deeper adult voice, occurs at a mean age of about 13.9 years. Peak height velocity, increased muscular strength, and worsening of acne typically occur around this same time.

Facial hair, usually starting with the upper lip, typically appears around the age of 15 years, but may not be of full adult quality until well past the teenage years.

Growth during puberty

Girls have their peak growth velocity early in puberty, typically beginning right before thelarche. Boys, in contrast, have their peak growth spurt during mid-puberty, at a mean age of 13.5 years, often corresponding to a testicular volume of 10 to 12 mL.

A common misconception is that the amount of growth remaining for a girl after menarche is only a couple of inches, which often leads to predictions of severe short stature in girls who have early normal menstruation.[12] In fact, the amount of growth remaining varies greatly depending upon when menarche occurs. Thus, a girl who has menarche at the age of 10 years grows, on average, an additional 4 in, while another girl who has menarche at the average of 12.7 years will grow on average another 3 in. The girl who has menarche at the age of 15 years may only grow 2 in more, but since she is already at a taller height by the time she has her first menstrual period, her final height is likely to be within her expected genetic potential.

PRECOCIOUS PUBERTY

Introduction

The first sign of clinically detectable puberty in girls is breast development in 85% of cases with pubic hair preceding thelarche in the other 15%. In actuality, ovarian enlargement is the first true sign of female puberty, but requires ultrasonography for detection. Analogously, testicular enlargement is the first sign in boys. Whether puberty is truly occurring earlier than was previously thought, especially in girls, is not universally accepted as some of the suggestive large-scale epidemiological data may be flawed because of ascertainment bias in subject selection, use of visual (as opposed to manual) determination of breast staging, and failure to perform diagnostic testing in children in the younger age ranges to definitively rule out pathological causes of precocity. That said, Danish Registry data suggest that 0.2% of all Danish girls and less than 0.05% of all Danish boys have some sort of precocious puberty.

Thus, the clinician must first determine in a child with "borderline" early puberty whether observed changes may represent normal variants or have a more serious organic basis. The next dilemma is when and if diagnostic testing is required since often nothing more than a bone age is required in clear examples of normal or slowly progressive variants. This decision may often be best left to the pediatric endocrinology consultant who can, in the most cost-effective manner, determine if, how (basally or after stimulation), where (noting tremendous variability in assays and clinical laboratories), and how often testing is required. Finally, decisions regarding the necessity for and type of treatment will usually require the specialist's input, noting that not all organic etiologies and certainly not the normal variants require treatment.

Presumed Normal Variants

Idiopathic isolated premature thelarche

Definition. Most commonly, premature thelarche begins around 2 years of age, but may be present from birth onward (Figure 7-8A). The observed tissue may be asymmetrical, unilateral, or bilateral. Although asymmetrical and/or unilateral breast tissue often causes parents to be concerned about the possibility of malignancy, this is rarely the case. In 30% to 60% of affected girls, the early breast tissue spontaneously regresses within an average of 18 months from its development. When it persists, the degree of breast development typically does not exceed Tanner stage 3.

Etiology. The etiology of typical isolated premature thelarche is unknown. Most studies have failed to show differences between basal and GnRH-stimulated gonadotropin levels in girls with simple premature thelarche *versus* age-matched normal girls (both of whom has an FSH-predominant response); in contrast, girls with true precocious puberty have an LH-predominant response. Conventional assays usually cannot detect elevated serum estradiol levels in girls with isolated premature thelarche, although higher mean levels compared to those in age-matched normal girls have been reported using an ultrasensitive recombinant cell bioassay, but with significant overlap between the two groups. By default, heightened sensitivity of breast tissue to estrogen has been invoked as a potential etiology. A causative role for environmental endocrine disruptors has also been suggested. In cases of either exaggerated isolated thelarche with advanced bone age and/or increased height velocity or self-limited recurrent episodes of isolated breast-budding that may be associated with advanced bone age and/or stepped-up height velocity, activating mutations of the $G_s\alpha$ gene have been reported in up to 25% of affected girls, akin to the mutation reported in full-blown McCune-Albright syndrome (see section "Idiopathic Isolated Precocious Menarche").

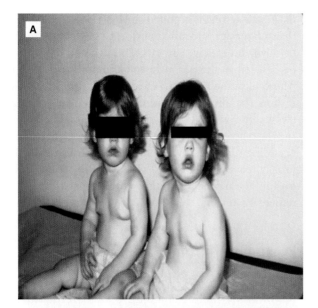
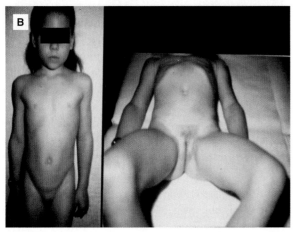
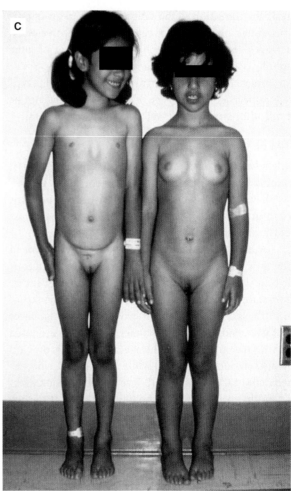

FIGURE 7-8 ■ **(A)** Twin 2-year-old females with idiopathic precocious thelarche and no other signs of puberty. **(B)** 5-year-old female with idiopathic precocious adrenarche and no other signs of puberty. **(C)** 3-year-old female (right) with idiopathic isosexual central precocious puberty characterized by both breast and pubic hair development, along with tall stature, contrasted to a normal 5-year-old prepubertal female child (left). (*A and C reproduced from: Geffner ME. Disorders of puberty. In: Kliegman RM, Greenbaum LA, Lye PS, eds.* Practical Strategies in Pediatric Diagnosis and Therapy. *Harcourt Health Sciences, 2005; with permission of Elsevier.*)

Diagnosis, evaluation, and natural history. For girls with "classical" precocious isolated thelarche, that is, starting at or prior to the age of 2 years, who, by definition, have no associated growth spurt and a bone age that is within 2 SD of their chronological age, no other diagnostic studies typically need to be performed. Such girls typically will go on to have menarche at a normal age and attain normal adult stature. Since a small subset of girls who present with precocious thelarche may progress to either a variant characterized by isolated progressive breast development in conjunction with accelerated linear growth and advancing bone age or to true precocious puberty, ongoing follow-up either by a pediatrician or a pediatric endocrinologist is mandatory with judicious use of additional/ongoing laboratory and radiological testing as dictated by the clinical course.

Treatment. Unless the condition progresses as noted earlier, no treatment is indicated.

Idiopathic isolated precocious adrenarche
Definition. This is another common pubertal variant that is characterized by the early development of pubic hair, axillary hair and odor, and/or a small amount of acne using the same age criteria defined previously (Figure 7-8B).

Etiology. It appears to result from increased production of adrenal androgens in both sexes at an earlier than normal age resulting from premature maturation of the zona reticularis of the adrenal cortex.[13] More specifically, it has been proposed that there is a reduction in 3β-hydroxysteroid dehydrogenase activity and induction of the 17,20-lyase component of the P450c17 enzyme complex in the zona reticularis through preferential hyperphosphorylation secondary to an autosomal dominant mutation of the kinase responsible for serine/threonine phosphorylation. Some subjects with precocious adrenarche have been reported to have heightened *androgen receptor* gene activity while others have been found to be more likely to harbor a specific polymorphism in the adrenocorticotropic hormone (ACTH) (melanocortin 2 receptor = MC2R) receptor promoter. Finally, etiological or permissive roles for corticotropin-releasing hormone, insulin, IGF-1, and leptin have also been proposed. Precocious adrenarche occurs much more commonly in girls than in boys (perhaps as much as tenfold), and appears to develop more often in obese and/or African-American girls. It also appears to occur more often in children with low birth weight.

Diagnosis, evaluation, and natural history. In both girls and boys, by definition, there is no clinical evidence of virilization, that is, no growth spurt, increase in muscle bulk, voice-deepening, or temporal hair recession (male pattern baldness). In addition, affected girls will not manifest clitoromegaly and boys will not have penile enlargement. Furthermore, there is no evidence of ovarian estrogen-mediated components of puberty in girls and no testicular enlargement or function in boys. If a child presents at a very young age, it is generally presumed that an organic cause is more likely to be found. However, in infant boys with isolated scrotal hair, typically no cause is found and the hair subsequently falls out within 12 months. In most cases of idiopathic precocious adrenarche, serum levels of DHEA and/or DHEAS are in the respective *pubertal* ranges for girls and boys, and the bone age is mildly, but not significantly, advanced. In girls with precocious adrenarche, serum levels of other adrenal steroids are usually normal or only slightly elevated for age, especially if measured after stimulation with ACTH, but normal after leuprolide administration. These observations suggest that precocious adrenarche in girls is associated with functional *adrenal* hyperandrogenism, but no biochemical evidence of *ovarian* hyperandrogenism. Yet it has also been demonstrated that girls with precocious adrenarche may have ultrasonographic and Doppler evidence of polycystic ovaries with an increase in ovarian volume, small-sized subcapsular follicle number, stromal echogenicity, and stromal vascularization over time. Thus, if a child presents with the classical phenotype, no other laboratory or radiological studies are usually warranted, unless there is significant rapidity of progression of symptoms. On rare occasion, children with more serious organic pathologies associated with hyperandrogenism (eg, nonclassical adrenal hyperplasia [NCAH], adrenal tumors, and gonadal

tumors) or true precocious puberty may initially present similarly to those with apparent idiopathic isolated premature adrenarche. Thus, in unclear situations, serum measurements of 17-hydroxyprogesterone (basally or after ACTH stimulation) and testosterone (early morning), along with ultrasounds of the adrenals and/or gonads, may need to be done. With the presence of isolated adrenarche in girls, measurement of LH, FSH, and estradiol is not indicated (as these should only be determined when there are isolated female changes of puberty or both female and male changes). Historically, this pubertal variant has been considered to be benign and self-limited, but recent epidemiological and biochemical data suggest that, at least in girls with associated low birth weight and rapid postnatal catch-up growth, precocious adrenarche may be followed by early onset and rapid progression of true puberty as well as by future development of functional ovarian hyperandrogenism/polycystic ovarian syndrome (PCOS). Additional features of this syndrome include early onset insulin resistance with a disturbance of the insulin-IGF-1 system, atherogenic lipid profiles, and hypertension (collectively known as the metabolic syndrome or syndrome X), and a positive family history of type 2 diabetes mellitus (T2DM), hypertension, PCOS, and anovulation beginning in late adolescence. Recently, it has been shown that boys with precocious adrenarche are also insulin-resistant. Thus, the adjective "benign" or term "normal variant" should not necessarily be applied to cases of premature adrenarche.

Treatment. Currently, there remains no proven treatment for idiopathic precocious adrenarche and no specific means by which to forestall future functional ovarian hyperandrogenism, although basic practices to limit weight gain, regulate cholesterol intake, and avoid smoking seem advisable. Investigative use of metformin in children with precocious adrenarche has been shown, in small cohorts, to improve body composition and delay the onset of true puberty, and, in so doing, perhaps improve adult height.

Idiopathic isolated precocious menarche
Definition. This is defined as menstruation without any other manifestations of puberty in a young girl prior to the age of 9 years.

Etiology. The cause is unknown, with the ultimate assignment of an idiopathic basis for its basis being a diagnosis of exclusion, so that one must also consider a foreign body, local masses, and McCune-Albright syndrome.

Diagnosis, evaluation, and natural history. In the setting of isolated early menarche, the situation is usually self-limited, albeit disturbing to parents and patients. In most cases, there is only one period, but there may be two or more. Adult height and subsequent menstrual patterns and fertility are usually normal.

Treatment. None is required.

Rapid tempo puberty[14]

Definition. No formal definition exists. Using a statistical approach, pubertal progression may be considered unduly fast if the start of puberty is within the normal range for gender and race, but subsequent milestones are achieved more than 2 SD ahead of their expected mean age of occurrence. As guidelines, in girls, the typical interval from breast budding (Tanner stage 2) to menarche (usually associated with at least Tanner stage 4 breasts) is 2.4 ± 1.1 years (mean $\pm$ 1 SD). In boys, the usual time from pubertal onset (Tanner stage 2 testes, ie, ≥ 3 mL in volume) to adult testicular volume (mean 20 mL) is 3.2 ± 1.8 years.

Etiology. The exact etiology is unknown. Factors that may modify the rate of pubertal maturation include: family genetics, a history of low birth weight (small for gestational age [SGA]), rapid and/or excessive growth in early childhood (especially if having been born SGA), diet, diminished physical activity, and an array of other factors (eg, treatment of hypothyroidism, adoption, and endocrine disruptors).

Diagnosis, evaluation, and natural history. Unfortunately, from a practical standpoint, the typically affected adolescent usually presents to medical attention nearly or even fully developed and having had marked height acceleration unduly early. In fact, such adolescents may already be in their postspurt height deceleration phase as a result of markedly advanced bone age that appears as a by-product of the phenomenon without yielding the requisite number of inches that would have occurred with a normal pubertal tempo. This process is often missed in a first affected child in a family because of the natural infrequency of visits to the primary care provider for well-child physical examinations in this age group.

Treatment. There are also no proven treatment strategies for rapid tempo puberty. In fact, when identified late as is often the case in the index case in a family, there is often no viable treatment option. When there is reasonable remaining growth potential, transient interruption of the hypothalamic-pituitary-gonadal axis, as is done in children with *bona fide* central precocious puberty, is usually considered using GnRH analogs without or with added GH. However, in the United States, use of either drug class to treat rapid tempo puberty is not FDA-sanctioned, so that their use may be moot because of an inability to obtain insurance company authorization. More importantly, there are no data demonstrating treatment efficacy in this situation, although, from a theoretical standpoint, combination therapy might be helpful. Use of other off-label agents, such as aromatase inhibitors in boys, may be considered, but once again this approach is based solely on a theoretical basis and anecdotal experience.[15]

Pathological Causes of Precocious Puberty

Isosexual central precocious puberty[16]

Definition. Central precocious precocity (CPP) results from activation of the hypothalamic-pituitary-gonadal axis at an earlier-than-normal age (Figure 7-8C). Although as noted above that the start of normal puberty may be occurring earlier than previously thought, most pediatric endocrinologists still consider 8 years in girls and 9 years in boys as general cut-points between early normal and early puberty, recognizing that an individualized approach needs to be taken for African-American girls between 6 and 8 years, Caucasian girls between 7 and 8 years, and all boys between 8 and 9 years (as pathological causes of precocity have occasionally been reported in this age range). Isosexual development refers to pubertal changes appropriate for the sex of the child, such as breast-budding in girls and testicular enlargement in boys. This contrasts with contrasexual development in which the pubertal features in females are male-hormone-directed, for example, clitoromegaly, or in males are female-hormone-directed, for example, breast development. In general, the presence of *both* female- and male-hormone-mediated features of puberty in females is a valuable clue to a central source for the precocity. However, on rare occasions, tumorous production of androgen by an adrenal tumor can provide sufficient substrate for either peripheral or intratumoral aromatization to estrogen, thereby confusing the clinical picture.

Etiology. In females, most cases (~80%) of CPP have been considered to be idiopathic. With the application of magnetic resonance imaging (MRI), a somewhat higher percentage of organic causes has been detected in girls (Table 7-2). In contrast, only about 10% of central cases are idiopathic in males, with the remainder being associated with an underlying lesion of the CNS. The most concerning causes of CPP are tumors that arise in the suprasellar region, which may also be present with other, usually anterior, pituitary hormone deficiencies. Tumor-associated *isolated* CPP can occur with histologically benign hypothalamic hamartomas, the most common cause of CPP in very young children (Figures 7-9A and 7-9B). They may trigger puberty through secretion of GnRH ("ectopic GnRH pulse generator") or transforming

Table 7-2.

Etiologies of Isosexual Central Precocious Puberty

- Idiopathic
- Hypothalamic hamartomas
- Other brain tumors (glial cell tumors, germ cell tumors, and, occasionally, craniopharyngiomas and pinealomas)
- "Idiopathic" isolated GH deficiency or multiple anterior pituitary hormone deficiencies, and ectopic neurohypophysis
- Congenital suprasellar brain defects (subarachnoid cysts, arachnoidoceles, and Rathke cleft cysts)
- Congenital mid-line anomalies (hydrocephalus, meningomyelocele, and optic nerve hypoplasia)
- Cranial irradiation
- Previous meningoencephalitis
- Major head trauma
- Perinatal insults
- Neurofibromatosis-1
- Untreated or undertreated peripheral causes of puberty (eg, congenital adrenal hyperplasia)
- "Overlap syndrome," in association with longstanding untreated primary hypothyroidism
- Hyperprolactinemia
- Adoption from abroad
- Activating mutation of the gene encoding *GPR54*, the G protein-coupled receptor mediating the effects of kisspeptin on stimulation of GnRH neurons

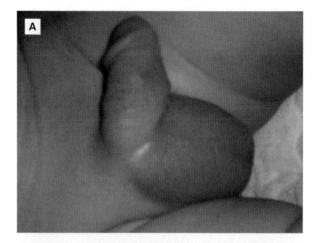

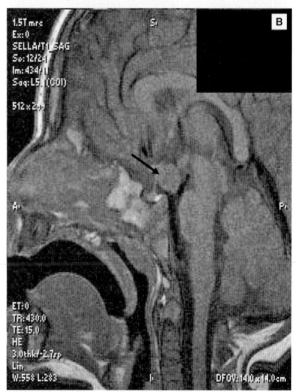

FIGURE 7-9 ■ **(A)** 9-month-old male who presented with 6-cc testes, Tanner stage 3 pubic hair, rapid linear growth, and a bone age of 3 years. **(B)** Sagittal T_1-weighted MRI demonstrating hypothalamic hamartoma (thin black arrow)

growth factor-β, another puberty-inducing factor. Hamartomas may, on occasion, be associated with gelastic (laughing) or other seizures. Other brain tumors that may cause CPP (with or without other pituitary hormone abnormalities) are glial cell tumors, germ cell tumors, and, occasionally, craniopharyngiomas and pinealomas. Recently, the occurrence of combined "idiopathic" isolated GH deficiency or multiple anterior pituitary hormone deficiencies, an ectopic neurohypophysis, and CPP has been described.

Other CNS causes include congenital brain defects that arise in the suprasellar region (eg, subarachnoid cysts, arachnoidoceles, and Rathke cleft cysts[17]); other congenital mid-line anomalies (eg, hydrocephalus, meningomyelocele, and optic nerve hypoplasia); cranial irradiation; previous meningoencephalitis; major head trauma (usually associated with loss of consciousness); and perinatal insult. The well-known association of CPP with neurofibromatosis-1 (Figure 7-10), characterized by associated smooth-bordered café-au-lait spots (resembling the coast of California), axillary and inguinal freckles, Lisch nodules, and neurofibromas, may result from the presence of a hypothalamic optic glioma, but may also have no detectable tumor on MRI. CPP may also occur in the setting of untreated or undertreated peripheral causes of puberty (see "Precocious pseudopuberty"),

such as CAH, in which premature activation of the GnRH pulse generator occurs, presumably as a result of prior or ongoing CNS exposure to high levels of androgens (or androgens aromatized to estrogens). Another cause of sexual precocity that begins outside of the hypothalamic-pituitary-gonadal axis is referred to as the "overlap syndrome," in which CPP develops in the setting of longstanding untreated primary hypothyroidism. The mechanism of this phenomenon is not

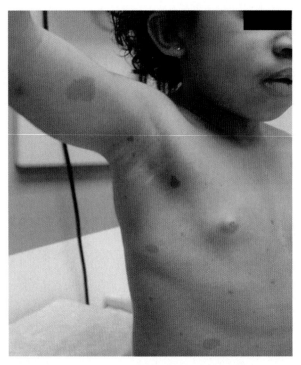

FIGURE 7-10 ■ Four-year-old female with neurofibromatosis demonstrating characteristic smooth-bordered ("coast-of-California") café-au-lait spots, axillary freckles, and Tanner stage 3 breast development. (Photograph courtesy of Erica Eugster, MD [Indiana University School of Medicine, Riley Hospital for Children]).

well-understood, although, in the past, it had been ascribed to both elevated thyrotropin-releasing hormone (TRH) levels that stimulate pituitary FSH/LH secretion and, more recently, to the hypothyroid state itself in which TSH promiscuously interacts with gonadotropin receptors in the gonads. Rarely, males with hyperprolactinemia may develop CPP (although hypogonadism is much more likely). A heightened risk of CPP has been reported in children adopted from abroad, although this association may be clouded by inaccurate birthdates.

The newest described etiology for CPP is an activating mutation of the gene encoding *GPR54*, the G protein-coupled receptor mediating the effects of its ligand, kisspeptin, on stimulation of GnRH neurons. This was recently reported as the mechanism for CPP in an adopted Brazilian girl with slow breast development beginning at birth. The frequency of such mutations is unknown, but it should be pointed out that there is a 27.5% prevalence of familial CPP. At the current time, there is not enough phenotypic information to make specific recommendations as to who should be considered for genetic testing which is currently only available in research laboratories.

Diagnosis, evaluation, and natural history. The initial evaluation of the child with precocious puberty is aimed at determining whether the process is normal or abnormal, has an idiopathic or pathological basis, what the rate of progression of the pubertal changes has been or will be, and whether the process originates centrally or peripherally (Figures 7-11 and 7-12). The initial test to perform is a bone age x-ray which provides an index of the potency of the process, although is not useful in delineating the source of the hormonal process. More specifically, if not significantly advanced (ie, within 20% of the chronological age in months) and not associated with acceleration in height velocity, this suggests either a normal variant, slow progression pattern, or a process of relatively short duration. If a girl with precocious puberty has a significantly advanced bone age, a laboratory workup must be initiated that is dictated by the findings on the physical examination. Measurement of free T_4 and TSH in both sexes is useful to rule out long-standing primary hypothyroidism which is usually apparent on clinical grounds.

If breast development is evident with or without androgen effects, measurement of random serum gonadotropins, using ultrasensitive assays for FSH and LH, and estradiol (using liquid chromatography tandem mass spectrometry or other methods to remove cross-reacting steroids) should be undertaken. Ultrasensitive bioassays for serum estrogenic bioactivity are under development. A pelvic ultrasound in this setting is often quite helpful. Noting that mean prepubertal ovarian volumes (calculated for an oblate ovoid by multiplying the measurements in millimeters of the three dimensions by 0.523) increase gradually with age (3 years: 0.51 mm^3; 5.0 years: 0.78 mm^3; 7 years: 1.14 mm^3; and 9 years: 1.31 mm^3), the presence of bilaterally enlarged ovaries for age suggests hypothalamic-pituitary activation (or, less likely, McCune-Albright syndrome). In addition, the maturation of the uterus can be determined simultaneously and is useful as another indicator of the potency of estrogenic action. Measurement of serum androgen levels in girls with breast development with or without concomitant androgen effects rarely adds any useful diagnostic information. Because of the pulsatile and initially preferential sleep-entrained secretion of serum gonadotropins, random daytime measurements of LH and FSH may be low in the setting of central activation. However, use of immunofluorometric (IFMA) and third-generation immunochemiluminescent (ICMA) assays for LH correlate much better with true CPP. However, if random gonadotropin levels are low, yet clinical suspicion suggests CPP, a GnRH stimulation test would next be performed. The most common protocol currently used for this test involves the subcutaneous administration of leuprolide acetate

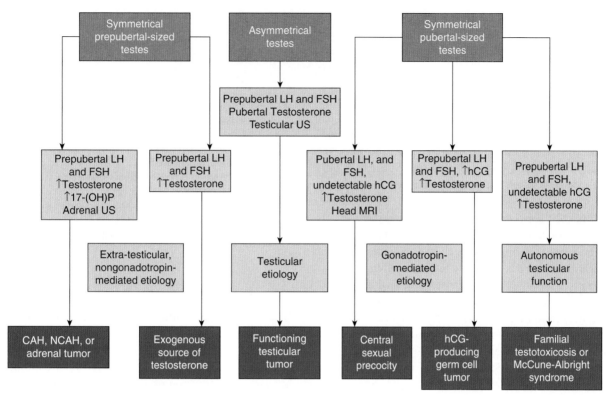

FIGURE 7-11 ▪ Simplified diagnostic algorithm for precocious puberty in boys.

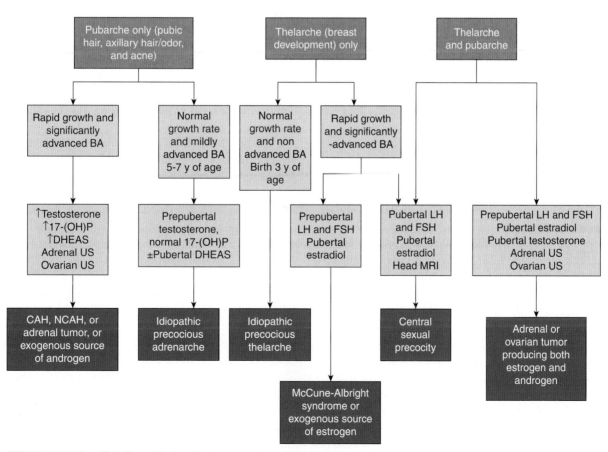

FIGURE 7-12 ▪ Simplified diagnostic algorithm for precocious puberty in girls.

(not the depot form) at a dose of 20 μg/kg with measurement of gonadotropins every 30 minutes for 2 hours and the sex steroid of interest 2 and 24 hours later. The results of these tests correlate remarkably well with those from multiple-sample, longer GnRH stimulation tests. The rationale for this interpretation is that, with central precocity, as with normal puberty, endogenous hypothalamic GnRH is being produced in a pubertal pattern that "primes" the pituitary gonadotrophs, so that, following administration of a single pharmacological dose of GnRH, there is abundant release of LH as typically occurs in teenagers. Measuring FSH levels during the test serves only to ensure biological activity of the leuprolide and the peak concentration attained tends to be overlap between the prepubertal and pubertal state. Regardless, if CPP is confirmed biochemically and is progressive, a head MRI—in a closed unit—with contrast (required for detailed assessment of hypothalamic-pituitary region anatomy) must be performed to look for potential lesions in the hypothalamic-pituitary region which are typically found in about 10% of girls with CPP. In cases of idiopathic CPP in girls, the MRI will frequently demonstrate exaggerated pituitary height (mean 6.2 ± 0.2 mm) as is typically seen in the adolescent female pubertal range.

The workup for a boy with isosexual precocity and a significantly advanced bone age is directed by the size of the testes. In cases of CPP, both testes are symmetrically enlarged for age, the degree to which will be governed by the potency and duration of the underlying etiology. Laboratory testing and the use of the leuprolide GnRH test are similar to that outlined above for girls, except for the substitution of testosterone for estradiol measurements. As with girls, if central precocity is confirmed biochemically, a contrast-enhanced head MRI must be performed as up to 50% of affected males will have demonstrable lesions of the CNS.

Treatment. As to general issues related to treatment of precocious puberty, not all cases, including not all cases of CPP, require treatment (Table 7-3). Children with CPP or early normal puberty with a strong familial basis may profit from a period of observation without treatment, especially if outcomes of affected family members have been unremarkable. In addition, not all children with *de novo* central precocious puberty require treatment as a significant number have either a slowly progressive and/or transient process. Unless clinical findings suggest a rapid progression and/or significant resultant psychosocial difficulties, most children with CPP should be observed for a 3- to 6-month period before a decision to initiate GnRH-agonist therapy is made.

The specific reasons that favor treatment include preservation of acceptable final stature based on family

Table 7-3.

Treatment of Central Precocious Puberty

Goal: inhibit secretion of gonadotropins and thereby reduce production of sex steroids by administration of GnRH analogs

Nafarelin acetate (Synarel-Syntex) given twice daily by intranasal route (rarely used)

Leuprolide acetate (Lupron-Abbott) given as a daily subcutaneous injection (rarely used)

Leuprolide acetate (Lupron Depot-Abbott) given as an intramuscular injection every 3-4 wk

Histrelin (Supprelin–Endo) as a 12-mo subdermal implant

height genetics, prevention of psychological trauma (eg, from menstruation at a young age), reversal of mature physical appearance and risk of pregnancy in girls (as others assume that affected children are older than they appear), and reduction of aggressiveness and preoccupation with sexuality. Of note, serious psychological effects of early puberty are not typically encountered and GnRH agonist treatment typically only halts, but not actually reverses, existing physical changes of puberty induced by gonadal steroids. Thus, the goal of therapy is to inhibit secretion of gonadotropins and thereby reduce production of sex-specific sex steroids. This is accomplished by the administration of GnRH agonists that behave antagonistically because of biochemical modifications that result in a prolonged reversible duration of action causing down-regulation of pituitary GnRH receptors (after initial stimulation for the first 1-2 months of use), ultimately eliminating responsiveness to endogenous GnRH and, thus, decreasing LH and FSH secretion. Verification of adequate suppression can be confirmed by demonstration of prepubertal LH levels as measured in one of the aforementioned ultrasensitive assays measured just before a dose of therapeutic GnRH agonist or 1 hour following its administration in which the therapeutic agent is simultaneously used as an acute gonadotropin stimulator. Ongoing documentation of axis suppression should be performed every 3 months. The available FDA-approved GnRH agonist formulations in the United States include: nafarelin acetate which is given twice daily by the intranasal route (but is rarely used), leuprolide acetate which is given either as a daily subcutaneous injection (also rarely used) or as an intramuscular depot injection every 3 to 4 weeks, and, most recently, implanted histrelin.[18] Because of the infrequent need for dosing, intramuscular leuprolide has been the most common formulation in the United States. Histrelin is a 12-month subdermal implant requiring surgical insertion and removal on an annual basis either under local or short-term general anesthesia. Three-year efficacy studies with the implant have been performed showing sustained suppression of the hypothalamic-pituitary-gonadal axis. Testing of a very long-acting formulation of leuprolide given every 3 months is underway. The clearest criteria for initiation of GnRH agonist treatment of children with sexual precocity include chronological age less than 6 years, a random LH level of more than 0.3 mIU/mL by ICMA in girls or boys, an LH response to leuprolide injection of more than 4.2 mIU/mL by IFMA and more than 3.3 mIU/mL by ICMA in girls or more than 3.3 by IFMA or more than 4.1 mIU/mL by ICMA in boys, a pubertal serum concentration of estradiol (in girls) or testosterone (in boys), advancement of bone age by more than 2 years over chronological age, the presence of an organic lesion or a pituitary height more than 6.0 mm on MRI, an abnormally low adult height prediction (eg, <152.5 cm in girls, <165 cm in boys, or <5 cm below predicted adult target height), and existing or anticipated psychological sequelae of precocious puberty. However, the ultimate decision to treat immediately, observe, and possibly treat later, or merely to observe must involve a careful analysis of all of the above criteria on a case-by-case basis. The implementation of treatment in cases of early normal, but rapid tempo puberty in females between 8 and 9 years and in boys between 9 and 10.5 years is often considered, but available data show that the GnRH agonists merely slow the pace of puberty without any significant effect on final adult height on average. Whether there may be a benefit in selected cases remains uncertain.

The optimal duration of GnRH agonist treatment also remains unclear, but, as a general guideline, most pediatric endocrinologists release or taper therapy beginning at about 11 years in girls and 12 years in boys.[19] From a clinical perspective, successful GnRH agonist treatment is associated with a stabilization of estrogen effects in girls (with no effect on androgen-mediated events) and androgen effects in boys. It is unusual that treatment results in complete reversal of physical changes to the prepubertal state. Height velocity and the rate of bone age maturation will slow down and, on some occasions, the linear growth rate actually becomes subnormal. This is not necessarily problematic as long as bone age maturation slows commensurately, but, on occasion, GH therapy must be added. Outcome data insofar as final height is concerned suggest that the best results occur in taller children at start of GnRH agonist therapy and when GnRH agonist therapy is initiated prior to the age of 6 years. Based on data from Japan and Italy, once GnRH analog therapy is discontinued, reactivation of the hypothalamic-pituitary-gonadal axis usually occurs within 12 months, with menarche or resumption

of menses occurring between 12 and 12.5 years on average and ovulation documented in 90% of girls at least 2 years after menarche, followed by subsequent fertility.[20] Unfortunately, there are limited long-term fertility data in individuals treated with GnRH agonists as children, with only a few reports of successful childbearing in this population. Other problems noted with leuprolide injections include sterile abscesses at the site of administration, as well as a tendency toward obesity. No specific side effects have been identified for the histrelin implant other than transient local discomfort and occasional breakage of the implant on removal. For large tumors in the hypothalamic-pituitary region, developmental anomalies, and hydrocephalus that are associated with CPP, surgical interventions are justified, although these are not for the purpose of treatment of precocious puberty. Finally, hypothalamic hamartomas are benign and tend to be very slow-growing and, therefore, surgical therapy is not usually recommended.

Precocious pseudopuberty[16]

Definition. The term, precocious pseudopuberty, refers to gonadal or adrenal sex steroid secretion not resulting from activation of hypothalamic-pituitary-gonadal axis (ie, pituitary-independent or peripheral in origin). This can involve isolated androgen, isolated estrogen, or combined androgen and estrogen production.

Etiology. Precocious and inappropriate androgen production in *girls*, including features of virilization, can be caused by ovarian arrhenoblastomas and hyperthecosis (Table 7-4). In *boys*, premature androgen production may result from Leydig cell tumors (some of which harbor activating mutations of the LH receptor); human chorionogonadotropin (hCG)-secreting tumors, such as hepatoblastomas (most common) or germ-cell tumors (sometimes seen in adolescent males with Klinefelter syndrome); McCune-Albright syndrome (although more often in girls); and familial testotoxicosis (also known as male LH-independent sexual precocity) (Figure 7-13). This rare condition involves gonadotropin-independent testicular maturation usually inherited in an autosomal-dominant, male-limited pattern with signs of puberty generally exhibited by 4 years of age. In boys with familial testotoxicosis, testosterone production and Leydig cell hyperplasia occur in the setting of prepubertal serum LH levels as a result of a mutation in the *LH receptor* gene resulting in its constitutive activation and gain-of-function. Affected males are fertile. Females who carry this mutation do not develop precocious puberty and apparently have normal reproductive function. Two unrelated boys with familial testotoxicosis have been described who also have pseudohypoparathyroidism type 1A owing to a tissue-specific temperature-sensitive mutation of the $G_s\alpha$ gene with activation in the testes

Table 7-4.

Causes of Precocious Pseudopuberty

Androgen overproduction: girls
  Ovarian arrhenoblastomas
  Ovarian hyperthecosis
Androgen overproduction: boys
  Leydig-cell tumors
  hCG-secreting tumors (eg, hepatoblastomas and germ cell tumors sometimes seen in boys with Klinefelter syndrome)
  McCune-Albright syndrome
  Familial testotoxicosis
Androgen overproduction: girls and boys
  Nonclassical (late-onset) adrenal hyperplasia
  Androgen-secreting adrenal tumors
  Generalized glucocorticoid resistance
  Some cases of Cushing syndrome
  Exogenous anabolic steroid abuse
Estrogen overproduction: girls
  Ovarian cysts
  Ovarian granulosa cell tumors
  Sertoli-Leydig cell tumors (isolated or as part of Peutz-Jeghers syndrome)
  McCune-Albright syndrome
Estrogen overproduction: boys
  Certain adrenal tumors
  Sertoli cell tumors (usually in the setting of Peutz-Jeghers syndrome)

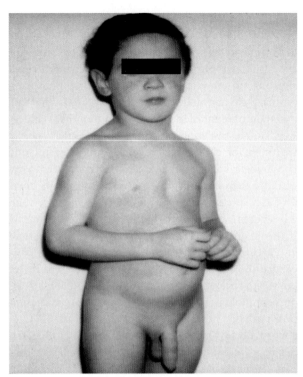

FIGURE 7-13 ■ A 3¹/₂-year-old male with Tanner stage 2 pubic hair, an enlarged penis, and 4-cc testes, rapid linear growth, basal LH and FSH <2 mIU/mL, testosterone 326 ng/dL, and bone age between 7 and 8 year. There was no increase of his gonadotropins levels in response to GnRH. He was diagnosed with familial testotoxicosis owing to an activating mutation of his *LH receptor* gene. His father was 4 ft 11 in tall and had been diagnosed with precocious puberty at age 2 year incorrectly thought to be secondary to congenital adrenal hyperplasia. (*From Geffner ME. Disorders of puberty. In: Kliegman RM, Greenbaum LA, Lye PS, eds. Practical Strategies in Pediatric Diagnosis and Therapy. Harcourt Health Sciences, 2005; owing with permission of Elsevier.*)

because of cooler temperature and loss-of-function at core temperature. Lastly, premature and inappropriate androgen production in *both sexes* may occur as a result of NCAH (Figure 7-14), androgen-secreting adrenal tumors, generalized glucocorticoid resistance, and some cases of Cushing syndrome (Figures 7-15A and 7-15B). A similar presentation can occur as a result of presumed unintentional exogenous anabolic steroid exposure (Figure 7-16).[21] On rare occasion, an adrenal tumor may produce both androgens and estrogens, thus mimicking the presentation of central sexual precocity.

Premature production of estrogen in *girls* may result from large (>2 cm) ovarian cysts, granulosa cell tumors, (30% of which contain activating mutations of the $G_s\alpha$ gene), and Sertoli-Leydig cell tumors. The latter are usually isolated occurrences, but may, on occasion, occur as part of Peutz-Jeghers syndrome (PJS) (oral melanosis and intestinal polyps). Another rare, but important, cause is McCune-Albright syndrome (Figures 7-17A and 7-17B). This disorder occurs much more commonly in girls than in boys and is characterized by the clinical triad of polyostotic fibrous dysplasia, irregularly bordered ("coast-of Maine") café-au-lait (brown pigmented) skin

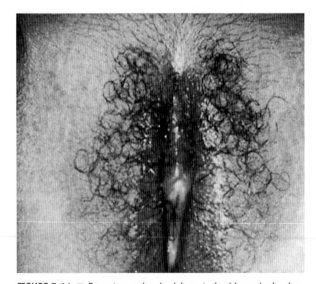

FIGURE 7-14 ■ Premature pubarche (characterized by early development of pubic hair and clitoromegaly) secondary to an adrenal adenoma in a 4-year-old female. (*From Muram D. Pediatric & adolescent gynecology. In: DeCherney AH, Nathan L, Goodwin TM, Laufer N, eds. Current Diagnosis & Treatment: Obstetrics & Gynecology 10th ed. New York, NY: McGraw-Hill; 2007:561. Originally published by Appleton & Lange. Copyright © 2007 by The McGraw-Hill Companies, Inc.*)

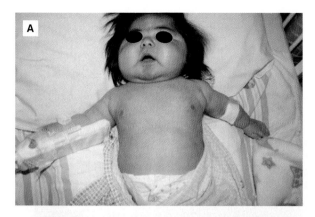

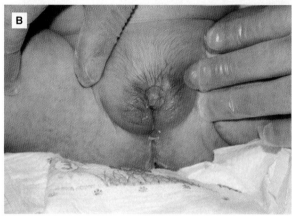

FIGURE 7-15 ■ A 5-month-old female with centralized obesity and moon facies owing to Cushing syndrome resulting from an adrenal tumor. **(A)** Note moustache, beard, and chest hair, and acne on chin. **(B)** Same child with clitoromegaly and Tanner 3 pubic hair.

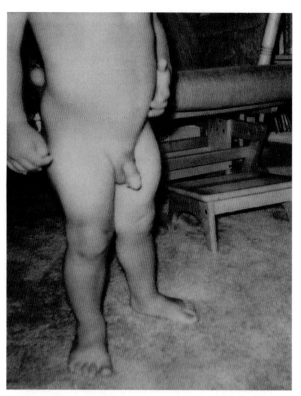

FIGURE 7-16 ■ A 2.67-year-old boy with an 8-month history of pubic hair (Tanner 3), penile enlargement, rapid linear growth, and increased muscle mass, in association with an elevated serum testosterone level of 361 ng/dL (normal <10 ng/dL) and unmeasurable gonadotropins. The boy's father subsequently admitted to prior use of anabolic steroids for bodybuilding and, to treat alleged hypogonadism, he was using a compounded testosterone cream topically, without attention to hand-washing after application or of the possibility of contact transmission to other family members. (*From Franklin SL, Geffner ME. Precocious puberty secondary to topical testosterone exposure. J Pediatr Endocrinol Metab. 2002; 16:107-110; with permission of Freund Publishing House, Ltd.*)

lesions, and multiple autonomous endocrinopathies (most commonly gonadotropin-independent precocious puberty, but also hyperthyroidism, acromegaly, and hypercortisolemia). Girls with McCune-Albright syndrome typically present with early occurrence of vaginal bleeding before or within a few months of breast development (secondary to the development of recurrent autonomous ovarian cysts) and then the existing skin findings are given due attention; bony lesions tend to present later. As occurs in a subset of granulosa cell tumors, McCune-Albright syndrome is owing to a mutation in the $G_s\alpha$ gene that occurs early in embryogenesis (somatic or postzygotic, rather than germ cell in origin) resulting in constitutive activation of adenylyl cyclase in multiple affected tissues; such mutations may also occur in the skin, bones, liver (cholestasis), heart (arrhythmias), and gastrointestinal tract, with affected tissues varying from patient to patient and presumed to be dependent on the exact timing of the mutation. This activation leads to autonomous function of affected tissues which, in the case of involved endocrine glands, results in unregulated production of hormone independent of the normal

stimulatory factors from the hypothalamus and/or pituitary gland. Affected patients appear to be at increased risk for cancer, including bone, breast, and thyroid. Precocious and inappropriate estrogen production in *boys* may occur in the setting of certain adrenal tumors that either overproduce both androgen and estrogen, or provide androgen substrate for subsequent aromatization by peripheral tissues or the tumor itself. Rarely, boys develop feminizing Sertoli cell tumors (usually occurring in the setting of PJS).

Diagnosis, evaluation, and natural history. Bone age in this group of disorders is usually moderately to markedly advanced at the time of diagnosis because of the presumed potency of the process (Figures 7-11 and 7-12). Laboratory testing should be targeted to explain the observed physical findings. Thus, if a girl with advanced bone age presents only with contrasexual

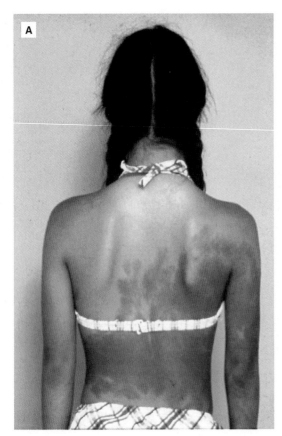 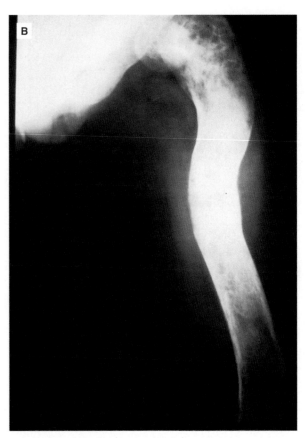

FIGURE 7-17 ■ A 12-year-old female with McCune-Albright syndrome with irregularly bordered ("coast-of-Maine") café-au-lait spot on the back **(A)** and representative lesion of fibrous dysplasia involving the left humerus **(B).** Presentation was at 8 months of age with breast development, vaginal bleeding, café-au-lait spots, and fibrous dysplasia involving long bones, pelvis, and skull. At 3.7 years of age, she developed autonomous hyperthyroidism. At 17.8 years of age was noted to have coarsening of her facial features and elevated serum levels of GH and prolactin owing to a pituitary adenoma which was treated with octreotide. (*From Geffner ME. Disorders of puberty. In: Kliegman RM, Greenbaum LA, Lye PS, eds. Practical Strategies in Pediatric Diagnosis and Therapy. Harcourt Health Sciences, 2005; with permission of Elsevier.*)

androgen-mediated development, that is, evidence of virilization, evaluation consists of measurement of serum total testosterone and 17-hydroxyprogesterone levels; the former provides an index of severity of the process (without localizing the source of the androgen) and the latter is the diagnostic test for 21-hydroxylase deficiency, the most common enzyme deficiency associated with NCAH. On occasion, an ACTH stimulation test may be required to determine the specific enzymatic deficiency. Screening for Cushing syndrome with a 24-hour urine free cortisol (and creatinine to document completeness of collection) may also be indicated if the appropriate body habitus and other features are present. If biochemical testing suggests an adrenal or ovarian tumor (arrhenoblastoma), performance of an abdominal/pelvic MRI is mandatory. Neither measurement of gonadotropins and estradiol nor a head MRI is indicated in the evaluation of virilization in girls.

The work-up for a boy with peripheral pseudopuberty and a significantly advanced bone age is directed by the size of the testes. If the testes are both prepubertal

in size, then the adrenal glands or exogenous administration is the source of the androgen. The same adrenal etiologies of androgen overproduction described earlier for girls also occur in boys and further testing would be performed as indicated earlier for girls. If, however, only one testis is enlarged, a radiological search (usually starting with an ultrasound) for an androgen-producing tumor within the larger testis is mandatory. If both testes are mildly enlarged for age, the etiology is most often central, although familial testotoxicosis must also be considered. These two entities can usually be distinguished by a combination of family history and the results of a GnRH stimulation test, as outlined earlier.

Finally, measurements of serum hCG (in males), prolactin, and free T_4 and TSH are important considerations in the child with unexplained sexual precocity. Tumors producing clinically relevant hCG only occur in males and should be suspected in the setting of disproportionately small testes for the degree of puberty that is present and in clinical situations predisposed to germ cell tumors such as Klinefelter syndrome. Measurement of prolactin would be crucial in the setting of galactorrhea along with manifestations of early puberty. Lastly, thyroid function tests should be considered in the setting of associated signs and symptoms of hypothyroidism, although these may be very subtle in childhood and, thus, their measurement should probably be included in the basic work-up of sexual precocity in all affected children.

Treatment. In cases of precocious pseudopuberty, treatment should, wherever possible, be targeted to the underlying etiology (Table 7-5). For example, androgen-producing ovarian arrhenoblastomas, estrogen-producing ovarian granulosa cell tumors, adrenal sex steroid-producing tumors, hCG-producing tumors, and tumors causing Cushing syndrome should be surgically extirpated. Additional treatment with chemotherapy and/or radiation therapy for specific tumors should be directed by an experienced pediatric oncologist. Large ovarian cysts can be drained under ultrasonographic guidance. Illicit or unintentional administration of exogenous estrogens or androgens should be exposed and eliminated. Familial testotoxicosis is best treated with the anti-fungal drug, ketoconazole, which, at moderately high doses, has the desirable and reversible side effect of interfering with sex steroid synthesis. This drug may also inhibit cortisol synthesis and has been associated with a reversible form of primary glucocorticoid

Table 7-5.

Treatment of Pseudoprecocious Puberty

Goal: target to specific cause

Surgical removal of tumors, for example, androgen-producing ovarian arrhenoblastomas, estrogen-producing ovarian granulosa cell tumors, adrenal sex steroid-producing tumors, hCG-producing tumors, and tumors causing Cushing syndrome

Additional treatment of tumors with chemotherapy and/or radiation therapy as indicated

Large ovarian cysts: drainage under ultrasonographic guidance

Illicit or unintentional administration of exogenous estrogens or androgens should be uncovered and eliminated

Familial testotoxicosis: ketoconazole (or combination of a non-steroidal anti-androgen and an aromatase inhibitor)

Nonclassical (late-onset) adrenal hyperplasia: exogenous glucocorticoid

Hypothyroidism: *levo*-thyroxine

McCune-Albright syndrome: tamoxifen

GnRH agonist therapy may need to be added to any of above therapies if central puberty concomitantly starts at an early age

insufficiency. Screening for hepatotoxicity is also required. Another approach to treat such boys is with a combination of a nonsteroidal antiandrogen and an aromatase inhibitor. NCAH is treated with exogenous glucocorticoids to prevent overproduction of androgens and hypothyroidism is corrected by administration of *levo*-thyroxine. Girls with precocious puberty secondary to McCune-Albright syndrome are most commonly treated with tamoxifen, an estrogen receptor blocker, to limit the effects of excess estrogen production on estrogen-sensitive tissues. The use of later-generation aromatase inhibitors in these girls has not been shown to be of consistent benefit despite the theoretical attraction of diminished estrogen synthesis. In cases of precocious pseudopuberty, GnRH agonist therapy is ineffective unless central puberty is concomitantly triggered.

When to refer. The criteria for referral of a child with precocious puberty to an endocrinologist are summarized in Box 7-1.

DELAYED PUBERTY

Introduction

Delayed puberty is defined as the lack of pubertal development by 2 SD above the mean age for the general population. In practical terms, this is a chronological age of 14 years for boys and 13 years for girls. In addition, an abnormality may be present if there is lack of the appropriate progression of puberty, if more than 4 years between the first signs of puberty and menarche in girls or between the onset and the completion of genital growth in boys. The goal of the assessment is to determine whether the delay or lack of development is as a result of a lag in normal pubertal maturation or represents an abnormality that must be investigated. Etiologies include: (1) constitutional delay of growth and development; (2) secondary or functional hypogonadotropic hypogonadism as a result chronic illness or malnutrition; (3) primary hypogonadotropic hypogonadism; and (4) hypergonadotropic hypogonadism.[22]

Constitutional Delay of Growth and Development

Definition. Constitutional delay of growth and development (CDGD) represents an exaggerated delay in onset and completion of puberty in an otherwise healthy boy or girl. It is often referred to as "late-blooming" and is usually diagnosed in boys, reflecting an ascertainment bias in referral patterns. In these children, puberty will occur spontaneously and progress normally beginning at an age later than the average.

Etiology. CDGD is considered a variant of normal in which there is a similar family history (usually in a parent or sibling) in approximately 50% of cases.[23] The exact etiology of CDGD is not currently known.

Diagnosis, evaluation, and natural history. Typically children with CDGD have a normal length and weight at birth and, after a period of normal growth, there is a decline in height velocity and weight gain typically occurring between 6 months and 2 to 3 years of age. Growth then returns to a normal rate and continues along a lower percentile than would be expected for the family height genetics for the remainder of the prepubertal years. At the expected time of puberty, the height of children with constitutional delay begins to drift further from the normal growth curve because of delay in the onset of the pubertal growth spurt. Confounding the issue is that the natural slowing of linear growth that occurs just before the onset of puberty may be exaggerated, magnifying the difference in size from peers who are beginning to show acceleration in their growth rate.

At the expected age of pubertal onset, children with CDGD demonstrate delayed bone ages and prepubertal levels of gonadotropins, initially making it difficult to distinguish this condition from primary or secondary gonadotropin deficiency. Periodic evaluation of height, weight, and stage of sexual maturation will help differentiate this normal variant from a pathological entity, eliminating the need for much if any laboratory testing. Since timing and tempo of sexual development appear to be delayed in accordance with the biological state of maturity (skeletal age), the height of a child with CDGD should be more or less appropriate for his or her genetic target height range when the height is plotted for bone age rather than chronological age (Figures 7-18A and 7-18B). There is a poorly understood subset of children with CDGD who have a blunted pubertal growth spurt relative to their peers and who may not reach their genetic target height. Unfortunately, it is not possible to prospectively identify which children with CDGD will fall into this category. As a result, it is important to monitor children with CDGD closely during puberty as they may require expedient intervention to maximize final height.

Treatment. There are many practitioners who would state that, if delayed puberty were not pathological, there is no proven medical necessity for initiating sex steroid replacement. However, there are adolescent boys with CDGD who are very short, significantly underdeveloped, and who feel psychologically compromised. These boys frequently request and will profit from a short course of testosterone therapy. The administration of testosterone to adolescent boys with CDGD has been controversial because of the possibility of premature epiphyseal closure and reduced final height. However, if administered in low doses for a short duration, testosterone therapy is effective and does not appear to adversely affect final adult height. Intramuscular testosterone enanthate or cypionate is typically provided in doses of 50 to 100 mg every 3 to 4 weeks, for a course of 3 to 12 months, depending on the needs of the patient. There are transdermal preparations, which have been used off label for this indication, but safety and efficacy have yet to be demonstrated. A pediatric endocrinologist experienced with prescribing testosterone is essential, as even short-term doses higher than appropriate may result in an accelerated advancement in skeletal maturity and significant short adult stature.

Functional Hypogonadotropic Hypogonadism

Definition. More than 30% of adolescents at one time or another suffer from a chronic disease. Such illnesses may have a significant impact on normal sexual development. In the face of poorly controlled or undiagnosed illnesses, children may not develop secondary sexual characteristics until the condition is identified and/or treated appropriately. These children are classified as having functional (or reversible) hypogonadotropic hypogonadism.

Etiology. Any underlying chronic illness, prolonged medical treatment requiring glucocorticoids, excessive emotional stress, intense physical activity, or inadequate nutritional state can result in reversible hypogonadism (Table 7-6). Examples include recurrent infections, immunodeficiency, gastrointestinal disease, cardiac disease, renal disturbances, respiratory illnesses, chronic anemia, endocrine disease, eating disorders, and excessive energy expenditure.[24] Pubertal delay associated with chronic illness is usually accompanied by a delay in

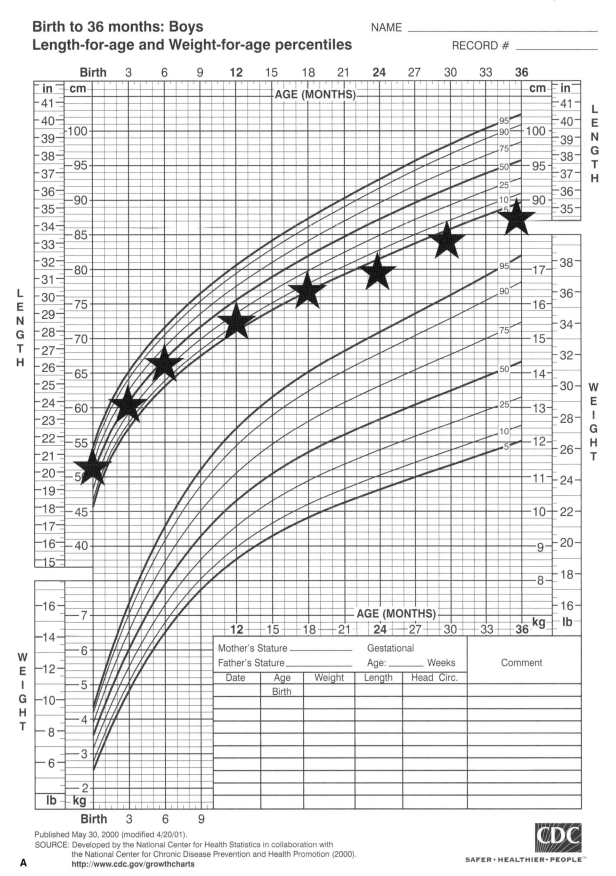

Birth to 36 months: Boys
Length-for-age and Weight-for-age percentiles

NAME _____

RECORD # _____

Published May 30, 2000 (modified 4/20/01).
SOURCE: Developed by the National Center for Health Statistics in collaboration with
the National Center for Chronic Disease Prevention and Health Promotion (2000).
http://www.cdc.gov/growthcharts

A

FIGURE 7-18 ■ Constitutional delay of growth and development (CDGD). **(A)** The infant-toddler male growth chart (birth—36 months) demonstrates the early height pattern of children with CDGD, that is, they have a normal length in the first few months of life, after which there is a steady decline in growth velocity between 6 months and 2 to 3 years of age. (*Continued*)

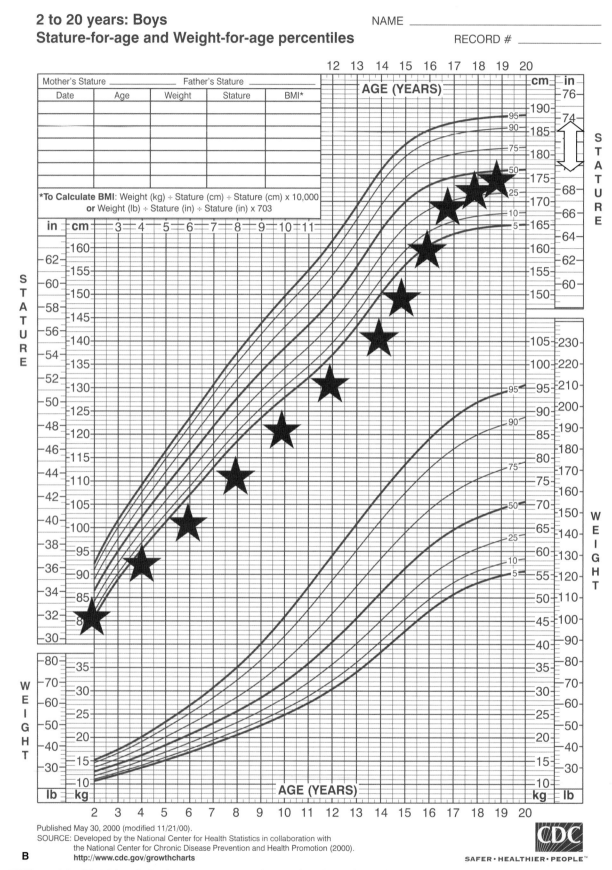

2 to 20 years: Boys
Stature-for-age and Weight-for-age percentiles

NAME _____

RECORD # _____

Published May 30, 2000 (modified 11/21/00).

SOURCE: Developed by the National Center for Health Statistics in collaboration with
the National Center for Chronic Disease Prevention and Health Promotion (2000).

http://www.cdc.gov/growthcharts

B

FIGURE 7-18 ▪ (B) Height velocity then returns to a normal rate and continues along a lower percentile curve than would be expected for the family height genetics with continued growth beyond the age that other boys complete their linear growth with ultimate attainment of a normal height for the family (mid-parental target height range indicated by two-headed arrow on far right of growth chart).(*From Centers for Disease Control and Prevention, Atlanta, Georgia.*)

Table 7-6.

Functional Hypogonadotropic Hypogonadism

Systemic illness
Recurrent infections
Immunodeficiency
Gastrointestinal disease
Cardiac disease
Renal disturbances
Respiratory illnesses
Chronic anemia
Endocrine disease
   Hypothyroidism
   Hyperprolactinemia
   Hypercortisolemia
Psychiatric disease
   Anorexia nervosa
   Bulimia
Chronic glucocorticoid use
Hemochromatosis

growth and by an absent or blunted pubertal growth spurt. The degree to which growth and pubertal development are affected in chronic illness depends upon the type of disease and individual factors, as well as on the age at illness onset, and its duration and severity. The earlier the onset and the longer and more severe the illness, the greater the repercussions for growth and pubertal development. The basis of abnormal puberty in children with a chronic illness is multifactorial.[25] Nutritional deficiency may contribute through insufficient food supply and/or malabsorption of nutrients. Moreover, increased energy supplies are often needed in patients with chronic disease, infection, or inflammation. More specific factors owing to the disease itself may be involved in growth and pubertal disorders. Abnormalities of the GH-IGF-1 axis and gonadotropin secretion have been described in patients with chronic renal failure, cystic fibrosis, and Crohn disease. More recently, it has been shown that cytokines produced during chronic diseases such as juvenile idiopathic arthritis may inhibit the normal function of the GH-IGF-1 axis. Finally, concomitant medications, such as glucocorticoids, which are often given to these patients, may contribute to delayed puberty and poor pubertal growth. Therefore, early diagnosis is essential and appropriate, and disease-specific therapy fundamental.

Malnutrition (resulting from malabsorption, anorexia, bulimia, and excessive athletic performance), chronic pain, and psychosocial factors can all disrupt the hypothalamic-pituitary-gonadal axis. Pituitary affinity

to iron deposition explains the high incidence of hypogonadism, pubertal delay, and growth retardation in hemochromatosis and in patients hypertransfused for chronic anemias.[26] Hypogonadism in males with HIV infection is an ongoing concern, even among patients whose viral replication is under control and who have normalized CD4+ cell counts.[27] Elevated lead levels have been shown to be associated with pubertal delay.[28]

Endocrinopathies such as hypothyroidism, hyperprolactinemia, and hypercortisolemia may also result in functional hypogonadotropic hypogonadism. Thyroid hormone deficiency impairs growth and development, perhaps through induction of transient reversible GH deficiency. Adolescents with poorly treated or undiagnosed hypothyroidism may also have significantly delayed sexual maturation. Prolactin is naturally synthesized and secreted by lactotroph cells in the anterior pituitary gland. Its primary function is during pregnancy to enhance breast development and induce lactation, but there is evidence to suggest that it also decreases gonadotropin secretion. Therefore, hyperprolactinemia should be considered in any teenager, boy or girl, with delayed sexual development and galactorrhea. Adolescents with hypercortisolemia demonstrate arrested pubertal development. Glucocorticoid excess inhibits gonadotropin release and also directly inhibits sex steroid secretion from the gonads.

Diagnosis, evaluation, and natural history. The initial approach in the diagnosis of delayed puberty requires a careful medical history, detailed growth history, complete family history, and physical examination (Table 7-7). The medical history should include a detailed search for a reversible etiology for delayed sexual development. A history of competitive athletics or dance should be a red flag for excessive energy expenditure and the likelihood of secondary hypothalamic dysfunction. Children with cardiac, gastrointestinal, rheumatological, renal, or pulmonary disease typically need no further examination. If significant medical history is absent, a simple laboratory search for occult chronic illness is appropriate. Initial testing should include the following: comprehensive chemistry panel, complete blood count and erythrocyte sedimentation rate, urinalysis, tissue transglutaminase antibody, TSH, and free T_4 (preferably by direct dialysis). The chemistry panel and complete urinalysis will help to assess hepatic and renal function, respectively, in addition to glucose status. The complete blood count will evaluate bone marrow function. The erythrocyte sedimentation rate is helpful to identify inflammatory disorders, such as systemic lupus erythematosis, juvenile rheumatoid arthritis, and inflammatory bowel disease. The tissue transglutaminase antibody is to identify celiac disease. Free T_4 and TSH will screen for thyroid dysfunction.

Table 7-7.
Hypogonadotropic *vs* Hypergonadotropic Hypogonadism

Hypogonadotropic
Congenital
  Isolated GnRH deficiency
    Kallmann syndrome
      KAL1, FGFR1, PROKR2
    Idiopathic hypogonadotropic hypogonadism
      GnRHR, FGFR1, GPR54, Leptin, FSH β-subunit, LH β-subunit
    Idiopathic hypogonadotropic hypogonadism
      associated with obesity
      Leptin, Leptin receptor, PC1
  Adrenal hypoplasia congenita
  Pituitary transcription factor deficiency
  Syndromes
    Prader-Willi syndrome
    Noonan syndrome
    CHARGE syndrome
    Bardet-Biedl syndrome
Acquired
  Suprasellar/sellar solid tumors
    Craniopharyngioma
  Trauma/surgery
  Infiltration
    Hypophysitis
      Lymphocytic
      Granulomatous
      Histiocytosis X
      Wegener
      Sarcoidosis
    Infectious—meningoencephalitis

Hypergonadotropic
Congenital
  Girls
    X chromosome abnormalities
      Gonadal dysgenesis
        Tuner syndrome (45,X)
        Swyer syndrome (46,XY)
        Mixed gonadal dysgenesis (46,XX/46,XY)
        Pure ovarian agenesis (46,XX)
      Fragile X permutation
    Galactosemia
    Blepharophimosis ptosis epicanthus inversus syndrome
    FSH β-subunit gene mutation
    FSH or LH receptor gene mutations
  Boys
    Klinefelter syndrome
    Anorchia
    LH receptor gene mutation
Acquired
  Anorchia
  Toxins
  Radiation
    Chemotherapy
  ETOH
  Trauma/surgery
  Inflammation
    Infections
    Autoimmunity

Treatment. Treatment of the underlying condition is the only therapy necessary although, if such treatment is unavailable or unsuccessful, sex steroid replacement may be required (see "Hypogonadotropic hypogonadism").

Hypogonadotropic hypogonadism

Definition. The lack of any clinical manifestation of puberty by the age of 13 years in girls and 14 years in boys, along with persistence of low LH and FSH levels, is indicative of hypogonadotropic hypogonadism.

Etiology. Etiologies of hypogonadotropic hypogonadism are divided into congenital and acquired forms (Table 7-7). Congenital deficiency states include isolated gonadotropin deficiency, adrenal hypoplasia congenita, and certain genetic syndromes. Acquired deficiency may result from an array of disorders affecting the brain, including tumors, malformations, head trauma, surgery, radiation, infections, and infiltrative disease.

Congenital

GnRH deficiency

GnRH-producing and olfactory neurons migrate together in embryological development so that disruption of this process can cause either isolated hypogonadotropic hypogonadism (IHH) or Kallmann syndrome. GnRH is released from neurons in the arcuate nucleus in a pulsatile fashion into the hypophyseal-portal circulation, the capillaries perfusing the anterior pituitary gland. GnRH binds to its receptors on the surface of gonadotrophs in the anterior pituitary gland, which then, in turn, synthesize and secrete LH and FSH into the circulation where they stimulate gonadal steroidogenesis and gametogenesis.

    IHH has clinical and genetic heterogeneity, multiple modes of inheritance, and variable association with other anomalies. IHH and Kallmann syndrome are both characterized by defects in hypothalamic GnRH secretion.[29] Impairment of both GnRH and olfactory neuron migration results in Kallmann syndrome, the combination of hypogonadotropic hypogonadism and anosmia (absent sense of smell). Normosmic patients are not diagnosed with Kallmann syndrome, but rather are labeled as IHH. Both Kallmann syndrome and IHH can occur in partial or complete forms. These disorders have been largely considered to be a monogenic disorder (although there is some recent literature to support digenic mutations) with several loci identified to date: *Kallmann syndrome 1 sequence (KAL1), FGF receptor 1 (FGFR1), prokineticin 2, and prokineticin receptor 2 (PROKR2)* underlie cases of Kallmann syndrome, while *gonadotropin-releasing hormone receptor (GnRHR),*

FGFR1, and G protein–coupled receptor 54 (GPR54) underlie normosmic IHH. Kisspeptin is the endogenous neuropeptide for GPR54 and is currently being aggressively studied to help better understand the genes important in the regulation of the hypothalamic-pituitary-gonadal axis. Additionally, nasal embryonic LHRH factor (NELF) has been implicated in the pathogenesis of Kallmann syndrome. All patients with Kallmann syndrome have either anosmia or severe hyposmia (reduced sense of smell), and may also exhibit unilateral renal agenesis, atrial septal defect, colorblindness, and synkinesia (mirror movements). The sense of smell can easily be confirmed by testing the recognition for common substances such as alcohol or coffee.

Other abnormal genes encoding members of the hypothalamic-pituitary-gonadal axis are also associated with early onset obesity. Mutations of genes encoding either *leptin* or the *leptin receptor* underlie cases of autosomally transmitted early onset obesity, hypogonadotropic hypogonadism, central hypothyroidism, and growth hormone deficiency presumably as the result of hypothalamic dysfunction. In one patient, a mutation in the *prohormone convertase (PC1)* gene led to hypogonadotropic hypogonadism, in addition to extreme obesity, hypocortisolemia, and deficient conversion of proinsulin to insulin.

Rarely, hypogonadotropic hypogonadism occurs as a result of isolated FSH deficiency owing to homozygous mutations in the *FSH β-subunit* gene. In one patient, isolated bioinactive LH was present because of a homozygous mutation in the *LH β-subunit* gene, which led to hypogonadotropic hypogonadism.

Transcription factors involved in pituitary development

Mutations of genes encoding various pituitary transcription factors may also result in hypogonadotropic hypogonadism. Pituitary development is governed by activation of a cascade of transcription factors that orchestrate both pituitary morphogenesis and differentiation of all five cell lineages of the anterior pituitary corticotrophs, gonadotrophs, thyrotrophs, somatotrophs, and lactotrophs. Of those pituitary transcription factors identified so far, defects of *HESX1, LHX3, LHX4, PROP1 (most common),* and *POU1F1 (Pit-1)* have been found to lead to the phenotype of multiple pituitary hormone deficiency in humans.[30] Endocrine phenotypes of *HESX1, LHX3, LHX4,* and *PROP1* defects tend to overlap and have been reported to include failure of up to all five cell lineages of the anterior pituitary. To make the understanding of phenotypes even more complex, the influences of these transcription factors on pituitary function seem to be dynamic with the potential to develop hormone deficiencies throughout the human lifespan.

Another cause of hypogonadotropic hypogonadism is adrenal hypoplasia congenita, caused by mutations found the *NROB1* gene (formally called *DAX1*). The *NROB1* gene encodes for DAX-1 protein, which is a transcription factor necessary for the development of the hypothalamus, pituitary gonadotroph, and the adrenal cortex. *DAX1* also appears to regulate gonadotropin secretion at both the hypothalamic and pituitary levels.[31] Children with *NROB1* mutations usually present with primary adrenocortical failure in infancy or childhood. Those adequately treated with gluco- and mineralocorticoids later present with delayed sexual development owing to hypogonadotropic hypogonadism.

Syndromes associated with hypogonadotropic hypogonadism

Prader-Willi syndrome (PWS), with a prevalence rate of 1:16,000, is the first human disorder attributed to genomic imprinting in which genes are expressed differentially based on the parent of origin. PWS results from the loss of imprinted genomic material within the *paternal* 15q11.2-13 locus. The loss of *maternal* genomic material at the 15q11.2-13 locus results in Angelman syndrome. The molecular events underlying the disorder include interstitial deletions (70%), uniparental disomy (25%), imprinting center defects (<5%), and rarely chromosomal translocations (<1%).[32] PWS is commonly associated with hypogonadotropic hypogonadism and small genitalia, although there are also rare reports of patients with hypergonadotropic hypogonadism. Characteristic facial features include narrow bifrontal diameter, almond-shaped palpebral fissures, narrow nasal bridge, and a down-turned mouth. Infants typically have poor tone, delayed development, and failure-to-thrive. By the age of 2 years, these children develop polyphagia and progressive obesity.

Noonan syndrome is an autosomal dominant, genetically heterogeneous disease of which approximately 50% of cases are caused by gain-of-function mutations in the *PTPN11* gene. The incidence is estimated to be 1:1000 to 2500 live births and it occurs equally in males and females (and, thus, should not be referred to as male Turner syndrome [TS]). The cardinal facial features are shown in Figure 7-19; affected individuals also manifest right-sided congenital heart disease (pulmonic stenosis) hypertrophic cardiomyopathy, and short stature. In affected males, testes are often small, cryptorchid, or both. Typical patients demonstrate hypogonadotropic hypogonadism, but there are also occasional reports of patients with elevated gonadotropins.

CHARGE syndrome is another autosomal dominant condition with genotypic heterogeneity. Most cases are owing to mutation or deletion of the *chromodomain helicase DNA-binding protein-7 (CHD7)* gene. The estimated incidence of CHARGE syndrome is 1:8500 to

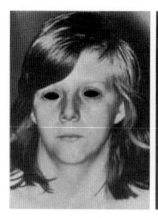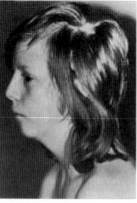

FIGURE 7-19 ■ The cardinal dysmorphic features of a patient with Noonan syndrome are demonstrated in this figure: triangular-shaped face, hypertelorism, down-slanting eyes, ptosis, low-set ears with thickened helices, high nasal bridge, and short webbed neck.

12,000 live births. It is associated with hypogonadotropic hypogonadism and olfactory bulb abnormalities similar to the abnormalities found in individuals with Kallmann syndrome.[33] Boys with CHARGE syndrome may have micropenis, cryptorchidism, and/or small testes. Girls may have small labia. The cardinal features of **C**oloboma (Figure 7-20), **H**eart anomalies, choanal **A**tresia, pre- and postnatal **R**etardation of growth, **G**enital hypoplasia, and **E**ar anomalies clinically define CHARGE syndrome.

Bardet-Biedl syndrome (BBS) is an autosomal recessive condition with a wide spectrum of clinical features.[34] BBS is a very rare disorder with an incidence in North America and Europe ranging from 1:140,000 to 1:160,000. However, in Kuwait and Newfoundland, the rate is much higher, with an estimated incidence of

1:13,500 and 1:17,500, respectively, suggesting a founder effect. BBS is genetically heterogeneous, with 12 potentially causative genes identified to date. Although the cellular mechanisms that underlie BBS remain unclear, it is now evident that all of the known BBS proteins are important for ciliary transport. BBS is characterized by early onset retinal dystrophy, obesity, postaxial polydactyly, and brachydactyly of the hands and feet (Figure 7-21), along with mental retardation, hypogonadism, and renal disease. Hypogenitalism (cryptorchidism and/or microphallus) is reported more frequently in BBS boys than in affected girls. Genital abnormalities encompass a wide range in girls, including hypoplastic fallopian tubes, uterus, and ovaries; partial and complete vaginal atresia; absent vaginal orifice; and absent urethral orifice. Hypogonadotropic hypogonadism has only been reported in BBS girls. Primary gonadal failure has also been described in both sexes.

Acquired

CNS lesions such as neoplasms, head trauma, surgery, radiation, infections, and infiltrative disease can disrupt hypothalamic-pituitary function resulting in hypogonadotropic hypogonadism.

Sellar and suprasellar tumors may alter pituitary function directly and/or disrupt the hypothalamic-pituitary stalk, leading to multiple pituitary hormone deficiencies. Craniopharyngiomas are the most common suprasellar tumors identified in children. These tumors have a benign histology with a malignant behavior, having the tendency to invade surrounding structures and to recur after what was thought to be complete resection. They frequently present as cystic structures (single or lobulated) filled with a turbid, proteinaceous

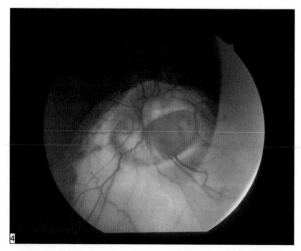

FIGURE 7-20 ■ Large coloboma involving the optic nerve in a child with CHARGE syndrome. (*Fundus photograph kindly provided by Mark Borchert, MD, Childrens Hospital Los Angeles.*)

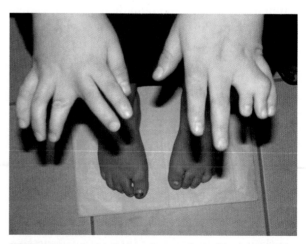

FIGURE 7-21 ■ Bardet-Beidl syndrome patient with postaxial skeletal malformations. Polydactyly (six digits) of both hands, partial syndactyly between fourth and fifth digits of the left hand, fifth digit clinodactyly. (*From Karaman A Bardet-Biedl syndrome: a case report.* Dermatol Online J. *2008;15(1)14:9.*)

material of brownish-yellow color that glitters and sparkles because of a high content of floating cholesterol crystals that has been compared to machinery oil. The tumor frequently arises in the pituitary stalk and projects into the hypothalamus. It extends voraciously along the path of least resistance (anteriorly into the prechiasmatic cistern and subfrontal spaces; posteriorly into the prepontine and interpeduncular cisterns, cerebellopontine angle, third ventricle, posterior fossa, and foramen magnum; and laterally toward the subtemporal spaces). Craniopharyngiomas account for 5% to 10% of intracranial tumors and 56% of suprasellar tumors in children and usually are diagnosed between the ages of 5 and 10 years. Affected patients present with characteristic symptoms of increased intracranial pressure (headache, nausea, and vomiting), pituitary dysfunction, and/or visual disturbance. Most children present with growth failure secondary to GH deficiency. Adolescents present with growth failure and delayed or absent sexual development, which can be overlooked until after symptoms of increased intracranial pressure develop. Some patients also have central hypothyroidism and adrenal insufficiency. The neurological examination is suggestive of increased intracranial pressure, in the form of papilledema and visual field deficits. The radiological hallmark of craniopharyngiomas is the appearance of suprasellar calcification on neuroimaging. If hypopituitarism were not present prior to therapy, resection of the tumor will likely disrupt the hypothalamic-pituitary communication fairly acutely. For this reason, children with a history of craniopharyngioma should be followed regularly by a pediatric endocrinologist.

Traumatic brain injury is, unfortunately, common in the adolescent population, especially in males. Necrotic, hypoxic, ischemic, and shearing lesions involving the hypothalamus and/or the pituitary are now being reported more frequently in adolescents with traumatic brain injury. Children at highest risk appear to be those who have suffered moderate or severe trauma. Clinical signs of anterior hypopituitarism are often subtle, including delayed puberty, and may be masked by the sequelae of traumatic brain injury. Therefore, posttraumatic anterior pituitary dysfunction may remain undiagnosed and, possibly, aggravate symptoms of brain injury. Moreover, it may, if undiagnosed, lead to a potentially fatal adrenal crisis.

Leukemia and brain tumors account for 53% of all cancers diagnosed among children younger than the age of 15 years and require CNS-targeted therapy. Because the peak incidence for both cancers is during a vulnerable neurocognitive developmental period, such therapy, in particular moderate- or high-dose cranial radiation therapy, often has significant long-term permanent consequences. Radiation-induced damage to the hypothalamic-pituitary axis is associated with a wide spectrum of subtle and frank abnormalities in anterior pituitary hormone secretion.[35] The frequency, rapidity of onset, and the severity of these abnormalities correlate with the total radiation dose delivered to the axis, as well as the fraction size, younger age, prior pituitary compromise by the tumor and/or surgery, and the length of follow-up. Although the hypothalamus is the primary site of radiation-induced damage, secondary pituitary atrophy evolves with time as a result of impaired secretion of hypothalamic trophic factors and/or time-dependent direct radiation-induced damage. Abnormalities in gonadotropin secretion are dose-dependent. Precocious puberty can occur after a radiation dose less than 30 Gy in girls and in both sexes equally with a radiation dose of 30 to 50 Gy. Gonadotropin deficiency is usually a long-term complication following a minimum radiation dose of 30 Gy. Radiation-induced anterior pituitary hormone deficiencies are irreversible and progressive. Regular testing is mandatory to ensure timely diagnosis and early hormone replacement therapy.

Inflammatory and infectious diseases of the pituitary gland are rare and diagnosis via imaging may be difficult. They encompass a wide spectrum of pathology, including autoimmune and granulomatous hypophysitis, local manifestations of systemic disease, and a multitude of infectious processes (HIV, herpes simplex virus, and *mycoplasma* to name just a few). Various degrees of hypopituitarism may ensue, including involvement of gonadotropins.

Diagnosis, evaluation, and natural history

Random LH and FSH measurements by the ultrasensitive ICMA method differentiate hypo- from hypergonadotropic hypogonadism (Table 7-8). However, it may be difficult to differentiate hypogonadotropic hypogonadism from simple delayed puberty since low gonadotropin levels are found in both situations. The serum LH response following administration of synthetic GnRH, or analogs thereof, was thought to differentiate between the two conditions with a significant rise expected in patients with simple physiologically delayed puberty whose pituitary has been primed with endogenous GnRH during the fetal and early postnatal period and little or no rise in true hypogonadotropic states. However, the results of several trials have yielded conflicting results insofar as their ability to ensure a certain difference between the two conditions. GnRH is administered at 2.5 μg/kg (maximal dose of 100 μg), with LH and FSH response measurements 30 minutes after the medication is administered. An LH level more than 8 IU/L indicates normal pituitary reserve and, thus, helps to identify patients who likely have constitutional delay rather than true hypogonadotropic hypogonadism.

If the patient is found to have permanent hypogonadotropic hypogonadism, the history and physician

Table 7-8.

Keys to Diagnosis of Absent/Delayed Puberty

Medical history
  Competitive athletics
  Chronic illness
  Glucocorticoid use
  Cancer history
    Radiation
    Chemotherapy
    Surgery
  Symptoms suggestive of occult disease
Growth history
  Growth velocity
Family history
  Constitutional delay in growth and development in ~50%
    of first-degree relatives
  Chronic illness
Perinatal history
  Growth parameters
  Cardiac defects
  Hypoglycemia
  Lymphedema
  Newborn screening abnormalities
Physical examination
  Auxological measurements
  Pubertal staging
  Neurological examination
    Visual fields
    Optic nerve evaluation
    Evidence of developmental delay or mental retardation
    Evaluation of the sense of smell
  Evidence of underlying/associated condition
    Thyroid
    Vitiligo
    Galactorrhea
Bone age
Laboratory tests
  Screening evaluation for occult disease
  Gonadotropins
  Estradiol or testosterone
  Karyotype if elevated gonadotropins are found
  Anti-ovarian antibodies
MRI for hypogonadotropic hypogonadism
Pelvic or scrotal ultrasound
Surgical exploration for gonadal tissue

examination should help to narrow the differential diagnosis. A patient or family history of hypogonadism and/or poor sense of smell suggests IHH or Kallmann syndrome. An abnormal perinatal history, with any of the following, should suggest the possibility of congenital hypopituitarism: micropenis, hypoglycemia, cleft lip/palate, bifid uvula, prolonged jaundice, and shock. History and physical examination will also help to

identify any of the syndromic etiologies for hypogonadotropic hypogonadism. Low tone with poor feeding during infancy, delayed development, along with rapid weight gain and polyphagia after 2 years, suggest a diagnosis of PWS. Pulmonic stenosis and short stature point toward Noonan syndrome. A perinatal history of choanal atresia or childhood history of coloboma are consistent with CHARGE syndrome. Progressive vision loss in a child with postaxial polydactyly or renal disease is indicative of BBS. Signs or symptoms of increased intracranial pressure strongly indicate the possibility of an intracranial tumor. A history of traumatic brain injury, especially with loss of consciousness, may result in pituitary insufficiency many years after the event, and should alert the physician to the possibility of hypopituitarism. Lastly, history of prior cancers, radiation, and/or chemotherapy also raise the possibility of gonadotropin deficiency.

Genetic analysis, if available, should definitively confirm some of the genetic syndromes. DNA methylation analysis for PWS is the diagnostic test of choice (not FISH). Evaluation of the *PTPN11* gene, which is abnormal in approximately 50% of Noonan syndrome patients, is commercially available.

An MRI of the brain with contrast dye enhancement in a closed tube system should be obtained in patients with hypogonadotropic hypogonadism. Abnormalities of the olfactory placode indicate Kallmann syndrome (Figure 7-22). Congenital malformations of the anterior or posterior pituitary, and congenital lesions of the septum pellucidum and corpus callosum, as well as acquired tumors or infiltrative lesions, may also be identified with MRI.

Treatment

The treatment of permanent hypogonadism, either hypo- or hypergonadotropic varieties, is the same.

Therapy for boys is aimed at replacement of testosterone in a stepwise fashion, targeted to mimic normal physiology. Therefore, in boys with hypogonadism, as well as for those with CDGD, intramuscular testosterone is begun in a similar manner, but, for those with permanent hypogonadism, there will be a need to continue administration with increases in 50-mg/month increments made over a 2- to 3-year period. Using this approach, most adult men receive 200 to 300 mg every 2 to 4 weeks. This dosing is based on the adult male testosterone production rate of 6 mg/day. Once at final adult height, older adolescent boys can take testosterone by patch or gel.

Therapy for girls with permanent hypogonadism is initiated with daily low-dose estrogen therapy alone for 1 to 2 years. This can be in the form of any number of equivalent estrogen preparations. Conjugated equine estrogens (eg, Premarin) have traditionally been utilized

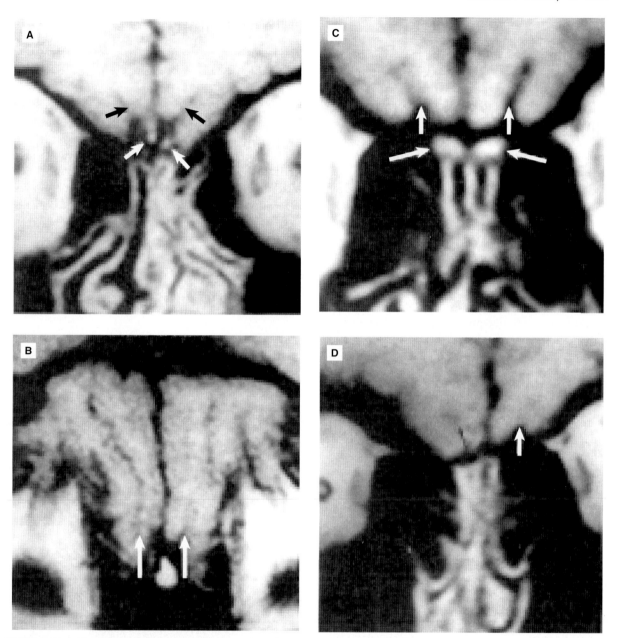

FIGURE 7-22 ■ Panel A is a coronal T$_1$-weighted image of a male with Kallmann syndrome (KS) showing (abnormal) medially oriented olfactory sulci (black arrows) and normal appearing olfactory bulbs (white arrows). Panel B is an axial T$_1$-weighted image of the same male with KS showing the presence of olfactory sulci (white arrows). Panel C is a coronal T$_1$-weighted image of a female with IHH showing normal olfactory bulbs (large arrows) and sulci (small arrows). Panel D is a coronal T$_1$-weighted image of a female with KS showing lack of olfactory bulbs with shallow olfactory sulci (arrows). *(From Quinton R, et al. The neuroradiology of Kallmann's syndrome: a genotypic and phenotypic analysis. J Clin Endocrinol Metab. 1996;81:3010-3017.)*

at 0.3 mg daily for the first 6 months, 0.625 mg daily for the second 6 months, followed by 0.6 to 1.2 mg starting in the second year. Ethinyl estradiol (eg, Estrace) has also been utilized as oral replacement with 0.02 mg daily for the first 6 months, followed by 0.1 mg for the second 6 months, and 0.2 mg thereafter. Transdermal estradiol preparations (eg, Vivelle) are also available and are initiated to provide 0.0625 mg daily, advancing slowly throughout the following 2 years to a total daily dose of 0.05 to 0.1 mg/day. Although it is not clear that patch-cutting to accomplish escalated dosing will reliably provide the equivalent amount of estradiol, this mode is currently being prescribed off-label. The initial duration of unopposed estrogen for 1 to 2 years does not appear to expose the uterus to any undue risk for endometrial hyperplasia and/or malignancy if not exceeded. At the end of the first few years, cyclic progesterone must be added. The two options include oral medroxyprogesterone at 10 mg/day (eg, Provera) and micronized progesterone at 200 mg/day (eg, Prometrium) on days 20 to 30 of the cycle. With this approach, withdrawal bleeding generally occurs in the following 3 to 10 days, although there can be some variability between patients. Another option is to provide continuous estrogen followed by progesterone on days 100 to 120 of the cycle to minimize menstruation, but provide uterine protection. Alternatively, at adult dosing, the aforementioned estrogen delivery methods are often abandoned in favor of a more conventional oral contraceptive or substituted with a weekly estrogen patch used in conjunction with oral progesterone. There are also oral contraceptive agents (eg, Seasonale) that decrease the frequency of menstruation to quarterly intervals.

Patients of either sex with hypogonadotropic hypogonadism are potentially fertile, but sex steroid therapy alone will not ordinarily be sufficient to initiate gametogenesis, although there are rare cases in men in which testosterone replacement alone has stimulated spermatogenesis, presumably by local intratesticular action on the seminiferous tubules. Thus, the typical approach to fertility induction is pump-administered GnRH therapy (assuming an intact pituitary gland) or parenteral combination gonadotropin treatment (synthetic LH/hCG and recombinant FSH) if the pituitary is nonfunctioning, in either case supervised by an experienced reproductive endocrinologist.

HYPERGONADOTROPIC HYPOGONADISM

Definition

Elevated serum LH and FSH levels in an adolescent being seen for delayed sexual development (see age criteria discussed earlier) are indicative of a primary defect in gonadal (testicular or ovarian) function. The hypergonadotropic state implies that the hypothalamic-pituitary component of pubertal signaling has been activated through lack of negative feedback that is normally exerted by the actions of sex steroids. Etiologies are classified as congenital *versus* acquired, and may be further segregated by the sex of the patient (Table 7-7).

Etiology

Boys

Congenital testicular failure. The most common cause of hypergonadotropic hypogonadism in males is Klinefelter syndrome, occurring in about 1:500 to 1000 live male births.[36] The term, Klinefelter syndrome, describes a group of chromosomal disorders in which

there is at least one extra X chromosome added to the normal male karyotype of 46,XY. The extra X chromosome is usually acquired through an error in meiosis (nondisjunction during parental gametogenesis) where a sperm or an egg carries an extra X chromosome in addition to the normal single sex chromosome. It also may result from an error in division during mitosis of the zygote.

Adult men with Klinefelter syndrome have traditionally been described as having a eunuchoidal body habitus with sparse body and facial hair, gynecomastia, increased fat mass, small testes and penis, and decreased verbal intelligence, in conjunction with biochemical testosterone deficiency, azoospermia, and elevated gonadotropins (Figure 7-23). During infancy, affected boys may have chromosomal evaluations done for

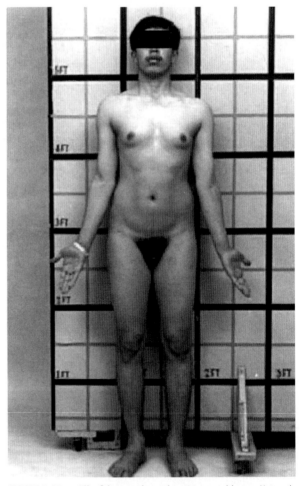

FIGURE 7-23 ■ Klinefelter syndrome in a 20-year-old man. Note relatively increased lower/upper body segment ratio, gynecomastia, small penis, and sparse body hair with a female pubic hair pattern. (*From Braunstein GD. Testes. In: Gardner DG, Shoback D, eds. Greenspan's Basic & Clinical Endocrinology, 8th ed. New York, NY: McGraw-Hill; 2007:483. Originally published by Appleton & Lange. Copyright © 2007 by The McGraw-Hill Companies, Inc.*)

hypospadias, small phallus, or cryptorchidism. The older boy or adolescent may be discovered during an evaluation for delayed or incomplete pubertal development with eunuchoidal body habitus, gynecomastia, and/or small testes despite relatively normal development of secondary sexual characteristics, such as pubic and axillary hair. Adult men, if previously undiagnosed may come to medical attention because of infertility or, rarely, breast malignancy.

There is an increased incidence of autoimmune disorders, such as hypothyroidism, systemic lupus erythematous, rheumatoid arthritis, and Sjögren syndrome, in patients with Klinefelter syndrome. There is a suggestion that this may be because of their lower testosterone and relatively higher estrogen levels, since androgens may protect against and estrogens promote autoimmunity. It is unclear at this time if early identification of Klinefelter syndrome and earlier initiation of androgen replacement will decrease the incidence of autoimmune conditions.

Acquired testicular failure. Acquired causes of primary testicular failure include congenital anorchia, exposure to toxins, orchitis, severe trauma, and autoimmunity.

Bilateral congenital anorchia is defined as the complete absence of testicular tissue with a normal male karyotype, phallus, and scrotum. The true prevalence of this condition is unknown because prospective studies have not been performed. However, it is estimated to occur in approximately 0.5 to 1.0 per 20,000 boys. The pathogenesis of congenital anorchia is poorly understood. The fetal testis and systemic testosterone must be present during the first 12 weeks of gestation for normal external male genitalia to develop. It follows that an anorchic boy with otherwise normal male external genitalia must have had, early in fetal life, functional testes that subsequently may have undergone torsion or atrophy. Clinical findings are not enough to make the diagnosis, which must be confirmed through endocrinological evaluation and provocative testing. Classically, an hCG stimulation test has been used to identify occult testicular tissue by assessing the serum testosterone response. Other hormones (inhibin B and anti-Müllerian hormone) released only by the gonad can now be measured in serum to search for the presence of occult tissue. The typical hormonal characteristics of congenital bilateral anorchia can be identified between 6 weeks and 6 months of life secondary to the mini-puberty of infancy. They include elevated concentrations of gonadotropins and a low concentration of testosterone. At any age, a lack of increase in serum testosterone after hCG is highly supportive of the diagnosis. With regard to imaging, neither ultrasonography nor MRI is generally very useful because these modalities

are insufficiently sensitive to differentiate between small testes and enlarged inguinal lymph nodes, and other pelvic/abdominal structures. Surgical exploration may be the only definitive option to identify any testicular tissue, but must be carried out with great care considering the small dimensions of the organs.

There is a large list of substances reported to have an adverse effect on testicular function. Chronic alcohol intoxication can result in testicular atrophy as seen in cirrhotic patients. Lead exposure may result in intoxication sufficient to cause systemic poisoning with testicular deposition and resultant hypogonadism. Cadmium damages testicular blood vessels causing ischemia and tubular necrosis. Alkylating chemotherapeutic agents (cyclophosphamide, busulfan, procarbazine, and etoposide) frequently cause dose-dependent testicular damage. Direct radiation, as used to treat leukemic infiltration of testes, is also quite toxic. Lastly, testicular infarction has been reported with sickle cell disease.

The most common microbial agent documented to cause orchitis and testicular damage is mumps; oöphoritis may occur in females. The hallmark of infection is swelling of the parotid gland. Laboratory diagnosis is based on isolation of virus, detection of viral nucleic acid, or serological confirmation (generally presence of IgM mumps antibodies). Mumps is vaccine-preventable and one dose of mumps vaccine is about 80% successful in preventing the disease.

Autoimmunity has also been linked to testicular damage, but is a more common cause of gonadal failure in girls than it is in boys.

Girls
Congenital ovarian failure

X chromosome abnormalities—Turner syndrome (TS) is the prototypical etiology of primary ovarian failure identified in childhood. It is a sporadic disorder defined by the complete or partial absence of the second X chromosome. X monosomy is the most commonly occurring sex chromosome anomaly (1%-2% of all female conceptions), with 90% or more of Turner conceptions spontaneously aborted. TS occurs with an incidence of about 1 in 2000 to 2500 live female births. Although not mandatory for the diagnosis of TS, phenotypic stigmata of short stature and delayed sexual development are the most frequent and, in 50% of girls with TS, are the only features. Girls with TS may present with short neck, webbed neck, left-sided cardiac anomalies (nonstenotic isolated bicuspid aortic valve, coarctation of the aorta, or hypoplastic left heart syndrome), low posterior hairline, epicanthal folds, ptosis, downslanting palpebral fissures, broad shield-like chest, hypoplastic nipples, cubitus valgus, nail hypoplasia, nail hypercovexity, low-set and/or malformed ears, hearing deficits, retrognathia, dental crowding, and/or a high-arched palate. Some of the features may be secondary to lymphedema during gestation. Girls with TS may present in childhood with short stature, declining growth velocity, mildly elevated levels of FSH, and/or any grouping of TS stigmata described earlier (Figure 7-24). Girls who present during adolescence with TS may come to medical attention with short stature, absence of breast development, pubertal arrest, primary or secondary amenorrhea, hypertension, and/or scoliosis.

Gonadal dysgenesis is a hallmark of TS. In most patients with TS, the ovaries at birth are already fibrous streaks. Ovarian deterioration appears to develop early in the second trimester with premature atresia complete before birth, although in some patients (up to 15%-20%) the atresia is not complete until adolescence of adulthood. It is this delayed rate of atresia that allows some girls with TS to have spontaneous pubertal development, an even smaller number

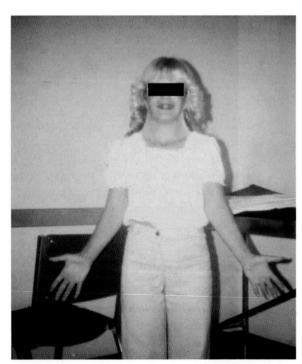

FIGURE 7-24 ■ A 16-year-old patient with Turner syndrome is shown. She demonstrates some of the characteristic stigmata of Turner syndrome, for example, short stature, webbed neck, low set ears, and cubitus valgus. (*From: Geffner ME. Disorders of puberty. In: Kliegman RM, Greenbaum LA, Lye PS, eds. Practical Strategies in Pediatric Diagnosis and Therapy. Harcourt Health Sciences, 2005; with permission of Elsevier.*)

spontaneous menarche, and, on rare occasion, spontaneous pregnancy. Therefore, the presentation of females with TS girls ranges from absence of any female pubertal development to mid-pubertal failure without progression to menarche, secondary amenorrhea, or early menopause in adulthood.

Premature ovarian failure has also been identified among heterozygous carriers of the fragile X mutation. Interestingly, only premutation carriers have been found to have an increased risk for premature ovarian failure, whereas full-mutation carriers and their noncarrier sisters appear to have the same risk that is seen in the general population. Approximately 16% of premutation heterozygotes have early ovarian failure. An observation that potentially explains the reduced penetrance is that paternally inherited premutations are more likely to give rise to premature ovarian failure than are maternally inherited permutations.

Delayed puberty in a phenotypic female can also be seen in pure gonadal dysgenesis (46,XY—Swyer syndrome) and mixed gonadal dysgenesis (45,X/46,XY). Complete gonadal dysgenesis is the result of a total lack of testicular function. Without testicular hormone production during gestation, the natural phenotypical default pathway is female. Girls with mixed gonadal dysgenesis may also have some somatic features typical of TS. Genital development ranges from female to ambiguous to male. Gonadectomy is clearly recommended in both conditions as dysgenetic gonads have an increased risk of developing dysgerminomas or gonadoblastomas.

In rare cases, pure ovarian agenesis with a 46,XX karyotype also occurs. Affected girls have normal or tall stature, no dysmorphic features, and normal female external genitalia, but hypoplastic or absent ovarian tissue.

Autosomal abnormalities—Autosomal abnormalities have also been identified as causing primary ovarian failure. Galactosemia is a rare (1: 50,000 live births) autosomal recessive disorder identified routinely by newborn screening. The condition results from impairment in galactose 1-phosphate uridyltransferase metabolism secondary to a mutation in the *GALT* gene. The resultant protein is a hepatic enzyme essential for the breakdown of lactose, which is commonly found in milk products. Galactosemia usually is asymptomatic at birth, but jaundice, diarrhea, vomiting, failure-to-thrive, and sepsis soon ensue. Secondary to the lethal nature of the condition if not identified early, galactosemia is one of the diseases checked in newborn screening programs. Despite adequate dietary control of the metabolic disorder with a soy-based formula, girls with galactosemia have lower intelligence, neurological dysfunction, dyspraxia, and delayed growth and sexual development, as well as primary ovarian failure. The prevalence of primary ovarian failure is 70% to 80% in girls with galactosemia. Ovarian damage has been attributed to a toxic effect of galactose or one of its metabolites on follicular structures during fetal life.

Blepharophimosis-ptosis-epicanthus inversus syndrome (BPES) is a very rare autosomal dominantly inherited disorder (exact incidence unknown), mapped to the long arm of chromosome 3. Classic BPES is a complex eyelid malformation invariably characterized by four major features: blepharophimosis, ptosis, epicanthus inversus, and telecanthus. Type 1 BPES includes the four major features and female infertility caused by premature ovarian failure and type 2 includes only the four major features.

Acquired ovarian failure

Autoimmune polyglandular syndromes— Autoimmune polyglandular syndrome (APS) can be categorized into types 1 and 2. APS 1 (**A**utoimmune **P**oly**E**ndocrinopathy-**C**andidiasis-**E**ctodermal **D**ystrophy or APECED) is an autosomal recessive disorder caused by mutations of the *autoimmune regulator (AIRE)* gene, which has been mapped to chromosome 21q22.3. The three major components of APS 1 are chronic mucocutaneous candidiasis, hypoparathyroidism, and adrenal insufficiency. In most cases of APS type 1, chronic candidiasis is the first manifestation of the disease, often occurring before the age of 5 years. It is typically followed by hypoparathyroidism, and then by adrenal insufficiency (Addison disease) that usually develops in adolescents. Glucocorticoid and mineralocorticoid deficiencies both occur. Antibodies to CYP21 (21-hydroxylase) and CYP17 (17-hydroxylase) seem to be the most commonly identified. Symptoms include weakness, fatigue, myalgias, weight loss, abdominal pain, anorexia, diarrhea, nausea, vomiting, dehydration, hypotension, and hyperpigmentation. Laboratory investigation demonstrates hyponatremia, hyperkalemia, metabolic acidosis, azotemia, and hypoglycemia in the presence of an elevated ACTH. APS 2 includes adrenal, thyroid, and/or pancreatic endocrine dysfunction. APS 2 occurs primarily in adulthood, usually in the third and fourth decades of life, especially in middle-aged women. It is associated with HLA-DR3 and/or -DR4 haplotypes, and the pattern of inheritance is autosomal dominant with variable expressivity. All APS 2 patients have adrenal insufficiency, more than half have thyroid disease (Hashimoto or Graves disease), and less than half have type 1 diabetes. Antibodies to each of the component organs are usually present. Other autoimmune diseases that are not the major components may also be present in both type 1 and type 2 APS, including hypergonadotropic hypogonadism. Primary ovarian failure occurs in approximately 60% in patients with APS type 1, but in only 10% to 25% of women with APS type 2.

OVARIAN TISSUE DAMAGE

With the increasing success of therapy for childhood cancers, there is a growing population of adolescent girls and women with ovarian failure. Approximately 50% of girls exposed to pelvic irradiation develop primary ovarian failure. The severity and likelihood is dependent on the dose delivered and age administered. Cytotoxic chemotherapy, as previously described for boys, may cause premature ovarian failure in many treated patients. The actively proliferating cells of the mature ovary appear to be especially sensitive to the effects of irradiation and cytotoxic agents. GnRH agonist therapy has been used successfully in an attempt to preserve ovarian function during chemotherapy with alkylating agents.

Diagnosis, evaluation, and natural history

As stated previously, random LH and FSH levels measured by the ultrasensitive ICMA method differentiate hypo- from hypergonadotropic hypogonadism (Table 7-8). Elevated gonadotropins, in the presence of low gonadal sex steroids, indicate the presence of hypergonadotropic hypogonadism. Such a biochemical profile is most apparent in the first few months of life and after the age of 10 years.

The history and physical examination are very helpful in narrowing the differential for this category. A history of poor school performance, in association with tall stature and small testes, is highly suggestive of Klinefelter syndrome. A history of absent testes at birth in an otherwise normal-appearing male suggests the presence of congenital anorchia. An unimmunized child may have had mumps exposure and gonadal insult. A perinatal history of lymphedema or congenital heart disease in a short girl suggests TS. A family history of fragile X may indicate a premutation carrier at risk for premature ovarian failure. A history of galactosemia or a special formula requirement in infancy may indicate toxic exposure to the ovaries resulting in premature ovarian failure. Eyelid abnormalities in a girl with delayed/absent puberty are suggestive of

BPES. The presence of other autoimmune conditions, such as thyroiditis, suggests the possibility of APS.

Measurement of serum estradiol levels in girls and testosterone levels in boys is also routinely obtained, but is not necessary as serum concentrations can usually be estimated by the degree of clinical pubertal development. Similarly, a pelvic ultrasound in girls is also frequently ordered although, in most cases, the size of the ovaries and uterus can be predicted from the clinical presentation.

Hypergonadotropic hypogonadism always warrants a karyotype to look for genetic syndromes. If normal in females, additional testing should include antiovarian antibodies to detect autoimmune ovarian failure. Galactosemia is typically detected on newborn screening.

Treatment

See section on Hypogonadotropic Hypogonadism discussed earlier for treatment strategies related to sex steroid replacement.

In contrast to patients with hypogonadotropic hypogonadism, patients with primary hypogonadism have intrinsic gonadal damage and, therefore, are, in almost all cases, infertile. There are promising projects looking at cryopreservation of oöcytes for females and intracytoplasmic sperm extraction for males which may afford these patients new options to allow fertility.

When to refer

The criteria for referral of a child with delayed puberty to an endocrinologist are summarized in Box 7-2.

GYNECOMASTIA[37]

Definition

Gynecomastia refers to the glandular proliferation of breast tissue in males.

Etiology

Physiological gynecomastia occurs most commonly around the age of 13 years in conjunction with Tanner stage 3 to 4 pubic hair and testicular volumes of 10 to 12 cc bilaterally. It is thought to result from a transient

---

Box 7-2. When to Refer

Delayed Puberty
- Statistically significant pubertal delay
  - No signs of puberty in girls more than 13 years
  - No signs of puberty in boys more than 14 years
- Pubertal arrest
  - Greater than 4 years between the first signs of puberty and menarche in girls or between the onset and completion of genital growth in boys
- Boys with constitutional delay and psychological compromise who might benefit from testosterone therapy

---

imbalance in the free androgen to free estrogen ratio that allows preferential estrogen effects on breast tissue during this time. However, typically there is often no demonstrable hormonal aberration that is detectable in serum. It has recently been suggested that the adipose tissue-derived hormone, leptin, may influence the pathogenesis of pubertal gynecomastia. With advancing puberty, serum androgen levels rise closer to adult levels resulting in a higher androgen-to-estrogen ratio so that, within 1 to 3 years, breast enlargement regresses in up to 90% of boys.

Pathological gynecomastia results from absolute or relative estrogen excess owing to exogenous estrogen administration, endogenous overproduction, or increased peripheral conversion of androgens to estrogens as is seen with excessive aromatase activity or androgen deficiency (Table 7-9). Since isolated prepubertal gynecomastia is quite rare, it should always be considered pathological. Even in this age group, the majority has age-appropriate, undetectable sex steroid levels and, thus, a specific cause is rarely identified. This suggests that the most common etiology of prepubertal gynecomastia (as with its pubertal counterpart) is idiopathic. That said, it also has been suggested that possible repeated exposures to environmental chemicals be considered as possible etiologies, including personal care products that contain lavender and tea tree oils. The list of common drugs and unintentional exposures associated with gynecomastia is shown in Table 7-10.

Gynecomastia can rarely be the presenting sign for testicular and adrenal cancer. Leydig cell tumors secrete estradiol directly, hCG-secreting tumors stimulate the testes to secrete estradiol (through its LH-like action on Leydig cells), and Sertoli cell tumors increase androgen-to-estrogen conversion via overexpression of aromatase activity. PJS is a rare autosomal dominant disorder that is characterized by multiple gastrointestinal polyps, mucocutaneous pigmentation, and an increased risk for various neoplasms. In recent years, Sertoli cell tumors have become increasingly recognized as a cause of prepubertal gynecomastia in children with PJS. Feminizing adrenocortical tumors are typically malignant and can secrete estrogens directly, but produce larger amounts of DHEA that are converted to estrone in peripheral tissues.

Similar to hCG-secreting, Sertoli cell, and feminizing adrenocortical tumors, several other conditions are associated with increased peripheral aromatization of androgens to estrogens leading to gynecomastia. The rare entity, aromatase excess syndrome, owing to an autosomal dominantly inherited gain-of-function mutation in the *CYP19 (aromatase)* gene, is characterized by accelerated early linear growth, prepubertal gynecomastia, and testicular failure in males and premature thelarche, macromastia, enlarged uterine size, and irregular

Table 7-9.

Differential Diagnosis of Gynecomastia

Etiology	Purported mechanism
Physiological (in adolescents)	Unknown (presumed increased estrogen-to-androgen ratio)
Idiopathic (prepubertal)	Unknown (presumed increased estrogen-to-androgen ratio)
Drugs and exposures	Direct or indirect estrogenic or estrogen-like stimulation
Leydig cell tumor	Secrete estradiol
Sertoli cell tumor	Increased androgen-to-estrogen conversion via overexpression of aromatase activity (Peutz-Jeghers syndrome)
hCG-secreting tumors	Stimulate testes to secrete estradiol
Adrenal tumors	Increased aromatase activity
Aromatase excess syndrome	Increased aromatase activity
Hyperthyroidism	Increased aromatase activity
Hypogonadotropic hypogonadism	Relative estrogen excess (decreased androgen) as occurs in Klinefelter syndrome
Hypergonadotropic hypogonadism	Relative estrogen excess (decreased androgen) as occurs in 17-ketoreductase deficiency
Hyperprolactinemia	Induction of hypogonadotropic hypogonadism

menstruation in females. In both sexes, there are elevated serum estrogen levels. Hyperthyroidism increases aromatization of androgens to estrogens and decreases free testosterone levels by increasing circulating SHBG levels. Reversible gynecomastia has been reported in 10% to 40% of hyperthyroid men.

Gynecomastia can be seen with any form of genetic or acquired hypogonadism associated with androgen deficiency. The primary defect in testicular failure is decreased serum testosterone levels, but, secondarily, because of absent central feedback, there is increased pituitary LH release and the remaining Leydig cells are stimulated to preferentially produce estradiol leading to relatively unopposed estrogenic effects on breast tissue. The most common chromosomal disorder associated with hypergonadotropic hypogonadism is Klinefelter syndrome. Affected men have about twice the usual amount of circulating estradiol resulting in elevated estradiol-to-testosterone ratios. Thus, 50% to 70% of men with Klinefelter syndrome have gynecomastia which also confers, in this population only, a significantly increased risk for breast cancer. Defects in testosterone synthesis (eg, 17-ketosteroid reductase deficiency) may also cause gynecomastia in association with

Table 7-10.

Medications/Exposures Associated with Gynecomastia

Mechanism of Action	Examples
Bind estrogen receptor or mimic estrogen	Oral estrogen or oral contraceptives, vaginal estrogen cream, digitalis, clomiphene, marijuana
Stimulate estrogen synthesis	Gonadotropins, growth hormone
Supply estrogen precursors that can be aromatized	Exogenous testosterone, androgen precursors (eg, androstenedione and DHEA)
Direct testicular damage	Busulfan, nitrosureas, vincristine, ethanol
Block androgen synthesis	Ketoconazole, spironolactone, metronidazole, etomidate
Block androgen action	Spironolactone, flutamide, bicalutamide, finasteride, cimetidine, ranitidine
Displace estrogen from SHBG	Spironolactone, ethanol
Unintentional exposures to estrogens or phytoestrogens	Essential (lavender and tea tree) oils (in personal care products), estrogen-containing anti-balding creams, licorice, meat and milk from estrogen-treated cows, nettle teas, soy

hypergonadotropic hypogonadism. Gynecomastia from central or secondary hypogonadism is unusual as, typically, all sex hormone levels are low, although continued peripheral aromatization of adrenal androgenic precursors to estrogen may favor a higher estrogen-to-androgen ratio that leads to breast tissue proliferation. Hyperprolactinemia may rarely cause gynecomastia by suppressing gonadotropin production and inducing hypogonadotropic hypogonadism (rather than by a direct effect on the breast).

Diagnosis, evaluation, and natural history

Appropriate examination requires the patient to be supine with hands behind the head following which the examiner brings his or her thumb and forefinger together from the periphery to the center of the breast. True gynecomastia is diagnosed by the presence of a palpable fibroglandular mass that measures more than or equal to 0.5 cm in diameter and is located concentrically beneath the nipple. It can develop as a unilateral, bilateral, and/or asymmetrical enlargement of the breasts, or as a painless or tender mass owing to the stretching of overlying tissues. The ability to distinguish true breast tissue from fat tissue under the nipples is often difficult and some patients have both.

Gynecomastia in *prepubertal* boys is uncommon and of potential concern, and, thus, should prompt an immediate search for an endogenous or exogenous source of estrogen, and a prompt referral should be made to a pediatric endocrinologist. Conditions to consider (see Box 7-3) include androgen- and estrogen-producing tumors, inherited disorders of sex steroid synthesis, aromatase excess, medications, and unintentional environmental exposures.

Conversely, gynecomastia in adolescents, especially during mid-puberty, is quite common. It is usually a physiological phenomenon typically followed by spontaneous regression within 1 to 3 years when adult testosterone levels are achieved. However, if there is evidence of underlying pathology, for example, macrogynecomastia (>4-cm breast diameter) with rapidly progressive enlargement (indicative of the magnitude of hormonal imbalance); galactorrhea (hyperprolactinemia); small testicles and lack of or reduced secondary male sexual characteristics (hypogonadism); an abdominal or testicular mass (tumor); eunuchoidal body habitus, behavioral problems, and firm testicles (Klinefelter syndrome); accelerated linear growth (excess aromatase); goiter (hyperthyroidism); and the like, diagnostic blood tests should be ordered. If the history and physical examination do not reveal a specific cause, checking an early morning blood sample for LH, testosterone, estradiol, DHEA, and hCG may be helpful. However, in a mid-adolescent-aged boy with an otherwise normal medical history and age-appropriate physical and sexual development, a diagnostic workup is usually unnecessary.

Box 7-3. When to Refer

Gynecomastia

- ■ In any affected prepubertal male
- ■ Rapid progression and undue amount of breast tissue regardless of age
- ■ In a pubertal-aged male with a disproportionate amount of secondary sexual development for the degree of testicular size (especially if <5 mL in volume) and/or if there are significant learning issues

---

Treatment

Correction of any underlying causative endocrinopathy or elimination of any offending medication or environmental exposure is the initial step in management. As gynecomastia results from a relative estrogen excess or androgen deficiency, medical treatment to block the effects of estrogen on the breast (clomiphene, tamoxifen, and raloxifene), diminish its production (aromatase inhibitors such as testolactone, letrozole, and anastrozole), or replace androgens (danazol) has been used (mostly in adult men) in an attempt to counterbalance the effects of the estrogens. Case reports and small clinical trials in adolescents have demonstrated some degree of breast size reduction in pubertal gynecomastia with most of the above agents. The only randomized, double-blind, placebo-controlled trial performed in the pediatric population to date found that anastrozole was no more effective than placebo in its ability to decrease gynecomastia by at least 50% over baseline. Thus, current data are insufficient to recommend routine medical treatment for idiopathic gynecomastia at this time. If spontaneous regression does not occur after 3 years, surgery is the only other option, and should be considered if there is persistent pain, embarrassment, or anxiety.

When to refer

The criteria for referral of a child with gynecomastia to an endocrinologist are summarized in Box 7-3.

HIRSUTISM/POLYCYSTIC OVARY SYNDROME[38]

Definitions

Hirsutism is defined as excessive hair growth on body parts influenced by androgen action, that is, sexual hair. Idiopathic hirsutism is not associated with other signs of hyperandrogenism, such as external genital virilization, increased muscle bulk, temporal hair recession, or voice-deepening. In contrast, hypertrichosis refers to non-androgen-mediated, excessive growth of lanugo hair over the entire body. The latter may have an ethnic basis, occurring more often in descendents from around the Mediterranean sea or result from the chronic use of certain medications, including diphenylhydantoin, cyclosporine, minoxidil, and diazoxide.

PCOS is the most common endocrine disorder affecting females of reproductive age, occurring in 5% to 10% of women worldwide, and, as defined by a 1990 NIH-sponsored consensus conference, is characterized by irregular or loss of menstrual disorders (oligo- or anovulation) *and* biochemical or clinical signs of hyperandrogenism, such as hirsutism, acne, or male pattern baldness. In 2003, the international Rotterdam Consensus Workshop expanded the above definition to include ovarian morphology, proposing that the diagnosis include at least two of the following criteria: oligo- or anovulation, biochemical or clinical signs of hyperandrogenism, and polycystic ovaries. However, inclusion of cystic ovarian morphology is controversial, as cystic ovaries may not be found when other criteria are clearly present and may be present in women of child-bearing age with no other manifestations of PCOS. Most recently, in 2006, the Androgen Excess Society suggested a definition of PCOS to include hyperandrogenism (hirsutism and/or hyperandrogenemia) and ovarian dysfunction (oligo-anovulation and/or polycystic ovaries). All definitions also require exclusion of related disorders (Table 7-11). In addition, obesity, insulin resistance, and metabolic syndrome occur in at least 50% of females with PCOS. Adolescents with PCOS manifest clinical, biochemical, and endocrine features similar to those of affected adult women.

Etiology

Idiopathic isolated hirsutism results from either overproduction of and/or increased hormonal action by androgens within the hair follicle, and requires elimination of related diagnoses, as noted below (Table 7-11).

The etiology of PCOS remains unclear and is probably multifactorial, involving a combination of ovarian and adrenal hyperandrogenism. A genetic basis seems likely with autosomal dominant familial clustering and a male phenotype associated with elevated DHEA sulfate levels. Linkage studies have shown associations to genes encoding various steroidogenic enzymes, the androgen receptor, SHBG, LH, insulin, the insulin receptor, leptin, adiponectin, and various inflammatory mediators. As such, the genesis of PCOS may actually begin *in utero* following exposure to a hyperandrogenic and/or insulin-resistant hormonal milieu. Known childhood risk factors for future PCOS include: congenital virilizing disorders; above average or low (small-for-gestational age) birth weight; precocious adrenarche; and severe obesity with acanthosis nigricans, metabolic syndrome, and glucose intolerance or T2DM. Women with PCOS manifest alterations in gonadotropin secretion characterized by increased LH pulse amplitude and, in some studies, increased pulse frequency, along with subnormal FSH induction of CYP19 aromatase activity in granulosa cells leading to a heightened androgen-to-estrogen ratio, although absolute estrogen levels tend to be elevated above normal. Additionally, both obese and thin women with PCOS tend to be resistant to the metabolic actions of insulin, with retention of responsiveness to its growth-promoting (mitogenic) actions so that the resultant compensatory hyperinsulinemia may lead to increased ovarian androgen secretion as well as to decreased hepatic SHBG production. Most recently, a unifying hypothesis has been invoked to explain both the overproduction of ovarian and adrenal androgens and diminished insulin action in which a single mutated serine kinase activates the P450C17 enzyme leading to

Table 7-11.

Differential Diagnosis/Evaluation of Irregular Menses and Hyperandrogenism

Disorder	Manifestation	Initial Evaluation*
Hypothyroidism	Irregular menses	Free T$_4$, TSH, ATA
Hyperthyroidism	Irregular menses	Free T$_4$, T$_3$, TSH, TSHRAb
Hyperprolactinemia	Irregular menses	Prolactin, head MRI
CAH/NCAH	Virilization/irregular menses	17OHP and T (pre- and post-ACTH stimulation)
Adrenal tumor	Virilization/irregular menses	T, DHEA sulfate, adrenal US
Ovarian tumor	Virilization/irregular menses	T, ovarian US
Cushing syndrome	Virilization/irregular menses	24-h urine free cortisol/Cr, T, adrenal US

ATA = antithyroperoxidase and antithyroglobulin antibodies
TSHRAb = TSH-receptor antibodies
17OHP = 17-hydroxyprogesterone
T = testosterone
US = ultrasound
Cr = creatinine
*17OHP and T levels should be measured at ~8:00 AM.

hyperandrogenism and inhibiting signaling through the insulin receptor β-chain causing insulin resistance. Greater derangements of insulin action are seen in obese subjects with greater adrenal contributions to hyperandrogenism in thin subjects with PCOS.

Diagnosis

Evaluation begins with a detailed menstrual history and exploration of the types and duration of hyperandrogenic symptoms. PCOS is typically associated with chronic menstrual abnormalities and slowly progressive features of hyperandrogenism. Abrupt changes in menstrual pattern and/or rapid onset and/or severe manifestations of hyperandrogenism should suggest alternate etiologies, such as hypo- or hyperthyroidism, hyperprolactinemia, CAH/NCAH, androgen-secreting tumors, and Cushing syndrome. Family history may be helpful regarding other women with PCOS or thyroid disease, and for the presence of consanguinity which would increase the chances for autosomally recessively inherited adrenal hyperplasia. Important physical findings include those associated with thyroid dysfunction (eg, presence of myxedema, brady- or tachycardia, and proptosis, with or without goiter), galactorrhea, Cushingoid features (eg, centralized obesity, buffalo hump, and moon facies), and generalized obesity (along with hypertension, acanthosis nigricans, and acrochordons [skin tags]).

Treatment

Girls with idiopathic hirsutism, normal menstrual cycles, and relatively normal hormonal values require only periodic examination; if obese, they should be encouraged to lose weight after which an amelioration of clinical manifestations may be noted (Table 7-12). However, if the condition worsens or menstrual cycles become irregular, further evaluation and possible medical treatment are warranted.

In teenagers and women with PCOS, treatment targets the components of the syndrome, that is, menstrual/reproductive, cutaneous, metabolic, and psychological. Since most affected females are overweight, basic therapy in this subset should target lifestyle modification involving diet and exercise which theoretically, if successful, could restore ovulatory cycles via reduction of insulin resistance.

Historically, administration of estrogen and progesterone (oral contraceptive) has been the mainstay of treatment for those not seeking pregnancy. This approach results in regular menses, reduced risk of endometrial hyperplasia and cancer, and improves androgenic manifestations such as acne and hirsutism. Estrogen acts by increasing hepatic production of SHBG which reduces availability of free testosterone while progesterone counteracts the neoplastic potential of

Table 7-12.

Therapeutic Approaches in the Treatment of Idiopathic Hirsutism/PCOS

Mechanism of action	Modality
Inhibition of androgen production and/ or action	Estrogen Spironolactone Flutamide
Improvement of insulin sensitivity	Weight loss (diet and exercise) Metformin Thiazolidinediones (rosiglitazone and pioglitazone)
Inhibition of LH production	Estrogen Progesterone GnRH analogs
Inhibition of ACTH production	Glucocorticoids
Mechanical hair removal: temporary	Shaving Waxing, Depilatory creams
Mechanical hair removal: permanent	Electrolysis Laser

unopposed estrogen acting on the uterus. However, it is important that the estrogen portion not be excessive (averaging about 30 μg/day of ethinyl estradiol) and that the progesterone component has low androgenicity or even be antiandrogenic (eg, drospirenone). Oral contraceptives decrease LH secretion, but do not appear to work by improving insulin sensitivity. Progestational agents alone are occasionally used for the purposes of inducing withdrawal bleeding, but will not aid hyperandrogenic symptoms. GnRH analogs are occasionally used to reduce LH secretion.

Antiandrogen drugs added to nonandrogenic oral contraceptives are often used adjunctively (and occasionally alone) in females with PCOS. The most commonly employed drug in the United States for this purpose, spironolactone, acts by binding to and blocking the androgen and may also interfere with (adrenal) steroidogenesis. This drug must be avoided during pregnancy because of teratogenic potential. Flutamide, with similar mechanisms of action to spironolactone, has been used, but concern regarding serious hepatotoxicity (seen with high doses) has limited its use. Occasionally, adjunctive glucocorticoid therapy is employed if there is a significant adrenal contribution to the prevailing hyperandrogenism. Outside the United States, cyproterone acetate is frequently used because it interferes with steroidogenesis and also possesses antigonadotropic effects. As pharmacological approaches to excess hair growth for the most part target only new hair

> **Box 7-4. When to Refer**
>
> Hirsutism/Polycystic Ovary Syndrome
>
> ■ Primary amenorrhea or secondary amenorrhea of more than or equal to 6 months duration
> ■ Progressive virilization, for example, clitoromegaly, cystic acne, increased muscle bulk, temporal hair recession, and/or voice-deepening
> ■ Presence of significant comorbidities, for example, morbid obesity, Cushingoid body habitus, hypertension, hyperlipidemia, and acanthosis nigricans

growth, mechanical hair removal remains a key approach to the removal of preexisting hair or for progressive hirsutism that is not responsive to drug therapy. Nonpermanent hair removal methods include shaving, waxing, and use of topical depilatory creams. Permanent methods, that is, electrolysis and laser therapy, are effective, but are more costly and may be painful.

Improvement of insulin sensitivity is now recognized as an important component of the therapeutic armamentarium. Weight loss and exercise can, in and of themselves, increase insulin sensitivity. In addition, medication may play a role in improving insulin resistance. Metformin monotherapy of obese adolescents with PCOS appears to improve insulin sensitivity, and, in so doing, to lower serum insulin and androgen levels, attenuate adrenal steroidogenic response to ACTH, and possibly increase the rate of ovulation. It has been suggested that the use of both antiandrogen and insulin-sensitizing treatments in young, nonobese women with hyperinsulinemic hyperandrogenism has additive benefits on insulin sensitivity, hyperandrogenemia, and dyslipidemia. Insulin-sensitizing agents of the thiazolidinedione class (rosiglitazone and pioglitazone) have also proven helpful in the treatment of women with PCOS leading to an improvement of ovulatory dysfunction, hirsutism, hyperandrogenemia, and insulin resistance, with minimal adverse effects. Note, however, that prescription of insulin sensitizer therapy in females with PCOS (unless diagnosed with T2DM) constitutes an off-label use for these drugs.

When to refer

The criteria for referral of a child with hirsutism/polycystic ovarian syndrome to an endocrinologist are summarized in Box 7-4.

REFERENCES

1. Popa SM, Clifton DK, Steiner RA. The role of kisspeptins and GPR54 in the neuroendocrine regulation of reproduction. *Annu Rev Physiol.* 2008;70:213-238.
2. Kaminski BA, Palmert MR. Genetic control of pubertal timing. *Curr Opin Pediatr.* 2008;20:458-464.
3. Euling SY, Herman-Giddens ME, Lee PA, et al. Examination of US puberty-timing data from 1940 to 1994 for secular trends: panel findings. *Pediatrics.* 2008;121(3):S172-191.
4. Juul A, Teilmann G, Scheike T, et al. Pubertal development in Danish children: comparison of recent European and US data. *Int J Androl.* 2006;29:247-255.
5. Louis GMB, Gray LE Jr, Marcus M, et al. Environmental factors and puberty timing: expert panel research needs. *Pediatrics.* 2008;121:S192-S207.
6. Kaplowitz PB. Link between body fat and the timing of puberty. *Pediatrics* 2008; 121(Suppl 3):S208-S217.
7. Bluher S, Mantzoros CS. Leptin in reproduction. *Curr Opin Endocrinol Diab Obes.* 2007;14:458-464.
8. Schoeters G, Hond ED, Dhooge W, van Larebeke N, Leijs M. Endocrine disruptors and abnormalities of pubertal development. *Basic Clin Pharmacol Toxicol.* 2008;102:168-175.
9. Herman-Giddens ME, Slora EJ, Wasserman RC, et al. Secondary sexual characteristics and menses in young girls seen in office practice: a study from the Pediatric Research in Office Settings Network. *Pediatrics.* 1997;99:505-512.
10. Kaplowitz PB, Oberfield SE. Reexamination of the age limit for defining when puberty is precocious in girls in the United States: implications for evaluation and treatment. *Pediatrics.* 1999;104:936-941.
11. Parent AS, Teilmann GE, Juul A, Skakkebaek NE, Toppari J, Bourguignon J-P. The timing of normal puberty and the age limits of sexual precocity: variations around the world, secular trends, and changes after migration. *Endocr Rev.* 2003;24:668-693.
12. Nakamoto JM. Myths and variations in normal pubertal development. *Western J Med* 2000;172:182-185.
13. Auchus RJ. The riddle of adrenarche. Many questions, not enough answers. *The Endocrinologist.* 2004;14:329-336.
14. Geffner ME. Variations in tempo of normal pubertal progression. *Pediatric Endocrinol Rev.* 2007;4:278-282.
15. Geffner ME. Aromatase inhibitors to augment height: have we lost our inhibitions? *Pediatr Endocrinol Rev.* 2008;5:756-759.
16. Carel JC, Léger J. Clinical practice. Precocious puberty. *N Engl J Med.* 2008; 29;358:2366-2377.
17. Monzavi R, Kelly D, Geffner ME. Rathke's cleft cyst in two girls with precocious puberty. *J Pediatr Endocrinol Metab.* 2004;17:781-785.
18. Hirsch HJ, Gillis D, et al. The histrelin implant: a novel treatment for central precocious puberty. *Pediatrics.* 2005;116:e798-802.
19. Pasquino AM, Pucarelli I, Accardo F, Demiraj V, Segni M, Di Nardo R. Long-term observation of 87 girls with idiopathic central precocious puberty treated with gonadotropin-releasing hormone analogs: impact on adult height, body mass index, bone mineral content, and reproductive function. *J Clin Endocrinol Metab.* 2008; 93:190-195.
20. Tanaka T, Niimi H, Matsuo N, et al. Results of long-term follow-up after treatment of central precocious puberty with leuprorelin acetate: evaluation of effectiveness of treatment and recovery of gonadal function. The TAP-144-SR Japanese Study Group on Central Precocious Puberty. *J Clin Endocrinol Metab.* 2005;90: 1371-1376.
21. Franklin SL, Geffner M. Precocious puberty secondary to topical testosterone exposure. *J Pediatr Endocrinol Metab.* 2003;16:107-110.

22. Seldmeyer IL, Palmert MR. Delayed puberty: analysis of a large series from an academic center. *J Clin Endocrinol Metab.* 2002;87:1613-1620.

23. Wehkalampi K, Widen E, Laine T, Palotie A, Dunkel L. Patterns of inheritance of constitutional delay of growth and puberty in families of adolescent girls and boys referred to specialist pediatric care. *J Clin Endocrinol Metab.* 2008;93:723-728.

24. Pozo J, Argente J. Delayed puberty in chronic illness. *Best Pract Res Clin Endocrinol Metab.* 2002;16:73-90.

25. Simon D. Puberty in chronically diseased patients. *Horm Res.* 2002;57:53-56.

26. De Sanctis V, Eleftheriou A, Malaventura C. Thalassemia International Federation Study Group on Growth and Endocrine Complications in Thalassemia. Prevalence of endocrine complications and short stature in patients with thalassemia major: a multicenter study by the Thalassemia International Federation (TIF). *Pediatr Endocrinol Rev.* 2004;2(2):249-255.

27. Cohan GR. HIV-associated hypogonadism. *AIDS Read.* 2006;16:341-345.

28. Selevan SG, Rice DC, Hogan KA, Euling SY, Pfahles-Hutchens A, Blethel J. Blood lead concentration and delayed puberty in girls. *N Engl J Med.* 2003;348:1527-1536.

29. Achermann JC, Jameson JL. Advances in the molecular genetics of hypogonadotropic hypogonadism. *J Pediatr Endocrinol Metab.* 2001:14;3-15.

30. Reynaud R, Gueydan M, Saveanu A, et al. Genetic screening of combined pituitary hormone deficiency: Experience in 195 patients. *J Clin Endocrinol Metab.* 2006:91:3329-3336.

31. Achermann JC, Gu Wx, Kotlar TJ, et al. Mutational analysis of DAX1 in patients with hypogonadotropic hypogonadism or pubertal delay. *J Clin Endocrinol Metab.* 1999;84:4497-4500.

32. Munce T, Simpson R, Bowling F. Molecular characterization of Prader-Willi syndrome by real-time PCR. *Genet Test.* 2008;12:319-324.

33. Pinto G, Abadie V, Mesnage R, et al. CHARGE syndrome includes hypogonadotropic hypogonadism and abnormal olfactory bulb development. *J Clin Endocrinol Metab.* 2005;90:5621-5626.

34. Beales PL, Elcioglu N, Woolf AS, Parker D, Flinter FA. New criteria for improved diagnosis of Bardet-Biedl syndrome: results of a population survey. *J Med Genet.* 1999;36:437-446.

35. Darzy KH, Shalet SM. Hypopituitarism as a consequence of brain tumours and radiotherapy. *Pituitary.* 2005;8:203-211.

36. Smyth CM, Bremner WJ. Klinefelter syndrome. *Arch Intern Med.* 1998;158:1309-1314.

37. Ma NS, Geffner ME. Gynecomastia in prepubertal and pubertal men. *Curr Opin Pediatr.* 2008;20:465-470.

38. Harwood K, Vuguin P, DiMartino-Nardi J. Current approaches to the diagnosis and treatment of polycystic ovarian syndrome in youth. *Horm Res.* 2007;68:209-217.

CHAPTER 8

Disorders of Sex Development

Peter A. Lee, Selma F. Witchel,
Alan D. Rogol, and
Christopher P. Houk

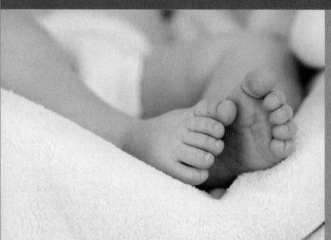

DEFINITIONS AND EPIDEMIOLOGY

A new nomenclature has been developed to describe conditions formerly known as "intersex." In this new nomenclature, the designation, *Disorders of Sex Development (DSDs)*, has been proposed to replace the word "intersex" and avoid the use of the term *hermaphrodite*.[1,2] DSDs are defined as congenital conditions in which there is inconsistency between chromosomal, gonadal, and/or anatomical sex. This classification includes not only conditions with ambiguous external genitalia, but also those conditions without ambiguity in which there is atypical gonadal or sex chromosome development. This system (Table 8-1) allows the incorporation of new information and more precise diagnostic labeling. The primary clinical advantage is to be able to use information obtained early in diagnostic evaluation—particularly karyotype and phenotype—to guide further etiological evaluation and management.

Diagnostic categories are listed in Table 8-2, but some conditions do not obviously fit into a single specific diagnostic category or may well fit into more than one category, such as forms of gonadal dysgenesis that may have a 46,XY, 46,XX, or 45,X/46,XY karyotype.

This classification purposefully avoids the terms, *hermaphroditism* and *pseudohermaphroditism* (Table 8-3), and attempts to be descriptive. This schema includes the genetic cause when known, but also allows for phenotypic variation within each etiological category. By definition, DSDs are not variations of normal sexual/reproductive development, but include those conditions that would impact reproductive or sexual function. While karyotype-specific labels may be useful in classification at the time of initial assessment of those with DSDs,

reference to genes rather than chromosomes is preferable as specific molecular etiologies are ascertained. The precise descriptive terminology used for DSDs is more helpful to promote understanding for clinical or research purposes, and hopefully avoids the risk of offending patients and families.

Accurate estimates regarding the incidence of DSDs are not readily available because of the multiple etiologies and the rarity of many of the etiologies. The most common cause of a DSD, classical adrenal hyperplasia (CAH) secondary to 21-hydroxylase deficiency, occurs in 1 in 5000 to 1 in 15,000 live births, but there is considerable variation among ethnic/racial backgrounds related to the frequency of the disease causing mutations in specific populations.

Although CAH secondary to 11-hydroxylase deficiency is rare, the incidence is high among Moroccan Jews in whom it occurs in approximately 1 in 6000. The incidence of 17-hydroxysteroid dehydrogenase deficiency is estimated at 1 in 147,000. The Smith-Lemli-Opitz syndrome, which is associated with multiple abnormalities, including urogenital anomalies, occurs with an estimated incidence of 1 in 20,000 to 60,000 live births. Many disorders are so rare that it has been difficult to estimate their incidence.

BACKGROUND INFORMATION CONCERNING PATHOGENESIS OF SEXUAL DIFFERENTIATION

Differentiation of the reproductive/sexual system can be divided into the components outlined in Table 8-4.

Table 8-1.

Nomenclature: Disorders of Sex Differentiation

Sex Chromosome DSD	46,XY DSD	46,XX DSD
45,X Turner syndrome	Aberrant testicular development	Aberrant ovarian development
47,XXY Klinefelter syndrome	Disorders of androgen synthesis or action	Disorders of androgen excess
45,X/46,XY Mixed gonadal dysgenesis	Disorders of MIH synthesis or action	Vaginal or uterine atresia
46,XX/46,XY Chimeric, ovotesticular	Other	Other

From Lee PA, Houk CP, Ahmed SF, Hughes IA and the International Consensus Conference on Intersex Working Group. Consensus statement on management of intersex disorders. Pediatrics. 2006;118:e488-e500.

Basics of Sexual Differentiation

Internal reproductive system differentiation

As occurs with most primordial reproductive structures, the paramesonephric/Müllerian and mesonephric/Wolffian ducts develop in both sexes. By the seventh week of gestation in those fetuses with testes, Sertoli cells begin to secrete Müllerian-inhibiting hormone (MIH) (also called anti-Müllerian hormone [AMH] and Müllerian-inhibiting substance [MIS]), which prohibits additional progression and causes regression of Müllerian duct development. Subsequently, testicular Leydig cells begin producing testosterone that promotes Wolffian duct development into the epididymis, vas deferens, and seminal vesicles. The lack of these testicular hormones in the developing female fetus permits Müllerian duct maturation into Fallopian tubes, uterus, cervix, and upper vagina, with no Wolffian duct development.

External reproductive system differentiation

The primordial bipotential genital structures, the genital tubercle, urethral folds, and labioscrotal swellings, differentiate into male and female external genitalia. The enzyme, 5α-reductase type 2, is expressed in these structures in the male fetus and converts testosterone, secreted by the fetal testis, into dihydrotestosterone (DHT). DHT induces male external genital differentiation. In the normal 46,XY human fetus, a cylindrical phallus approximating 2 mm in length with genital swellings develops by 9 weeks of gestation. By 12 to 14 weeks of gestation, the urethral folds fuse to form the

Table 8-2.

Examples of Diagnoses using DSD Classification[1]

A. XY DSD
1. Disorders of testicular development
   a. Complete gonadal dysgenesis (Swyer syndrome)
   b. Partial gonadal dysgenesis
   c. Gonadal regression syndrome
   d. Ovotesticular DSD
2. Disorders in androgen synthesis or action
   a. Androgen biosynthesis defects
      i. 5α-reductase deficiency
      ii. 17-hydroxysteroid dehydrogenase deficiency
      iii. StAR mutations
   b. Defects in androgen action
      i. Partial androgen insensitivity
      ii. Complete androgen insensitivity
   c. LH receptor defects (Leydig cell aplasia/hypoplasia)
   d. Disorders of AMH (MIH) and AMH receptors (persistent Müllerian duct syndrome)
3. General categories
   a. Hypospadias not associated with hormone defect
   b. Cloacal exstrophy

B. 46,XX DSD
1. Disorders of gonadal (ovarian) development
   a. Ovotesticular DSD
   b. SRY+, dup *SOX9* testicular DSD
   c. Gonadal dysgenesis
2. Androgen excess
   a. Fetal adrenal
      i. 21-hydroxylase deficiency
      ii. 11-hydroxylase deficiency
   b. Fetoplacental
      i. Aromatase deficiency
      ii. Cytochrome P450 oxidoreductase deficiency
3. General categories
   a. Cloacal exstrophy
   b. Vaginal atresia (Mayer-Rokitansky-Küster-Hauser Syndrome)
   c. MURCS Association (Müllerian hypoplasia/aplasia, renal agenesis, and cervicothoracic somite abnormalities)

C. Sex chromosome DSD
1. 45,X – Turner syndrome and variants
2. 47,XXY – Klinefelter syndrome and variants
3. 45,X/46,XY – Mixed gonadal dysgenesis, ovotesticular DSD
4. 46,XX/46,XY (Chimeric, ovotesticular DSD)

cavernous urethra and corpus spongiosum. The genital tubercle develops into the corpora cavernosa of the penis and the labioscrotal folds fuse from posterior to anterior to form the scrotum. By 14 weeks, the external genitalia are clearly masculine except for lack of testicular descent. It is thought that placental hCG stimulates the fetal testes to produce testosterone before the fetal pituitary begins to secrete luteinizing hormone (LH)

Table 8-3.

New DSD Nomenclature Compared with Earlier Classifications[1]

New Nomenclature Disorder of Sex Development (DSD)	Previous Classification Intersex
46,XY DSD	Male pseudohermaphrodite
	Undervirilized/undermasculinized XY male
46,XX DSD	Female pseudohermaphrodite
	Overvirilized/overmasculinized XY male
Sex chromosome DSD	Gonadal dysgenesis
Ovotesticular DSD	True hermaphrodite
46,XX testicular DSD	XX male/XX sex reversal
46,XY complete gonadal dysgenesis	XY sex reversal

around the 12th week of gestation. Fetal phallic growth after genital differentiation is a result of fetal pituitary LH secretion, which promotes testosterone production by testicular Leydig cells.

Deficient testosterone production, inadequate testosterone action, or other factors can result in incomplete fusion of the genital components as illustrated in Figure 8-1 which shows the spectrum as Prader stages. This figure depicts genitalia along the spectrum from female to male and such may occur in a 46,XX fetus with excessive androgen stimulation or in a 46,XY fetus with deficient androgen levels. The high prevalence of hypospadias in boys suggests that urethral fusion is a

delicate and finely regulated process that may be impacted by numerous other factors in addition to androgen.

The critical role of DHT to promote full differentiation of male external genitalia is illustrated by the incomplete differentiation of male external genitalia among boys with 5α-reductase deficiency. Affected boys have normally functioning testes and normal testosterone production, but are unable to convert testosterone to DHT in target tissues, that is, external genital structures and prostate.

In the absence of androgens or androgen action, the urethral folds and labioscrotal swellings in the 46,XX (or 46,XY) fetus remain unfused and develop into the labia minora and labia majora, respectively. The genital tubercle forms the clitoris and canalization of the vaginal plate creates the lower portion of the vagina. By 11 weeks of gestation, the clitoris is prominent and the lateral boundaries of the urogenital sulcus have separated. The separation of vagina and urethra, which is not hormone-dependent, is completed by 12 weeks. However, high levels of androgen, as seen in CAH, prevent this separation as evidenced by high insertion of the urethra into the vagina. At 20 weeks of gestation, the clitoris has grown minimally, the labia majora are well-defined, the labia minora remain hypoplastic, and separate vaginal and urethral perineal openings are present. As indicated above, in the female fetus, excessive androgen stimulation during the period of genital differentiation prior to 12 weeks of gestation results in a varying extent of labial fusion and phallic urethral development (Figure 8-1). Androgen excess later during gestation stimulates excessive clitoral growth and scrotalization of the unfused labial folds. Since no fusion occurs beyond the window of differentiation, the gestational age of androgen excess can be estimated by the genital anatomy.

Table 8-4.

Embryological Origins of Internal and External Reproductive Structures

Precursor	Male	Female
1. Internal duct systems		
a. Mesonephric (Wolffian)	Epididymis, vas deferens and seminal vesicles	Regression
b. Paramesonephric (Müllerian)	Regression	Fallopian tubes, uterus, upper part of vagina
	Prostatic utricle	
2. Urogenital sinus	(Urethra)	Lower portion of vagina (and urethra)
3. External genitalia		
a. Genital tubercle	Corpora cavernosa of penis	Clitoris
b. Labio-scrotal folds	Scrotum	Labia majora
c. Labio-urethral folds	Penile urethra, glans, and corpus spongiosum	Labia minora
4. Undifferentiated gonad	Testis	Ovary

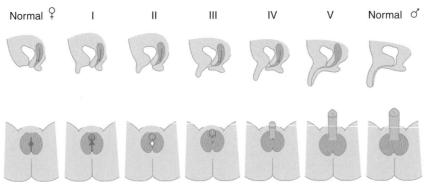

Normal ♀   I   II   III   IV   V   Normal ♂

FIGURE 8-1 ■ Shows lateral and *en face* views of external genitalia of the fully differentiated female on the left, increasing amounts of virilization (excessive for a female and inadequate for a male) going from left to right, with complete male differentiation on the right.[3]

Gonadal differentiation

The urogenital ridges, the primordial structures that form the gonads, reproductive tract, kidneys, and adrenal cortices, are an outgrowth of coelomic epithelium (mesothelium) and are present by 6 weeks of gestation. Proximity to the mesonephros as a source of endothelial cells is required for gonadal differentiation. The primitive gonad has a cortex and a medulla. Testicular differentiation occurs earlier than does ovarian development. Around the seventh week of gestation, testicular development begins in the medullary portion of the urogenital ridge. Ovarian development begins in the cortex of the primitive gonad at a later gestational age.

The SRY protein is a nuclear high-mobility group (HMG) domain protein expressed in pre-Sertoli cells where it triggers a molecular switch to initiate the process of male sexual differentiation. In fact, the first evidence of testicular differentiation is the appearance of primitive Sertoli cells (induced by the SRY protein) at 6 to 7 weeks of gestation in the human fetal testis. This is followed by migration of endothelial cells from the mesonephros and the appearance of peritubular myoid cells, steroid-secreting Leydig cells, and germ cells. The development of the testicular cords occurs by interaction of the primitive Sertoli cells and endothelial cells. These cords develop into the seminiferous tubules containing mature Sertoli and germ cells. Cell proliferation rates increase. Testicular germ cells enter a state of mitotic arrest.

Germ cell meiosis in the ovary begins at 10 to 11 weeks of gestation. Approximately 10 weeks pass between the appearance of oögonia to the presence of structured follicles. The primary oöcyte is adjacent to granulosa cell precursors to form the primary follicle which is first evident at 20 weeks of gestation. The large number of oöcytes present at mid-gestation begins to degenerate and approximately 2 million are present at birth. This process of follicular atresia appears to be accelerated in the streak gonads of fetuses with X monosomy.

Time Course of Sexual Differentiation

The sequence of the development of the components of the reproductive system development (Figure 8-2) involves differentiation of the bipotential primordial structures discussed earlier.

Differentiation of the testis with discernible Sertoli and Leydig cell lines beginning around the 7th to 8th week precedes ovarian differentiation in which oögonia do not appear until the 10th week of gestation. Fetal Leydig cell testosterone secretion begins concomitantly with differentiation of the Wolffian ducts; Müllerian duct regression in the male is evident slightly later. Male external genital differentiation begins around the 8th week of gestation and is completed by the 12th to 14th week. Virilization continues with penile growth and, in the presence of excessive androgen, clitoral enlargement proceeds. Vaginal development occurs during this period with the lower two-thirds arising from an invagination of the epidermal layers and merging with the upper third which develops from a downward extension of the Müllerian ducts.

Molecular/Genetic Overview

Genes known to be involved in the differentiation of the gonad, external genitalia, and internal genitalia are depicted in Figure 8-3.

The *sex-determining region on the Y chromosome (SRY)* gene encodes a transcription factor which initiates the formation of the testes. Subsequently, the *SOX9* gene, which is necessary for Sertoli-cell differentiation and type 2 collagen production, is expressed in the testes.[5] Mutations of *SOX9* are associated with sex-reversal. Haploinsufficiency of *SOX9* results in campomelic dysplasia, a disorder showing skeletal dysplasia that is associated with sex reversal in the majority of affected XY individuals (XY sex-reversal). Duplication of *SOX9* is a cause of a male phenotype and an XX karyotype (XX sex reversal).

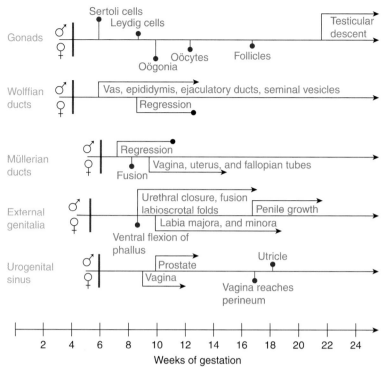

FIGURE 8-2 ■ Shows the age (in weeks of gestation) of the onset of anatomical changes and differentiation allowing for comparison of relative age of onset. Male differentiation is shown above the line for each primordial structure with female below.[4] (*From White PC, Speiser PW. Congenital adrenal hyperplasia due to 21-hydroxylase deficiency. Endoc Rev. 2000;21:245-291. With permission.*)

Other molecular factors involved in gonadal differentiation include steroidogenic factor 1 (SF1), a transcription factor necessary for steroidogenesis, male sexual differentiation, and fertility. Mutations of SF-1 have been identified in patients with agonadism, adrenal hypoplasia, hypogonadotropic hypogonadism, cryptorchidism, micropenis, and XY sex reversal.[6]

A gonad-specific transcription factor upregulated in the ovary called DAX1 (**D**osage-sensitive **A**drenal hypoplasia congenita region on the **X** chromosome *that is encoded by the NROB1 gene*), although not required for normal testicular development, appears to function as an antitestis factor in the XX ovary (Figure 8-4).

Duplication of DAX1 in the 46,XY fetus is thought to represses SRY resulting in XY sex reversal and *NROB1* mutations are associated with a syndrome of adrenal hypoplasia and hypogonadotropic hypogonadism (adrenal hypoplasia congenita [AHC]).

Thus, a threshold level of SRY activity is necessary for male sexual differentiation. Sequential expression of several other genes, including *SRY-related HMG box-containing-9 (SOX9), MIH, NROB1, steroidogenic factor-1 (SF1), Wilms' tumor 1 (WT1), GATA-binding-4 (GATA4), desert hedgehog (DHH), patched (PTC), wingless-related mouse mammary tumor virus (MMTV) integration site 4 (WNT4),* and *WNT7a,* are required for normal male sexual differentiation.

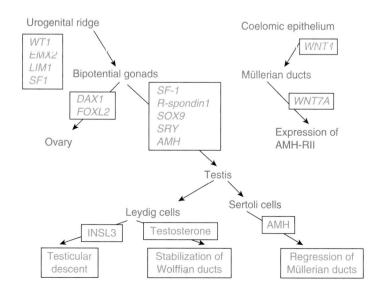

FIGURE 8-3 ■ Genes involved in genital differentiation are shown in black boxes in italics at steps shown. Hormonally directed differentiation of the testes is shown. Note AMH is also called MIH or MIS. AMH-RII = Anti-Müllerian hormone receptor type II.

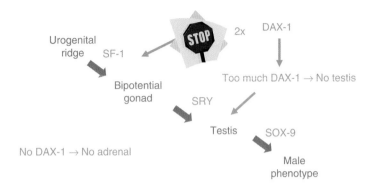

Effects of DAX-1 are highly dosage-sensitive
DAX-1 is located at Xp21

FIGURE 8-4 ■ Depicts the normal developmental sequence along with the impact of duplication or deletion of DAX-1 on testicular and adrenal development.[7] (*From Meeks JJ, Weiss J, Jameson JL. DAX1 is required for testis determination. Nat Genet. 2003;34:32-33.*)

Cells, mostly endothelial in origin, migrate from the mesonephros and interact with the pre-Sertoli cells to promote development of the testicular cords.

Although it has generally been considered that ovarian differentiation is constitutive, recent evidence suggests that specific genes are required for normal ovarian development. Primordial germ cells migrate from their origin in the hindgut and colonize in the genital ridges under the influence of fragilis proteins 1 and 3 (IFITM1 and IFITM3), stromal cell-derived factor 1 (SDF1 or CXCL12), and its receptor CXCR4.

Disorders Associated with Ambiguous Genitalia

Steroidogenesis-metabolic pathways

Mutations of steroidogenic enzyme genes are a frequent cause of genital ambiguity caused by alterations in sex steroid biosynthesis. Such enzymes are expressed in the placenta, gonads, and adrenal cortex. In the 46,XY fetus, specific proteins necessary for testosterone and DHT biosynthesis include steroidogenic factor-1 (SF-1), steroidogenic acute regulatory peptide (StAR), 17α-hydroxylase/17,20-lyase (CYP17), 3β-hydroxysteroid dehydrogenase type 2 (HSD3B2), 17α-hydroxysteroid dehydrogenase type 3 (HSD17B3), P450-oxidoreductase, and 5α-reductase type 2 (SRD5A2) (Figure 8-5). In the 46,XY fetus, defective testosterone biosynthesis can lead to ambiguous genitalia.

The steroidogenic pathways of the adrenal cortex, ovary, and testis are depicted in Figure 8-5. Differences in enzyme expression are indicated by the specific boxes showing androstenedione as the endpoint of sex steroid synthesis in the adrenal (zona reticularis), testosterone in the testis, and estradiol in the ovary. Other steroid endpoints in the adrenal cortex are aldosterone (zona glomerulosa) and cortisol (zona fasciculata).

Virilizing disorders (defects in steroidogenesis) impacting 46,XX fetuses

21-hydroxylase deficiency. 21-hydroxylase deficiency caused by mutations in the *21-hydroxylase (CYP21A2)* gene is the most common cause of CAH. This autosomal recessive disorder is responsible for more than 95% of the cases of 46,XX genital ambiguity. Deficient 21-hydroxylase activity results in decreased cortisol biosynthesis, secondary to insufficient conversion of 17-hydroxyprogesterone to 11-deoxycortisol in the zona fasciculata, and decreased aldosterone biosynthesis from impaired conversion of progesterone to deoxycorticosterone in the zona glomerulosa. The loss of negative feedback inhibition from cortisol leads to increased ACTH secretion with subsequent increased adrenal androgen secretion (Figure 8-6).

46,XX patients with severe 21-hydroxylase deficiency manifest genital ambiguity at birth. Virilization of the external genitalia exists along a spectrum ranging from mild clitoromegaly and mild posterior labial fusion to, although rare, a genital appearance consistent with a normal male with bilateral cryptorchidism. Clitoromegaly results from any source of excessive fetal androgen and, hence, the various causes are listed in Box 8-1. Despite the excessive prenatal androgen exposure, affected females have normal internal reproductive anatomy with a uterus, normally positioned ovaries, fallopian tubes, and upper vagina (Müllerian derivatives). Because of glucocorticoid and mineralocorticoid deficiencies, untreated infants develop hyponatremia, hyperkalemia, and dehydration around 7 to 10 days of life. The serum 17-hydroxyprogesterone (17-OHP) concentrations are usually more than 5000 ng/dL and are often considerably higher. Serum androstenedione and progesterone concentrations are also elevated, but to a lesser degree than are those of 17-OHP. Measurement of plasma renin activity (PRA) is necessary to assess mineralocorticoid status. Newborn screening programs

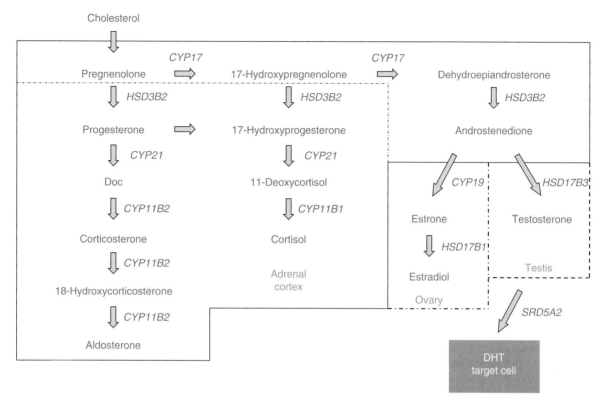

FIGURE 8-5 ■ Depicts the steroidogenic pathways of the adrenal cortex, ovary, and testis. Common pathways of both the adrenals and gonads are shown across the top of the figure. The steroids and enzymes present in the adrenal cortex are within the solid line, while enzymes and steroids not present in the adrenal cortex, but unique to the ovary and testis, are shown within the broken lines. CYP17-17α hydroxylase/17,20 lyase, HSD3B2-3β hydroxysteroid dehydrogenase type 2, CYP21-21α hydroxylase, CYP11B2-11β hydroxylase type 2, CYP11B1-11β hydroxylase type 1, CYP19-aromatase, HSD17B1-17α hydroxysteroid dehydrogenase type 1, HSD17B3-17α hydroxysteroid dehydrogenase type 3, and SRD5A2-5α reductase type 2.

measure whole blood 17-OHP concentrations obtained on filter paper with the primary goal of permitting early detection in affected male infants. Newborn screening programs generally do not detect children with nonclassical adrenal hyperplasia (NCAH), who do not present with genital ambiguity.

The degree of impairment of 21-hydroxylase activity varies depending upon the compromise of

Pathophysiology of the Virilizing forms of CAH

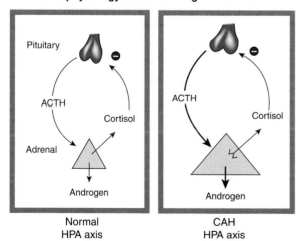

Normal HPA axis   CAH HPA axis

FIGURE 8-6 ■ Pathophysiology of classic adrenal hyperplasia (CAH). This cartoon illustrates the loss of negative feedback owing to impaired glucocorticoid biosynthesis associated with virilization of the 46,XX fetus. Insufficient cortisol concentrations lead to ACTH excess resulting in androgen overproduction.

Box 8-1.

Clitoromegaly in a 46,XX infant usually results from excess androgen exposure as occurs in patients with:

- 21-hydroxylase deficiency
- 11-hydroxylase deficiency
- 3β-hydroxysteroid dehydrogenase deficiency
- Placental aromatase deficiency
- Oxidoreductase deficiency
- Ovotesticular DSD
- Testicular DSD
- Maternal androgen exposure

Also, rarely results from inclusion of other tissues, such as neurofibromatosis.

enzyme function associated with specific mutations. In general, complete loss-of-function mutations are associated with more severe virilization of the external genitalia in affected females and clinically relevant salt-wasting. The simple-virilizing form of CAH is associated with a 1% to 2% level of residual enzyme activity whereas that of NCAH generally has a 20% to 60% level of enzyme activity. Over 100 mutations of the *21-hydroxylase gene, CYP21A2,* have been reported. A limited number of mutations accounts for the majority of the affected alleles and there appears to be reasonable genotype-phenotype correlation.

11β-hydroxylase deficiency. CAH caused by 11β-hydroxylase deficiency is associated with glucocorticoid deficiency, hypertension (excessive concentrations of salt-retaining hormones), and excessive androgen secretion. Curiously, some infants with 11β-hydroxylase deficiency may manifest salt loss and hypotension in the neonatal period. Affected female infants may present with ambiguous genitalia. In contrast to patients with 21-hydroxylase deficiency, those with 11β-hydroxylase deficiency have a hormonal profile with elevated 11-deoxycortisol and relatively less elevation in 17-hydroxyprogesterone, androstenedione, and testosterone. PRA concentrations are typically suppressed. Mutations in the *11β-hydroxylase (CYP11B1)* gene, located on chromosome 8q22, have been identified in patients with 11β-hydroxylase deficiency.

3β-hydroxysteroid dehydrogenase deficiency. CAH caused by deficiency of 3β-hydroxysteroid dehydrogenase, type 2, may result in genital ambiguity in *both* 46,XX and 46,XY fetuses. In this autosomal recessive disorder, increased DHEA synthesis leads to virilization in the 46,XX fetus and deficient testosterone production results in undervirilization in the 46,XY fetus. The condition is characterized by elevated serum concentrations of the Δ^5 steroids (pregnenolone, 17-hydroxypregnenolone, and DHEA) because of a reduced ability to convert them to their corresponding Δ^4 steroids (progesterone, 17-OHP, and androstenedione) (Figure 8-5). Impaired biosynthesis of mineralocorticoids, glucocorticoids, and sex steroids is associated with acute adrenal insufficiency which may occur in the newborn period. Mutations in the *HSD3B2 gene,* located on chromosome 1p13.1 and expressed in the adrenal cortex and gonads, have been documented in affected individuals.

Placental aromatase deficiency. The enzyme, aromatase, catalyzes the biosynthesis of estrogens from androgens. Aromatase deficiency is a rare autosomal recessive disorder in which inactivating mutations of the *aromatase (CYP19A1)* gene result in increased serum androgen levels. Since this enzyme promotes estrogen biosynthesis, there are distinct phenotypes in males and females.[8] Aromatase is active in the placenta,

where it normally protects the mother from the potential virilizing effects of the fetal androgens (predominantly DHEA and DHEAS). In placental aromatase deficiency, 46,XX fetuses are virilized and manifest variable degrees of labio-scrotal fusion, clitoromegaly, and perineoscrotal hypospadias. Often, there is a history of progressive maternal virilization during pregnancy characterized by acne, hirsutism, clitoral hypertrophy, acne, and frontal balding. During the pregnancy, maternal concentrations of testosterone, DHT, and androstenedione are elevated and decline rapidly after delivery. Affected 46,XX children have delayed pubertal development secondary to hypergonadotropic hypogonadism with poor breast development, primary amenorrhea, and cystic ovaries. Affected 46,XY infants have normal internal and external genital development, but, at the age of puberty, may have tall stature and continued growth (asymmetrical with relatively long legs) because estrogen is required to fuse the growth plates of the long bones. The estrogen deficiency found in men with aromatase deficiency is associated with abdominal obesity, insulin resistance, dyslipidemia, and relative infertility.

Oxidoreductase deficiency. Recently, another disorder affecting steroidogenesis has been described that is characterized by decreased 17α-hydroxylase and 21-hydroxylase activities. The phenotype includes genital ambiguity in males and females, craniosynostosis, mid-face hypoplasia, radio-humeral synostosis, and glucocorticoid deficiency. The skeletal manifestations are reminiscent of those seen in the Antley-Bixler syndrome, an autosomal dominant disorder caused by mutations in the *fibroblast growth factor receptor-2 (FGFR-2)* gene. Affected males may be undervirilized and females may be virilized. Signs of androgen excess, including acne, hirsutism, and clitoromegaly, may develop during pregnancy in mothers carrying affected fetuses. Typically, postnatal virilization does not occur. The 17-OHP levels are elevated, sex steroid levels are low, and mineralocorticoid concentrations are normal.

This disorder is caused by loss-of-function mutations in the *cytochrome P450 oxidoreductase (POR)* gene which is located on chromosome 7q11-12. This gene encodes a protein that functions as a cofactor for several steroidogenic enzymes.[9] It has been suggested that an alternative pathway of androgen biosynthesis, with conversion of 17-OHP to 5α-pregnane-3α,17α-dio-20 one to androstenedione, may be seen in this disorder.[10]

Defects in testosterone synthesis impacting the 46,XY fetus

17β-HSD deficiency. The *17β-hydroxysteroid dehydrogenase type 3 (HSD17B3)* gene is expressed in the Leydig cells of the testes where it catalyzes conversion of androstenedione to testosterone (Figure 8-7). Loss-of-function mutations in this gene are inherited in

17β-Hydroxysteroid Dehydrogenase Deficiency
5α-Reductase Deficiency

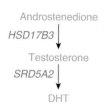

At birth, affected 46,XY infants have perineal hypospadias with a blind-ending vaginal pouch. Testes are present and may be located in labioscrotal folds or incompletely descended.

At gonadarche, affected 46,XY males virilize.

hCG stimulation tests may be required to confirm diagnosis.

FIGURE 8-7 ■ Note similar phenotypes occur in these two forms of 46,XY DSD.

an autosomal recessive manner and result in testosterone deficiency and undervirilization of 46,XY fetuses. In some instances, affected males are thought to be females at birth. The external genital phenotype in the 46,XY infant with 17β-hydroxysteroid dehydrogenase deficiency may range from a completely female (Figure 8-1) appearance with a blind-ending vaginal pouch to variable degrees of genital ambiguity with gonads palpable in the labio-scrotal folds, labio-scrotal fusion, and hypospadias.[11] Internal male reproductive structures derived from the Wolffian ducts are usually present. Underproduction of androgen in females with this mutation appears to confer no obvious phenotype.

Elevated basal or hCG-stimulated androstenedione-to-testosterone ratios are consistent with this enzyme defect. When LH and FSH secretion increase during puberty, virilization may occur because of conversion of androstenedione to testosterone by the other unaffected isoforms of 17β-hydroxysteroid dehydrogenase present in extra-testicular tissue. Affected children raised as females have been reported to change gender assignment at puberty. Thus, male gender assignment should be made in infancy for affected children. Breast development may result from increased conversion of androstenedione to estrogens.

5α-reductase deficiency. The *5α-reductase type 2 (SRD5A2)* gene is expressed in androgen target tissues such as the prostate and the primordial external genital tissue This enzyme converts testosterone to DHT (Figure 8-7), the hormone responsible for virilization of the external genitalia. The external genitalia of affected males are characterized by a small phallus, a urogenital sinus with perineal hypospadias, and a blind vaginal pouch. Internally, male (Wolffian) structures are *partially* differentiated and female (Müllerian) ducts are absent. Serum testosterone levels may be elevated, whereas DHT levels are typically low. Elevated basal or hCG-stimulated testosterone-to-DHT ratios are consistent

with the diagnosis of 5α-reductase deficiency. In patients whose testicles are left intact, significant virilization often begins during puberty with development of penile growth, male physique, and voice change. In general, male ducts are inadequately developed to deliver mature sperm. Although this autosomal recessive condition is rare, there are clusters of affected individuals in the Dominican Republic, Papua New Guinea, Turkey, and the Middle East.[12]

Congenital lipoid adrenal hyperplasia (StAR mutations). Congenital lipoid adrenal hyperplasia (Box 8-2) is an autosomal recessive disorder caused by loss-of-function mutations in the *steroidogenic acute regulatory protein (StAR)* gene. The StAR protein functions to move cholesterol from the outer to inner mitochondrial membrane[13] resulting in impaired conversion of cholesterol to pregnenolone, the first step in steroid synthesis.

Both 46,XY and 46,XX infants have essentially female external genitalia, because external virilization is impaired as a reslut of decreased testosterone production. All adrenal and gonadal steroid hormone levels are low or undetectable, including 17-hydroxypregnenolone and pregnenolone, because steroidogenesis in both the adrenal cortex and in the gonads is deficient. Thus, affected infants also have mineralocorticoid and glucocorticoid deficiencies. In addition to the defective steroidogenesis, lipids accumulate in the steroidogenic cells ultimately resulting in their destruction. Although congenital lipoid adrenal hyperplasia has been considered to be a disease affecting infants, later presentations have also been described.[14]

Steroid action

Androgen insensitivity is an X-linked recessive disorder caused by mutations in the *androgen receptor (AR)* gene which is located on the proximal long arm of the X chromosome.

Affected, 46,XY children with complete androgen insensitivity syndrome (CAIS) present in infancy with inguinal or labial gonads, inguinal herniae, but otherwise normal external female genitalia. It has been estimated that 1% to 2% of girls with bilateral inguinal herniae

---

Box 8-2. Congenital Lipoid Adrenal Hyperplasia

Consequence of a "Two-hit mechanism"

Autosomal recessive disorder owing to inactivating mutations in the *steroidogenic acute regulatory protein (StAR)* gene. The consequence is impaired transport of cholesterol into mitochondria leading to loss of ability to synthesize glucocorticoids, mineralocorticoids, and sex steroids.

Associated with accumulation of cholesterol esters and other cholesterol metabolites that alter cell cytostructure, leading to cell destruction.

have androgen insensitivity. Some affected individuals present in adolescence with primary amenorrhea. Findings in partial AIS (PAIS) include ambiguous genitalia with perineo-scrotal hypospadias, microphallus, bifid scrotum, and testes located in the scrotum or undescended. Müllerian derivatives such as the uterus are not present in androgen insensitivity because testicular MIH secretion results in regression of these structures.

Testosterone and LH levels may be elevated in infancy. However, the usual LH surge and increased testosterone concentrations expected during the first few months of life may be absent. In affected children more than 10 years of age, elevated serum LH and testosterone concentrations occur. This loss-of-function mutation results in loss of hypothalamic-pituitary feedback inhibition leading to increased LH and testicular testosterone synthesis. In contrast, FSH concentrations may be normal or only mildly elevated because inhibin secretion by Sertoli cells is intact.

Infants with PAIS may require a trial of androgen administration to promote phallic enlargement. Over 300 *AR* gene mutations have been described in AIS. Generally, but not always, CAIS results from complete loss-of-function mutations such as deletions, insertions, or deletions associated with frameshifts and premature termination codons. In contrast, PAIS is associated with partial loss-of-function mutations.[15] Although phenotype generally correlates with genotype, phenotypic heterogeneity can occur even among family members carrying the identical mutation. In addition to hormone determinations, DNA sequence analysis of the *AR* gene is commercially available (www.genetests.org and www.androgendb.mcgill.ca) and may be diagnostic.

Because of the presence of a Y chromosome, the risk for gonadal tumors, particularly carcinoma *in situ* (CIS) and seminomas, is increased. The decision must be made concerning the need for and timing of gonadectomy. For CAIS, but not PAIS, it can be argued that leaving the testes in place until pubertal feminization is complete is preferable. For those raised male, it can be argued that the testicles could be left intact as long as they are partially descended in the hopes of providing some fertility, function, and cosmesis. Gonads should be carefully monitored for development of malignancy. One series reported that only 2 of the 44 (<5%) patients with CAIS who underwent gonadal biopsy had testicles with CIS.[16]

Luteinizing hormone defects

Leydig cell hypoplasia. This autosomal recessive disorder arises from a loss-of-function mutation in the *LH receptor (LHCGR)* gene. In the absence of effective LH stimulation because of LHCGR loss-of-function mutations, fetal Leydig cells fail to develop leading to deficient testosterone production. The phenotype ranges from complete male-to-female sex reversal or 46,XY undervirilization. Those with the female phenotype frequently have palpable labial gonads. Müllerian duct-derived structures are absent because MIH is normally secreted. Thus, the findings on physical examination are reminiscent of CAIS. Testes contain immature Sertoli cells, lack mature Leydig cells, but have rare spermatogonia.

Serum hormone levels include elevated LH, low testosterone, and normal FSH concentrations. There is no significant testosterone response to hCG stimulation. The *LHCGR* gene encodes for a seven-transmembrane domain G protein-coupled receptor, which is expressed in fetal and adult Leydig cells. Family studies have indicated that sisters who carry *LHCGR* gene mutations on both alleles have normal female genital differentiation and normal pubertal development, but may have primary amenorrhea and infertility.

Hypogonadotropic hypogonadism. Male infants with hypogonadotropic hypogonadism (see Chapter 7) generally present with microphallus and/or cryptorchidism, but not genital ambiguity. Genetic etiologies of hypogonadotropic hypogonadism include inactivating mutations in the *KAL1, FGFR1, GPR54, PROKR2, PROK2, GNRHR,* and *LHβ* genes.[17] X-linked Kallmann syndrome is often associated with anosmia and olfactory bulb hypoplasia on MRI. Although affected individuals may show pubertal development and improvements in fertility in response to pulsatile/intermittent therapy with LH, hCG, or GnRH, most patients are treated with sex steroid replacement.

Gonadal differentiation

The karyotype of the primordial gonad directs development into a testis or an ovary. Subsequently, other factors such as transcription factors and hormones influence differentiation of the internal and external genital structures. Although ovarian differentiation has long been considered to be the "default" pathway, specific genetic factors contributing to ovarian differentiation, as previously noted, have been described.[18]

Following migration from the hindgut to the developing gonadal ridges, local factors predominantly influence germ cell differentiation. Germ cell differentiation into male or female germ cells is also governed by cell cycle decisions between mitosis and meiosis.[19] Germ cell meiosis begins at approximately 10 to 11 weeks gestation in the developing ovary. Following the first meiotic division, the primary oöcyte becomes associated with granulosa cells to constitute the primary follicle. In the developing testis, the developing germ cells undergo mitotic arrest.

Disorders of gonadal differentiation, both general categories and specific forms, resulting in gonadal dysgenesis are listed in Table 8-5.

Table 8-5.

Disorders of Gonadal Differentiation (Selected Specific Forms Discussed in Text)

Disorders of Gonadal Differentiation

General categories
  Gonadal dysgenesis
    SRY mutations (pure gonadal dysgenesis)
  Vanishing testes
  Ovotesticular DSD
  Mixed gonadal dysgenesis (45X, 46XY)
Specific forms
Wnt4 mutations
Smith-Lemli-Optiz
I MAGe syndrome
Denys-Drash syndrome (WT1)
Frasier syndrome (WT1)
SF1 mutations
DAX1 mutations
SOX9 mutations
FOXL2 mutations
R-spondin[1]

Wnt4. The secreted protein encoded by this gene, located on chromosome 1p31-1p35, binds to members of the frizzled receptor family. Duplication of Wnt4 in 46,XY patients results in ambiguous genitalia with hypospadias with remnants of both Wolffian and Müllerian ducts. Histological examination of the gonad shows differentiation of interstitial cell lineage, but suppression of Leydig cell development. Women carrying loss-of-function mutations may present in adolescence with primary amenorrhea secondary to Müllerian duct abnormalities and hyperandrogenism.[20]

Smith-Lemli-Opitz. This autosomal recessive disorder is characterized by multiple malformations that include urogenital anomalies, mental retardation, failure-to-thrive, facial abnormalities including cleft palate, developmental delay, and behavioral abnormalities. The urogenital abnormalities include hypospadias, cryptorchidism, and male-to-female sex reversal. These anomalies are a consequence of mutations in the *7-dehydro-cholesterol reductase (DHCR7)* gene resulting in low cholesterol and high serum concentrations of 7-dehydrocholesterol and other sterol intermediates that accumulate as a result of defective enzyme activity. Decreased cholesterol concentrations, the precursor for steroid synthesis, result in reduced steroid synthesis (glucocorticoid, mineralocorticoid, sex steroids).[21]

IMAGe syndrome. In 46,XY infants, the IMAGe syndrome is characterized by urogenital anomalies (including micropenis and cryptorchidism), adrenal hypoplasia, intrauterine growth retardation, and other congenital anomalies including metaphyseal dysplasia.

46,XY sex reversal

WT1 gene. Denys-Drash and Frasier syndromes are both associated with mutations in the *WT1* gene. Denys-Drash syndrome is characterized by 46,XY sex reversal, Wilms tumor, and renal failure caused by focal or diffuse mesangial sclerosis. Genetic females with Denys-Drash syndrome generally have normal female external genitalia. Frasier syndrome is characterized by 46,XY sex reversal, gonadal dysgenesis, gonadoblastoma, and renal failure caused by glomerular sclerosis. The majority of cases of Frasier syndrome are caused by a specific mutation in intron 9 of the *WT1* gene.

Steroidogenic factor 1. SF1 plays a role in gonadal differentiation, development of the ventro-medial hypothalamus, steroidogenesis, and expression of *MIH* gene. The phenotype of 46,XY patients with loss-of-function *SF1/NR5A1* gene mutations is female internal and external genitalia, and streak gonads. The condition may be lethal in the neonatal period owing to profound adrenal insufficiency. There is also impaired gonadotrophic expression of LH, FSH, and GnRH receptors, and absence of the ventro-medial hypothalamic nucleus. Normal ovarian morphology has been reported in 46,XX individuals with adrenal hypoplasia. Undervirilization of 46,XY fetuses without overt adrenal insufficiency has been reported in newborns with haploinsufficiency of *SF1.*[22] Heterozygous *SF1/NR5A1* mutations were identified in 5/27 (18.5%) of 46,XY DSD patients; none of these patients had adrenal insufficiency.[23]

DAX1 mutations or duplication. The *DAX1 (NROB1)* gene is located on the short arm of the X chromosome and encodes for an orphan nuclear receptor. Loss-of-function mutations in 46,XY individuals are associated with the syndrome of AHC and hypogonadotropic hypogonadism (Figure 8-4). AHC can occur as a component of a contiguous gene deletion disorder In association with glycerol kinase deficiency, Duchenne muscular dystrophy, ornithine transcarbamylase deficiency, and mental retardation.

In 46,XY fetuses, duplication results in XY sex reversal. The presumed mechanism is that the increased dosage of DAX-1 expression represses SRY expression.

SOX9. SOX9 is a HMG-box protein expressed in high levels in the fetal testis. In addition to 46,XY male-to-female sex reversal, haploinsufficiency of SOX9 caused by heterozygous mutations is associated with campomelic dwarfism. Features of campomelic dwarfism include congenital bowing of the long bones, hypoplastic scapulae,

11 pairs of ribs, clubfeet, micrognathia, and cleft palate. Respiratory insufficiency often results in neonatal death.

46,XX gonadal dysgenesis

FOXL2 mutation. Mutations in *FOXL2*, a gene located on chromosome 3q23, are associated with the Blepharophimosis-Ptosis-Epicanthus Inversus syndrome (BPES) (see Chapter 7). Premature ovarian failure is the most common phenotype for this autosomal dominant condition. Data obtained from the investigation of transgenic mouse models suggest that the ovarian failure associated with BPES is caused by aberrant granulosa cell function during follicle formation.[24] Mutations in this gene have also been found in association with XX female-to-male sex reversal.

46,XX sex reversal (46,XX males)

Mutations in the *R-spondin1 (RSPO1)* gene. In this autosomal recessive disorder, the phenotype includes absence of Müllerian duct derivatives, masculinization of internal and external genitalia, and palmoplantar keratoderma. The dermatological features include a predisposition for squamous cell carcinoma.[25]

Ovotesticular DSD. Ovotesticular DSD (formerly known as true hermaphroditism) is defined as presence of ovarian tissue with follicles and testicular tissue with seminiferous tubules in the same individual. The most commonly identified gonad is an ovotestis, but there can be an ovary on one side and a testis on the other. In most ovotestes, ovarian and testicular tissue show distinct separation in an end-to-end arrangement. The majority of affected individuals have a 46,XX karyotype.

45,X/46,XY gonadal dysgenesis (formerly known as mixed gonadal dysgenesis). Individuals with sex chromosome DSDs caused by "mixed gonadal dysgenesis" generally present with asymmetrical genital ambiguity. Short stature, webbed neck, cubitus valgus, gonadal failure, and other features of Turner syndrome may be present. Although the most common karyotype is 45,X/46,XY, mosaic karyotypes with multiple cell lines, including a monosomic X cell line, may be detected. There is much phenotypic heterogeneity in that internal and external genital differentiation can range from ambiguous to normal male or female.[26]

Environmental causes. Although it has been hypothesized that synthetic and natural compounds in the environment can be "endocrine disruptors," such molecules have not been clearly shown to cause DSDs. Genital ambiguity in three 46,XY infants born in heavily agricultural areas has been reported and attributed to fetal exposure to endocrine disruptors, since no other cause or known mutations were found.[27] Exposure to endocrine disrup-

tors in the environment has also been implicated as a cause of the reported increased frequency of both cryptorchidism and poor semen quality.[28] Hence, while causality has yet to be verified, it should be recognized that some compounds have estrogenic or anti-androgenic properties, such as organochlorine pesticides, polychlorinated biphenyls (PCBs), and alkylpolyethoxylates. A possible mechanism by which hydroxylated PCB metabolites cause ambiguity is that they may bind to estrogen sulfotransferase with greater affinity than does estradiol. It has been known for some time that prenatal exposure to the non-steroidal synthetic estrogen, diethylstilbesterol, is associated with urogenital abnormalities in both sexes, including cryptorchidism in the male fetus. Further, some pesticides may inhibit placental aromatase activity.

Müllerian duct abnormalities. MIH, a member of the TGF-β family, signals through two different interacting membrane-bound serine/threonine receptors. Abnormalities are associated with either a mutation in the *MIH* or in the *MIH (AMH) receptor (AMH-RII)* gene[29] and a common phenotype with autosomal recessive inheritance. Patients with mutations in the *MIH* gene have low serum concentrations of AMH, whereas levels are elevated or normal among those with *AMH-RII* gene mutations.

Features of the persistent Müllerian duct syndrome (PMDS) usually include cryptorchidism, testicular ectopia associated with inguinal hernia, and *hernia uteri inguinalis*. Although testicular differentiation occurs normally, the male excretory ducts may be incompletely developed and are embedded within remnants of the Müllerian ducts. Since the poorly developed *vasa deferentia* are trapped within the uterine wall and the excretory ducts are not adequately connected to the testes, natural fertilization may be precluded. When diagnosed in childhood, it is frequently discovered during either an inguinal herniorrhaphy or orchiopexy when a uterine cervix is identified within the hernia sac. Testicular torsion may also occur when the testes are not fully attached to the *processus vaginalis*. Females who carry mutations on both *AMH* alleles have normal fertility.

Müllerian duct abnormalities may also occur in 46,XX patients, usually associated with other abnormalities. The Mayer-Rokitansky-Küster-Hauser syndrome involves congenital absence of the vagina and uterine hypoplasia or aplasia. It often is not diagnosed until the age of puberty when a nonpatent vagina or primary amenorrhea is evaluated. Associated renal anomalies, including unilateral agenesis, and skeletal malformations are also identified in affected individuals. Hence, evaluation for skeletal malformations and renal sonography is part of the evaluation of women with abnormal development of the Müllerian duct system.[30] The association of Müllerian duct aplasia with renal aplasia and cervico-thoracic somite dysplasia is called the MURCS syndrome and the association of Müllerian duct hypoplasia with facio-auriculo-vertebral anomalies constitutes the Goldenhar syndrome. While not specifically a Müllerian duct abnormality, transverse vaginal septae may occur, sometimes in association with the McKusick-Kaufman syndrome.

Testicular descent. Testicular descent occurs in two phases: intra-abdominal and inguino-scrotal. The cranial suspensory ligament and the gubernaculum develop on either side of the developing gonad. The former becomes the suspensory ligament of the ovary while, in the male, it regresses in response to testosterone secretion. The latter connects the testis and the internal inguinal ring by 14 weeks of fetal life.[31] The intra-abdominal phase of descent appears to be a result of the testis staying near the pelvis as the abdomen elongates so that, in a relative manner, it becomes located much more distally in the abdomen. Factors important during this first phase of testicular descent include INSL3 and its receptor, LGR8. The second phase of descent through the inguinal canal, also related to the gubernaculum, occurs at the beginning of the third trimester of pregnancy with descent into the scrotum completed in most by the middle of the third trimester. Androgens play a role in influencing the second or inguino-scrotal phase of testicular descent. Usually, testicular descent is completed by the 35th week of gestation. Increased androgen levels in the 46,XX fetus which occur with virilizing CAH are not associated with ovarian descent.

Cryptorchidism (undescended testes) is associated with many syndromes and other endocrine disorders. Approximately 3% of male infants have cryptorchidism at birth. The prevalence decreases by 6 months of age because of spontaneous late testicular descent. Incomplete testicular descent occurs in some instances of DSD, as in CAIS in which the intra-abdominal phase is usually completed, but not the inguino-scrotal phase which is presumably related to lack of androgen action and underdevelopment of a scrotal sac. Mutations in the INSL3 and LGR8 genes have been identified among boys with cryptorchidism.[32]

CLINICAL PRESENTATION AND DIFFERENTIAL DIAGNOSIS

An algorithm, based on gonadal symmetry, for the differential diagnosis of DSDs is shown in Figure 8-8.

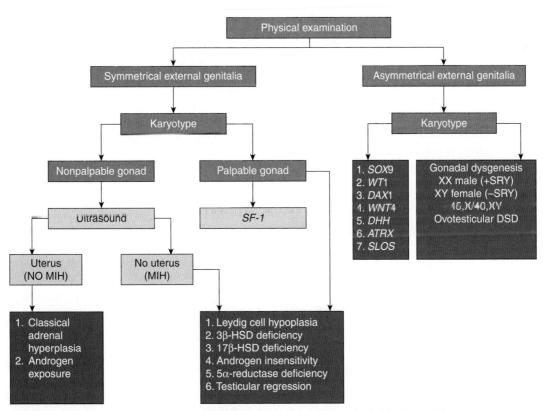

FIGURE 8-8 ■ Algorithm for differential diagnosis of specific DSDs based upon physical findings and karyotype.

Initial Evaluation

The initial evaluation involves verifying that there is not a medical emergency, such as adrenal insufficiency, renal failure, or other systemic life-threatening illness. Adrenal insufficiency, associated with CAH secondary to 21-hydroxylase deficiency, is the most common emergency. Hence, when a neonate presents with symmetrically ambiguous genitalia without palpable gonads, the initial testing should include measurement of serum levels of 17-OHP, androstenedione, and cortisol, and, until these results are available, monitoring serum sodium and potassium levels should be done after 48 to 72 hours of life.

The infant with genital ambiguity who has one or two palpable gonads is unlikely to have adrenal insufficiency. The 46,XY infant with 21-hydroxylase deficiency has normal genital anatomy, except for hyperpigmentation of the genitals and nipples, but may present with adrenal insufficiency after several days of age. Newborn screening for this form of CAH should minimize this occurrence through earlier disease detection and appropriate treatment. Prenatal diagnosis of fetuses at risk for CAH is now possible. Suppression of fetal ACTH and adrenal androgens via high-dose dexamethasone treatment of pregnant mothers can reduce the extent of genital ambiguity in female fetuses with 21-hydroxylase deficiency. However, therapy must be begun before the diagnosis of 21-hydroxylase deficiency can be confirmed or refuted. Although long-term safety data of this prenatal therapy are not available, this form of therapy is felt to be safe and worthwhile.[33]

The initial assessment (Box 8-3) can be approached from the perspective that identification of the etiology of the child's genital ambiguity will be helpful. This assessment should include immediate consultation with specialists in the fields of pediatric endocrinology, urology, psychology, and social services. When available, a team of health care providers representing these subspecialties and experienced with DSD management issues should delegate a leader to supervise the evaluation. Pertinent findings should be carefully recorded.

The steps of the initial evaluation (performed as soon as possible) involve a medical history with emphasis on familial disorders, a physical examination including a careful description of the genitalia, a karyotype or more rapid assessment for sex chromosome complement, hormone determinations, and a pelvic ultrasound.

Based upon the findings from history and physical examination, appropriate serum hormone levels should be obtained which include adrenal and gonadal steroid hormones, gonadotropins, and other peptide hormones.

History

Pertinent facts from history should include items listed in Box 8-4.

A detailed family history should include asking about siblings with ambiguous genitalia, deaths during infancy, and the presence of infertile aunts or partially virilized uncles in the maternal family.

Physical examination

A basic guide to items to be included in the genital examination is outlined in Box 8-5.

A thorough physical examination should be performed. Particular attention should be paid to the genitalia, including symmetry, with measurements as outlined in Box 8-6. Examples of asymmetrical and symmetrical genital are shown in Figures 8-9 and 8-10, respectively. The extent of skin pigmentation of the genitalia and nipples should be noted as dark pigmentation suggests excessive ACTH stimulation. If transabdominal ultrasound is readily available, it should be done to provide a reliable assessment of the presence of a uterus.

The extent of fusion (virilization) of the labio-scrotal and labio-urethral folds should be carefully described, in comparison with the standards of Prader (Figure 8-1). It should be documented whether a single or double opening can be visualized and whether the single opening is a consequence of the presence of a urogenital

---

Box 8-3. Initial testing
For infants with symmetrical genital ambiguity (most likely having the diagnosis of CAH secondary to 21-hydroxylase deficiency), initial testing should include a karyotype and measurement of serum 17-hydroxyprogesterone (17-OHP), androstenedione, testosterone, and cortisol levels. Other hormones, including renin, and electrolytes, as discussed in the text, can be assayed if blood samples are readily available.
For infants with asymmetrical genital ambiguity and one or two palpable gonads, testing should include karyotype, and measurement of LH, FSH, and testosterone concentrations.

Box 8-4. Important Information from Medical History
■ Family history of females who are childless or have amenorrhea
■ Current and any previous pregnancies
■ Maternal virilization
■ Exposure to androgens
■ Exposure of either parent to endocrine disruptors such as phenytoin or aminoglutethimide
■ Any unexplained infant deaths (especially neonatal)
■ History of consanguinity

Box 8-5. Genital Examination and Description

■ Symmetry or asymmetry of the external genitalia
■ Palpability and location of apparent gonads on both sides
■ Verified measurement of phallic (corporal) length and diameter
■ Visualization of one or two openings
■ Location of urethral meatus with notation of whether voiding has been witnessed
■ Extent of fusion and rugation of the labia/scrotum
■ Genital pigmentation

It should be noted whether the anatomy is consistent with lack of virilization or excessive virilization of the expected process of differentiation or suggestive of pathology other than abnormal hormonal stimulation, as found in cloacal extrophy, penoscrotal transposition, or other anomalies such as neurofibromatosis.

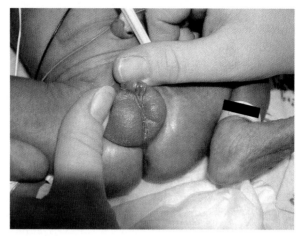

FIGURE 8-9 ■ Shows symmetrical virilization.

Box 8-6. Findings in Infant with Ambiguous Genitalia and Significance

■ Symmetrical genitalia with
  ■ Phallic development greater than clitoris in volume, but without full configuration of a penis
  ■ Varying extent of posterior fusion of the primordial labio-scrotal folds from posterior to anterior, with varying amount of rugation of the skin
  ■ Extension of the primordial labio-urethral folds from the hood of the phallus extending toward the orifice(s); when overlaid by excessive fusion of labial-scrotal folds
  ■ Orifice, if single, extends posteriorly beneath the uro-genital sinus created by the fusion of labio-scrotal folds
  ■ No palpable gonads within the labio-scrotal folds
    ■ Suggestive of virilization of female genitalia
      ■ 46,XX DSD
        ■ Most common-21 hydroxylase deficiency CAH (Figure 8-10)
■ Asymmetrical genitalia with
  ■ Midline phallus with chordee or anchored ventrally
  ■ Single opening on perineum or at base of phallus
  ■ Hemi-scrotal structure on one side with palpable gonad-like structure unilaterally (Figure 8-11)
  ■ Labial-like structure on contralateral side containing no palpable structure
    ■ Suggestive of partial or unilateral testicular differentiation
      ■ 46,XY DSD or sex chromosome DSD
■ Symmetrical female genital differentiation with palpable gonadal structures within labia
  ■ Suggestive of complete androgen insensitivity syndrome or LH receptor-inactivating mutation
■ Symmetrical male genital differentiation
  ■ With coronal or mid-shaft hypospadias
    ■ Unlikely to have identifiable cause
  ■ Bilaterally undescended testes
    ■ Unlikely to be a DSD
      ■ Rarely may be fully virilized 46,XX DSD

sinus or whether it appears as a urethral meatus. Partial fusion of the labio-urethral folds results in the urethral opening being at various points along the underside of the phallus, with lack of fusion resulting in the opening on the perineum. With the presence of a urogenital sinus resulting from partial fusion of the labio-scrotal folds, two separate openings, urethral and vaginal, may be present, but not visible by inspection. With virilization of the female fetus, as occurs with CAH, the vagina may open into this sinus or into the urethra. The internal anatomy

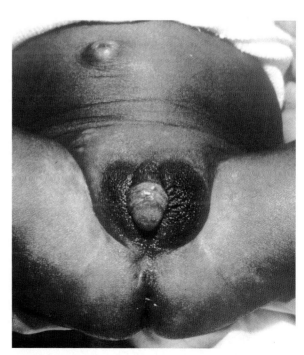

FIGURE 8-10 ■ Shows asymmetrical virilization, with less development of the labio-scrotal fold on the right and a palpable gonad on the left.

cannot be confirmed by physical examination. Hence, the urinary and reproductive system tract anatomy must be visualized using available radiographic, ultrasonographic, and cystoscopic modalities.

Phallic size should be carefully measured. The extended length, in the nonerect state, should be measured along with the dorsal surface from the tip of the glans, excluding the prepuce, to as close to the underlying pubic bone as possible and compared with published standards, with recognition that there are some minor racial differences. In general, a stretched length of less than 2 cm is considered abnormal for a term infant. The criteria for premature children are listed in Table 8-6.

It is important to realize that the clitoris is prominent in the premature or very lean infant girl because of the lack of surrounding subcutaneous tissue. Both length and width can be reliably estimated. The length is measured from the palpable base to the tip of the glans; normal length ranges from as low as 9 mm, that is, less than 1 cm.[34] The width is measured by spreading surrounding tissues; usual dimensions are generally less than 6 mm. Box 8-6 lists some of the causes of clitoromegaly.

The ano-genital ratio,[35] an estimate of degree of masculinization, is the distance between the anus and posterior fourchette divided by the distance between the anus and the base of the clitoris. This ratio is greater with male than with female differentiation and, because it is a ratio, it can be used in the premature or term infant regardless of body size. A ratio of greater than 0.5 suggests posterior labial fusion and virilization.

To ascertain the presence, size, and location of gonads, the inguinal area and the partially or fully developed scrotum and labia majora should be carefully palpated. Mobility, size, consistency, and location of the gonads should be carefully noted. If gonads are present within the labio-scrotal structures, they are probably testes. When there is asymmetry of labio-scrotal development, the more virilized half (hemi-scrotum) is more likely to contain a palpable gonad, either a testis or, rarely, an ovotestis. The contralateral gonad is usually nonpalpable and likely to be a dysgenetic testis, an ovary, or an ovotestis. When there is symmetry of the labio-scrotal structure, at any Prader stage, and no palpable gonads, the most frequent diagnosis is virilizing CAH in a 46,XX virilized female. The fully virilized patient with an empty scrotum, however, is more commonly a 46,XY male with bilateral cryptorchidism or anorchia (vanishing testis/testicular regression syndrome).

Differential diagnosis. Disorders have been discussed earlier in this chapter that constitute the various DSD conditions that present with genital ambiguity. They are listed in Box 8-7.

Genital ambiguity most often results from excess androgen production in genetic females than from inadequate androgen production in genetic males. Excess production most commonly is a consequence of deficient enzyme activity in the adrenal glands. Diminished androgen production can be a result of inhibited production along the sex steroid biosynthetic pathway or from decreased action. Figure 8-11 provides a reference to visualize the pattern of steroid levels in relation to compromised conversion resulting in impaired steroidogenesis. In general, steroids proximal to the enzyme block (depicted with arrows) are produced in excessive amounts while those distal to the enzyme block are produced in diminished concentrations. Hence, profiles of steroid intermediates commonly suggest the sites of compromised synthesis. Steroid profile panels are available from the major contract laboratories

Table 8-6.				

Normal Penis and Clitoris Size at Birth

Sex	Population	Age	Stretched Penile Length, Mean ± SD, cm (Males), or Clitoral Length, Mean ± SD, mm (Females)	Penile Width, Mean ± SD, cm (Males), or Clitoral Width, Mean ± SD, mm (Females)
M	United States	30-wk GA	2.5 ± 0.4	
M	United States	Term	3.5 ± 0.4	1.1 ± 0.1
M	Japan	Term	2.9 ± 0.4	
M	Australia	24-36- wk GA	2.3 ± 0.16	
M	China	Term	3.1 ± 0.3	1.07 ± 0.09
M	India	Term	3.6 ± 0.4	1.14 ± 0.07
F	United States	Term	4.0 ± 1.24	3.32 ± 0.78
F	Korea	Term	4.9 ± 1.89	2.55 ± 1.48
F	Jewish	Term	5.87 ± 1.48	
F	Bedouin	Term	6.61 ± 1.72	

Box 8-7.

Differential Diagnosis of Genital Ambiguity (More frequent)

A. Virilizing disorders (defects in steroidogenesis) impacting 46,XX fetuses
   a. *21-hydroxylase deficiency*
   b. 11β-hydroxylase deficiency
   c. 3β-hydroxysteroid dehydrogenase deficiency
   d. Placental aromatase deficiency
   e. Oxidoreductase deficiency (POR)

B. Defects in testosterone synthesis or action impacting 46,XY fetuses
   a. Defect in testicular testosterone biosynthesis
      i. 17β-HSD deficiency
      ii. 5α-reductase deficiency
      iii. Congenital lipoid adrenal hyperplasia (StAR)
   b. Leydig cell hypoplasia (LH receptor mutation)
   c. LH deficiency
   d. Androgen insensitivity

C. Disorders of gonadal differentiation
   a. Gonadal dysgenesis
      i. Wnt4 duplication in 46,XY
      ii. Smith-Lemli-Opitz syndrome
      iii. IMAGe syndrome
      iv. 46,XY sex reversal
         ■ Denys-Drash syndrome
         ■ Frasier syndrome
         ■ *Steroidogenic factor 1 (SF1)* mutations
         ■ *NROB1* mutations
         ■ *SOX9* mutations
      vi. 46,XX gonadal dysgenesis
         ■ FOXL2
      vii. 46,XX sex reversal (46,XX males)
         ■ *r-spondin1 (RSPO1)* mutations
      viii. *Ovotesticular DSD (true hermaphroditism)*
      ix. *45,X/46,XY (mixed) gonadal dysgenesis*

which can help pinpoint the location of the specific enzyme defect.

Diagnostic tests

Even when the patient is expected to be referred imminently, it is helpful to obtain a blood sample for a "stat" karyotype for sex determination and hormone levels as outlined later. Generally, if the virilized genitalia are symmetrical and no gonads are palpable, samples for 17-OHP, androstenedione, and testosterone should be obtained and emergently assayed in a specialized reference laboratory.

If the virilized genitalia are not symmetrical and either one or two gonads are palpable, LH, FSH, and testosterone levels should be obtained.

A karyotype and/or a Y chromosome fluorescent *in situ* hybridization (FISH) should be ordered as soon as possible, the initial sample using peripheral blood leukocytes, while realizing that, in some instances, further testing may be necessary, mosaic patterns may be present, and karyotyping of gonadal tissue may not match that of circulating leukocytes.

An abdominal/pelvic ultrasound can be used to determine the presence or absence of a uterus, and sometimes determine the presence, size, and location of the gonads and adrenal glands. A genitourethrogram is useful in determining the interconnection of the genital and urinary tract cavities and ducts, but can be delayed until later. Cystoscopy provides even more information, but is invasive. One or both is required when surgery is being planned.

The choice of initial hormone tests depends upon the physical findings present:

1. Symmetrical partially virilized external genitalia with no palpable gonads, particularly if a normal uterus is present. Additional studies should be directed towards causes of virilization of a female infant. This is because CAH secondary to 21-hydroxylase deficiency is the most likely diagnosis (Figure 8-12). Serum 17-OHP, androstenedione, testosterone, 11-deoxycortisol, and cortisol levels should be obtained. Even though adrenal insufficiency with hyponatremia and hyperkalemia may be associated with this diagnosis and may be life-threatening, this does not usually develop until approximately 7 to 10 days of life. Hence, testing of sodium, potassium, and renin levels, normally higher in the newborn than in older children, may be delayed and is only useful at this point to determine baseline values.

2. When one or both gonads are palpable, screening tests should be focused on gonadotropin and sex steroid hormone concentrations to assess androgen synthesis and action. Serum LH, FSH, testosterone, and DHT concentrations can be obtained to assess the hypothalamic-pituitary-gonadal axis and testicular function. These values may change remarkably just after parturition since hCG possesses LH-like stimulating properties.

The relative levels of steroid hormone and gonadotrophin concentrations provide the basis to assess a functional hypothalamic-pituitary-gonadal axis and specific defects in steroidogenesis (Figure 8-11). While 17-OHP concentrations more than 5000 ng/dL are highly suggestive of CAH caused by 21-hydroxylase deficiency, markedly elevated values more than 10,000 ng/dL (~300 nmol/L) are felt to be diagnostic. 17-OHP concentrations are also elevated, but generally not to the same degree, in the much less common form of CAH, 11β-hydroxylase deficiency. In contrast to CAH caused by 21-hydroxylase deficiency, 11β-hydroxylase deficiency

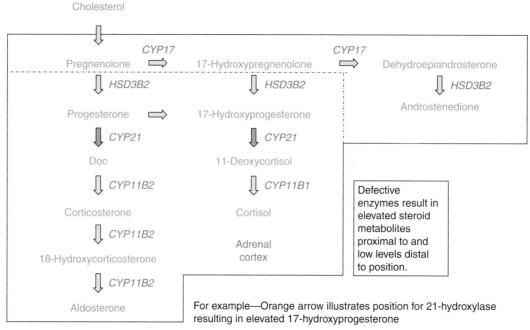

FIGURE 8-11 ■ Metabolic pathways of adrenal mineralocorticoid, glucocorticoid, and androgen steroidogenesis. The respective endpoints are aldosterone, cortisol, and androstenedione, respectively. CYP17-17α hydroxylase/17,20 lyase, HSD3B2-3, hydroxysteroid dehydrogenase type 2, CYP21-21α hydroxylase, CYP11B2-11β hydroxylase type 2, and CYP11B1-11β hydroxylase type 1.

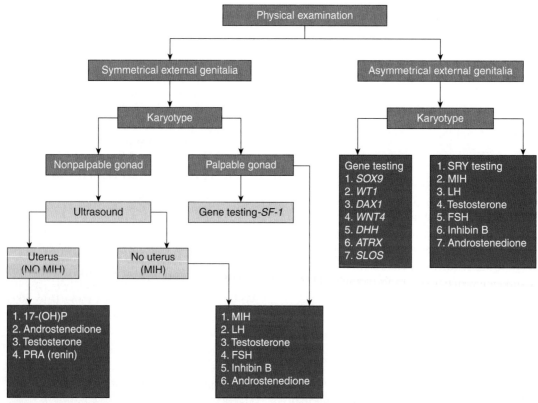

FIGURE 8-12 ■ Suggested hormonal and genetic testing based upon physical findings and karyotype.

is diagnosed by showing elevated 11-deoxycortisol concentrations. Although hypertension is a classical finding in this form of CAH, it may not be present in the neonatal period. Children with another rare type of CAH, caused by 3β-hydroxysteroid dehydrogenase deficiency, typically have elevated pregnenolone, 17-hydroxypregnenolone, and DHEA concentrations.

Referral of all infants born with genital ambiguity to a center that can offer a team approach to DSDs is mandatory and should be made during the first day of life, before sex-of-rearing is discussed in detail. It is appropriate to inform the parents that there has been a developmental problem involving the reproductive organs and that their child needs to be evaluated by a team of experts to determine the cause as well as to determine potential sexual and reproductive function before they make any decision about further evaluation, treatment, and sex assignment.

Referral should not be delayed pending the results of initial testing. Obtaining a blood sample for karyotype and hormone levels, with careful notation of age when samples are obtained, generally can be done without delay and will accelerate key decision-making by the referral team. Ultrasonography and invasive radiological examinations should be done only by an individual experienced in studying infants.

Treatment

Interactions with parents. The parents play obligatory and vital roles in medical decisions after they have been fully informed. Parents must be made aware of all available information even though there are often inadequate outcome data to provide absolute guidelines for gender assignment and for timing and complexity of surgery. Suggestions for how to discuss the situation with parents are outlined in Box 8-8. Parents must be provided available data concerning surgical outcome, even though such data may be based upon older surgical techniques that have become much more refined over time. For example, the neurovascular complex supplying the clitoris[36] is carefully spared during modern feminizing surgery. Even though the outcomes of current procedures can be expected to be more favorable cosmetically and functionally, actual data will not be available for decades. Regardless, sharing the current knowledge of psychological and biological factors related to gender and sexual development provides parents with information on which to base their decisions. The ultimate responsibility of the child's care falls to the parents. With input from the care team and understanding of factors involved concerning the evaluation of their child, they should be equipped to make the best possible decisions. Providing them with an overall understanding of the complex interplay between biological, social, and psychological/psychosexual factors,

based upon clear scientific data, provides them with a basis by which to form their own decisions, including the decision of whether to and when to have surgery.

Information impacting the approach to management of the infant with genital ambiguity. For a small portion of the diagnoses, considerations of gender assignment should be guided by outcome data. These are listed in Box 8-9, although, for most diagnoses, these data are not yet available. Thus, considerations are based upon factors including those listed here.

The perspective concerning consideration of psychosexual development as it relates to gender assignment is that the relative role of factors leading to an established gender identity remains unknown. It is unclear in these situations how factors such as male levels of androgen exposure during fetal life, family and social environment, and genital anatomy interact to impact upon gender development.

Although there was, in the past, a likelihood of a female gender assignment to a 46,XY individual if the penis were judged to be inadequate, studies are much needed in relation to the current shift of raising all those as male who have a 46,XY karyotype, even if a penis cannot be surgically created. While there is evidence that such a child can grow up with a male gender identity and content even with physical limitations of sexual activity,[37] it is not clear that such persons will be free of significant psychological problems related to underdeveloped genitalia and inability to participate in usual male sexual activities. This may be particularly true for the person

---

Box 8-8. Patient and Family Education

Enhance open interactions with parents
- Do NOT refer to their child as "IT, HE, or SHE". Rather, talk about "your baby."
- Discuss the process of sexual differentiation in words that the parents understand, using illustrations such as those in this chapter.
  - Sex determination as the process through which the male or female structures (phenotype) develop.
  - All parts, the gonads, internal genital ducts, and external genital structures develop from the same beginning (bipotential) embryological structures.
  - Differentiation of these structures reflects regulated expression and interaction of specific genetic direction (genes and gene products).
- Show the child's genitalia to the parents, pointing out structures while discussing how they developed.
- Inform the parents that they will be involved with a team of doctors in the process to determine which gender is appropriate for their child and that these doctors will be involved in future care.
- Unless sex of rearing is obvious, suggest that they delay naming the child and completion of the birth certificate.

Box 8-9.

Gender assignment recommendations for newborn

- Female
  - 46,XY complete androgen insensitivity syndrome
  - 46,XX classical adrenal hyperplasia with significant virilization (note that there are inadequate data for those with complete male genitalia)
- Male
  - 5α-reductase deficiency
  - 17β-hydroxysteroid dehydrogenase (17β-HSD) deficiency
- Based upon gonadal and internal ductal formation
  - Ovotesticular DSD
- Insufficient data
  - Partial androgen insensitivity syndrome
  - Cloacal exstrophy
- Phallic size must be considered, but is only one of many factors
  - Normal variations of male and female genital size must be considered with those within +2.5 SD generally being considered clearly acceptable
  - It is pertinent to realize currently that a 46,XY individual with functional testes is currently almost never considered for a female assignment even when the penis is incompletely fused and small

Box 8-10. When to Refer to a Specialist: Includes Multiple Disciplines

Referral pattern for child with ambiguous genitalia

- Initial referral to tertiary care center with specialists AFTER
  a. Initial discussion with parents concerning basics of sexual differentiation so that they understand how ambiguous genitalia can form, that studies need to be done to ascertain the most appropriate sex assignment, and that their child has the potential for a fulfilling life
  b. Initial laboratory studies have been obtained including karyotype and 17-OHP
- At tertiary care center, referrals should include
  A. Pediatric endocrinologist who is most commonly the team leader
  B. Surgeon experienced with genital reconstruction surgery
  C. Psychologist or behavioral scientist experienced with DSD and gender identity issues
  D. Others from Figure 8-13 with experience to contribute to the goals of the management team

having surgery during puberty who previously experienced the associated pleasurable genital sensations.[38]

Referral to a tertiary care center, preferably with an experienced multidisciplinary team specializing in DSDs, should be made after initial blood samples and discussions with the parents have been completed (Box 8-10). This should generally be accomplished during the first 24 hours of life.

Algorithm of treatment plan (includes multiple disciplines). The current approach requires a specialized team, a further reason for early referral of such patients to a tertiary care clinic where all aspects of management may be considered. Such an expert team includes endocrinologists, geneticists, and surgeons from pediatric, urological, or gynecological subspecialties, along with psychologists, social workers, and specialized nurses (Figure 8-13). The charge to the team is to verify the phenotype, determine as specific a diagnosis as possible, including, when appropriate, a recommendation

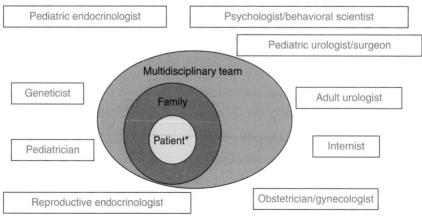

FIGURE 8-13 ▪ Members of the multidisciplinary team required to care for the patient with a DSD include those listed above. Usually a designee from this team serves as the primary interactor with the family. Continuation of management by the team as the child grows allows coordinated ongoing care and counseling.

for gender assignment. One or more team members should provide counseling to the parents, providing background information and treatment options, including, but not limited to, surgery for genital reconstruction and, when appropriate, biopsy to make a more specific diagnosis and gonadectomy to preclude malignant change as appropriate.

REFERENCES

1. Lee PA, Houk CP, Ahmed SF, Hughes IA and the International Consensus Conference on Intersex Working Group. Consensus statement on management of intersex disorders. *Pediatrics*. 2006;118(2):e488-e500.

2. Houk CP, Hughes IA, Ahmed SF, Lee PA on behalf of the LWPES/ESPE Working Group. Summary of consensus statement on intersex disorders and their management. *Pediatrics*. 2006;118(3):753-757.

3. Ogilvy-Stuart AL, Brain CE. Early assessment of ambiguous genitalia. *Arch Dis Child*. 2004;89(5):401-407.

4. White PC, Speiser PW. Congenital adrenal hyperplasia due to 21-hydroxylase deficiency. *Endoc Rev*. 2000;21(3):245-291.

5. Clarkson, MJ, Harley, VR. Sex with two SOX on: SRY and SOX9 in testis development. *Trends Endocrinol Metab*. 2002;13(3):106.

6. Ozisik, G, Achermann, JC, Meeks, JJ, Jameson, JL. SF1 in the development of the adrenal gland and gonads. *Horm Res*. 2003;59(1):94.

7. Meeks JJ, Weiss J, Jameson JL. DAX1 is required for testis determination. *Nat Genet*. 2003;34(1):32-33.

8. Jones ME, Boon WC, McInnes K, Maffei L, Carani C, Simpson ER. Recognizing rare disorders: aromatase deficiency. *Nat Clin Pract Endocrinol Metab*. 2007 May;3(5):414-421.

9. Scott RR, Miller WL. Genetic and clinical features of p450 oxidoreductase deficiency. *Horm Res*. 2008;69(5):266-275.

10. Ghayee HK, Auchus RJ. Basic concepts and recent developments in human steroid hormone biosynthesis. *Rev Endocr Metab Disord*. 2007 Dec;8(4):289-300.

11. Lee YS, Kirk JM, Stanhope RG, et al. Phenotypic variability in 17beta-hydroxysteroid dehydrogenase-3 deficiency and diagnostic pitfalls. *Clin Endocrinol (Oxf)*. 2007 Apr 27; [Epub ahead of print].

12. Imperato-McGinley J, Zhu YS. Androgens and male physiology the syndrome of 5α-reductase-2 deficiency. *Mol Cell Endocrinol*. 2002;198(1-2):51-59.

13. Miller WL. StAR search—what we know about how the steroidogenic acute regulatory protein mediates mitochondrial cholesterol import. *Mol Endocrinol*. 2007 Mar;21(3):589-601.

14. Chen X, Baker BY, Abduljabbar MA, Miller WL. A genetic isolate of congenital lipoid adrenal hyperplasia with atypical clinical findings. *J Clin Endocrinol Metab*. 2005 Feb;90(2):835-840.

15. Hughes IA, Deeb A. Androgen resistance. *Best Pract Res Clin Endocrinol Metab*. 2006 Dec;20(4):577-598.

16. Hannema SE, Scott IS, Rajpert-De Meyts E, Skakkebaek NE, Coleman N, Hughes IA. Testicular development in the complete androgen insensitivity syndrome. *J Pathol*. 2006 Mar;208(4):518-527.

17. Herbison AE. Genetics of puberty. *Horm Res*. 2007;68(5):75-79.

18. Cederroth CR, Pitetti JL, Papaioannou MD, Nef S. Genetic programs that regulate testicular and ovarian development. *Mol Cell Endocrinol*. 2007 Feb;265-266:3-9.

19. Kimble J, Page DC. The mysteries of sexual identity. The germ cell's perspective. *Science*. 2007 Apr 20;316(5823):400-401.

20. Philibert P, Biason-Lauber A, Rouzier R, et al. Identification and functional analysis of a new WNT4 gene mutation among 28 adolescent girls with primary amenorrhea and müllerian duct abnormalities: a French collaborative study. *J Clin Endocrinol Metab*. 2008 Mar;93(3):895-900.

21. Porter FD. Smith-Lemli-Opitz syndrome: pathogenesis, diagnosis and management. *Eur J Hum Genet*. 2008 May;16(5):535-541.

22. Lin L, Philibert P, Ferraz-de-Souza B, et al. Heterozygous missense mutations in steroidogenic factor 1 (SF1/Ad4BP, NR5A1) are associated with 46,XY disorders of sex development with normal adrenal function. *J Clin Endocrinol Metab*. 2007 Mar;92(3):991-999

23. Köhler B, Lin L, Ferraz-de-Souza B, et al. Five novel mutations in steroidogenic factor 1 (SF1, NR5A1) in 46,XY patients with severe underandrogenization but without adrenal insufficiency. *Hum Mutat*. 2008 Jan;29(1):59-64.

24. Moumné L, Batista F, Benayoun BA, et al. The mutations and potential targets of the forkhead transcription factor FOXL2. *Mol Cell Endocrinol*. 2008 Jan 30;282(1-2):2-11.

25. Parma P, Radi O, Vidal V, et al. R-spondin1 is essential in sex determination, skin differentiation and malignancy. *Nat Genet*. 2006 Nov;38(11):1304-1309.

26. Telvi L, Lebbar A, Del Pino O, et al. 45,X/46,XY mosaicism: report of 27 cases. *Pediatrics*. 1999;104(2 Pt 1):304.

27. Paris F, Jeandel C, Servant N, Sultan C. Increased serum estrogenic bioactivity in three male newborns with ambiguous genitalia: a potential consequence of prenatal exposure to environmental endocrine disruptors. *Environ Res*. 2006 Jan;100(1):39-43.

28. Weidner IS, Moller H, Jensen TK, et al. Cryptorchidism and hypospadias in sons of gardeners and farmers. *Environ Health Perspect*. 1998;106(12):793-796.

29. Josso N, Belville C, di Clemente N, Picard JY. AMH and AMH receptor defects in persistent Mullerian duct syndrome. *Hum Reprod Update*. 2005 Jul-Aug;11(4):351-356.

30. Oppelt P, von Have M, Paulsen M, et al. Female genital malformations and their associated abnormalities. *Fertil Steril*. 2007 Feb;87(2):335-342.

31. Virtanen HE, Cortes D, Rajpert-De Meyts E, et al. Development and descent of the testis in relation to cryptorchidism. *Acta Paediatr*. 2007;96(5):622.

32. Tomboc M, Lee PA, Mitwally MF, Schneck FX, Bellinger M, Witchel SF. Insulin-like 3/relaxin-like factor gene mutations are associated with cryptorchidism. *J Clin Endocrinol Metab*. 2000 Nov;85(11):4013-4018.

33. de Vries A, Holmes MC, Heijnis A, et al. Prenatal dexamethasone exposure induces changes in nonhuman primate offspring cardiometabolic and hypothalamic-pituitary-adrenal axis function. *J Clin Invest*. 2007 Apr;117(4):1058-1067.

34. Oberfield SE, Mondok A, Shahrivar F, et al. Clitoral size in full-term infants. *Am J Perinatol*. 1989;6(4):453.

35. Callegari C, Everett S, Ross M, Brasel JA. Anogenital ratio: measure of fetal virilization in premature and full-term newborn infants. *J Pediatr.* 1987;111(2):240.

36. Baskin LS. Anatomical studies of the female genitalia: surgical reconstructive implications. *J Pediatr Endocrinol Metab.* 2004;17(4):581-587.

37. Mazur T. Gender dysphoria and gender change in androgen insensitivity or micropenis. *Arch Sex Behav.* 2005;34(4):411-421.

38. Lee PA, Houk CP. Outcomes studies among men with micropenis. *J Pediatr Endocrinol Metab.* 2004;17(8):1043-1053.

CHAPTER 9

Obesity

Lisa D. Madison and
Bruce A. Boston

INTRODUCTION

Obesity is an increasingly common condition in childhood and adolescence, and has emerged as one of the most serious public health concerns in the 21st century. With the growing prevalence of childhood obesity has come an increase in the incidence of obesity-related comorbid disease prior to adulthood. The profound personal and economic impacts of childhood obesity should compel us to understand this complex topic in the hope that successful efforts can be made at prevention and early intervention.

DEFINITIONS AND EPIDEMIOLOGY

Definitions of Overweight and Obesity in Children

Any discussion of this topic must begin with a consensus as to how overweight and obesity are to be defined in the pediatric population. Multiple different indices and techniques can be used to estimate the degree of adiposity. The most commonly used measure is body mass index (BMI), defined as kilograms (kg) of body weight per height in square meters (m^2). Adults are defined as overweight if their BMI is 25.0 to 29.9 kg/m^2 and obese if more than 30.0 kg/m^2. This index of adiposity, however, is less accurate in children that have not yet achieved full adult height. The number of children defined as obese using the adult criteria would be greatly underestimated. Therefore, the BMI percentile (%ile) is a more accurate index of body mass in the pediatric age group. BMI percentile curves have been generated using data from the National Health and Nutrition Examination

Survey (NHANES) and take into account both age and gender (Figure 9-1). The Centers for Disease Control define children as overweight if the BMI is more than 95th %ile and, at risk for overweight, if the BMI is between the 85th to 95th %ile. The BMI percentile graphs only include children older than 2 years of age. For children less than 2 years of age, standard weight-for-length curves can be used to assess body mass.

Prevalence of Overweight and Obesity in Children

Multiple national surveys indicate a significant increase in the frequency of overweight children over the past 30 years. With current prevalences of overweight and obese children ranging from 12% to 30% in developed nations and from 2% to 12% in the developing world, this has become one of the most common health problems in childhood.[1] The most recent NHANES data indicate that 33.6% of American children and adolescents aged 2 to 19 year have a BMI more than 85th %ile, with 17.1% having a BMI more than 95th %ile.[2] The risk of overweight and obesity is not evenly distributed, with low income groups and minorities most affected in industrialized societies. In the United States, for example, childhood obesity rates approach 25% among African American and Hispanic populations *versus* 10% to 12% among Caucasians.[1]

Progression of Childhood Obesity into Adulthood

Obese children tend to become obese adults. Those at highest risk are adolescents in the highest weight categories who come from families with at least one obese

2 to 20 years: Boys
Body mass index-for-age percentiles

NAME _____

RECORD # _____

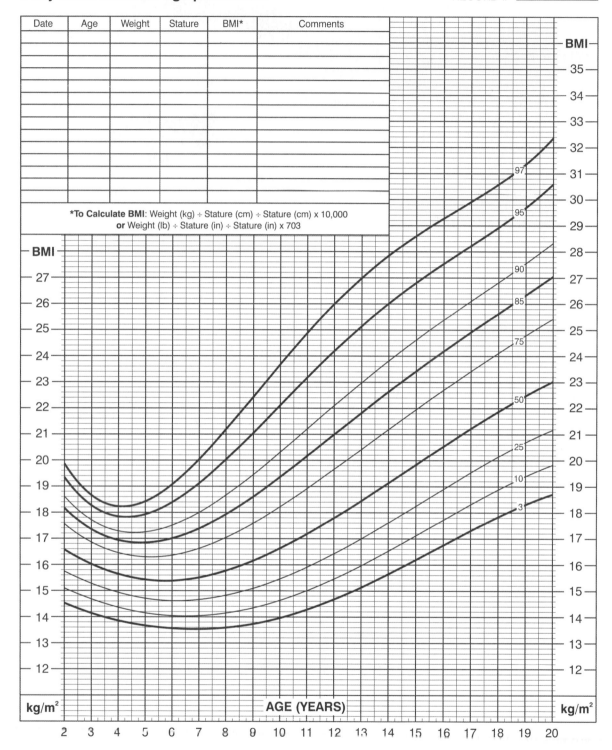

*To Calculate BMI: Weight (kg) ÷ Stature (cm) ÷ Stature (cm) x 10,000
or Weight (lb) ÷ Stature (in) ÷ Stature (in) x 703*

Published May 30, 2000 (modified 10/16/00).
SOURCE: Developed by the National Center for Health Statistics in collaboration with
the National Center for Chronic Disease Prevention and Health Promotion (2000).
http://www.cdc.gov/growthcharts

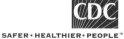

FIGURE 9-1 ■ BMI percentile curves. Age- and gender-specific curves generated using data from the National Health and Nutrition Examination Survey (NHANES). (*Source: National Center for Chronic Disease Prevention and Health Promotion, Centers for Disease Control and Prevention, Atlanta, Georgia.) A = boys and B = girls. (http://www.cdc.gov/growthcharts*)

2 to 20 years: Girls
Body mass index-for-age percentiles

NAME _____

RECORD # _____

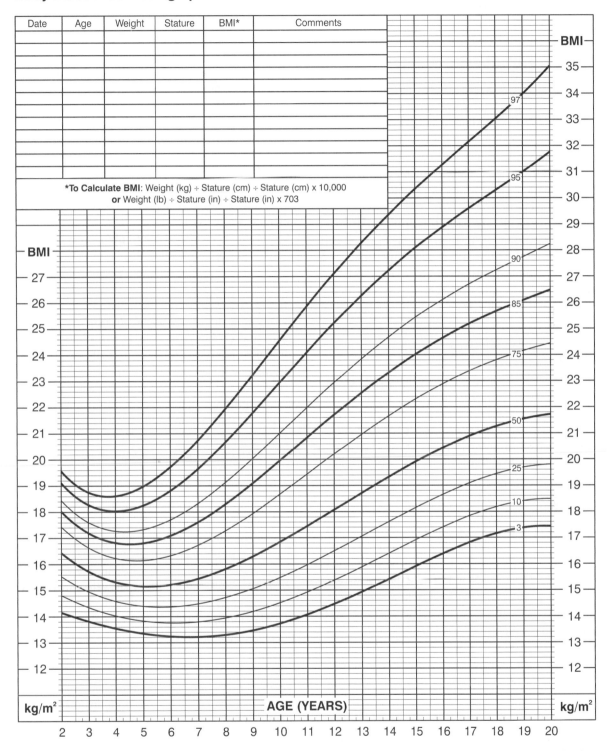

Date	Age	Weight	Stature	BMI*	Comments

*To Calculate BMI: Weight (kg) ÷ Stature (cm) ÷ Stature (cm) x 10,000
or Weight (lb) ÷ Stature (in) ÷ Stature (in) x 703

Published May 30, 2000 (modified 10/16/00).
SOURCE: Developed by the National Center for Health Statistics in collaboration with
    the National Center for Chronic Disease Prevention and Health Promotion (2000).
    http://www.cdc.gov/growthcharts

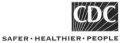
SAFER · HEALTHIER · PEOPLE™

FIGURE 9-1 ■ *(Continued)*

parent.[1,3] The probability of adult obesity (BMI >30 kg/m^2) is more than 50% among children older than 13 years of age whose BMI percentiles meet or exceed the 95th %ile for age and gender.[3]

Prevalence of Obesity-Related Disease

Increased adiposity can lead to both immediate complications in children and adolescents and long-term health consequences as adults. Insulin resistance almost always accompanies obesity and is directly related to the degree of adiposity. Many of the consequences of obesity, including impaired glucose tolerance (IGT) and type 2 diabetes mellitus (T2DM), dyslipidemia, hypertension, polycystic ovarian syndrome (PCOS), and acanthosis nigricans, are related to insulin resistance. Other consequences of obesity not related to insulin resistance include pulmonary, gastrointestinal, and orthopedic complications. In addition, obese children often suffer from psychosocial complications including depression and low self-esteem.

Impaired glucose tolerance and type 2 diabetes mellitus

The prevalence of T2DM is increasing in parallel with the epidemic of childhood obesity. Previously considered an adult disease, a recent survey conducted in 2001 found that T2DM accounted for approximately 15% of diabetes cases among youths aged 10 to 19 years. The overall prevalence of T2DM in this age group was 0.42 per 1000.[4] Prediabetes or impaired glucose tolerance (IGT), defined as a fasting glucose more than 100 mg/dL or a 2-hour post-oral glucose load level between 140 and 200 mg/dL, is also becoming increasingly common in children and adolescents. In one study of children referred to an obesity clinic, a high prevalence of IGT was noted affecting 25% of 4- to 10-year-olds and 21% of 11- to 18-year-olds.[5] Other population-based studies, however, demonstrate a lower incidence (approximately 4%-4.5%) of IGT in overweight children.[6] The discrepancy between these studies is likely related to the degree of obesity in the study subjects with a tendency toward cases with more severe obesity being seen in obesity clinics.

Hypertension

Once considered rare, hypertension in children has become increasingly common in association with obesity and other risk factors. When screening children in school settings, the rate of hypertension is as high as 10% among children with BMI more than the 97th %ile.[7] Similarly, a meta-analysis of blood pressure data gathered in children aged 8 to 17 years participating in multiple population-based studies showed an increase in the prevalence of pediatric hypertension with the authors concluding that the rise in blood pressure was significantly associated with the increase in childhood obesity.[7]

Hyperlipidemia

Hyperlipidemia is common in overweight children and may occur as part of the metabolic syndrome. The observed hyperlipidemia usually consists of increased serum LDL-cholesterol and triglycerides, and decreased HDL-cholesterol levels. A number of large childhood health surveys has documented cholesterol levels more than 200 mg/dL in 10% to 13% of school-aged children.[8]

Metabolic syndrome

The metabolic syndrome is a strictly defined as a group of factors related to insulin resistance that predicts increased risk for T2DM and cardiovascular disease. Classically characterized as a combination of abdominal obesity, glucose intolerance, hypertension, and dyslipidemia, definitions initially developed for adults have been extended to adolescents[9,10] (Table 9-1). Long-term prospective studies to demonstrate a connection between the presence of metabolic syndrome in adolescents and cardiovascular disease as adults have to be designed. However, adolescents with metabolic syndrome tend to become adults with metabolic syndrome. Therefore, until conclusive studies are available, metabolic syndrome-related risk of future cardiovascular disease is inferred and may warrant early aggressive interventions to increase insulin sensitivity in adolescents with metabolic syndrome.

Polycystic ovary syndrome

Adolescent females with obesity often present with signs and symptoms consistent with hyperandrogenism and ovarian dysfunction, including amenorrhea or oligomenorrhea, acne, and hirsutism. Hyperandrogenism appears to primarily result from hyperinsulinemia. PCOS affects approximately 5% of adult women, primarily those who are overweight or obese, with most women first becoming symptomatic during adolescence (see Chapter 7 for more information on PCOS).[11]

Other obesity-related complications

Gastrointestinal disease, including fatty infiltration of the liver and cholelithiasis may occur in overweight children and correlates with the severity of adiposity. In studies of obese children, 10% to 25% have been found to have elevation of liver enzymes and approximately 50% to 75% have evidence of fatty infiltration of the liver on ultrasound.[12] Although uncommon, this condition can progress to liver fibrosis and cirrhosis. The duration of obesity, but not its severity, is correlated with the extent of fibrosis. Obesity is also a risk factor for cholelithiasis and gall bladder disease. Although these are collectively rare in children, almost 50% of

Table 9-1.

Definitions of Pediatric Metabolic Syndrome

International Diabetes Federation Criteria[9,10]

Central obesity (required feature)

Waist circumference	>90th %ile for age, gender, and ethnicity* *or*
	Male ≥94 cm
	Female ≥80 cm

Plus any two of the following:

Raised triglycerides	≥150 mg/dL
Reduced HDL cholesterol	< 40 mg/dL (<50 mg/dL in females >16 y)
Raised blood pressure	Systolic :≥130 mm Hg *or*
	Diastolic: ≥85 mm Hg
Elevated fasting plasma glucose	Fasting plasma glucose ≥100 mg/dL *or*
	Previously diagnosed type 2 diabetes

Modified Adult Treatment Panel (ATP III) Criteria[9]

Any three or more of the following criteria:

Waist circumference	>75th %ile for age and gender*
Raised triglycerides	>100 mg/dL
Reduced HDL cholesterol	<50 mg/dL, except in boys aged 15 to 19 y, in whom the cut-point is <45 mg/dL
Raised blood pressure	Systolic >90th %ile for gender, age, and height†
Raised fasting plasma glucose	Fasting plasma glucose >110 mg/dL

*Reference for age-, gender-, and ethnic-specific waist circumference. Fernandez JR, Redden DT, Pietrobelli A, Allison DB. Waist circumference percentiles in nationally representative samples of African American, European American, and Mexi an American Childen and Adolescents. J Pediatr. Oct 2004;145(4):439-444.

†Reference for age-, gender-. and height-specific blood pressures. National High Blood Pressure Education Program Working Group on Hypertension Control in Children and Adolescents. Update on the 1987 Task Force Report on High Blood Pressure in Children and Adolescents: A Working Group Report from the National High Blood Pressure Education Program. Pediatrics. Oct 1996;98(4):649-658.

cases of cholecystitis in adolescents are associated with obesity.

Pulmonary disease, including both asthma and obstructive sleep apnea, is common in overweight children. The incidence of sleep apnea in obese children is 4 to 5 times that seen in non-obese children.[13] Severe sleep apnea may ultimately lead to *cor pulmonale.*

Obesity is a risk factor for the development of orthopedic disorders, including both Blount disease and slipped capital femoral epiphysis (SCFE). Blount disease, also termed tibia vara, occurs when the inner part of the tibia just below the knee fails to develop normally, causing angulation of the tibia. Unlike benign tibia vara which tends to correct with age, Blount disease is progressive and can cause severe bowing of one or both legs. Adolescent-onset Blount disease affects African American males almost exclusively, with a prevalence of 2.5% among the obese adolescent black male population.[14]

SCFE occurs when the epiphysis of the proximal femur begins to slip off the corresponding metaphysis. SCFE presents as a limp combined with hip pain and/or referred pain to the knee. The affected limb appears to be externally rotated on examination and there is pain with passive manipulation. Data from a number of studies indicate that 51% to 72% of SCFE cases occur in obese individuals.[14]

Psychosocial effects of obesity

The most prevalent consequence of childhood obesity may be the stigmatization experienced by the obese child. Teasing is common by both peers and family members, and even healthcare professionals may display negative biases in their interactions with obese children and adolescents.[15] Multiple studies have shown poor body image, low self-esteem, depression, and even suicidal ideation in children and adolescents teased about their weight.[16] Severely overweight children have demonstrated health-related quality-of-life scores comparable to children with cancer.[17] The social and economic impacts of childhood obesity may be far-reaching, with at least one study showing that women with a history of overweight in adolescence ultimately completed less schooling, were less likely to be married, had lower household incomes, and had higher rates of poverty than matched controls who had not been overweight.[18]

Economic impact

The growing economic impact of childhood obesity is staggering. In youth aged 6 to 17 years, financial costs related to treatment of obesity-associated diseases more than tripled from a cost-of-living adjustment of 35 million dollars in 1979 to 1981 to 127 million dollars in 1997 to 1999.[19] A recent study estimated that approximately 9% of annual US health-care spending (or 92.6 billion dollars) was related to costs of treatment for overweight, obesity, and their sequelae in both children and adults (NIH Fact Sheet, June 2007).

Pathogenesis

Genetic and environmental components

Obesity is clearly a "genetic" disorder that is heavily influenced by environmental factors. Twin studies indicate that 50% to 80% of the tendency to gain weight is genetically determined.[20,21] The adiposity of a child's parents also has a profound effect on the adiposity of the child.[22] Furthermore, data from the Bogalusa heart study indicate that the increase in BMI observed in children over the past few decades is not evenly distributed amongst the population.[23] When age-, sex-, and race-adjusted data collected from children in the 1970s is compared to a cohort of children in the 1990s, the adjusted BMI that defines the lower percentiles (ie, the thinnest individuals) changes very little. However, there is a significant further increase in adiposity in individuals already at higher body mass in BMI percentiles (Figure 9-2). Data from the National Health and Examination Survey (NHES) and

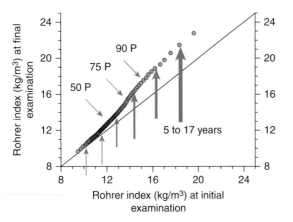

FIGURE 9-2 ■ Bogalusa heart study. Graph compares body mass index (BMI) percentiles in cross-sectional studies from 1973 to 1976 (initial examination) and 1992 to 1994 (final examination). Arrows demonstrate a greater effect of environmental changes on weight gain in segment of population with higher BMI. Environmental changes have had less effect on the population genetically predisposed to thinness. (*Adapted from Freedman DS, Srinivasan SR, Valdez RA, Williamson DF, Berenson GS. Secular increases in relative weight and adiposity among children over two decades: the Bogalusa Heart Study. Pediatrics. 1997;99:420-426.*)

NHANESIII studies demonstrate a similar phenomenon. In summary, there has been little change over the years in adiposity in those individuals genetically predisposed to thinness. Adverse environmental changes in our society appear to have the greatest impact on individuals with a genetic predisposition to obesity.

There is no question that changes in our environment have had a profound effect on the prevalence of overweight children. These changes have adversely impacted energy balance, particularly in the genetically susceptible individual. The typical modern western diet emphasizes high-fat, calorie-dense foods with larger portions. Physical activity has declined in parallel with the increase in the incidence of overweight children.[24] Television, computers, and video games have changed how children entertain themselves, with more time spent in sedentary activities. The result is a profound decrease in caloric expenditure combined with an increase in caloric intake.

The "Thrifty" Gene Hypothesis

Genetic traits predisposing to obesity likely evolved as these genes provided a selective advantage for survival. Individuals with a genetic predisposition toward obesity shunt consumed calories toward storage in adipose tissue and further protect energy stores during starvation with a decrease in energy expenditure.[25] Food-seeking behaviors are also more pronounced. Obese individuals have a "thrifty" phenotype that optimizes utilization of energy resources, a selective advantage during famine.

Contrast individuals with a "thrifty" phenotype to thin individuals who are inefficient with caloric resources. Individuals with a "wasteful" phenotype store less energy as adipose tissue and have less intense food-seeking behaviors. Since genes that comprise the "thrifty" phenotype confer selective advantage during times of famine, these genes would become more prevalent in populations subjected to starvation. There are many historical examples of enrichment of "thrifty" genes that exist in populations.[26] Unfortunately, the emergence of a western diet and sedentary lifestyle has resulted in profound increases of obesity-related complications in these ethnic populations.

Weight Set Point and Regulation of Energy Homeostasis

Physiological mechanisms exist that tightly regulate food intake and energy expenditure, even in most overweight and obese individuals. The existence of a tightly regulated feedback system can be demonstrated in long-term clinical studies of weight loss. Weight loss induced by very low calorie diets and/or behavior modification is rarely maintained

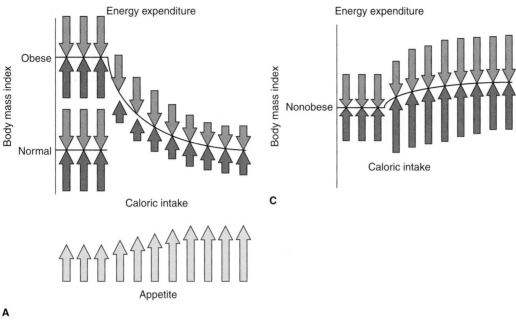

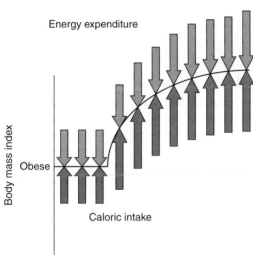

FIGURE 9-3 ■ Weight set point. Changes in caloric intake result in compensatory changes in metabolic rate and appetite as a function of adiposity. **(A)** If caloric intake decreases, metabolic rate decreases with decreasing adiposity until a new weight set point is achieved that balances caloric intake with energy expenditure. Obese individuals may achieve a normal body mass, but often with a lower than "normal" metabolic rate and will require a decreased caloric intake despite increased appetite. **(B)** Small increases in caloric intake have a profound effect on body mass in individuals predisposed to obesity. **(C)** In contrast, individuals predisposed to "thinness" robustly defend body mass.

over time.[27] Most individuals tend to gain weight back to a point at or near the prestudy weight. A similar phenomenon can be demonstrated in individuals that are overfed and forced to gain weight.[28] These subjects gain adipose mass, but are unable to maintain this degree of adiposity when the study is stopped. They rapidly lose weight and, as a group, end up near their prestudy weight. These observations imply that most individuals have a genetically determined "weight set point."

The weight set point is maintained in most individuals by adjustments to metabolic rate in response to changes in body mass. Total energy requirements to maintain weight stability in both non-weight-reduced obese and nonobese subjects are very similar. Obese individuals that have undergone weight loss, however, require 10% to 15% fewer calories to maintain weight stability than a "non-weight-reduced" person of similar body composition and weight.[25] Further weight loss results in further decline in total energy expenditure in an attempt by the individual to protect adipose stores. A sustained decrease in caloric intake in overweight subjects eventually results in a new steady-state body weight, rather than continued weight loss, as the decline in daily energy expenditure equilibrates with the decline in energy consumption (Figure 9-3A). Furthermore, the diet-reduced adipose mass leads ultimately to an increased appetite and difficulty in maintaining the lower caloric intake. A resumption of the "prediet" caloric intake will almost certainly result in a return to the previous obese body weight set point.

A tightly regulated feedback system that controls body weight is absolutely necessary to keep an individual's weight relatively stable over time. Thin and normal-weight individuals have feedback systems that regulate appetite and metabolic rate tightly in response to changes in adiposity (Figure 9-3B & C). Feedback systems in individuals genetically predisposed to obesity are not

as tightly regulated allowing for greater increases in body mass. If these homeostatic mechanisms did not exist, small, but persistent, increases in caloric intake would result in significant obesity. It has been estimated that approximately 1 lb of adipose tissue is added for every

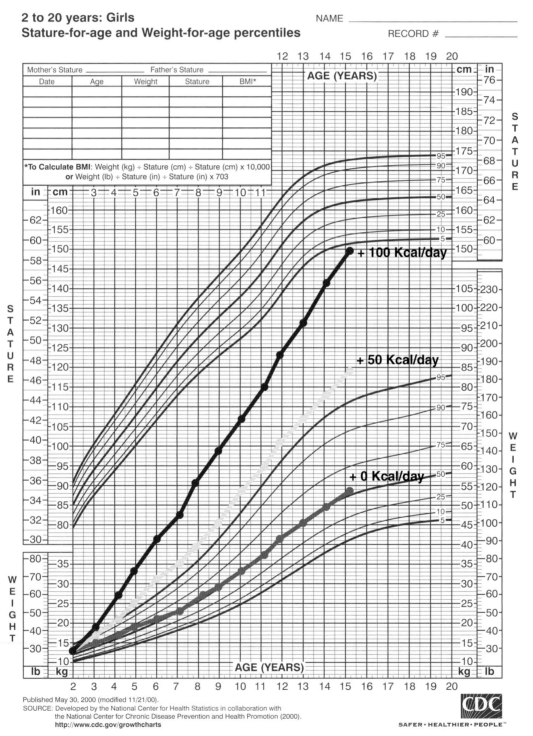

FIGURE 9-4 ◼ Estimated weight gain from excess caloric consumption. Projected weight gain assumes all calories consumed in excess of growth and development requirements are converted to body mass and no compensatory adjustments occur in energy expenditure. Lines represent projected weight gain from age 2 to 15 years with 0 kcal/day, 50 kcal/day, and 100 kcal/day in excess of requirements for normal growth and development. (*Source: Centers for Disease Control and Prevention, Atlanta, Georgia.*)

3500 kcal consumed in excess of caloric requirement for energy expenditure and growth. As little as 50 extra kcal/day for 10 years would result in a 50-lb gain in adipose mass. A caloric intake of 200 kcal/day in excess of caloric expenditure would result in a 100-lb weight gain in as little as 5 years (Figure 9-4). Fortunately, most individuals defend "ideal weight" by alteration of both energy expenditure and food intake. Therefore, the weight of most children tends to follow standard published growth curves. However, if the homeostatic mechanisms are not intact, dramatic weight gain can occur.

The Neuroendocrinology of Weight Regulation

Energy balance and weight set point regulation are accomplished by a complex feedback system. Adequacy of energy stored in the adipocyte is communicated centrally by the adipocyte-derived hormone, leptin. Secreted from adipocytes in proportion to the degree of adiposity, leptin acts at the hypothalamus to inhibit feeding behavior, decrease insulin secretion, and increase metabolic rate.[29] As an animal gains weight, leptin levels rise resulting in decreased appetite and increased metabolic rate. Likewise, weight loss leads to a decline in leptin levels and an increase in food-seeking behavior with a decrease in basal metabolic rate.

Leptin signaling in the hypothalamus is primarily via receptors located in the arcuate nucleus.[30] The arcuate nucleus lacks a blood-brain barrier allowing direct communication of peripheral "metabolic" signals including both nutrients and hormones. Leptin signals centrally by inhibiting neurons that contain neuropeptides (NPY and agouti-related peptide [AgRP]) that stimulate appetite/ decrease metabolic rate, while stimulating neurons that contain neuropeptides that inhibit appetite/increase metabolic rate including proopiomelanocortin (POMC) (Figure 9-5A).

Peripheral signals other than leptin also appear to play a role in appetite regulation and energy homeostasis. Ghrelin, a hormone secreted by the stomach, stimulates NPY/AgRP neurons centrally.[31] Ghrelin levels rise in the fasted state and decrease with feeding. Another gastrointestinal peptide, Peptide YY (PYY), is secreted from the intestine.[32] In contrast to ghrelin, PYY appears to be upregulated with feeding. PYY inhibits NPY/AgRP neurons while stimulating POMC neurons. It is theorized that, while leptin serves as a more general indicator of energy stores, ghrelin and PYY modulate leptin signaling to provide short-term feedback on caloric intake (Figure 9-5B). Insulin also appears to signal satiety via central nervous system (CNS) mechanisms similar to leptin. Therefore, postprandial increases in insulin in response to a carbohydrate meal may also act to decrease further food intake.

This complex interplay between peripheral signals of "energy status" and central control of feeding and metabolism must be intact to maintain normal weight homeostasis. If it is loosely regulated or interrupted by genetic defects or hypothalamic injury, significant obesity can result.

CLINICAL PRESENTATION AND DIAGNOSIS

Signs and Symptoms

In order to properly monitor for the development of overweight and obesity, all children should have height and weight measured and weight for length (prior to age 2 years) or BMI (after age 2 years) plotted on the growth curve at every health maintenance visit. Children and adolescents at risk for overweight, with BMI greater than the 85th %ile, should receive a medical evaluation. Even before the BMI reaches the 85th %ile, primary care physicians should consider initiating a workup for children demonstrating rapid weight gain with upward crossing of weight percentiles and particularly for those children who show a concomitant decrease in linear growth velocity. Simple caloric excess is expected to fuel both weight gain and linear growth, so the absence of appropriate height gain in the face of excessive weight gain should trigger an investigation of possible pathologies.

Children with hypothyroidism may report increased fatigue, excessively dry skin, constipation, or cold intolerance. Striae, easy bruising, and central fat distribution are potentially consistent with glucocorticoid excess. Those individuals with a CNS lesion affecting the hypothalamus or pituitary might report severe nocturnal headaches and emesis, vision changes, polyuria and polydipsia, poor illness tolerance, and precocious or delayed puberty. Finally, children with genetic syndromes linked to obesity may be noted to have dysmorphic features, hypotonia, and developmental delay.

In the assessment of overweight children, with BMI greater than the 95th %ile, attention is warranted to signs and symptoms of comorbid conditions. Patients may report polydipsia, polyuria, nocturia, and nocturnal enuresis as clues to the development of diabetes mellitus. Patients who report snoring, sleep disruption, and daytime somnolence may require workup for obstructive sleep apnea. Female adolescent patients may complain of menstrual irregularity, acne, and hirsutism as indicators of possible polycystic ovary syndrome. Overweight children may also report orthopedic complaints such as hip, knee, and/or back pain, and lower extremity deformity.

History and physical

A careful history and physical examination can largely distinguish individuals with familial obesity from those with obesity secondary to hormone disorders, CNS lesions, or genetic syndromes (Figure 9-6). Significant findings in the prenatal history include decreased fetal

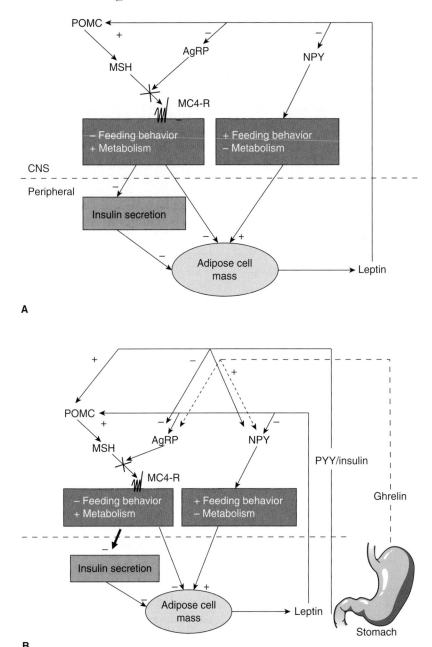

FIGURE 9-5 ■ Neuroendocrinology of weight and energy homeostasis. **(A)** Chronic regulation: Increased leptin secretion in proportion to adipose mass stimulates POMC and inhibits AgRP/NPY neurons. These neurons signal increased feeding behavior, decreased metabolic rate, and decreased insulin secretion. The result is decreased energy storage in adipose tissue and decreased leptin secretion. **(B)** Acute regulation: Nutrient intake results in increased PYY, increased insulin, and decreased ghrelin levels. These hormones may modulate leptin signals to alter energy homeostasis acutely in response to a meal. AGRP = Agouti Related Peptide; MC4-R = Melanocortin 4 Receptor; MSH = Melanocyte Stimulating Hormone; NPY = Neuropeptide Y; POMC = Proopiomelanocortin; PYY = Peptide YY

movement which might predict postnatal hypotonia consistent with Prader-Willi syndrome (PWS). Birth history may reveal traumatic aspects of delivery possibly associated with an early CNS insult. Important elements of the neonatal history include hypoglycemia and micropenis and/or cryptorchidism which may be associated with growth hormone (GH) deficiency. Failure-to-thrive in infancy and early childhood is associated with Prader-Willi syndrome. Delayed achievement of

milestones, learning disabilities, and mental retardation may be associated with a number of genetic syndromes linked to obesity.

In terms of the more immediate history, overweight children should be questioned about severe headaches, visual changes, and recurrent vomiting to look for evidence of a CNS lesion. The physician should inquire as well about signs and symptoms of hypothyroidism, diabetes mellitus, and obstructive sleep apnea as noted earlier.

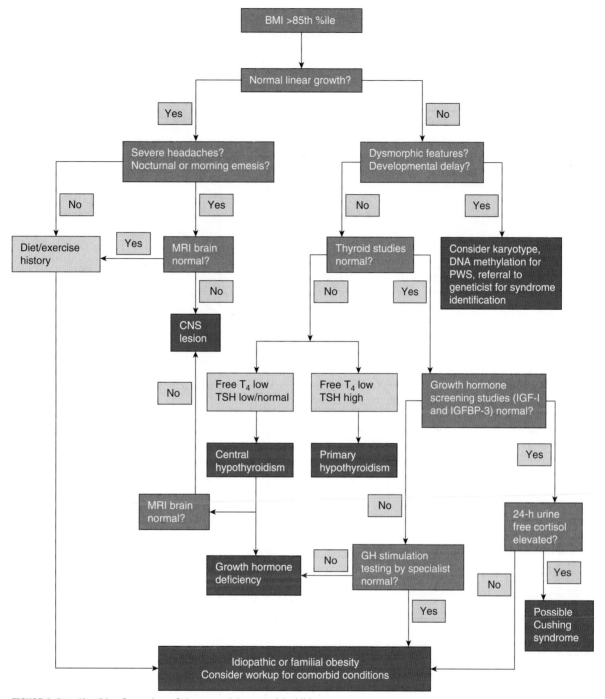

FIGURE 9-6 ■ Algorithm for workup of the overweight or at-risk child.

Menstrual history should be reviewed in adolescent girls, keeping in mind that both primary and secondary amenorrhea may be manifestations of hyperandrogenism.

The history should include a review of any available previous growth records. A history of poor growth velocity despite increased weight gain is more consistent with hormonal disorders and genetic syndromes, while normal or increased growth velocity suggests familial obesity (Figure 9-7).

The final component of the obesity evaluation is an assessment of caloric intake, feeding behaviors, and energy expenditure. A nutritionist can obtain a diet history that details both nutrient composition and total caloric intake. Identifying maladaptive behaviors is the key to designing an effective treatment plan. Questions regarding food-seeking behaviors, appetite, eating habits, exercise, television-watching, and the like are all important in identifying areas for behavioral intervention. It is

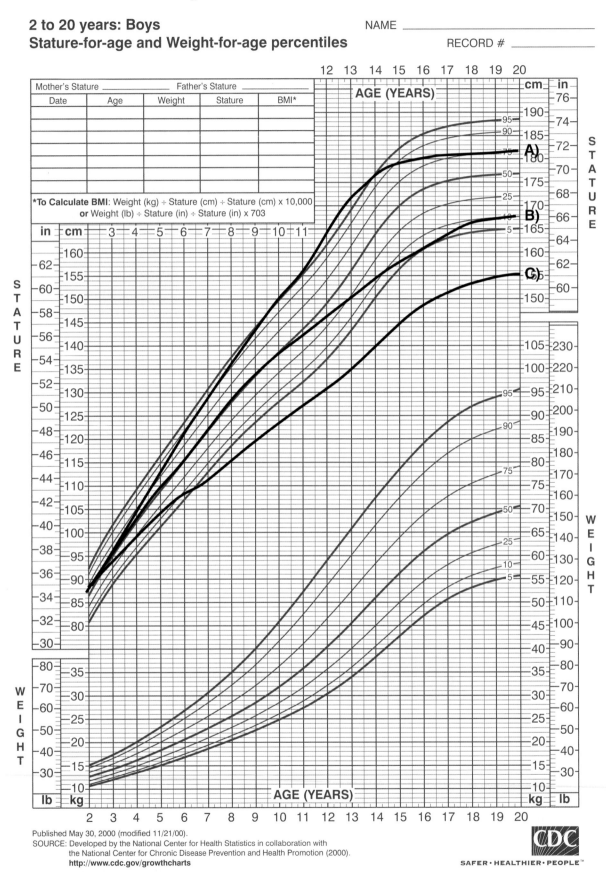

2 to 20 years: Boys
Stature-for-age and Weight-for-age percentiles

NAME _____

RECORD # _____

Published May 30, 2000 (modified 11/21/00).
SOURCE: Developed by the National Center for Health Statistics in collaboration with
the National Center for Chronic Disease Prevention and Health Promotion (2000).
http://www.cdc.gov/growthcharts

CDC
SAFER · HEALTHIER · PEOPLE™

FIGURE 9-7 ■ Typical obesity-related growth curves. **(A)** Slightly increased growth velocity and growth percentile typical of "familial" obesity. **(B)** Normal growth with subsequent growth failure consistent with acquired growth hormone deficiency, thyroid hormone deficiency, or cortisol excess. **(C)** Genetic obesity syndromes often associated with decreased growth velocity and lower growth percentiles. (*Source: Centers for Disease Control and Prevention, Atlanta, Georgia.*)

important to define these behaviors in the context of the family, rather than just the child. Frequently, problems with obesity exist within the entire family. Interventions with the pediatric patient only are unlikely to be successful unless family behavioral patterns are changed.

The physical examination of the overweight child or adolescent should include blood pressure measurement at every visit, using an appropriately sized cuff. General body habitus should be noted, including a description of body fat distribution (apple *versus* pear body shape), as well as the presence of moon facies, buffalo hump, or any dysmorphic features. On head and neck examination, an obstructed oropharynx (eg, enlarged tonsils) suggests an increased risk for obstructive sleep apnea. The abdominal examination may be difficult depending upon the degree of adiposity, but a concerted effort should be made to palpate the liver, as hepatomegaly may be noted in obese patients with fatty infiltration of the liver. Tanner staging should be performed with attention to evidence of either precocious or delayed puberty. While precocious pubertal development might suggest the presence of a CNS lesion, delayed puberty is often seen in obese adolescent boys. Skin examination should include a search for acanthosis nigricans and skin tags (acrochordons) seen primarily on the posterior neck (nape) and in the axillae (and both reflecting insulin resistance), as well as documentation of striae or excessively dry skin. Finally, a neurological examination, including assessment of visual fields by confrontation, is important if the history suggests the possibility of a CNS lesion.

Diagnostic Tests

The basic evaluation of all overweight children and adolescents should include a multichemistry panel containing a random glucose, transaminases, and a bicarbonate (CO_2) measurement (Table 9-2). If blood is being drawn, a free T_4 and TSH should be checked to rule out hypothyroidism. While hypothyroidism alone generally leads to only modest weight gain and does not result in severe obesity, suboptimal thyroid function will complicate a child and family's best efforts at weight loss and should be identified and treated.

Fasting glucose and hemoglobin A1C can be used to screen for T2DM, but an oral glucose tolerance test (OGTT) provides considerably more information as this may reveal glucose intolerance, a precursor to the development of frank diabetes mellitus that may not be appreciated with other screening modalities (Table 9-2). These tests should be considered especially if there is a history of polydipsia and polyuria, but asymptomatic T2DM can also occur. Repeat screening should be considered annually, particularly in children over 10 years of age.

Total cholesterol should also be measured in all overweight children (Table 9-2). Based on recommendations by the American Academy of Pediatrics,[33]

a random total cholesterol more than 200 mg/dL should be followed by a fasting lipid profile. Levels between 170 and 200 mg/dL should be repeated. If the average of two measurements remains in the borderline (170-200 mg/dL) or elevated range, then a fasting lipid profile should be obtained. Individuals with cholesterol levels less than 170 mg/dL should have lipid levels rechecked every 5 years.

Additional laboratory work-up might include a fasting insulin level and free testosterone level if there is suspicion of polycystic ovary syndrome, gonadotropins and sex steroids if there is concern about precocious or delayed puberty, a 24-hour urine for free cortisol and creatinine if there is a suggestion of glucocorticoid excess, and a karyotype or other genetic testing if there is suspicion that a syndrome may exist.

Excessive daytime sleepiness and severe snoring may indicate sleep apnea. If the history is consistent with sleep apnea, or if an elevated serum CO_2 is detected on a venous blood gas or multichemistry panel, polysomnography is strongly recommended. Other studies such as videotaping and nocturnal pulse oximetry are helpful if positive, but are of poor predictive value if negative. If sleep apnea is present, an electrocardiogram should be obtained to evaluate for the presence of right ventricular hypertrophy followed up by an echocardiogram and cardiology referral if indicated.

Assessment of actual body composition (lean mass *versus* fat mass as well as fat distribution) provides much richer data than does height, weight, and BMI alone. Indices such as BMI percentile and weight-for-height percentile are only indirect measures of adiposity. Individuals with increased muscle mass may have a BMI greater than 95th %ile despite a normal amount of adiposity. "Direct" measures of adiposity are available, although many of these methods are primarily used in a research setting. These methods vary from less accurate techniques easily performed in a clinic (ie, skinfold thickness and bioelectrical impedance) to very accurate techniques (ie, DEXA scanning, isotope dilution, magnetic resonance spectroscopy, and underwater weighing), most of which are only available in clinical research centers. Although this information is interesting and potentially useful, it is generally not practical for the general pediatric practice setting.

Laboratory Values

Standards for interpretation of fasting plasma glucose and the 2-hour OGTT

A fasting plasma glucose level more than 126 mg/dL or a glucose level of more than or equal to 200 mg/dL after oral glucose administration is suggestive of diabetes. The American Diabetes Association recommends repeating glucose levels suggestive of diabetes on a different day to confirm the diagnosis. Given the higher likelihood and

Table 9-2.

Laboratory Testing in the Work-Up of the Overweight Child

Test	Indication	Intepretation
Glucose (random)	All overweight	>140 mg/dL—possible impaired glucose tolerance >200 mg/dL—possible diabetes mellitus
AST/ALT	All overweight	Elevated AST/ALT suggest fatty infiltration of liver
CO_2	All overweight	Elevated CO_2 may be consistent with obstructive sleep apnea
Free T$_4$/TSH	Slowing of growth velocity Excessively dry skin Constipation Cold intolerance Oligoamenorrhea	Decreased free T$_4$ and/or elevated TSH diagnostic of hypothyroidism
2-h oral glucose tolerance test	Polyuria/polydipsia Nocturia Acanthosis nigricans Elevated fasting insulin Random glucose >140 mg/dL Fasting glucose >100 mg/dL	See Table 9-3
Total cholesterol	All overweight	>200 mg/dL—requires follow-up with fasting lipid panel 170-200 mg/dL—should be repeated at close intervals <170 mg/dL—should be repeated every 5 y
Fasting lipid panel	Total cholesterol >200 mg/dL Family history including early cardiac disease	LDL >190 mg/dL—consider pharmacological therapy
Fasting insulin Free testosterone	Hirsutism Acne Secondary amenorrhea Oligoamenorrhea	Elevated values suggest polycystic ovary syndrome
24-h urine free cortisol	Slowing of growth velocity Hypertension Striae Central fat distribution	Elevated value suggests glucocorticoid excess
Karyotype FISH DNA Methylation studies Other genetic studies	Dysmorphic features Short stature Significant developmental delay	
Polysomnography	Increased CO_2 on chemistry panel Severe snoring Daytime somnolence Observed apnea	Interpretation by a sleep disorders specialist

more acute nature of type 1 diabetes in children and adolescents, it may be more prudent to check urine ketones when an abnormal glucose result is first noted and proceed immediately to initiation of therapy if urine ketones are positive. In the absence of urine ketones, rechecking an abnormal glucose result within a matter of days to confirm the diagnosis of diabetes may be acceptable.

Fasting glucose levels between 100 and 126 mg/dL and postprandial plasma glucose levels between 140 and 200 mg/dL indicate some impairment of normal glucose homeostasis, as further defined in Table 9-3.

DIFFERENTIAL DIAGNOSIS

Increased adiposity in childhood and adolescence is not always the result of a genetic predisposition toward weight gain superimposed on a calorie-rich environment (Tables 9-4 and 9-5). Although endocrine disorders and syndromes associated with obesity are found in less than 5% of children referred for evaluation of obesity, it is important to consider these etiologies in the evaluation of the overweight child. Hypothyroidism, GH deficiency, and glucocorticoid excess all may result

Table 9-3.

Definitions of Abnormal Glucose Metabolism

	Fasting Glucose (mg/dL)	2-h glucose (following 1.75 g/kg glucose load; maximum 75 g)
Normal glucose tolerance	<100	<140
Impaired fasting glucose (IFG)	100-125	
Impaired glucose tolerance (IGT)	—	140-200
Diabetes mellitus	>126	>200

in an increase in adiposity. In addition, some boys with hypogonadism and low testosterone levels have a body composition that favors fat deposition over development of lean body mass. In contrast to most children with obesity who tend to be tall with advanced bone ages, children with the above hormone deficiencies or with glucocorticoid excess tend to have significantly decreased height velocities and delayed bone ages.

A number of genetic syndromes are also associated with increased weight gain. PWS, a result of uniparental disomy of the maternal allele or deletion of the paternal allele at the chromosomal region 15q:11-13, is a syndrome characterized by obesity, hypogonadism, developmental delay, short stature, and hypotonia. Affected children frequently fail thrive because of feeding problems within the first year of life, but rapidly gain weight thereafter. Bardet-Biedl syndrome is characterized by obesity, postaxial polydactyly, retinitis pigmentosa, hypogonadism, developmental delay, and short stature. This is an autosomal recessive trait which is caused by at least three separate genes that have been mapped to chromosomes 3, 15, and 16. Other genetic disorders, including Carpenter, Cohen, Alström, Albright hereditary osteodystrophy, and Down syndromes, are also associated with excessive weight gain.

Table 9-4.

Differential Diagnosis—Common Conditions

Idiopathic or Familial Obesity

Genetic syndromes	Down syndrome
Endocrine	Growth hormone deficiency
	Hypogonadism
	Hypothyroidism
Single gene mutations	MC4R

Table 9-5.

Differential Diagnosis—Rare Conditions

Hypothalamic lesions	Tumor
	Anoxic brain injury
	Meningitis
	Head trauma
Genetic syndromes	Prader-Willi
	Bardet-Biedel
	Carpenter
	Cohen
	Alström
	Albright hereditary osteodystrophy
Endocrine	Glucocorticoid excess
Single gene mutations	Leptin
	Leptin receptor
	Proopiomelanocortin
	Prohormone convertase-1

As with endocrine disorders leading to obesity, these syndromes are generally associated with short stature. Many are also characterized by developmental delay.

Hypothalamic injury may also result in rapid weight gain and obesity. Lesions involving the arcuate nucleus and/or the paraventricular nucleus of the hypothalamus can disrupt the ability of the brain to detect peripheral adiposity signals. Individuals with the hypothalamic obesity syndrome develop increased food-seeking behavior with lack of satiety. Furthermore, they still tend to gain weight even with "normal" caloric intake, suggesting a decrease in energy expenditure. Craniopharyngiomas are the most common lesions associated with the hypothalamic obesity syndrome. Although occasionally the tumor itself directly damages the circuits that control hunger, satiety and energy expenditure, surgical removal of these lesions more commonly results in obesity. Other forms of traumatic brain injury, including anoxic brain injury, meningitis, and severe head trauma can, on occasion, result in varying degrees of obesity.

The majority of cases of obesity, however, have an "idiopathic" basis, although it is clear that there are major genetic influences that determine body size. The tendency toward developing "idiopathic" or "familial" obesity is polygenic. Despite the fact that many of the genes that regulate weight and energy homeostasis are known, at present it is unclear how often defects in these genes contribute to common obesity. Only a minority of single gene mutations have been found in the coding regions of the known weight regulatory genes that could account for obesity. Genome scans looking for obesity genes, however, have uncovered a number of genetic loci that may contribute to the obesity tendency. There is a strong association between body fat and specific DNA markers on chromosomes 1p, 2p, 3p, 6p, 7q, and 11q.[34] If human syntenic regions corresponding to mouse quantitative train locus (QTL) maps are included, all human chromosomes, except 9, 18, 21, and Y, have at least one candidate locus for genes regulating weight homeostasis. The large number of obesity loci in the human genome emphasizes that fact that the cause of most human obesity is likely to be polygenic.

At present, single gene mutations account for less than 10% of all cases of obesity. By far the most common of these single gene mutations are defects in the *melanocortin 4 receptor (MC4R)* gene, accounting for approximately 6% of cases of severe obesity with onset during childhood.[35] While all individuals with homozygous defects have severe obesity, detailed family studies of heterozygous individuals indicate a variable penetrance of the *MC4R* gene mutation. In one study, only 68% of individuals with heterozygous mutations were classified as obese,[36] indicating a large effect of other genetic and environmental modifiers on the actual degree of adiposity in heterozygous individuals.

The onset of obesity in subjects with *MC4R* mutations occurs in early childhood. Affected individuals tend to have increased lean body mass and increased bone density. Increased linear growth is also observed although no changes in GH secretion have been noted. Thyroid function is normal. Unlike what is seen in leptin deficiency, puberty is not affected and fertility is preserved.

Severe hyperinsulinemia occurs in all obese individuals with *MC4R* defects.[36] In addition, subjects with MC4R deficiency appear to be hyperphagic when compared to unaffected siblings.[35,36] Many of these individuals exhibit food-seeking behaviors. Unlike the MC4R knockout mouse, humans with *MC4R* gene mutations exhibit no deficits in energy expenditure.[36] However, it remains possible that differences in energy expenditure are either too small to detect or would only be apparent after caloric restriction and a decrease in percent body fat to normal.

The obesity and hyperinsulinemia phenotype in MC4R deficiency appears to improve with age.[36] The decrease in insulin levels parallels an improvement in the hyperphagia. The effect of the *MC4R* gene defect on long-term obesity-associated morbidity and mortality is presently unknown.

Single gene mutations other than *MC4R* that are known to result in obesity are collectively quite rare. Mutations have been described in leptin and in the leptin receptor resulting in early onset obesity, hyperphagia, hyperinsulinemia, delayed puberty, and short stature.[35] *POMC* gene mutations result in childhood-onset obesity, adrenal insufficiency, and red hair.[35] Finally, *prohormone convertase* gene mutations have been shown to result in extreme childhood obesity, abnormal glucose homeostasis with very low insulin levels, hypogonadotropic hypogonadism, and adrenal insufficiency.[37]

Treatment

Treatment of overweight and obese children and adolescents remains a difficult and challenging proposition. Inherited weight set points resist efforts to change body composition. Loss of adipose tissue brings about compensatory decreases in metabolic rate and increases in appetite. Nevertheless, the primary focus of treatment in obese children is decreased caloric intake in combination with increased energy expenditure through increased activity (Figure 9-8). In children who are still growing, it is important that any limit in caloric intake be carefully determined to allow enough calories for adequate growth. Treatment should begin early before the development of severe obesity. The treatment plan should involve the entire family and progress in a stepwise manner as habits are changed and skills are learned.

Lifestyle Change

There remains considerable debate regarding whether fats or carbohydrates should be the primary nutritional component limited in the diet to achieve decreased caloric intake. Energy expenditure and body composition do not appear to change with isoenergetic constant protein meals even with extreme changes in the fat-to-carbohydrate ratio.[38] When limiting caloric intake to induce weight loss, however, some studies suggest a benefit of limiting carbohydrate instead of limiting fat to achieve target calorie goals. Although reported weight loss between low-carbohydrate and low-fat diets is similar, paradoxically the low-fat diet results in a less favorable result on lipid profiles.[39] Diets high in carbohydrate result in increased hepatic lipogenesis and increased triglycerides.[40] There may also be a shift to smaller more atherogenic LDL particles with low-fat diets.

Alternatively, low-fat diets may have some advantages over low-carbohydrate diets.[41] Fat consumption may be less satiating than carbohydrate and a high fat-to-carbohydrate ratio in the diet may promote overconsumption. This would result in a positive energy balance and weight gain in susceptible individuals. Fat is more easily absorbed from the intestine than is carbohydrate and fecal energy loss is lower in diets with a higher percentage of dietary fat. Fatty foods are calorically more dense with a greater amount of calories per gram than are carbohydrates. Thus, more calories can be consumed over a short period of time with fatty foods than with high-carbohydrate foods. These findings would suggest a benefit of low-fat diets. Conflicting results of various studies make it difficult to recommend one method of

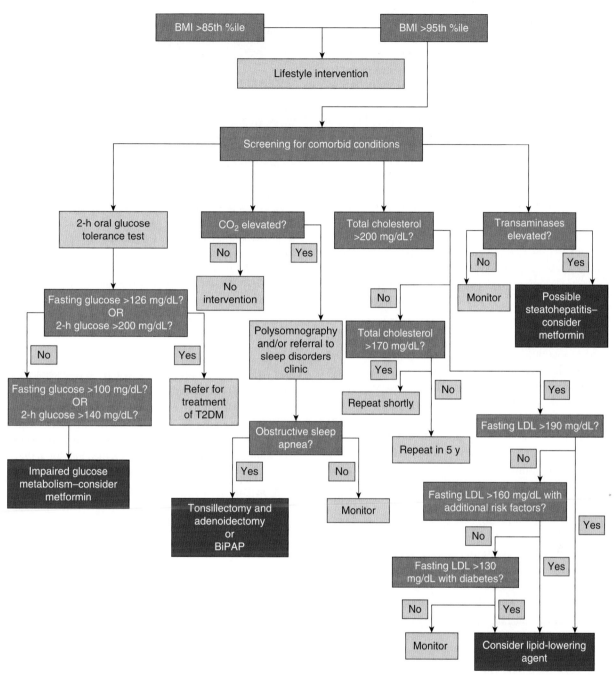

FIGURE 9-8 ■ Treatment algorithm for obesity and comorbid conditions.

decreased caloric intake over another. Regardless of the actual composition of the diet, any decrease in caloric intake should be of some benefit to the overweight patient provided adequate protein is supplied to allow for growth.

The type of carbohydrate consumed may also be an important mediator of increased weight gain. High intake of fructose has been implicated in mediating obesity in children. Most of the soft drinks on the market today contain high-fructose corn syrup. Both fructose and glucose are metabolized via glycolysis and the Krebs cycle to form energy. Alternatively, these compounds can form substrate for lipogenesis and, therefore, energy storage as adipose tissue. Glucokinase, catalyzing the rate-limiting enzyme for glycolysis, is inhibited by increased ATP generation. Inhibition of glucokinase tends to limit the entry of glucose into the cell when energy stores are sufficient and, therefore, less substrate is available for lipogenesis. Fructokinase, however, is not limited by increased energy stores. Therefore, fructose is available to be used and easily converted into triglycerides regardless of the energy state of the cell.

The actual recommended daily caloric intake will vary from patient to patient depending on age and degree of adiposity. Furthermore, total daily energy expenditure required for normal growth and development in each individual varies. Depending on the severity of the obese condition, the daily recommended caloric intake in an overweight child should allow for either weight maintenance or a rate of weight gain less than normal for age. This allows the child to gradually approach a healthier weight without the adverse effects on growth that can be seen with severe caloric restriction. In general, actual weight loss is not recommended in growing children unless life-threatening comorbid conditions exist.

One approach to calculating daily recommended caloric intake is to estimate the total average daily caloric intake in excess of that needed for normal growth and development. This can be estimated using the equation that, for every 3500 kcal of food consumed and not used for growth and development, 1 lb of fat is stored. If a child has gained more weight during a period of time than would have been expected using standard growth charts, that child has likely consumed excessive calories and converted the calories into adipose tissue. The excessive calories consumed can be calculated by determining the total excess weight gained over a defined number of days (in pounds), multiply by 3500, and divide by the number of days. This daily caloric excess can be subtracted from the patient's current daily caloric intake as estimated by a nutritionist using dietary recall. In theory, a diet based on these calculations should provide caloric intake equal to that required for normal growth and development. In practice, it serves as a starting point. Repeat monthly weight measurements, assuming full compliance, will provide more information regarding the ideal caloric intake required for weight maintenance or weight loss in any obese child.

Exercise is also critical to successful weight loss or weight maintenance. The benefit of exercise is twofold. Increased activity increases energy expenditure. In addition, increased activity may result in increased muscle mass. Increased muscle mass will result in an increase in the resting energy expenditure. Overweight children need to be encouraged to become more active. Studies have shown that simply targeting sedentary behaviors (ie, decreasing television-viewing and video-game-playing), rather than enforcing physical activity, is enough to result in an improvement in body composition.[42] Any recommendation to exercise should emphasize activities that are fun. If the activities are uncomfortable or are uninteresting to the child, they are unlikely to be sustained.

Behavioral modification is necessary to achieve and maintain long-term weight loss (Table 9-6). Habits

Table 9-6.

Suggestions for Positive Changes in Behavior

Eat meals as a family.

Eat slowly. Take at least 20 min for satiety cues to take effect.

Increase consumption of water rather than soft drinks, sport drinks, *etc.*

Do not use food as a reward. Do not limit food as a punishment.

Do not eat while watching TV, playing computer games, *etc.*

Limit sedentary activities to less than 2 h per day.

Walk 20-30 min per day.

Walk to neighborhood stores and parks.

Park further away from destination (*i.e.,* malls, church, school, *etc.*) and walk the last few blocks.

Take stairs instead of escalators or elevators.

that encourage a sedentary lifestyle need to be changed. In addition, behaviors that result in increased consumption of calories should be altered. Any changes in behaviors should be targeted to the family if long-term weight loss and maintenance are the goal. Behavioral interventions aimed at the patient alone are unlikely to achieve long-term success. Indeed, the only weight loss intervention studies that demonstrate long-term success in maintaining weight loss are those targeted to changing behaviors in the entire family.[43]

Anorectic Medications and Bariatric Surgery

Intensive intervention, either medical or surgical, should be discouraged except in very limited situations. Only in patients that have documented life-threatening comorbid conditions should aggressive intervention be considered. These patients should have failed prolonged attempts at nutritional management and behavioral counseling. Orlistat, a lipase inhibitor, is the only FDA-approved weight loss drug for children aged 12 years and more. It has a modest effect on weight and compliance is limited by gastrointestinal side effects. Essentially no controlled clinical studies exist that provide information on the safety and efficacy of other anorectic medications in pediatric patients. The short-term effects on growth and the long-term effects on general health of these medications in children are unknown. Weight loss induced by any of these medications would require lifelong administration of these drugs for weight maintenance. Therefore, long-term potential side effects need to be considered and balanced against current health problems resulting from the overweight condition of the patient.

Bariatric surgery has been performed on a limited number of obese adolescent patients and has been associated with some success. Patients need to be carefully selected and surgery should be performed only at centers experienced in adolescent bariatric surgery. Close follow-up with a weight loss team is essential for long-term success. As with anorectic medications, the long-term consequences of these procedures in adolescents are unknown and, therefore, bariatric surgery should be cautiously considered only in cases in which significant comorbid conditions exist and where diet and exercise have failed.

Treatment of Comorbidities

Treatment of comorbidities related to insulin resistance

Many of the obesity-related comorbid conditions are related to insulin resistance and associated elevated insulin levels. Weight loss and exercise remain the primary treatments for insulin resistance-related complications. However, metformin, a biguanide drug that improves insulin sensitivity, is approved for use in children 10 years of age and older for treatment of T2DM. Although metformin is not specifically indicated for the treatment of obesity, glucose intolerance, metabolic syndrome, polycystic ovarian syndrome, hyperlipidemia, or nonalcoholic steatohepatitis in children and adolescents, there is literature to support a positive effect of metformin in all of these conditions. One study demonstrated a 1.3% reduction in BMI, 11% reduction in fasting glucose, and 38% reduction in fasting insulin levels following 6 months of modest-dose metformin therapy in adolescents aged 12 to 19 years with hyperinsulinemia and a family history of T2DM. None of the adolescents in this study had glucose intolerance or PCOS.[44] A study of obese adolescent girls with evidence of PCOS showed that the addition of metformin to a treatment regimen consisting of lifestyle intervention +/− oral contraceptives further reduced serum testosterone levels, decreased waist circumference, and increased HDL cholesterol.[45] Another study demonstrated a significant decrease in triglycerides and total cholesterol with metformin and low-calorie diet over only 8 weeks of intervention.[46] Finally, an open-label pilot study of metformin in children with biopsy-proven nonalcoholic steatohepatitis showed significant improvement in both serum aminotransferase levels and hepatic fat content assessed by MR spectroscopy, prompting a randomized controlled trial that is still underway.[12]

On a practical level, while metformin is considered a first-line agent for the treatment of pediatric T2DM, pediatric endocrinologists differ as to when they consider the addition of metformin therapy in the management of the nondiabetic obese child or adolescent. In light of evidence in the adult population that metformin therapy may decrease the progression of impaired glucose tolerance to frank diabetes mellitus by as much as one-third,[47] many pediatric providers are now using metformin in children and adolescents with glucose intolerance (Figure 9-7). Likewise, the use of metformin in female patients with evidence of PCOS is becoming more common. Further research in the pediatric population is necessary, however, before this therapy should be considered routine.

Treatment of hyperlipidemia

The most recent policy statement of the American Academy of Pediatrics recommends the following thresholds for consideration of lipid-lowering medications (Figure 9-7). For patients 8 years and older with an LDL concentration of greater than or equal to 190 mg/dL, pharmacological intervention should be considered. If there are two or more coexisting risk factors for early heart disease (ie, family history, obesity, physical inactivity, smoking, or hypertension), the recommended threshold for pharmacological intervention decreases to an LDL concentration of 160 mg/dL and, if diabetes is present, to 130 mg/dL. The initial goal is to lower the LDL concentration to 160 mg/dL. However, targets as low as 130 mg/dL or even 110 mg/dL may be warranted when there is a strong family history of cardiovascular disease, especially with other risk factors including obesity, diabetes mellitus, the metabolic syndrome, and other higher-risk situations.[8]

Treatment of pulmonary complications

Both reactive airway disease and sleep apnea respond positively to weight loss. Asthma should be aggressively treated with pharmacological agents, including inhaled steroids if needed. The lowest possible dose of inhaled steroids should be used as multiple studies have demonstrated a systemic effect of inhaled glucocorticoids at moderate to-high doses. Systemic absorption can increase weight gain and worsen insulin resistance. Sleep apnea should be suspected in individuals with severe snoring, morning headaches, or daytime somnolence. A sleep study should be obtained and treatment with BiPAP (bi-level positive airway pressure) considered in confirmed cases (Figure 9-7). If sleep apnea is severe, consider performing an electrocardiogram (ECG) and referring to a cardiologist if right-sided cardiac hypertrophy is detected.

When to refer

The only therapy that has shown long-term success in the treatment of obese children is family based behavior modification therapy. Unfortunately, such programs are not widely available or financially accessible. When attempts to manage pediatric obesity fail in the primary care setting, many children are referred to pediatric endocrinologists. However, in a retrospective study of 587 children referred to pediatric endocrinologists for obesity evaluation and treatment, the mean percentage overweight increased over the follow-up interval of 1.9 years. While 38% of children showed improvement in percentage overweight, only five subjects (<1%) reduced their BMI to less than 95th %ile.[48] As such, referral should be reserved for those likely to have an etiology other than idiopathic familial obesity, and, of course, for those demonstrating obesity-induced comorbidity.

Referral to endocrinologists. Primary care physicians should consider referral to a pediatric endocrinologist for patients who meet any of the criteria in Box 9-1.

Referral to other subspecialists. Referral to subspecialists other than pediatric endocrinologists is warranted if the initial workup of follow-up of obese patients reveals any of the findings listed in Box 9-2.

Box 9-2. Findings Warranting Nonendocrine Subspecialty Referral	
Clinical Findings	**Recommended Referral**
Signs/symptoms of increased intracranial pressure	Neurosurgery
CNS lesion by imaging	
Dysmorphic features	Genetics
Developmental delay	
Hypotonia	
History of early failure-to-thrive	
Short stature without evidence of endocrinopathy	
Non-restorative sleep/daytime somnolence	Pulmonology or Otolaryngology or Sleep disorders clinic
Loud snoring	(choice dependent on
Observed respiratory pauses during sleep	availability/local referral pattern)
Inability to sleep fully supine	
CO_2 retention	
Persistent hip pain	Orthopedics
Persistent knee pain	
Lower extremity deformity	

Box 9-1. Referral Criteria—Pediatric Endocrinology	
Abnormalities of insulin/glucose homeostasis	Acanthosis nigricans
	Elevated fasting insulin
	Impaired fasting glucose (>100 mg/dL)
	Glucose intolerance (2-hr post-Glucola >140 mg/dL)
	Type 2 diabetes mellitus (2-hr postglucola or random >200 mg/dL)
Ovarian hyperandrogenism	Hirsutism
	Acne
	Oligomenorrhea
	Secondary amenorrhea
	Delayed menarche
Evidence of growth hormone deficiency	Short stature
	Declining linear growth velocity
	Low IGF-I and/or IGFBP-3
Evidence of hypogonadism	Delayed puberty
	Delayed menarche
	"Stalled" pubertal development
Evidence of cortisol excess	Short stature or slowing of linear growth velocity
	Delayed or "stalled" puberty
	Hypertension (less reliable)
	Violaceous striae (less reliable)
Hyperlipidemia (criteria are for children 8 y and older)	LDL >190 mg/dL
	LDL >160 mg/dL + family history of early heart disease
	LDL >130 mg/dL + diabetes mellitus

CONCLUSIONS

Although positive results can sometimes be obtained in the treatment of overweight children, successful resolution of the childhood obesity epidemic will not be accomplished at the individual level. Profound changes within our society have resulted in the dramatic increase in the number of children classified as overweight. It will take equally profound changes to reverse this trend. Changes need to occur at every level within our society. Governments should support research programs into the causes and treatment of obesity. Insurance companies should be required to recognize obesity as a disorder and provide coverage for evaluation and long-term treatment of overweight children. Schools should have adequate resources to provide physical education to all children from kindergarten through high school. Adequate funding for school lunch programs would allow nutritious low-fat and lower-calorie meals to be provided to all students. Families should be encouraged to alter their lifestyles by eating healthier, consuming less fast food, and getting more exercise. Providing a safe environment with adequate parks, bike paths, and the like for these endeavors will certainly help promote a more active lifestyle. The genetic make-up of our population will not change over short periods of time. Therefore, the problem of childhood obesity will always remain. Positive changes within our society, however, can have a profound effect on the prevalence of childhood obesity and result in a much healthier population now and in the future.

REFERENCES

1. Flynn MA, McNeil DA, Maloff B, et al. Reducing obesity and related chronic disease risk in children and youth: a synthesis of evidence with 'best practice' recommendations. *Obes Rev.* 2006;1:7-66.
2. Uli N, Sundararajan S, Cuttler L. Treatment of childhood obesity. *Curr Opin Endocrinol Diab Obes.* 2008;15:37-47.
3. Whitlock EP, Williams SB, Gold R, Smith PR, Shipman SA. Screening and interventions for childhood overweight: a summary of evidence for the US Preventive Services Task Force. *Pediatrics.* 2005;116.
4. Mayer-Davis EJ. Type 2 diabetes in youth: epidemiology and current research toward prevention and treatment. *J Amer Diet Assoc.* 2008;108.
5. Sinha R, Fisch G, Teague B, et al. Prevalence of impaired glucose tolerance among children and adolescents with marked obesity. *N Engl J Med.* 2002; 346:802-810.
6. Uwaifo GI, Elberg J, Yanovski JA. Impaired glucose tolerance in obese children and adolescents. [comment]. *N Engl J Med.* 2002;347:290-292.
7. Flynn JT. Pediatric hypertension: recent trends and accomplishments, future challenges. *Am J Hypertens.* 2008;21:605-612.
8. Daniels SR, Greer FR, Committee on N. Lipid screening and cardiovascular health in childhood. *Pediatrics.* 2008;122:198-208.
9. de Ferranti SD, Gauvreau K, Ludwig DS, Neufeld EJ, Newburger JW, Rifai N. Prevalence of the metabolic syndrome in American adolescents: findings from the Third National Health and Nutrition Examination Survey. *Circulation.* 2004;110:2494-2497.
10. Zimmet P, Alberti G, Kaufman F, et al. The metabolic syndrome in children and adolescents. *Lancet.* 2007;369:2059-2061.
11. Leibel NI, Baumann EE, Kocherginsky M, Rosenfield RL. Relationship of adolescent polycystic ovary syndrome to parental metabolic syndrome. *J Clin Endocrinol Metab.* 2006;91:1275-1283.
12. Patton HM, Sirlin C, Behling C, Middleton M, Schwimmer JB, Lavine JE. Pediatric nonalcoholic fatty liver disease: a critical appraisal of current data and implications for future research. *J Pediatr Gastroenterol Nutr.* 2006;43:413-427.
13. Redline S, Tishler PV, Schluchter M, Aylor J, Clark K, Graham G. Risk factors for sleep-disordered breathing in children. Associations with obesity, race, and respiratory problems. *Am J Resp Crit Care Med.* 1999;159:1527-1532.
14. Wills M. Orthopedic complications of childhood obesity. *Pediatr Phys Ther.* 2004;16:230-235.
15. Schwartz MB, Chambliss HO, Brownell KD, Blair SN, Billington C. Weight bias among health professionals specializing in obesity. *Obes Res.* 2003;11:1033-1039.
16. Hayden-Wade HA, Stein RI, Ghaderi A, Saelens BE, Zabinski MF, Wilfley DE. Prevalence, characteristics, and correlates of teasing experiences among overweight children vs. non-overweight peers. *Obes Res.* 2005;13:1381-1392.
17. Schwimmer JB, Burwinkle TM, Varni JW. Health-related quality of life of severely obese children and adolescents. *JAMA.* 2003;289:1813-1819.
18. Gortmaker SL, Must A, Perrin JM, Sobol AM, Dietz WH. Social and economic consequences of overweight in adolescence and young adulthood. *N Engl J Med.* 1993; 329:1008-1012.
19. Wang G, Dietz WH. Economic burden of obesity in youths aged 6 to 17 years: 1979-1999.[erratum appears in Pediatrics 2002 Jun;109(6):1195]. *Pediatrics.* 2002;109: E81.
20. Allison DB, Kaprio J, Korkeila M, Koskenvuo M, Neale MC, Hayakawa K. The heritability of body mass index among an international sample of monozygotic twins reared apart. *Int J Obes Rel Metab Dis.* 1996;20:501-506.
21. Faith MS, Pietrobelli A, Nunez C, Heo M, Heymsfield SB, Allison DB. Evidence for independent genetic influences on fat mass and body mass index in a pediatric twin sample. *Pediatrics.* 1999;104:61-67.
22. Dorosty AR, Emmett PM, Cowin S, Reilly JJ. Factors associated with early adiposity rebound. ALSPAC Study Team. *Pediatrics.* 2000;105:1115-1118.
23. Freedman DS, Srinivasan SR, Valdez RA, Williamson DF, Berenson GS. Secular increases in relative weight and adiposity among children over two decades: the Bogalusa Heart Study. *Pediatrics.* 1997;99:420-426.
24. Kimm SY, Glynn NW, Kriska AM, et al. Longitudinal changes in physical activity in a biracial cohort during adolescence. *Med Sci Sports Exer.* 2000;32:1445-1454.
25. Leibel RL, Rosenbaum M, Hirsch J. Changes in energy expenditure resulting from altered body weight. *N Engl J Med.* 1995; 332:621-628.
26. Diamond JM. Human evolution. Diabetes running wild. *Nature.* 1992;357:362-363.
27. Wadden TA. Treatment of obesity by moderate and severe caloric restriction. Results of clinical research trials. *Ann Int Med.* 1993;119:688-693.
28. Pasquet P, Apfelbaum M. Recovery of initial body weight and composition after long-term massive overfeeding in men. *Am Jour Clin Nutr.* 1994;60:861-863.
29. Friedman JM, Halaas JL. Leptin and the regulation of body weight in mammals. *Nature.* 1998;395:763-770.
30. Baskin DG, Hahn TM, Schwartz MW. Leptin sensitive neurons in the hypothalamus. *Horm Metab Res.* 1999;31:345-350.
31. Nakazato M, Murakami N, Date Y, et al. A role for ghrelin in the central regulation of feeding. *Nature.* 2001;409:194-198.
32. Batterham RL, Cowley MA, Small CJ, et al. Gut hormone PYY(3-36) physiologically inhibits food intake. *Nature.* 2002;418:650-654.
33. American Academy of Pediatrics. Committee on N, American Academy of Pediatrics. Committee on Nutrition. Cholesterol in childhood. *Pediatrics.* 1998;101:141-147.
34. Bouchard C. Genetics of human obesity: recent results from linkage studies. *J Nutr.* 1997;127:S1887-S1890.
35. Farooqi S. Insights from the genetics of severe childhood obesity. *Horm Res.* 2007;5:5-7.
36. Farooqi IS, Keogh JM, Yeo GS, Lank EJ, Cheetham T, O'Rahilly S. Clinical spectrum of obesity and mutations in the melanocortin 4 receptor gene. *N Engl J Med.* 2003; 348:1085-1095.

37. Jackson RS, Creemers JW, Ohagi S, et al. Obesity and impaired prohormone processing associated with mutations in the human prohormone convertase 1 gene. *Nat Genet.* 1997;16:303-306.

38. Leibel RL, Hirsch J, Appel BE, Checani GC. Energy intake required to maintain body weight is not affected by wide variation in diet composition. *Am J Clin Nutr.* 1992;55: 350-355.

39. Samaha FF, Iqbal N, Seshadri P, et al. A low-carbohydrate as compared with a low-fat diet in severe obesity. *New Engl J Med.* 2003;348:2074-2081.

40. Schwarz JM, Linfoot P, Dare D, Aghajanian K. Hepatic de novo lipogenesis in normoinsulinemic and hyperinsulinemic subjects consuming high-fat, low-carbohydrate and low-fat, high-carbohydrate isoenergetic diets. *Am J Clin Nutr.* 2003;77:43-50.

41. Astrup A. The role of dietary fat in the prevention and treatment of obesity. Efficacy and safety of low-fat diets. *Int J Obes Rel Metab Dis.* 2001;25:S46-S50.

42. Epstein LH, Paluch RA, Gordy CC, Dorn J. Decreasing sedentary behaviors in treating pediatric obesity. *Arch Pediatr Adol Med.* 2000;154:220-226.

43. Epstein LH, Valoski A, Wing RR, McCurley J. Ten-year outcomes of behavioral family-based treatment for childhood obesity. *Health Psychol.* 1994;13:373-383.

44. Freemark M, Bursey D. The effects of metformin on body mass index and glucose tolerance in obese adolescents with fasting hyperinsulinemia and a family history of type 2 diabetes. *Pediatrics.* 2001;107.

45. Hoeger K, Davidson K, Kochman L, Cherry T, Kopin L, Guzick DS. The impact of metformin, oral contraceptives and lifestyle modification, on polycystic ovary syndrome in obese adolescent women in two randomized, placebo-controlled clinical trials. *J Clin Endocrinol Metab.* 2008.

46. Kay JP, Alemzadeh R, Langley G, D'Angelo L, Smith P, Holshouser S. Beneficial effects of metformin in normoglycemic morbidly obese adolescents. *Metab Clin Exp.* 2001;50:1457-1461.

47. Knowler WC, Barrett-Connor E, Fowler SE, et al. Reduction in the incidence of type 2 diabetes with lifestyle intervention or metformin. *N Engl J Med.* 2002;346:393-403.

48. Quattrin T, Liu E, Shaw N, Shine B, Chiang E. Obese children who are referred to the pediatric endocrinologist: characteristics and outcome. *Pediatrics.* 2005;115:348-351.

CHAPTER 10

Diabetes Mellitus

THE EDITORS

The inclusion of "diabetes mellitus" as part of pediatric endocrinology is a relatively recent concept. The first two editions (1950 and 1957) of Lawson Wilkins' classic text "The Diagnosis and Treatment of Endocrine Disorders in Childhood and Adolescence" only mentioned diabetes mellitus in pregnancy in the context of neonatal hypoglycemia. Wilkins' third edition, published just after his death in 1965 devoted less than a page to diabetes.

Later, we began to recognize "juvenile onset" diabetes as a pediatric-appropriate inclusion in textbooks, and now we realize that that designation includes many subtypes of diabetes, including classic Type 1 but also MODY and other forms. What was known at one time as "adult-onset" or "non-insulin-dependent" diabetes is neither limited to adults, nor is necessarily non-insulin dependent, and is now more appropriately designated Type 2 diabetes.

The editors therefore enlisted a village of experts in the various aspects of "Diabetes Mellitus" to contribute to this chapter, which, of necessity, is given in four parts: (A). Introduction; (B). Type 1 Diabetes; (C). Type 2 Diabetes; and (D). Other specific types of diabetes and causes of hyperglycemia.

Selected Readings will be listed at the end of each part.

Part A. Introduction to Diabetes

David W. Cooke, Leslie Plotnick, Dana Dabelea, Georgeanna J. Klingensmith, Lisa Gallo, Janet H. Silverstein, and William Winter

A majority of cases of diabetes mellitus fall into one of two categories: (1) type 1 diabetes, which is most commonly caused by autoimmune destruction of the pancreatic islet cells resulting in β-cell failure and an absolute deficiency of insulin (type 1 A diabetes, T1DM), and (2) type 2 diabetes (T2DM), which results from a combination of insulin resistance in target tissues and a lack of an adequate compensatory insulin response to overcome this resistance. The American Diabetes Association (ADA)[1] recognizes more than 50 other specific types of diabetes (Table 10-1). All of these disorders collectively account for only 1% to 5% of cases of diabetes (see "Part D" of this chapter later on).

Ensuring a correct diagnosis and defining the correct type of diabetes is important for choosing the most appropriate therapy, managing the expected complications, anticipating associated disorders, and predicting disease risk in relatives or reoccurrence in offspring. Although clinical differences at the time of diagnosis usually allows the presumptive classification of patients as T1DM or T2DM, the classification is not always clear-cut. Likewise, it is important to know when to consider one of the more unusual forms of diabetes, as differentiating them from the more common type 1 and type 2 diabetes can present a significant diagnostic challenge.

A complete discussion of the different types of diabetes is presented in the subsequent parts of this chapter. Part B: Type 1 Diabetes and Part C: Type 2 Diabetes present the epidemiology, specific clinical presentations, and

Table 10-1.

Classification of Diabetes Mellitus

Initial presentation in patients < 6 mo old
Neonatal diabetes
 Transient
 Permanent
Genetic defects in insulin action
 Rabson-Mendenhall syndrome
 Donahue syndrome (Leprechaunism)

Initial presentation in patients > 6 mo old
Type 1 diabetes
 Immune-mediated
 Slowly progressive type 1 diabetes
 Non-immune-mediated
Type 2 diabetes
Monogenic diabetes
Atypical diabetes (Flatbush)
Maturity onset diabetes of youth (MODY)
 MODY1
 MODY2
 MODY3
 MODY4
 MODY5
 MODY6
Mitochondrial diabetes
Genetic defects in insulin action
 Type A insulin resistance
 Lipoatrophic diabetes
Diseases of the exocrine pancreas
 Cystic fibrosis
 Trauma/pancreatectomy
 Neoplasia
 Pancreatitis
 Hemochromatosis
Endocrinopathies
 Acromegaly
 Cushing syndrome
 Glucagonoma
 Pheochromocytoma
 Hyperthyroidism
 Somatostatinoma
 Aldosteronoma
Drug- or chemical-induced
 Corticosteroid-induced
 Others
Infections/critical illness
Uncommon forms of immune-mediated diabetes
 "Stiff man" syndrome
 Type B insulin resistance
 Autoimmune hypoglycemia
Genetic syndromes associated with diabetes
 Down syndrome
 Klinefelter syndrome
 Turner syndrome
 Wolfram syndrome
 Friedreich ataxia
 Huntington chorea

(Continued)

Table 10-1. (Continued)

Classification of Diabetes Mellitus

 Laurence-Moon-Biedl syndrome
 Myotonic dystrophy
 Porphyria
 Prader-Willi syndrome
 IPEX
Gestational diabetes mellitus

treatments of type 1 and type 2 diabetes, respectively. Part D: Other Specific Types of Diabetes Mellitus and Causes of Hyperglycemia, discusses diabetes in infants less than 6 months at diagnosis as well as the differential diagnosis of patients with an autosomal dominant or maternally transmitted patterns of diabetes inheritance as well as diabetes associated with medication or other endocrine disorders.

DIAGNOSTIC CRITERIA FOR DIABETES

The criteria for making the diagnosis of diabetes are the same, regardless of the etiology. The diagnostic criteria are presented in Table 10-2. Type 1 and type 2 diabetes mellitus are, by far, the most common forms, but atypical presentations or clinical course should alert the clinician that one of the less common forms may be the actual diagnosis.

Table 10-2.

Criteria for the Diagnosis of Diabetes Mellitus

Any of the following findings on two separate occasions*:
 Random plasma glucose concentration ≥ 200 mg/dL in the absence of symptoms of hyperglycemia
 OR
 Fasting plasma glucose ≥ 126 mg/dL
 OR
 2-h post-prandial glucose ≥ 200 mg/dL after a 75 g glucose load (or 1.75 g/kg)

In the presence of unequivocal symptoms of hyperglycemia, a random laboratory plasma glucose ≥ 200 mg/dL is adequate to diagnose diabetes, or if a patient presents in DKA or hyperosmolar nonketotic coma make a diagnosis of diabetes mellitus.
In the absence of unequivocal hyperglycemia, elevated plasma glucose concentrations should be confirmed by repeat testing on a different day.
A 2-h plasma glucose is obtained after 1.75 g/kg of glucose (maximum of 75 g) is ingested orally in the fasting state.
Adapted from American Diabetes Association. Diagnosis and classification of diabetes mellitus. Diabetes Care. 2008; 31:S55-S60.

In the absence of a preceding history of polydipsia and polyuria, a diagnosis of diabetes mellitus should not be made based on hyperglycemia documented during a serious illness. This stress-induced hyperglycemia is usually moderate in degree, typically no higher than 200 to 250 mg/dL, although levels above 600 mg/dL have been reported. Typically, the glucose rapidly normalizes in these patients as the illness resolves. If blood glucose testing after resolution of the intercurrent illness does not confirm the presence of hyperglycemia or diabetes, the risk that such a child will develop diabetes in the future is very low, unless the child has measurable diabetes-associated antibodies, or is an adolescent with high risk factors for type 2 diabetes.

CLASSIFICATION OF DIABETES TYPES

The differential diagnosis of hyperglycemia and diabetes mellitus is listed in Table 10-1 and Figures 10-1 and 10-2. While this is an extensive list, the vast majority of children have type 1 diabetes, up to 50% of newly diagnosed teens in minority groups may have type 2 diabetes, and the other forms are rare. Nevertheless, it is important to recognize unusual presentations or an atypical clinical

course for childhood diabetes and look further for these rarer forms of diabetes. When generating a differential diagnosis it is important to discriminate between diseases in which diabetes is the primary abnormality and those where diabetes is a secondary abnormality presenting as a symptom of another disorder or syndrome (Figure 10-3). It is also important to recognize the different causes of diabetes in patients who develop diabetes before versus after 6 months of age (See Part D).

CLINICAL PRESENTATION

Signs and Symptoms

As β-cell function declines the serum glucose level rises. The symptoms of **hyperglycemia** are similar regardless of the underlying cause and include polyuria, polydipsia, polyphagia, and (in cases of severe insulin deficiency) weight loss, blurry vision, and fatigue. Patients may be asymptomatic if mild hyperglycemia is present. Once the blood glucose concentration exceeds the capacity of the kidneys to reabsorb glucose, which is at approximately 180 mg/dL, some of this glucose is lost in the urine. This glucosuria serves as an osmotic force that increases water excretion. As urinary fluid losses

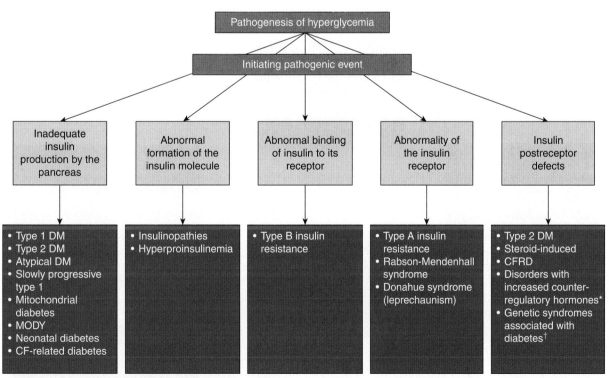

*Acromegaly, Cushing syndrome, Glucagonoma, etc.
†Down syndrome, Klinefelter syndrome, Turner syndrome, etc.

FIGURE 10-1 ■ Pathogenesis of hyperglycemia.

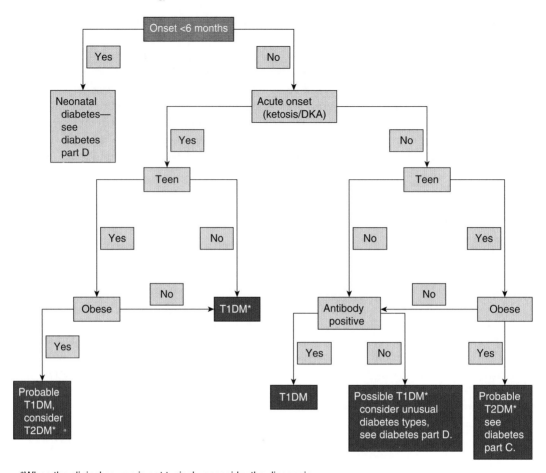

*When the clinical course is not typical, reconsider the diagnosis.
Additional testing may be required, see diabetes parts B–D.

FIGURE 10-2 ■ Diagnostic algorithm when primary presentation is diabetes mellitus.

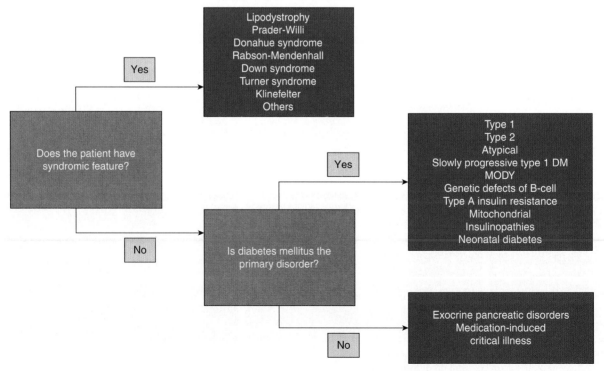

FIGURE 10-3 ■ Patient presentation as an aid in differentiating the different causes of diabetes.

increase, the thirst center is activated to work to maintain normal hydration. The glucosuria also leads to a loss of calories, this combined with the loss of the anabolic actions of insulin results in weight loss. This physiology explains the signs and symptoms of diabetes: polydipsia, polyuria, polyphagia, and weight loss.

Typical complaints that suggest polyuria include the reemergence of bedwetting, new or increased nocturia, and disruption of class work in school for frequent visits to the bathroom or requests to get water to drink. These symptoms are typically only present for less than a month. This acute presentation is most common in T1DM, however, T2DM and several of the more unusual forms of diabetes can also present acutely.

In evaluating a child for diabetes it is important to obtain a thorough history and review of symptoms and to perform a full physical examination to ensure that the diagnosis of diabetes type is made as accurately as possible. The history should focus on the acuity of the symptoms, as patients with diabetes resulting from insulin resistance often have an insidious course whereas diabetes owing to insulin insufficiency is usually more acute in onset. Insulin resistant adolescents may exhibit other signs of insulin resistance such as obesity, acanthosis nigricans of the neck, axillary area, knees, or inguinal creases, hypertension, and, in females, a history of oligomenorrhea or even amenorrhea. (If sexually active, pregnancy should be ruled out if amenorrhea is present.) Calculation of the body mass index (BMI* = kg/m^2) may help to quantify the degree of overweight/obesity and percentiles for age, gender, and ethnicity are published (Figures 10-4 and 10-5).[1] Stress-induced diabetes and medication-induced hyperglycemia are not usually associated with symptoms of polyuria, polydipsia, or weight loss before the precipitating event resulted in elevated blood glucose concentrations.

It is important to obtain a list of the patient's prescribed and over-the-counter (OTC) medications to determine if the diabetes is as a result of to medication use (See "Diabetes Part D" for medications causing hyperglycemia). In addition, a detailed family history will allow detection of similarly affected family members, which becomes especially important when trying to ascertain if type 2 diabetes, maturity onset diabetes of the young (MODY) (autosomal dominant), or mitochondrial diabetes (maternal transmission) are possible diagnoses. In all patients, but especially in infants, close attention

should be given to the presence or absence of dysmorphic features or prototypical features which can be seen in the various genetic and endocrine disorders that have diabetes as one of their manifestations (Figure 10-3).

If severe hyperglycemia is left untreated, the patient can develop nonketotic hyperosmolar syndrome or ketoacidosis, so inquiries regarding the presence of nausea, vomiting, abdominal pain, volume of urine output, fluid intake, difficulty breathing, and alterations in mental status should be made. *If type 1 diabetes is suspected, laboratory confirmation of diabetes should be obtained urgently.* The initial physical assessment should include vital signs, with specific attention paid to the heart rate and blood pressure, as these may be abnormal if dehydration is present. If tachycardia is present in the setting of suspected fluid depletion, the blood pressure should be taken with the patient in both a supine and upright position to assess hydration status. Orthostatic hypotension in adults is defined as a decrease in blood pressure in the upright position of more than 20/10 mm Hg. In a child that presents with nausea and vomiting, diabetic ketoacidosis (DKA) should be considered if there is a preceding history of polydipsia and polyuria, particularly in the absence of supportive evidence of a viral illness, such as lack of sick contacts, diarrhea, and fever. Additionally, the history of polyuria in a dehydrated appearing child should alert the clinician to the possibility of diabetes with DKA as the etiology of the vomiting. The presence of Kussmaul respirations can serve as indicators of the patient's acid/base balance and suggest the presence of a significant metabolic acidosis (see Part B later in this chapter).

Laboratory Findings and Diagnostic Tests

In the presence of a history indicating polydipsia and polyuria, a single random, or casual, plasma glucose concentration greater than 200 mg/dL confirms the diagnosis of diabetes. However, there are situations when glucosuria or hyperglycemia are identified as an incidental finding in an individual without symptoms of diabetes. In these situations, the diagnosis of diabetes is based on finding an elevated plasma glucose level (Table 10-2): a fasting level of greater than 125 mg/dL, a random value greater than 199 mg/dL, or a level greater than 199 mg/dL at 2 hours during an oral glucose tolerance test (OGTT). Only in the absence of symptoms should an abnormal value should be confirmed on a second day. A hemoglobin A1c value may be useful as additional confirmation of diabetes, but at this time is not a diagnostic test for diabetes.

Glycosuria and ketonuria are highly indicative of diabetes but a serum glucose level of greater than 200 mg/dL

---

*The body mass index (BMI) is a measure of adiposity, and an abnormal BMI confers increased morbidity in general, including an increased risk for the development of type 2 diabetes. BMI is calculated as (weight in kg/height [in meters squared]). Charts of BMI versus age for boys and for girls are shown in Figures 10-4 and 10-5.

2 to 20 years: Boys
Body mass index-for-age percentiles

NAME _____

RECORD # _____

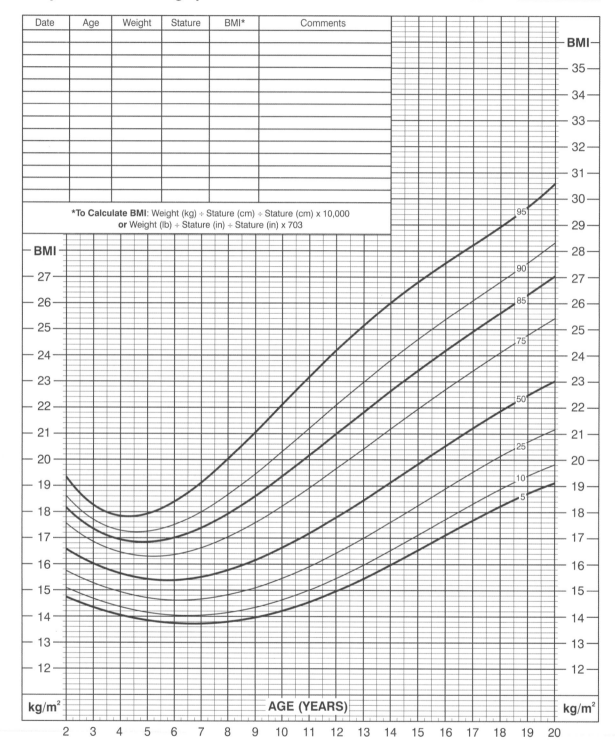

*To Calculate BMI: Weight (kg) ÷ Stature (cm) ÷ Stature (cm) x 10,000
or Weight (lb) ÷ Stature (in) ÷ Stature (in) x 703

AGE (YEARS)

Published May 30, 2000 (modified 10/16/00).

SOURCE: Developed by the National Center for Health Statistics in collaboration with
the National Center for Chronic Disease Prevention and Health Promotion (2000).
http://www.cdc.gov/growthcharts

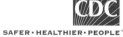

SAFER · HEALTHIER · PEOPLE™

FIGURE 10-4 ■ Body mass index (BMI)-for-age percentiles for boys aged 2 to 20 years. (*From Centers for Disease Control and Prevention, Atlanta, Georgia.*)[2]

2 to 20 years: Girls
Body mass index-for-age percentiles

NAME _____

RECORD # _____

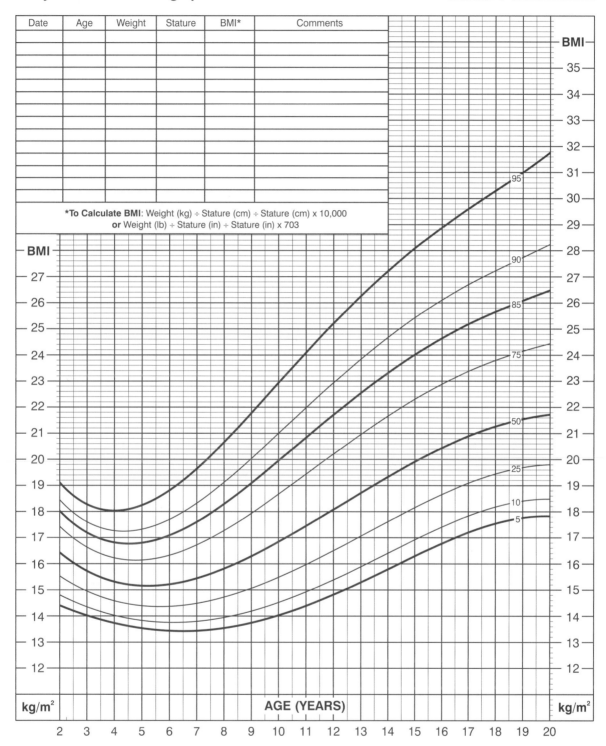

*To Calculate BMI: Weight (kg) ÷ Stature (cm) ÷ Stature (cm) x 10,000
or Weight (lb) ÷ Stature (in) ÷ Stature (in) x 703

Published May 30, 2000 (modified 10/16/00).
SOURCE: Developed by the National Center for Health Statistics in collaboration with
the National Center for Chronic Disease Prevention and Health Promotion (2000).
http://www.cdc.gov/growthcharts

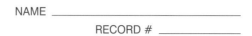

SAFER · HEALTHIER · PEOPLE™

FIGURE 10-5 ■ Body mass index (BMI)-for-age percentiles for girls aged 2 to 20 years. (*From Centers for Disease Control and Prevention, Atlanta, Georgia.*)[2]

is required to confirm a diagnosis of diabetes, while documentation of acidosis (venous pH < 7.3) and ketonemia or ketonuria document DKA.

In an individual with evolving type 1 diabetes, the period of time prior to the development of symptoms of diabetes during which there are abnormalities of glucose control is usually relatively brief. Therefore, it is not useful to screen for type 1 diabetes except within a research trial.

Differential Diagnosis of Type 2 and Type 1 Diabetes

In the past, a diagnosis of diabetes mellitus in a child rarely involved consideration of causes other than type 1 diabetes. However, there are now increasing numbers of children and adolescents identified with type 2 diabetes. Therefore, there are clinical scenarios where etiologies other than type 1 diabetes must be considered, including children with risk factors for type 2 diabetes (Figure 10-2).

Clinical differences at the time of diagnosis, more completely discussed in parts B and C, usually do allow presumptive classification of most patients as T1DM or T2DM. However, classification is not always clear-cut. Obese and minority pubertal children and adolescents, those with a parent with type 2 diabetes and those with signs of insulin resistance (acanthosis nigricans, hypertension, or hyperlipidemia) are more likely to have T2DM. However, the weight distribution of children with T1DM is proportionate to the weight distribution in the general population. Thus, approximately 25% of children with T1DM would be expected to be overweight, although rarely as overweight as most patients with T2DM. Additionally, while family history is important in identifying the possibility for T2DM, the family history of diabetes alone is not sufficient to differentiate the two.

Glycated hemoglobin (HbA1c) levels are not helpful in differentiating between the two diabetes types.

Ketosis or ketoacidosis is more common with T1DM, however, up to 33% of type 2 patients have ketosis at disease onset and 10% may present with DKA because of hyperglycemia-induced β cell toxicity, resulting in very low insulin levels. Owing to this suppressed β cell function, C-peptide levels may not be helpful in classification at onset of diabetes since they may be low at diagnosis of T2DM and normal during the honeymoon phase of T1DM. Individuals who do not follow the typical course expected for T2DM may be tested for C-peptide levels 2 years following diagnosis of diabetes. The C-peptide level at this time may be helpful in differentiating diabetes type since T2DM patients generally still have modestly elevated insulin levels while T1DM individuals usually have low insulin levels 2 years after diagnosis.

Further discussion of the differentiation of T1DM versus T2DM is presented in Part C: Type 2 Diabetes.

Differential Diagnosis of Other Genetic Forms of Diabetes

In young infants or children with a family history suggesting an autosomal dominant or maternally inherited pattern of diabetes, a diagnosis of neonatal diabetes, MODY, or maternally inherited diabetes could be considered (Table 10-1). These forms of diabetes are not autoimmune mediated, generally are not associated with increased insulin resistance, and have characteristic clinical presentations and findings. A definite diagnosis requires specific genetic testing. The clinical presentations and diagnostic tests are described in more detail in Part D.

REFERENCE

1. American Diabetes Association: Diagnosis and classification of diabetes mellitus. *Diabetes Care.* 2008;31(1):S55-S60.
2. National Center for Health Statistics. 2000 CDC Growth Charts. Hyattsville, MD:Centers for Disease Control and Prevention; 2009. http://www.cdc.gov/GrowthCharts/

Part B. Type 1 Diabetes Mellitus*

David W. Cooke and Leslie Plotnick

EPIDEMIOLOGY

The prevalence of type 1 diabetes in children 0 to 19 years of age in the United States is approximately 2 per 1000.[1] The incidence of type 1 diabetes varies substantially across the globe, with rates near 1 per 100,000 person-years in China and parts of South America, while rates above 30 per 100,000 person-years are found in Sweden, Finland, and Sardinia. The most recent data indicate that the incidence of type 1 diabetes in non-Hispanic white children in the United States is now greater than

*This part is reproduced with permission in part from Cooke DW, Plotnick L. Type 1 diabetes in pediatrics. *Pediatr Rev.* 2008;29:374-84; and Cooke DW, Plotnick L. Management of diabetic ketoacidosis in children and adolescents. *Pediatr Rev.* 2008;29:431-5.

20 per 100,000 children per year.[2] Prior estimates have been lower; for example a study from Allegheny County Pennsylvania in the early 1990s found a rate of 16.5 per 100,000 person-years. This increase is consistent with evidence of a world-wide trend of an increase in the incidence of type 1 diabetes over the past few decades—albeit a less dramatic increase than that of type 2 diabetes.

The incidence of type 1 diabetes in the United States is highest in non-Hispanic white children. The incidence in African American and Hispanic children 0 to 14 years of age is only approximately one-half that of non-Hispanic white children, although the difference is less in children 15 to 19 years of age. The incidence is lowest in American Indian and Asian/Pacific Islander children.

Males and females have an equal incidence of type 1 diabetes. There are two peaks in the age-specific incidence of type 1 diabetes: the largest is at 10 to 14 years of age, with a smaller peak in earlier childhood. There is some seasonal variation in the onset of type 1 diabetes, with fewer cases presenting during the summer months; this seasonal variation has decreased over the past 10 years.

PATHOGENESIS AND NATURAL HISTORY OF TYPE 1 DIABETES

Type 1 diabetes is owing to an absolute deficiency of insulin. In almost all cases, this is owing to an autoimmune process that results in the destruction of the insulin-producing β-cells of the pancreatic islets. This type 1A diabetes is what is traditionally referred to when discussing "type 1" diabetes. A rare form of insulinopenic

diabetes, type 1B, can occur without evidence of autoimmunity; these patients are most often of African or Asian ancestry. The cause of type 1B diabetes is not known. It is strongly inherited, but does not share the same genetic linkage to the HLA locus as type 1A diabetes.

Type 1 diabetes is felt to occur when an environmental trigger initiates an autoimmune response to the pancreatic β-cells in a genetically susceptible individual.[3] Once initiated, immune-mediated destruction of the β-cells ultimately leads to a degree of insulinopenia that prevents normal glucose homeostasis, and the patient develops hyperglycemia (Figure 10-6). The inhibition of lipolysis is sensitive to low amounts of insulin, so that initially hyperglycemia exists without significantly disordered lipid metabolism. However, if the diabetes is unrecognized for a period of time, the insulinopenia worsens and the patient is at risk of developing ketoacidosis from the combined effects of unrestrained lipolysis and hyperglycemia.

Greater than 80% of the pancreatic β-cells must be lost before a patient becomes sufficiently insulinopenic to develop hyperglycemia. The time from the initiation of the autoimmune response to diabetes can vary from months to years. In general, the process appears to be more rapid in infants and younger children, and to be more gradual in older children and adolescents. Similarly, the time after diagnosis during which significant insulin production persists can vary from weeks to years, with the duration generally being inversely related to the age at presentation. This persistence of insulin secretion results in a "honeymoon" period, where exogenous insulin requirements and glucose fluctuations are both smaller compared to the situation once no or minimal insulin secretory activity remains.

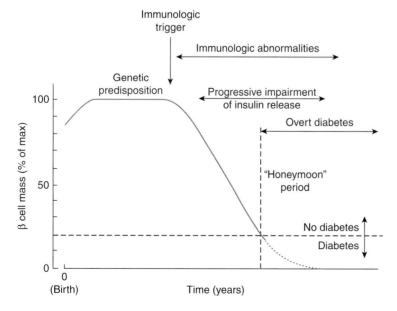

FIGURE 10-6 ■ Evolution of Type 1 diabetes mellitus. An immunologic trigger from the environment initiates an autoimmune response to pancreatic β-cells. This leads to the destruction of β-cells, ultimately resulting in sufficient insulinopenia to cause diabetes. The rate of decline in β-cell mass varies among individuals, with diabetes developing once greater than 80% of β-cell mass is lost. During the "honeymoon" period, some β-cell function remains, somewhat mitigating exogenous insulin requirements. (*From: Skyler JS, ed. Medical Management of Type 1 Diabetes. 3d ed. Alexandria, VA: American Diabetes Association; 1998.*)

Table 10-3.

Risk of Developing Type 1 Diabetes for the General Population and for Individuals with a Relative with Type 1 Diabetes

General population	0.2%
Individuals with a relative with type 1 diabetes:	
Sibling	6%
Identical twin	30%-40%
HLA	
Identical	15%
Haploidentical	6%
Nonidentical	1%
Offspring	5%
Father with IDDM	6%
Mother with IDDM	2%

Genetic Predisposition

There is a clear genetic component to the risk of type 1 diabetes, as indicated by the increased risk of diabetes in relatives of individuals with diabetes (Table 10-3). It is important to note, however, that most children diagnosed with diabetes are the first individual in their family with diabetes: only 10% to 20% of individuals with type 1 diabetes have a family member with type 1 diabetes.

The strongest contributor to the genetic risk of type 1 diabetes is the major histocompatibility complex (MHC) on chromosome 6—more specifically the genes encoding the class II antigens DR and DQ. These genes are felt to alter type 1 diabetes risk by affecting the ability of these class II molecules to bind to and present β-cell protein peptide fragments to T-cells and therefore to activate an autoimmune reaction.

The risk associated with the MHC is complicated by both the extensive allelic variation of these genes as well as the genetic linkage between MHC genes.

There are specific histocompatibility loci antigens (HLAs) that confer an increased risk of type 1 diabetes and others that confer a decreased risk.[4] In general, HLA-DR3 and HLA-DR4 are associated with an increased risk of type 1 diabetes. In addition, the absence of aspartate as the amino acid in the 57th position in the HLA-DQB chain generally increases the risk of type 1 diabetes (being homozygous non-Asp/non-Asp, having an amino acid other than aspartate at position 57 of both HLA-DQB chains, increases the risk of diabetes 100-fold, although this is found in 20% of the nondiabetic population in the United States). There are, however, HLA-DQB alleles with aspartate at the 57th position that are

associated with an increased risk of type 1 diabetes, emphasizing the complexity of this risk association. Up to 90% of individuals with type 1 diabetes carry either the DR3/DQ2 or the DR4/DQ8 haplotypes (both DQ2 and DQ8 are non-Asp alleles). In contrast, while 20% of the population carry the DQ6.2 allele (with aspartate at position 57) this allele is rare in individuals with type 1 diabetes, marking this as a dominantly protective allele. While only 10% of individuals with diabetes lack both the DR3/DQ2 and the DR4/DQ8 haplotypes, 50% of the general population lack both DR3 and DR4 with an additional 8% that have DR4 but lack DQ8. However, the importance of other genes—and factors other than genes—in the development of type 1 diabetes is indicated by the fact that most individuals with a predisposing haplotype do not develop the disease: while 2% of the population carry the high risk DR3-DR4/DQ8 genotype, only 1 in 20 of these individuals will develop type 1 diabetes.

A site of a variable number of tandem repeats (VNTR) upstream of the insulin and IGF2 genes on chromosome 11 contributes approximately 10% to the genetic risk of type 1 diabetes. Class I alleles, with 20 to 63 repeats, are associated with susceptibility to type 1 diabetes, while Class III alleles, with 140 to 210 repeats are associated with protection. Studies have demonstrated that class III alleles are associated with an increase in expression of the insulin gene in the fetal thymus, and it has been proposed that this leads to improved recognition of insulin as a self-antigen, inhibiting autoimmune recognition of β-cells. In addition, imprinting of this region, or alternatively, unequal parental transmission of class III versus class I alleles may be responsible for the increased risk of diabetes in offspring of fathers with type 1 diabetes compared to offspring of mothers with type 1 diabetes.

The loci in the MHC on chromosome 6 and near the insulin gene on chromosome 11 together confer approximately 50% of the genetic risk of type 1 diabetes. Numerous other loci have been identified as confirmed or potential contributors to the remainder of the genetic risk for type 1 diabetes.

Environmental Influences

The finding that the concordance for type 1 diabetes in monozygotic twins is only 30% to 40% implicates something other than genetic risk in the development of type 1 diabetes. This could be owing to differences that exist in monozygotic twins, including differences in immunologic repertoire through the process of T- and B-cell receptor gene rearrangements, somatic mutations, or other such processes. Alternatively, environmental factors may play a role in the pathogenesis of type 1 diabetes, and a number of such factors have been proposed.

Viruses, including mumps, rubella, and coxsackievirus, have been implicated in the pathogenesis of type 1 diabetes.[5] However, except for congenital rubella infection, where up to 20% of such individuals will develop type 1 diabetes, the involvement of other viruses as significant contributors to the causation of type 1 diabetes remains unproven. Exposure to the rodenticide Vacor can lead to diabetes, and other environmental toxins such as nitrosoureas have been proposed as triggers for β-cell autoimmunity, but none have been conclusively linked to the development of type 1 diabetes. Some studies have found that individuals who were exclusively breast-fed as infants are at lower risk of developing type 1 diabetes. Early exposure to cow's milk and an immunologic reaction to bovine milk proteins have been proposed to explain this finding. Mechanisms hypothesized to explain the role of these environmental factors in triggering β-cell autoimmunity include exposure of β-cell antigens after cellular injury owing to toxins or infection, induction of a superantigen response, and molecular mimicry whereby the immune system is triggered by a foreign antigen that shares common or similar immunologic epitopes with a β-cell antigen.

Vitamin D has been implicated in regulating the immune system and having involvement in autoimmune diseases, including type 1 diabetes. Indeed, the geographic variation in type 1 diabetes incidence, with higher prevalence in northern latitudes where there is less sunlight-induced vitamin D synthesis, supports such a role. Other data also implicate lower vitamin D levels as increasing the risk for type 1 diabetes, including association studies showing lower vitamin D levels in patients with newly diagnosed diabetes compared with controls, and observational studies showing a lower risk of type 1 diabetes in infants who had been supplemented with vitamin D compared to controls.

Autoimmunity

The immune reaction in type 1 diabetes includes the development of antibodies and T lymphocytes targeted to β-cells and β-cell antigens as well as cytokine release within the pancreatic islets. While β-cell autoantibodies are found in greater than 80% of patients at the time of diagnosis of type 1 diabetes, they do not appear to play a direct role in β-cell destruction, which is a T-cell mediated process. The most compelling evidence for this is that transfer of T-cells, but not of antibody, can induce autoimmune diabetes in experimental animal models. The β-cell destruction is thought to be caused by a combination of direct CD8+ T-cell attack of the β-cell, along with cytotoxicity from free radicals and cytokines (principally IL-1, TNFα, TNFβ, and IFNγ) released from macrophages and CD4+ and CD8+ T-cells.

Diabetes-associated autoantibodies can be identified in the serum of patients months to years before the development of diabetes, indicating the prolonged preclinical course of the autoimmune process. Commercially available assays exist for the detection of antibodies against whole islets (islet cell antibodies [ICAs]), and antibodies against insulin, the 65-kd isoform of glutamic acid decarboxylase (GAD-65), and insulinoma associated protein 2 (IA-2, also identified as islet cell antigen 512 [ICA512]). Notably, of the specific protein targets identified as diabetes-associated autoantibodies, insulin is the only protein unique to β-cells. With the exception of insulin autoantibodies, each of these autoantibodies is detected in approximately 70% to 80% of patients at the time of diagnosis of diabetes. Insulin autoantibodies (IAAs) are often the first diabetes autoantibody detected, although the prevalence of IAAs at the time of diagnosis is somewhat lower than that of the other autoantibodies. It is unclear if all individuals with positive diabetes-associated autoantibodies will develop diabetes, but their presence identifies individuals at higher risk of diabetes.

Measuring diabetes-associated antibodies in children in the general population has not been proven to be sufficiently predictive or cost effective to justify widespread screening. While one study did find that positive ICAs indicated a 45% 7-year risk of type 1 diabetes, other studies have found ICAs in 3% to 4% of children, and an observed or predicted risk of only 6% to 7% in such children. In contrast, the presence of diabetes-associated antibodies in individuals with a family member with diabetes can be highly predictive for the development of diabetes. The risk of developing diabetes is highest in individuals with multiple β-cell autoantibodies, with a risk of developing diabetes within 5 years greater than 25% in those with two autoantibodies, and greater than 50% in those with three or more autoantibodies.

Prevention

As more is learned about the pathophysiology underlying type 1 diabetes, as well as information learned from studies of its epidemiology, consideration is being given to whether it is possible to prevent its development. Certainly it can be justified to endorse interventions with little or no risk that provide benefits beyond the potential to prevent type 1 diabetes—such as prolonged breast feeding and optimizing vitamin D intake. For other interventions, it is necessary to understand the risks, and to balance them against the likelihood and benefits of success. Research is ongoing on studies aimed at either primary or secondary prevention of type 1 diabetes.

Primary prevention studies seek to interrupt the natural history of the development of type 1 diabetes at some time prior to its clinical presentation. These studies could in theory involve interruption prior to the initiation of the autoimmune attack of β-cells, or after the initiation of the autoimmune reaction, but at a time when sufficient β-cells remain to allow normal glucose homeostasis. A critical aspect to primary prevention is to identify individuals at increased risk of developing type 1 diabetes compared to the low risk in an unselected population (~0.2% in the United States). By evaluating genetic risk (through family history and/or HLA-typing), measuring diabetes-associated autoantibodies, and characterizing insulin secretion and glucose control, such individuals can now be identified and can be accurately stratified into groups with defined risk. Studies are ongoing, although no successful primary prevention has been identified. Because of this, except for within research studies, there is no indication to screen individuals to identify those at risk.

Secondary prevention studies seek to terminate the autoimmune process at or shortly after the individual presents with clinically diagnosed diabetes—a time when as much as 10% to 20% of normal β-cell function remains. Because optimal control of diabetes is more successfully achieved when the individual retains residual, albeit subnormal, endogenous insulin secretion (as is seen during the "honeymoon" period), successful secondary prevention would be of great benefit to patients. Successful secondary prevention has not yet been demonstrated, although a number of approaches to modulating the immune system at the time of diagnosis have shown potential for success to this approach.

CLINICAL PRESENTATION AND DIAGNOSIS

Signs and Symptoms

Tables 10-4A and B outline the presenting findings of type 1 diabetes and of ketoacidosis. As described in the section "Introduction to Diabetes," the hallmark signs and symptoms of diabetes are polydipsia, polyuria, polyphagia, and weight loss. Typical complaints that suggest polyuria include the reemergence of bedwetting, new or increased nocturia, and disruption of class work in school for frequent visits to the bathroom or requests to get water to drink. These symptoms are typically only present for less than a month.

Up to 40% of children with type 1 diabetes present in DKA. The development of DKA requires a greater degree of insulin deficiency than that which causes hyperglycemia, so that these children often will have a preceding history of the classic symptoms of diabetes. Ketoacidosis results in abdominal pain, nausea, and vomiting. The nausea and vomiting impair fluid intake, which combines with the ongoing glucosuria-driven osmotic diuresis to cause dehydration. The stress of the evolving physiologic deterioration results in an increase in circulating levels of the counterregulatory hormones glucagon, cortisol, growth hormone, and epinephrine. The more significant insulin deficiency, along with these counterregulatory hormones cause a greater rise in blood glucose level, as well as the production and accumulation of ketoacids. The acidosis stimulates the respiratory center, resulting in deep Kussmaul respirations;

Table 10-4A.

Signs and Symptoms Associated with the Metabolic Derangements of Diabetes

Hyperglycemia	Ketoacidosis	Dehydration	Insulin Resistance
Asymptomatic	Nausea	Tachycardia	Obesity
Polyuria	Vomiting	Normotensive or hypotensive (late finding)	Acanthosis nigricans
Polydipsia	Abdominal Pain		Hirsutism*
Polyphagia	Tachypnea	Sunken eyes	Irregular menses or amenorrhea*
Weight loss	Kussmaul respirations	Poor skin turgor	
Blurry vision	Sweet-smelling/fruity breath (acetone odor)	Dry mucous membranes	Acne*
Fatigue	Altered mental status	Cool extremities	Hepatic steatosis
Nocturia	Lethargy	Delayed capillary refill	
Secondary enuresis	Coma		
Candidiasis —oral and/ or cutaneous			

Associated with hyperandrogenism resulting from hyperinsulinemia.

Table 10-4B.

Laboratory Findings of Diabetes, Diabetic Ketoacidosis and Insulin Resistance

Hyperglycemia	Ketoacidosis	Insulin Resistance
Glycosuria	Glucosuria	Elevated insulin
Ketonuria	Ketonuria/ketonemia	Elevated C-peptide
	Anion gap acidosis	Elevated adrenal androgens
	Decreased pH	Elevated liver enzymes
	Decreased pCO$_2$	

the patient may have a sense of respiratory distress. There is a further rise in the serum glucose and accumulation of ketoacids in the blood as excretion of these compounds is impaired owing to a decrease in glomerular filtration with the developing dehydration. The resulting hyperosmolarity and acidosis produce an impairment of consciousness that can progress from lethargy to coma.

Laboratory Findings and Diagnostic Tests

The diagnostic criteria for diabetes are given in Table 10-2. In the presence of a history indicating polydipsia and polyuria, a plasma glucose concentration greater than 200 mg/dL confirms a diagnosis of diabetes.[6] In a child that presents with nausea and vomiting, DKA should be considered if there is a preceding history of polydipsia and polyuria, particularly in the absence of supportive evidence of a viral illness, such as lack of sick contacts, diarrhea, and fever. Documentation of acidosis (venous pH < 7.3) and ketonemia or ketonuria confirm DKA.

When glucosuria or hyperglycemia are identified in an individual without symptoms of diabetes, the diagnosis of diabetes is based on an elevated plasma glucose level, that is, a fasting level greater than 125 mg/dL, or a level more than 199 mg/dL at 2 hours during an OGTT.

Differential Diagnosis

In certain clinical scenarios, a cause of diabetes other than type 1 diabetes should be considered. In adolescents type 2 diabetes should be considered. In infants less than 6 months of age or in children with specific family histories of diabetes mellitus, genetic forms of diabetes should be considered. See Parts C and D for detailed discussions of when to consider and how to evaluate for causes of diabetes other than type 1.

TREATMENT

Optimal treatment of type 1 diabetes requires the expertise of a number of health professionals, so that patients with type 1 diabetes mellitus are best managed by an experienced diabetes team that can work together to coordinate the various aspects of care. This team is usually led by a pediatric endocrinologist or other physician with experience managing pediatric patients with diabetes, and ideally also includes a nurse educator, dietitian, and mental health professional. Diabetic ketoacidosis should be treated in pediatric emergency departments or in hospitals with expertise in managing critically ill children.

Goals of Treatment

The goals of treatment for children and youth with type 1 diabetes are to:

1. achieve as close to metabolic normalcy as possible with currently available technology
2. avoid acute complications
3. minimize the risk of long-term microvascular and macrovascular complications
4. allow the child and family to achieve normal psychological maturity and independence and a normal lifestyle

To reach these goals the physician and the family will need to set glycemic goals for the individual patient guided by American Diabetes Association (ADA) targets,[7] and provide the patient and family with the educational resources and treatment options needed to reach this goal. Patients and their families should be seen by the diabetes team about every 3 months. At these appointments, it is important to review individual goals and glycemic control, acute complications occurring since the last appointment and discuss strategies to avoid recurrence of these problems, and to monitor for and treat complications and comorbidities.

One fundamental and important goal in diabetes care is independent self management. Families who are well-educated about diabetes and its management are equipped with the knowledge to make independent decisions about care. This ability can enhance independence and self esteem. Day-to-day decisions about hypoglycemia, hyperglycemia, ketonuria, sick-days, erratic meal, and sports schedules are well handled by knowledgeable families.

Decisions about which insulin regimen to use should consider the needs, abilities, and resources of the child and the family. The meal plan should be designed using sound nutritional principles as well as consideration of the family's food preferences and habits. Children with type 1 diabetes should be able to participate in any activities appropriate to their age and interest and their diabetes regimen can be adapted to allow this flexibility.

Box 10-1 lists the circumstances in which a patient suspected of having type 1 diabetes should be referred to an emergency department or to a specialist.

Insulin Regimens

At the time of the diagnosis of diabetes, patients have some residual β-cells. Their function may improve with insulin treatment when the toxic effect of hyperglycemia on β-cells is removed. Thus, there is often a temporary decrease in insulin requirements 1 to 3 months after diagnosis. This is called the honeymoon period. Insulin requirements may decrease to well below 0.5 units/kg/day. The honeymoon period may last several months and sometimes persist as long as 12 or more months. Over time, however, the majority of patients with type 1 diabetes will have no residual insulin production. Except during this honeymoon period, most prepubertal children need about 0.5 to 1.0 units/kg/day of insulin, with even lower doses in young children.[8] Adolescents usually need insulin doses that are about 25% higher, or about 0.8 to 1.2 units/kg/day. This increased dose requirement is owing to less insulin sensitivity during puberty.

Recombinant DNA technology is used to manufacture all currently available types of insulin and is based on the amino acid sequence of human insulin. Insulin preparations are listed here by timing of action.

Rapid-acting analogs

1. Lispro (Humalog, Eli Lilly)
2. Aspart (NovoLog, Novo-Nordisk)
3. Glulisine (Apidra, Sanofi-Aventis)

After subcutaneous injection, analogs are absorbed and cleared more rapidly than regular insulin. Thus, they more closely mimic the timing of pancreatic insulin secretion. They can be given after a meal in children when food intake is unpredictable, although this may be associated with more postprandial hyperglycemia than if given at the start of the meal.

Short-acting insulin: Regular (several manufacturers) Regular is also used in intravenous infusions to treat DKA.

Intermediate-acting insulins

1. Neutral protamine Hagedorn (NPH) (several manufacturers)
2. Detemir (Levemir, NovoNordisk)

NPH has intermediate timing for peak and duration of action. Detemir can be considered either intermediate or long-acting. Its time of action is dose-related.

Long-acting insulins

1. Detemir (Levemir, NovoNordisk)
2. Glargine (Lantus, Sanofi-Aventis)

Glargine is peakless and has a duration of action of about 20 to 24 hours or more and can usually be given once per day. Detemir has a shorter duration of action than glargine and may require two injections per day. There may be less variability in the effect of detemir compared with that of glargine.

Insulin pharmacodynamics are summarized in Table 10-5 and Figure 10-7. With all the insulin formulations currently available, many options exist for insulin treatment regimens.

1) *NPH-based or split/mixed regimens.*

These are two or three injection regimens based on NPH, an intermediate-acting insulin. See Figure 10-8A and Table 10-6. Two shots of NPH are given, per day: one in the morning shortly before breakfast and a second shot in the evening, either at dinner or at bedtime. Then either regular or a rapid-acting analog is given at breakfast and dinner and sometimes at lunch. Absorption may vary from different injection sites and is more rapid in exercised sites and at higher temperatures. Injection into hypertrophied sites may slow absorption.

Table 10-5.

Timing of Action of Available Insulins in Hours (Times are Approximate)

	Onset	Peak	Duration
Lispro, Aspart, Glulisine	0.25	0.5-1.0	3-4
Regular	0.5-1.0	2-3	4-6
NPH	2-4	6–10	14-16
Detemir	Slowly	6-8	6-24*
Glargine	2-3	No peak	20-24

*dose-related.
Several different mixes are available which combine different percents of short- or rapid-acting insulin with intermediate-acting insulin.

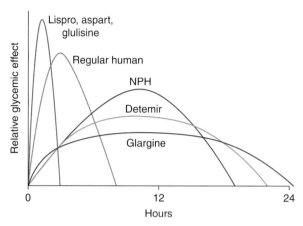

FIGURE 10-7 ■ Timing of action of insulin preparations.

These regimens may use NPH and regular together at breakfast and again at dinner. The total daily dose is split into two shots and each shot is a mix of NPH and regular which may be given in the same syringe. With one variation, the evening dose is divided so regular insulin is given at dinner and NPH at bedtime. This allows the NPH to last until morning. The peak actions of insulin used in these NPH-based, split/mixed regimens do not correlate well with usual mealtimes nor with nutrient absorption. Because of this there is significant between-meal insulin action and to counter this, specific mealtimes and meal amounts, including snacks, are needed to avoid hypoglycemia. The risk of nocturnal hypoglycemia appears to be greater with NPH and regular than with glargine or detemir and with rapid-acting analogs.[9] Split/mixed regimens may use rapid-acting insulin in place of regular insulin. Like regular, rapid-acting insulins can be mixed with NPH in the same syringe and given as a single injection. The use of rapid-acting insulin decreases the problem of between-meal insulin peaks when regular is used. However, the peak with NPH occurs several hours after injections (see Table 10-5 and Figure 10-7) and can be variable. Thus, achieving glycemic targets without causing hypoglycemia using split/mixed regimens may be unachievable.

Traditional dose recommendations, when split/mixed regimens are used, are to give about two-thirds of the total daily dose in the morning and one-third in the evening. These doses usually are split between one-third regular/rapid-acting insulin and two-thirds NPH to closer to one-half/one-half (see Table 10-6). More regular/rapid-acting insulin may be required in the morning than at dinner. This is because of the dawn

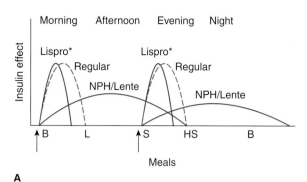

A

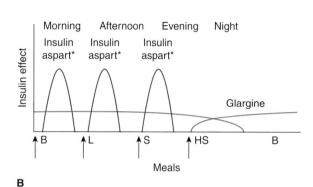

B

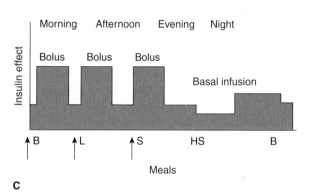

C

FIGURE 10-8 ■ Three insulin regimens. For each panel, the y-axis shows the amount of insulin effect and the x-axis shows the time of day. B, breakfast; L, lunch; S, supper; HS, bedtime; CSII, continuous subcutaneous insulin infusion. An asterisk indicates that either lispro or insulin aspart can be used. The time of insulin injection is shown with a vertical arrow. The type of insulin is noted above each insulin curve. **(A)** The injection of two shots of intermediate-acting insulin (NPH or lente) and short-acting insulin (lispro, insulin aspart, or regular). Only one formulation of short-acting insulin is used. **(B)** A multiple-component insulin regimen consisting of one shot of glargine at bedtime to provide basal insulin coverage and three shots of lispro or insulin aspart to provide glycemic coverage for each meal. **(C)** Insulin administration by insulin infusion device is shown with the basal insulin and a bolus injection at each meal. The basal insulin rate is decreased during the evening and increased slightly prior to the patient awakening in the morning. (*From: Farkas-Hirsch R, ed.* Intensive Diabetes Management. *2nd ed. Alexandria, VA: American Diabetes Association; 1998.*)

Table 10-6.

Example of Split/Mixed Insulin Regimen for a 40-kg Child on a Diet with a Fixed Number of Carbohydrate Grams per Meal (60 for Meals and 30 for Snacks)

Morning (before breakfast): 16 NPH
Before dinner or at bedtime: 6 NPH
Sliding scale regular or rapid-acting dose:

Blood glucose	Breakfast	Dinner
<50	6	4
50-100	7	5
100-150	8	6
150-200	9	7
200-250	10	8
250-300	11	9
>300	12	10

Table 10-7.

Example of a Basal Bolus Regimen for a 40-kg Child on a Diet without Fixed Carbohydrates

Total daily insulin dose = 32 units (0.8 units/kg)
Basal insulin = 50% of total daily dose = 16 units given as either 16 units glargine per day OR 0.6 units per hour of rapid-acting insulin (lispro, aspart, or glulisine) as pump basal rate.
Bolus doses for food: Insulin to carbohydrate ratio for meals and snacks determined by the 450-500 rule:
450-500 divided by total daily insulin dose (450-500/32 = 14-15). Use 1 unit per 15 carbohydrate grams to start.
Bolus doses for high glucose correction: determined by 1800 rule:
1800 divided by total insulin dose (1800/32 = 56). Use 1 unit per 56 (round to 60) blood glucose points (or 0.5 unit per 30 blood glucose points) above target.
Target blood glucose: generally 120 in the daytime and 150 at night, usually somewhat higher for young children and those with hypoglycemia unawareness.

phenomenon, a decrease in insulin sensitivity in the morning owing to normal nocturnal increases in some counter regulatory hormones.

While most children are now using basal/bolus regimens, it is useful to know how to convert a patient from a two or three shot regimen with NPH to a basal/bolus regimen. Recommendations are to use 50% to 80% of the NPH dose for the initial basal insulin dose, with the lower percentages for younger children.

2) Basal/bolus regimens.

The goal of basal/bolus insulin regimens is to provide more physiologic insulin levels so that peak levels coincide with nutrient absorption and basal levels occur between meals so that there is less between meal insulin action. The basal insulin component provides baseline, between meals, or fasting insulin needs. The bolus component provides insulin to cover food requirements and to correct hyperglycemia. The basal component may be provided by either rapid-acting insulin given by the basal rate using an insulin pump, or with once or twice daily injections of detemir or glargine. (Per labeling, unlike NPH insulin, detemir and glargine cannot be mixed with any other insulin, requiring that they be given as additional injections.) The bolus insulin is provided by rapid-acting insulin which may be given by injections, or by the bolus function through an insulin pump. Figure 10-8B shows a diagram of a basal bolus regimen.

Estimated dose calculations are shown in Table 10-7. These calculations are based on clinically determined empiric formulas. Modifications to initial calculations will often need to be made once individual patient responses to starting doses are assessed. Usual basal requirements are about 50% of total daily insulin requirements. Bolus doses have two parts: first, the dose of insulin needed to cover the amount of carbohydrate grams in the meal or snack, and second, the dose of insulin needed to correct for blood glucose levels which are outside of the individual's blood glucose target range. Insulin to carbohydrate ratios differ for different individuals and can also differ for different times of day in a given individual. The insulin to carbohydrate ratio is the amount of insulin needed to cover each gram of ingested carbohydrate, specified as 1 unit per each X carbohydrate grams (eg, 1 unit per 10 carbohydrate grams). The correction or sensitivity factor refers to the amount that an individual patient's blood glucose will decrease when given 1 unit of insulin.

The amount of the premeal bolus dose, therefore, is the sum of: first, the insulin to carbohydrate ratio multiplied by (planned or ingested) grams of carbohydrate and second, the correction or sensitivity factor multiplied by the amount that the blood glucose needs to fall from the blood glucose level determined preprandially to achieve the target range. Target ranges are individualized and may be set for example at 70 to 110 for daytime and 100 to 150 at the child's bedtime.

A disadvantage of glargine or detemir for basal insulin compared to insulin pumps is that pumps offer flexibility in basal rate (Figure 10-8C). With pumps, the basal rate can be set differently at different times of day. Pumps also allow administration of insulin with snacks and for blood glucose levels above target range without additional injections. Children using an injection-based basal/bolus regimen may resist additional needle sticks.

Combining long-acting insulin by subcutaneous injections with insulin pump use can be done. This regimen replaces most of the pump basal rate with long-acting insulin given by a subcutaneous injection. This plan can be used to allow pump users to disconnect from the pump for several hours for swimming or for sports, or for a prom, for example.

MEDICAL NUTRITION MANAGEMENT

It is important for children and adolescents with type 1 diabetes to have a nutritionally balanced diet with adequate calories and nutrients for normal growth. Recommendations usually include about 50% to 55% as carbohydrate calories, 20% protein, and approximately 30% fat. The majority of carbohydrate calories are complex carbohydrates, and the fat component should be "heart healthy" emphasizing low levels of cholesterol and saturated fats. For patients who are using NPH-based split/mixed insulin regimens, constancy in the timing and the carbohydrate amount of meals is important as this will help minimize blood glucose variability. In addition to the usual three meals, midafternoon snacks are necessary. This is because the timing of this snack coincides with the typical peak of the patient's morning NPH insulin dose and with most after-school sports activities. Bedtime snacks are important for most children receiving evening NPH doses and help avoid nocturnal hypoglycemia. Midmorning snacks are useful in preschool-aged children. However, school-aged children often find that midmorning snacks are disruptive to their school schedule. Midmorning snacks are usually not recommended after a child begins elementary school. The child's meal plan should allow occasional treats. Patients and their families can learn how to adjust insulin doses to accommodate times of increased caloric intake, such as holidays and birthdays. For patients using basal/bolus regimens, either with pumps of with a glargine or detemir-based regimen, near total flexibility in timing, amount, and content of meals is possible. The ability for patients and families to achieve this flexibility requires the ability to understand and execute accurate carbohydrate counting and insulin dose calculation based on an insulin to carbohydrate ratio, and a correction/sensitivity factor based on blood glucose level (Table 10-7).

Overweight and obese patients will require calorie control. Meal plans that fit with the child and family's food preferences and that provide satiety are necessary for realistic adherence to the nutritional recommendations. Clearly meal plans need to be individualized for each child and family.

An increased frequency of eating disorders, particularly in adolescent girls with type 1 diabetes has been reported at some centers. When this occurs, metabolic consequences can be devastating. Serious intervention, such as inpatient admission to an eating disorders unit, is indicated.

Nutritional management is complex, and is best guided by regular evaluations with a nutritionist who has expertise in diabetes management. This becomes especially important when using sophisticated regimens based on carbohydrate counting.

EXERCISE

Physical fitness and regular exercise are to be encouraged in all children with type 1 diabetes. Metabolic control, self-esteem, and body image may be better in the physically fit child. Exercise in a child with diabetes, however, requires specific attention. During periods of exercise, extra calories or lower insulin doses may be needed to prevent hypoglycemia.[10] Some patients have a delayed hypoglycemic response to exercise, sometimes hours later. Blood glucose monitoring to assess the effects of exercise and the response to interventions on blood glucose levels should be done to determine an effective regimen for the individual child. The stress of exercise when metabolic control is poor (eg, during hyperglycemia, especially with ketosis) may worsen metabolic control, so that it may be necessary to delay exercise at these times.

MONITORING

Self-monitoring of blood glucose is fundamental to diabetes management. More frequent monitoring has been shown to correlate with improved glycemic control. Glucose meters are small, portable, and accurate, and many have memory storage of several hundred readings. Some meters allow patients to record carbohydrate amounts and insulin doses. The ability to download the information to computers with specific software programs and to organize the data in different formats is available and can be very helpful in achieving good metabolic control. Some meters can communicate the glucose level to an insulin pump.

Blood glucose traditionally is monitored before meals, at bedtime, and overnight. Some children also monitor before snacks, especially those receiving bolus insulin with all carbohydrate intake. Basal/bolus regimens require a blood glucose level each time one ingests any calories so accurate dose decisions can be calculated. Postprandial levels can be helpful in assessing whether the selected dose was satisfactory. Many people monitor at least 8 to 10 times per day, more often with sports, when ill, or during periods of metabolic instability. Fasting and preprandial blood glucose readings in the 100 to 180 mg/dL range for preschool aged children, 90-180 mg/dL for school-aged children and 90 to 130 mg/dL for teenagers are reasonable goals. Bedtime or overnight levels of 110 to 200 mg/dL in preschoolers, 100 to 180 mg/dL in school-aged children, and 90 to 150 mg/dL in teenagers are also reasonable.

New continuous glucose sensors are available that read interstitial glucose levels and send the readings every few minutes to a display.[11] These devices also display rate and direction of change and have alarms which can be set to alert for low or high glucose levels or impending levels in these ranges. Acceptability of these in children and youth, improvement in metabolic control, and insurance coverage remain to be determined.

Glycated hemoglobin (HbA1c) is an objective level that measures average blood glucose concentration over approximately the previous 2 months, and should be measured regularly, usually every 3 months. While the ideal goal is to achieve a HbA1c level as close to normal as possible, goals that most patients should achieve vary with age: for toddlers and preschoolers (under 6 years old) 7.5% to 8.5%; for school-aged children (6-12) less than 8%; and for adolescents and young adults (13-19) less than 7.5 %. However, hypoglycemia may limit the ability to achieve these goals. Indeed, with the limitations of current insulins and methods of administration, reaching these target levels is often not achievable, especially in adolescents. The high risk and vulnerability of young children to hypoglycemia are why blood glucose and HbA1c goals are higher for younger children.

Urine or blood ketones also should be monitored when the blood glucose levels are elevated (eg, above 250-300 mg/dL), when children have a fever, when they feel nauseous or are vomiting, or when they are not feeling well. This monitoring is important in achieving the goal of aborting DKA episodes by treating early ketosis. Checking ketones may be forgotten by patients and families and reminders are often necessary.

EDUCATION

Living with and managing diabetes is complex and demanding and requires initial and ongoing education. Education is fundamental to diabetes management and metabolic control. Patients and families need to understand all aspects of diabetes, including acute and long-term complications. They must understand details of insulin action, including duration and timing and dose adjustments, injection and insertion techniques, electronics and mechanics of insulin pumps, dietary information including carbohydrate counting, blood glucose monitoring and interpretation, and urine ketone checks and appropriate interventions. They must gain skills in integrating the demanding clinical regimen into their schedules so that they can achieve emotional stability and ongoing psychological growth.

Education must be appropriate to the child's age and the family's educational background, and it must be ongoing. Shifting responsibility from parent to child for diabetes self-care skills (eg, insulin injections) should be done gradually and when the child shows interest and readiness to do so. Premature shifting of responsibility may be a cause of deterioration in metabolic control. Management of diabetes involves the whole family even as responsibility is shifted primarily to the adolescent. The life of the entire family is affected by having a child with type 1 diabetes. Sharing responsibilities and attending support groups and camps for type 1 diabetes children can help with psychological adjustment.

Teaching about diabetes management is best handled by a diabetes management team, including a physician, nurse educator, dietitian, and mental health professional. Excellent comprehensive educational manuals for children and families are available and several comprehensive websites are exceptional (see selected resources at the end of this part). Diabetes education is lifelong for patients, families, and for the diabetes team.

COMPLICATIONS

A major goal of treatment in type 1 diabetes is to avoid both acute and chronic complications. DKA and hypoglycemia are the most significant acute complications of diabetes and its treatment—both with a significant risk of morbidity and mortality. Diabetes mellitus leads to damage to the microvascular circulation that results in tissue and organ damage, most notably in the retina, kidneys, and nerves. Because of these microvascular complications, diabetes mellitus is a leading cause of blindness, end-stage renal disease, and neuropathy. There is also a significant increase in the risk of atherosclerotic vascular disease in individuals with diabetes. This macrovascular disease results in strokes and heart attacks which are the most common cause of death in patients with diabetes.

Recombinant insulin analogs, insulin pumps, and newer devices for home monitoring have drastically improved our ability to control glucose levels in patients with diabetes. However, the feedback control in the healthy state that allows minute-to-minute regulation of insulin secretion cannot be recapitulated with current diabetes therapies, so full metabolic normalization is not yet possible. Thus, some degree of hyperglycemia persists in virtually all patients with diabetes. Long-term complications, including renal failure, retinopathy, neuropathy, and cardiovascular disease are related to and likely caused by the hyperglycemia.

Decreasing the Risk of Long-Term Complications

It is now firmly established that both the microvascular and macrovascular complications of diabetes are related to the hyperglycemia that persists even with treatment of the disease.[12-15] The development of chronic complications is also dependent on the duration of diabetes, generally taking decades for clinically significant complications to appear. Therefore, while some late adolescents with early onset of diabetes may show early evidence of complications (eg, nonproliferative retinopathy, microalbuminuria [urinary albumin excretion of 30-300 mg/day], or changes in nerve conduction), it is extremely uncommon for a child to have significant diabetic microvascular or macrovascular complications. Nonetheless, it is necessary to maximize glycemic control in children with diabetes to minimize their risk of future long-term complications.

Clinical trials, including the Diabetes Control and Complications Trial (DCCT) demonstrated that the lower the hemoglobin A1c (HbA1c) that a patient maintains, reflecting a lower average blood glucose level, the lower the risk of microvascular complications. Recent data from the DDCT indicate that the A1c level explains nearly all the difference in complication risk in this study. An improvement in HbA1c of 1% (reflecting a decrease in mean glucose levels of 30-35 mg/dL) decreases the risk of long-term complications by approximately 20% to 50%. There was no threshold for this effect—that is, a lower HbA1c is always better in terms of lowering the risk of long-term complications. However, the absolute risk reduction is less at lower HbA1c levels, and lower average glucose levels may increase the risk of the acute complication of hypoglycemia. Therefore, diabetes management involves balancing the long-term benefit of lowering the average glucose level with avoiding the acute complication of hypoglycemia.

Hypoglycemia

Hypoglycemia, a blood glucose level less than 60 mg/dL, is a frequent occurrence in children treated for type 1 diabetes. It is caused by the inability to perfectly match the minute-to-minute changes in insulin requirements with current therapy, resulting in periods when insulin action exceeds insulin requirements. Patients with lower average blood glucose levels may have more frequent episodes of hypoglycemia. The severity of symptoms of hypoglycemia depends on both the degree of hypoglycemia, as well as the rapidity of its development. The adrenergic symptoms of hypoglycemia include sweating, trembling, hunger, and palpitations; the neuroglycopenic symptoms include headache, lightheadedness, dizziness, diplopia, and confusion. With severe hypoglycemia coma and seizures can occur.

Mild to moderate hypoglycemia is treated by ingesting 10 to 15 g of glucose (eg, 4 oz of juice or nondiet soft drink). Hypoglycemia in infants and young children, and moderate reactions resulting in confusion in older children, require that caregivers, including teachers and coaches, and the like, be prepared to assist in the recognition and treatment of hypoglycemia. Severe reactions require treatment with intramuscular or subcutaneous glucagon (0.5-1 mg, except for infants less than 10 kg, where 0.5 mg is given). Because hypoglycemia can occur away from home, a source of glucose to treat it (eg, a tube of cake frosting) and a glucagon emergency kit should always be available.

Hypoglycemia unawareness

Hypoglycemia unawareness is defined as having blood glucose values less than 65 mg/dL without the adrenergic symptoms of hypoglycemia caused by decreased epinephrine and/or glucagon output. This may result in altered cognition without self-identified symptoms of hypoglycemia. Hypoglycemia unawareness is an important cause of severe hypoglycemia (36% of the hypoglycemia during the DCCT occurred while subjects were awake). Since the blood glucose threshold for adrenergic release will vary with the recent level of blood glucose control (higher blood glucose values, higher blood glucose threshold), one hypoglycemic event can lead to significant decrease in counter-regulatory responses and cause an unawareness of hypoglycemia for the subsequent 24 hours leading to a "snow-ball" effect with increasing frequency of hypoglycemia. Additionally moderate exercise may result in a decrease in symptoms of hypoglycemia caused by decreased adrenergic release the next day. Also, the blood glucose threshold is reduced during sleep.

Since hypoglycemia unawareness is a strong predictor for a severe hypoglycemia event, a detailed history of the glucose threshold for hypoglycemia symptoms should be obtained at each visit. Patients and families should be counseled to contact a diabetes provider if hypoglycemia unawareness develops. There is evidence that loss of awareness of hypoglycemia can be reversed by avoiding hypoglycemia for 2 to 3 weeks.[16] This is accomplished by setting higher blood glucose targets during this time, decreasing the insulin dose and increasing the frequency of blood glucose testing, including some middle of the night tests.

Ketonemia/Ketonuria and Sick Day Management

The presence of urine or blood ketones is an indication of significant insulin deficiency. Urine ketones should never be measurable and blood ketones should not be elevated in a patient with type 1 diabetes. Whenever persistent, significant hyperglycemia occurs (eg, blood glucose >250 mg/dL in spite of corrective doses of insulin being given), urine or blood ketones should be tested. Urine or blood ketones should also be tested whenever the child feels ill, particularly with nausea and vomiting. Aggressive treatment with additional insulin is necessary once ketosis develops in order to prevent deterioration to ketoacidosis. In a patient whose diabetes is managed with an insulin pump, insulin doses to correct persistent hyperglycemia or ketosis should be given by injection with needle and syringe, as pump malfunction is a possible cause of the insulin deficiency. Rapid-acting insulin at doses of 10% to 20% of the total daily requirement should be given every 3 to 4 hours until ketones are cleared. In a child who is not able to take sufficient caloric intake because of illness, care must be given to avoid causing hypoglycemia.

Management of diabetes during even simple illnesses can be challenging, more so in illnesses that interrupt oral intake. While uncertain oral intake puts the patient at risk of insulin-induced hypoglycemia, insulin treatment must be continued to prevent deterioration into DKA; indeed, total insulin requirements may increase during illness because of the insulin-antagonizing effects of inflammation and stress hormones. Management of diabetes during an illness will usually require guidance from the patient's diabetes team. Basal insulin should be continued, generally at the usual dose but sometimes at a slightly decreased dose based on blood glucose levels. Blood glucose and ketone measurements should be performed frequently (at least every 3-4 hours). Extra fluids are given to maintain hydration, which also helps excrete excess glucose and ketoacids. If solid foods cannot be eaten, sugar-containing liquids such as soda, juice, jello, and popsicles can be given to maintain some caloric intake to prevent hypoglycemia. During some illnesses, the usual daily insulin doses, adjusted for intake and glucose levels, can be continued. For illnesses where oral intake is more disrupted, when ketones have developed, or for more significant illnesses, it may be best to treat with more frequent, small doses of insulin; typical doses may be 5% to 10% of the total daily dose every 3 to 4 hours, increasing to 10% to 20% of the total daily dose every 3 to 4 hours if ketones are present. Persistent vomiting, or a refusal or inability to take fluids or food orally requires an emergency department or office visit.

Glucagon must be available to treat hypoglycemia during an illness. The dose of glucagon to maintain glucose values within the normal range or treat mild hypoglycemia owing to poor intake is lower than that required to treat severe hypoglycemia:[17] 10 mcg/year of age (minimum 20 mcg, maximum 150 mcg); if there is no response at 30 minutes, a repeat dose at twice the initial dose can be attempted. The usual dose (0.5-1 mg for weight > 10 kg; 0.5 mg for weight ≤ 10 kg) is given for severe hypoglycemia. The higher doses of glucagon frequently cause significant nausea and vomiting, further compromising the ability to ingest food, so should be avoided if possible when treating milder hypoglycemia associated with poor oral intake.

Diabetic Ketoacidosis

Diabetic ketoacidosis (DKA) represents the most severe derangement of insulin-regulated metabolism. It is responsible for most deaths in children with type 1 diabetes, with a mortality risk of up to 0.3%. DKA is characterized by hyperglycemia (>200 mg/dL), and acidosis (serum pH < 7.3, bicarbonate < 15mmol/L), along with evidence of an accumulation of ketoacids in the blood (measurable serum or urine ketones, increased anion gap—see Tables 10-4A and B). The metabolic derangements of DKA lead to dehydration, electrolyte loss, and hyperosmolality. The best treatment of DKA is its prevention, through early recognition and diagnosis of diabetes in a child with polydipsia and polyuria, and through careful attention to management in children with known diabetes, particularly during illnesses.

DKA in a known diabetic patient is usually caused by missed insulin doses. Causes for this include failure of an insulin pump, and the improper discontinuation of insulin during an illness associated with poor oral intake. Indeed, intercurrent illnesses can increase insulin requirements, and a failure to match this increased requirement can lead to ketoacidosis in a child with diabetes. In an older child given responsibility for management of their diabetes without oversight, DKA is most often caused by missed insulin doses that are forgotten. Recurrent DKA is almost always caused by intentional omission of insulin.

Presentation

The acidosis and ketosis of DKA creates an ileus, causing patients to develop nausea and vomiting. Occasionally the ileus will produce pain severe enough to raise concern for an acute abdomen. The ketosis can give patients a fruity breath. As the DKA becomes more severe, the patients will develop lethargy that can progress to coma.

Treatment

Successful treatment of DKA corrects the metabolic abnormalities while avoiding complications that can

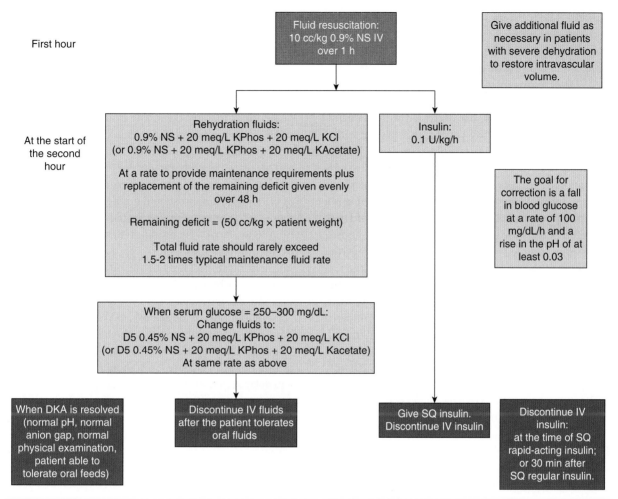

FIGURE 10-9 ■ Outline of therapy that may be required for a child presenting with moderately severe DKA (6% dehydration). No patient with DKA should be considered "typical"—each requires determination of their specific individual requirements for treatment, with adjustments in treatment made based on careful monitoring. (*From Cooke DW, Plotnick L. Management of diabetic ketoacidosis in children and adolescents.* Pediatr in Rev. 2008 [in press]).

occur during the correction. Management of DKA consists of fluid and electrolyte replacement, insulin treatment, and careful ongoing monitoring of clinical and laboratory factors.[18-20] Figure 10-9 outlines the major aspects of the management of DKA.

Fluid and electrolyte replacement. The osmotic diuresis produced by glucosuria results in large water and electrolyte losses, exacerbated by compromised intake from nausea and vomiting. Intravenous fluid replacement is begun as soon as the diagnosis of DKA is established. Initial fluid resuscitation can be started with 10 cc/kg of 0.9% NaCl (normal saline) given over 1 hour. In more critically ill children, where there is concern over impending cardiovascular collapse, additional resuscitation fluid given more rapidly will be needed.

After the initial fluid resuscitation, the remainder of the fluid deficit is replaced evenly over 48 hours. Most patients with DKA are approximately 6% dehydrated

(10% for children <2 years). In patients presenting with more severe DKA (serum glucose levels > 600-800 mg/dL and pH < 7.1) fluid losses are approximately 9% of body weight (15% for children <2 years). Maintenance fluid requirements are added to this deficit replacement to give the total fluid requirements, which should rarely exceed 1.5 to 2 times the usual daily fluid requirement. At presentation, the osmotic diuresis driven by the hyperglycemia can represent a significant ongoing fluid loss. These urinary fluid losses decline in the first hours of treatment as the glucose level decreases, and so, in an effort to avoid excessively rapid fluid delivery, they are generally not specifically replaced. However, careful attention to the fluid balance during DKA is necessary in order to identify the patients who will need additional fluid. This is particularly true in the first hours after presentation. IV infusion of 0.9% saline (with added potassium) is continued as the hydration fluid until the blood glucose level declines to less than 250 to 300 mg/dL. At that time, the fluid is changed to D5 0.45% saline (with added potassium). If the blood glucose level declines below 100 to 150 mg/dL, it may be necessary to increase the dextrose content to 10% or even 12.5%.

DKA results in total-body potassium depletion. However, depending on the degree to which the glomerular filtration rate has decreased with the dehydration that is part of DKA, patients may present with a high, normal, or low serum potassium level. During treatment of DKA, the insulin that is given, as well as correction of the acidosis that occurs, both cause potassium to move intracellularly. Because of this hypokalemia is a potentially fatal complication during treatment of DKA. Therefore, unless the patient is hyperkalemic or anuric, potassium is added to the intravenous fluids at the beginning of the second hour of therapy; otherwise it is added as soon as urine output is established or the hyperkalemia abates. If the patient presents with hypokalemia, potassium replacement should be initiated immediately. Most patients will require 30 to 40 mEq/L of potassium in the replacement fluids, adjusted based on serum potassium levels measured every 1 to 2 hours.

DKA results in significant phosphate depletion, and serum phosphate levels will decrease during treatment of DKA. Clinical studies have not shown benefit from phosphate replacement during the treatment of DKA, although phosphate replacement should be given if the level drops less than 1 mg/dL. In the absence of severe hypophosphatemia, phosphate may be provided by giving half of the potassium replacement as potassium phosphate. This practice decreases chloride delivery to the patient, minimizing the hyperchloremic metabolic acidosis that will occur in most patients. This hyperchloremia is generally of no clinical significance, although it can confound the clinician's interpretation of DKA resolution. Use of potassium acetate to provide the other half of the potassium replacement further decreases the chloride load. The serum calcium level must be monitored if phosphorus is given owing to the risk of hypocalcemia. If hypocalcemia develops, phosphate administration should be stopped.

Bicarbonate losses are large in DKA. However, during the treatment of DKA, substantial bicarbonate can be produced by the patient, as insulin stimulates the generation of bicarbonate from the metabolism of ketones. Consistent with this, clinical trials have failed to show any benefit of bicarbonate use during the treatment of DKA. Potential risks of bicarbonate therapy include paradoxical central nervous system (CNS) acidosis and exacerbation of hypokalemia. Bicarbonate treatment has also been associated with cerebral edema, the most common cause of mortality for children with DKA. Therefore, bicarbonate treatment should only be considered in cases of extreme acidosis, such as those with pH less than 6.9 when the acidosis may impair cardiovascular stability, or

as treatment of life-threatening hyperkalemia. If bicarbonate is felt to be necessary, 1 to 2 mmol/kg (added to 0.45% saline) should be given over 1 to 2 hours.

Insulin

Insulin treatment is begun at the beginning of the second hour of therapy. Beginning insulin treatment at the same time as initiating fluid resuscitation increases the risk of severe hypokalemia and of decreasing the serum osmolarity excessively rapidly. It is best given as a continuous intravenous infusion of regular insulin at a rate of 0.1 U/kg/h; a bolus should not be given at the start of therapy. The infusion tubing should be prepared by running 30 to 50 cc of the insulin solution through it to saturate binding sites. Short- or rapid-acting insulin injected intramuscularly or subcutaneously every 1 or 2 hours can be used if intravenous administration of insulin is not possible.[22]

Resolution of the acidosis in DKA invariably takes longer than normalization of the blood glucose level. The temptation to decrease the rate of insulin administration based on glucose levels should be resisted, as this will delay resolution of the acidosis. The dose of insulin should remain at 0.1 U/kg/h until the acidosis resolves (pH > 7.3, bicarbonate > 18). The insulin dose should only be decreased if hypoglycemia or a fall in serum glucose persists after maximal dextrose concentrations are used. If the acidosis is not resolving, the dose of insulin should be increased to 0.15 or 0.20 U/kg/h.

Monitoring

The initial assessment of a patient with DKA includes evaluation of vital signs and physical examination, including a mental status evaluation and neurologic examination. These serve as a baseline, and along with results of laboratory testing, allow treatment to be given if evidence of an infection is found, and allows adjustment to the initial fluid resuscitation based on the degree of dehydration and the cardiovascular status that is found. (Note that the elevated levels of epinephrine and cortisol that are present in DKA can lead to an elevation in the white blood cell. Thus, while infection can be a precipitant of DKA so that careful evaluation for an infection is important, leukocytosis during DKA is not a reliable indicator of infection.)

If the patient is markedly obtunded, a nasogastric tube should be placed to decrease the risk of aspiration. Vital signs and mental status are then monitored frequently, at least every hour. The balance of total fluid intake and fluid output should also be calculated each hour. The goal is to see changes indicating rehydration and improving mental status with resolution of the DKA.

Serum glucose, electrolytes (including blood urea nitrogen and creatinine) and pH and urine ketones should be obtained at presentation. Subsequently, serum glucose and pH should be measured hourly, with serum electrolytes and urine ketones measured every 2 to 3 hours. If phosphate is given, serum calcium concentrations must be monitored. The goal for correction of hyperglycemia is a fall of 100 mg/dL per hour. The persistence of severe hyperglycemia suggests inadequate rehydration (or incorrectly mixed insulin), while too rapid a fall may be an indicator of too rapid a rate of rehydration. After the first hour, the pH should increase at least 0.03 units per hour. A slower rise suggests a need for a higher insulin dose or a need for increased hydration.

Hyperglycemia causes the osmotic shift of water into the intravascular compartment, causing dilutional hyponatremia. The calculation for the corrected sodium concentration accounts for this effect:

$$[\text{Na}^+]_{corrected} = [\text{Na}^+]_{measured} + 1.6 \times ([\text{glucose}] - 100)/100$$

Both the measured and the corrected serum sodium levels should increase as the serum glucose level decreases during treatment of DKA. A failure of the corrected sodium level to rise, or even more significantly a fall in either sodium level, suggests overly rapid rehydration.

Cerebral Edema

Cerebral edema is responsible for the majority of deaths realted to DKA in children, and significant neurologic morbidity persists in many of the survivors. While it typically presents 4 to 12 hours after treatment is begun, it can present later, or earlier, including before treatment is initiated. The cause of cerebral edema in DKA is not known, although a number of mechanisms have been proposed. These include cerebral ischemia and hypoxia, fluid shifts caused by inequalities in osmolarity between the extravascular and intravascular intracranial compartments, increased cerebral blood flow, and altered membrane ion transport. Risk factors that have been identified for the development of cerebral edema include[21]: young age; DKA in an undiagnosed diabetic child; factors indicating a more severe presentation (pH < 7.2 and lower serum bicarbonate concentration, higher serum glucose concentration, higher blood urea nitrogen concentration, a calculated serum sodium concentration in the hypernatremic range, and hypocapnia); a lack of rise of the corrected sodium concentration during rehydration; and treatment with bicarbonate. Earlier uncontrolled studies had suggested that a higher rate of rehydration increased the risk of cerebral edema. While subsequent controlled studies have not found the rate of fluid administration to be a factor in the risk of cerebral edema, current recommendations for more gradual, even fluid replacement during the treatment of DKA are related to this concern.

The signs and symptoms of cerebral edema include: severe headache; sudden deterioration in mental status; bradycardia (or a sudden, persistent drop in heart rate not attributable to improved hydration); hypertension; cranial nerve dysfunction; and incontinence. If suspected, immediate treatment should be initiated with 0.25 to 1.0 g/kg of intravenous mannitol. If the patient requires intubation, hyperventilation should be avoided, as it has been shown to be associated with worse outcomes.[22]

Resolution

When the ketoacidosis has resolved, the patient may be transitioned from intravenous fluids and intravenous insulin to oral intake and subcutaneous insulin. Criteria for this transition include a normal sensorium and normal vital signs, an ability to tolerate oral intake, and resolution of the acidosis, reflected by a normal pH, a serum bicarbonate level greater than 18, and a normal anion gap. Because of the excess in chloride delivered with the intravenous fluids during the treatment of DKA, many patients will develop a hyperchloremic metabolic acidosis. Because of this, the pH and serum bicarbonate level may not completely normalize in spite of resolution of the ketoacidosis. These patients, with a normal anion gap, should also be transitioned off of intravenous fluids and insulin.

The action of intravenous insulin dissipates in minutes. Therefore, the intravenous insulin should not be discontinued until a dose of insulin is given subcutaneously. For rapid-acting insulin analogs, this can be just before the intravenous infusion is stopped; for regular insulin, the subcutaneous injection should be given 30 minutes before the infusion is stopped. It is easiest to make this transition at the time of a meal.

Chronic Complications and Comorbidities

Associated Autoimmune Disease

Associated autoimmune disease, particularly thyroid dysfunction, occurs with greater frequency with type 1 diabetes. TSH should be measured shortly after diagnosis and may then be measured every 1 to 2 years. TSH should also be measured anytime any thyroid-related signs or symptoms occur. T_4 and thyroid antibodies may also be obtained. Although rare, autoimmune adrenal hypofunction can occur, and symptoms to suggest this should prompt appropriate testing.

Celiac disease also occurs more frequently in children with type 1 diabetes. Thus, all patients should be screened for this at least once, perhaps every few years, and any time poor growth or gastrointestinal (GI) symptoms, including poor weight gain, occur. Tissue transglutaminase and antiendomysial antibodies are more sensitive and specific than antigliadin antibodies.

Also, since these are IgA antibodies, it is important to ensure that the individual patient is not IgA deficient by obtaining an IgA level.

Growth Disturbance

Linear growth is negatively affected by poor diabetic control. Decreased growth velocity, crossing height and weight percentiles downward on the growth curve, eventual short stature, and delayed skeletal and sexual maturation are associated with chronic undertreatment with insulin. An extreme form of this—the Mauriac syndrome, or diabetic dwarfism—occurs rarely and usually is associated with hepatomegaly. Careful height and weight measurements should be obtained at every appointment and plotted on growth curves so that deviations from normal can be detected early. Alternatively, treatment with excessive insulin doses often leads to excessive weight gain, causing the weight curve to cross percentiles upward. The maintenance of normal growth curves for height and weight is an important part of diabetes management.

Retinopathy

Retinopathy usually is not seen before 5 to 10 years of diabetes duration.[23] Recommendations (ADA) are for the first ophthalmological examination to be done once the child is 10 years old or more and has had diabetes for 3 to 5 years.[7] Yearly follow-up is generally recommended. Poor metabolic control, elevated blood pressure, smoking, albuminuria, and elevated lipids are all risk factors for retinopathy. Diabetes duration and pregnancy also are associated with increased risk.

Nephropathy

A significant minority of patients with type 1 diabetes eventually develop end-stage renal disease and need dialysis or transplantation. All patients with type 1 diabetes should be monitored by urine microalbumin at least annually beginning after the child is 10 years of age and has had diabetes for 5 years.[7] Hypertension accelerates the progression of nephropathy. Therefore, blood pressure should be monitored several times a year, and hypertension should be aggressively treated. Angiotensin-converting enzyme inhibitors and angiotension receptor blockers are recommended for treatment of hypertension. If hypertension, overt proteinuria, or elevation in serum creatinine or urea nitrogen is found, monitoring of renal function several times each year and consultation with a nephrologist is warranted. Microalbuminuria (30-299 mg/g creatinine on a spot urine) is a marker for early nephropathy. Two out of three urine specimens with elevated levels done on different days are needed for confirmation. Whether using angiotensin-converting enzyme inhibitors in normotensive individual prevents or retards nephropathy is not known. Patients should avoid other risk factors for nephropathy, such as smoking.

Neuropathy

Symptomatic diabetic neuropathy, peripheral or autonomic, is uncommon in children and adolescents with type 1 diabetes. Changes in nerve conduction, however, may be seen after 4 to 5 years diabetes duration. Overall, neuropathy is a common type 1 diabetes complication, and its frequency increases with the duration of disease and degree of hyperglycemia. Improvements in glycemic control may help neuropathic symptoms.

Macrovascular Complications/Lipids

Patients with type 1 diabetes tend to have coronary artery, cerebrovascular, and peripheral vascular disease more often, at an earlier age, and more extensively than the nondiabetic population. A prominent cause of macrovascular disease appears to be hyperglycemia. Hypertension, elevated blood lipid levels, and cigarette smoking are other risk factors for developing macrovascular complications. Risk factor assessment, including lipid panels, blood pressure measurements, and determination of smoking status should be done, and treatment should be instituted as indicated. A strong admonition against smoking and referral to an appropriate program for patients who are already smokers is indicated. Studies continue to show that lower LDL (low density lipoprotein) levels are beneficial in decreasing the risk of vascular disease and recommendations continue to evolve. Screening with fasting lipids should begin in children at age 12 years if there is no concerning family history and at diagnosis (after establishing metabolic control) when there is a positive family history of lipid abnormalities or early cardiovascular events.[7] Some clinicians begin lipid screening at earlier ages.

Recommendations at the current time are to treat children above age 10 years with LDL cholesterol at or above 160 and to consider treatment if LDL is at or above 130 if other risk factors are present. Treatment goals are to achieve an LDL below 100. While bile acid sequestrants may be recommended as the first-line treatment in children, they are poorly tolerated and effective therapeutic data is lacking. Thus, statins should be considered with appropriate monitoring. Dietary counseling and blood glucose control are important parts of lipid management.

REFERENCES

1. SEARCH for Diabetes in Youth Study Group. The burden of diabetes mellitus among US youth: prevalence estimates from the SEARCH for Diabetes in Youth Study. *Pediatrics.* 2006;118:1510-8.
2. The Writing Group for the SEARCH for Diabetes in Youth Study Group. Incidence of Diabetes in Youth in the United States. *JAMA.* 2007;297:2716-24.

3. Jahromi MM, and Eisenbarth GS. Cellular and molecular pathogenesis of type 1A diabetes. *Cell Mol Lif Sci.* 2007;64:865-872.

4. Emery LM, Babu S, Bugawam TL, et al. Newborn HLA-Dr, DQ genotype screening: age- and ethnicity-specific type 1 diabetes risk estimates. *Pediatr Diabetes.* 2005;6:136-144.

5. Peng H, Hagopian W. Environmental factors in the development of type 1 diabetes. *Rev Endocr Metab Disord.* 2006;7:149-162.

6. Expert Committee on the Diagnosis and Classification of Diabetes. Diagnosis and classification of diabetes mellitus. *Diabetes Care.* 2007;S1:S42-S47.

7. Silverstein J, Klingensmith G, Copeland K, et al. Care of children and adolescents with type 1 diabetes: a statement of the American Diabetes Association. *Diabetes Care.* 2005;28:186.

8. Weigand S, Raile K, Reinehr T, et al. Daily insulin requirement of childrena and adolescents with type 1 diabetes: effect of age, gender, body mass index and mode of therapy. *Eur J Endocrinol.* 2008;158:543-549.

9. Chase HP, Dixon B, Pearson J, et al. Reduced hypoglycemic episodes and improved glycemic control in children with type 1 diabetes using insulin glargine and NPH. *J Pediatr.* 2003;143:737-740.

10. Diabetes Research in Children Network (DirecNet) Study Group, Tsalikian E, et al. Prevention of hypoglycemia during exercise in children with type 1 diabetes by suspending basal insulin. *Diabetes Care.* 2006;29:2200-2204.

11. JDRF Continuos Glucose Monitor Study Group, Tamborlane WV, et al. Continuous glucose monitoring and intensive treatment of Type 1 diabetes. *N Eng J Med.* 2008:359.

12. DCCT Research Group. The effect of intensive diabetes treatment on the development and progression of long-term complications in IDDM: the DCCT. *N Engl J Med.* 1993;329:977-986.

13. DCCT Research Group. The effect of intensive diabetes treatment on long-term complications in adolescents with IDDM: the DCCT. *J Pediatr.* 1994;125:177-188.

14. White NH, Cleary PA, Dahma W, et al. Beneficial effects of intensive therapy of diabetes during adolescence: outcomes after the conclusion of the DCCT. *J Pediatr.* 2001;139:804-812.

15. Lachlin JM, Genuth S, Nathan DM, et al. Effect of glycemic exposure on the risk of microvascular complications in the DCCT-revisited. *Diabetes.* 2008;57:995-1001.

16. Fanelli CG, Epifano L, Rambotti AM, et al. Meticulous prevention of hypoglycemia normalizes the glycemic thresholds and magnitude of most of neuroendocrine responses to, symptoms of, and cognitive function during hypoglycemia in intensively treated patients with short-term IDDM. *Diabetes.* 1993;42:1683-1689.

17. Haymon M, Schreiner B. Mini-dose glucagon rescue for hypoglycemia in children with Type 1 diabetes. *Diabetes Care.* 2001;24;634-645.

18. American Diabetes Association. Diabetic ketoacidosis in infants, children, and adolescents. *Diabetes Care.* 2006;29:1150-1159.

19. Wolfsdorf J, Glaser N, Sperling MA. Diabetic ketoacidosis in infants, children, and adolescents. *Diabetes Care.* 2006;29:1150-1159.

20. Dunger DB, Sperling MA, et al. ESPE/LWPES consensus statement on diabetic ketoacidosis in children and adolescents. *Arch Dis Child.* 2004;89(2):188-194.

21. Glaser N, Barnett P, McCaslin I, et al. Risk factors for cerebral edema in children with diabetic ketoacidosis. *N Engl J Med.* 2002;344:264-269.

22. Marcin JP, Glaser N, Barnett P, et al. Factors associated with adverse outcomes in children wiht diabetic ketoacidosis-related cerebral edema. *J Pediatr.* 2002;141:793-797.

23. Lueder GT, Silverstein J, et al. Screening for retinopathy in the pediatric patient with Type 1 diabetes. *Pediatrics.* 2005; 116:270.

Websites

American Diabetes Association: www.diabetes.org
Children with Diabetes: www.childrenwithdiabetes.com
Diabetes TrialNet: www.diabetestrialnet.org/
Juvenile Diabetes Research Foundation: www.jdrf.org/
Immune Tolerance Network: www.immunetolerance.org/
International Society for Pediatric and Adolescent Diabetes diabetes guidelines: www.ispad.org

Part C. Type 2 Diabetes Mellitus

Dana Dabelea and Georgeanna J. Klingensmith

INTRODUCTION

Historically, young children and teenagers with diabetes have had type 1 diabetes (T1DM), caused by an autoimmune destruction of the β cells of the pancreas leading to absolute insulin deficiency, while those over 30 have been considered to have type 2 diabetes (T2DM), defined as diabetes resulting from insulin resistance, with a concomitant insulin secretory defect. However, childhood diabetes, as adult diabetes, is now acknowledged to be a complex and heterogeneous disorder. An increasing proportion of youth have apparent T2DM, especially in minority populations. Nonetheless, population-based data on the incidence of pediatric T2DM are still limited.

EPIDEMIOLOGY

The incidence of type 2 diabetes is increasing in youth. The increase began in the United States in the early 1990, although in retrospective analysis[1] T2DM was recognized in Native American youth in the early 1980s.[2] The true magnitude of T2DM in youth may be underestimated since most data come from reviews of diabetes clinics with differing definitions of type 2 diabetes resulting in potential for misclassification of diabetes type. There is a need for large population-based studies using standardized case definitions to more accurately define the magnitude of childhood T2DM. However, it is clear that T1DM remains the predominant form of diabetes in youth.

Prevalence

Population-based studies, where all individuals within a geographical area undergo diabetes screening, are ideal to determine prevalence, as they capture even undiagnosed cases. However, very few such studies in youth exist. The most comprehensive epidemiologic studies of prevalence and incidence of T2DM in youth show the following.

The NHANES survey of US youth from 1999 to 2002, found the prevalence 0.3%, or 3 per 10,000 youth in the general population.[3] This included self-report of 2DM and those treated with both insulin and oral medications, hence probably having T2DM.

SEARCH for Diabetes in Youth is a large, multicenter, multiethnic collaborative US study of physician-diagnosed diabetes in youth less than 20 years of age in the US. In 2007, SEARCH found a similar T2DM prevalence of 02.2 per 10,000 in the general population.[4] SEARCH also documented that T2DM is rare in children under 10. Among the 1349 diabetes cases in children age 0 to 9 years, only 11 had T2DM Among the 6030 cases in youth age 10 to 19 years, T2DM accounted for about 6% of diabetes diagnosed in non-Hispanic whites, but 22% in Hispanics, 33% in African Americans, 40% in Asian/Pacific Islanders, and 76% in Native American youth.

T2DM is very common among Native North American adolescents. Thirty years of data collected among the Pima Indians of Arizona have shown increasing rates of antibody negative diabetes among children, with a female preponderance. From 1967-1976 to 1987-1996 the T2DM prevalence in Pima youth increased from 2.4% to 3.8% in males, and from 2.7% to 5.3% in females, the highest rates reported in youth to date.[2] In 2001, one in 359 (28/10,000 youth) Navajo youth age 15 to 19 years participating in the SEARCH study had diabetes. Among other Southwest Indians, Alaskan Native, Canadian First Nation youth, T2DM prevalence was also very high, and reportedly increasing.

T2DM has now been reported in youth of almost all countries worldwide with T2DM appearing to be the leading cause of childhood diabetes in Asia.

Incidence and Temporal Trends

Clinic-based studies

Many studies rely on data collected from diabetes clinics. A strength of such studies is that pediatric endocrinologist assignment of DM type is likely to be more accurate (though not always uniform) than in population-based studies. However, a particular clinic population may not accurately represent the general U.S. population and may suffer from referral bias.

Clinic-based studies were the first to report an increased incidence of T2DM in youth. In Chicago, T2DM incidence rates rose by 9% per year from 1985 to 1994, in African American and Latino children. With a higher incidence in African Americans than Latinos (15.2 vs 10.7/100,000/year), and a female predominance. Similarly, in Cincinnati T2DM incidence increased tenfold, from 3% to 4% of new cases of diabetes in 1982 to 20% in 1994 (Figure 10-10).[1] Similar trends are reported from centers around the country. Significant predictors of T2DM are older age at diagnosis, Hispanic or African-American race/ethnicity and female gender. An analysis of the U Indian Health Service outpatient database revealed a 68% increase in the prevalence of diabetes between 1990 and 1998 among adolescents aged 15 to 19, from 3.2 per 1000 to 5.4 per 1000. During this period, the rate for those less than 15 years old remained stable and relatively low at 1.2 per 1000. Studies from England and Australia reflect similar trends with adolescents with females and minority youth at increasing risk for type 2 diabetes.[5] However, the overall incidence of T2DM compared with the incidence of T1DM indicates that T2DM is still relatively infrequent.

Population-based studies

SEARCH for Diabetes in youth is the first population-based US study to provide comprehensive estimates of T2DM incidence in youth according to race/ethnicity. In 2002 and 2003, a total of 2435 youth with newly diagnosed diabetes were ascertained covering over 10 million person-years. Among children age less than 10 years, most had T1DM, regardless of race/ethnicity, with only 19 children with T2DM. Overall, T2DM was relatively infrequent, except among 10 to 14 and 15 to 19 year old minority groups. The rates of T2DM were the highest among Native Americans (25.3/100,000/year and 49.4/100,000/year for ages 10-14 and 15-19 years, respectively), followed by African Americans (22.3 and 19.4), Asian/Pacific Islanders (11.8 and 22.7) and Hispanic youth (8.9 and 17.0), and were low (3.0 and 5.6) among non-Hispanic whites.[6] Thus, while T2DM is relatively uncommon in white youth, T2DM contributes considerably to the overall diabetes incidence among minority youth age more than or equal to 10 years, and rates are approximately 60% higher in females than in males.

While there is evidence supporting an increasing incidence and prevalence of T2DM among youth, it is possible that the rise world wide is mainly a feature of high-risk ethnic groups although increasing prevalence rates of obesity in all population groups has been associated

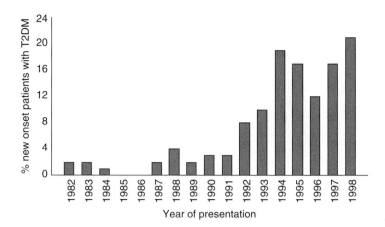

FIGURE 10-10 ■ Changing frequency of Type 2 diabetes mellitus in new onset youth (0-19 years at diagnosis).[1]

with increased rates of type 2 diabetes in all population groups in the United States. Well-designed studies of youth in Germany, Austria, France, and the UK all indicate that T2DM remains a rarity in these populations, accounting for only 1% to 2% of all diabetes cases.[7] In contrast, while the U SEARCH data support the notion that T2DM in youth is predominantly occurring in high-risk ethnic groups, T2DM accounts for 14.9% of all diabetes cases among NHW adolescents age 10 years and older. Although differences in obesity rates between US and European youth are likely contributors, the full explanation for these discrepancies remains uncertain.

PATHOGENESIS

Whereas T1DM is owing to β-cell destruction, T2DM is caused by a combination of insulin resistance and the inability of β-cells to maintain adequate compensatory insulin secretion (Figure 10-11). T2DM in youth typically occurs during puberty and is thought to coincide with a physiologic rise (as high as 50%) in insulin resistance. Healthy adolescents are able to compensate for the peri-pubertal rise in insulin resistance with a compensatory increase in insulin secretion.[8] However, in some adolescents pancreatic β-cells cannot overcome this rise in insulin resistance with a compensatory increase in insulin secretion, and thus a relative insulin deficiency develops, eventually leading to T2DM. In addition, as in adults, both overall obesity and central obesity have been associated with increased insulin resistance. In obese adolescents, the additive effects of obesity-related and pubertal-related insulin resistance create additional stress on the pancreas, and may tip the balance over to T2DM. Since puberty occurs on average a year earlier in females than males, pubertal insulin resistance also begins earlier in females. This may partly explain the earlier age of onset in females, and the female predominance in adolescent T2DM.

Insulin resistance occurs primarily in liver, muscle, and fat cells, and has effects on glucose, protein, and lipid metabolism, as well as on vascular endothelial function. As insulin secretion diminishes, postprandial hyperglycemia develops, and finally fasting hyperglycemia occurs. Over time, there is continued decrease in insulin secretory capacity and need for exogenous insulin replacement. Data from adult studies suggest that by the time of diagnosis there is already a 50% reduction in β-cell secretory capacity and after 6 or 7 years there is inadequate insulin secretion, even with oral secretagogues, and exogenous insulin is required. There is concern that this time course may be accelerated in teens.

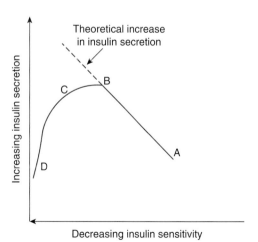

FIGURE 10-11 ■ Type 2 diabetes: decreased insulin sensitivity with inadequate compensatory insulin secretion over time. **(A)** Normal insulin sensitivity/balanced insulin secretion (normal glucose tolerance). **(B)** Decreased insulin sensitivity/compensatory insulin secretion (normal glucose tolerance) **(C)** Continued decrease in insulin sensitivity/relative lack of compensatory insulin secretion (impaired glucose tolerance). **(D)** Markedly decreased insulin sensitivity/absolute lack of compensatory insulin secretion (Type 2 DM).

RISK FACTORS

Race and Ethnicity

Race/ethnicity is widely recognized as an important risk factor in the development of T2DM in adults. The influence of race/ethnicity appears to be even stronger for youth-onset T2DM. Higher prevalence rates have been seen in Asians, Hispanics, African Americans, and indigenous peoples (USA, Canada, Australia), with the highest rates in the world being observed in Pima Indians.

Racial/ethnic differences in the prevalence of T2DM in youth may reflect differences in genetic susceptibility for insulin resistance. Even when controlling for body weight, there appear to be ethnic differences in insulin resistance, with African American youth having more hyperinsulinemia and insulin resistance than those of European ancestry. African American children have increased insulin resistance when compared to weight, age, sex, pubertal stage, and BMI matched Caucasian controls.[9] In addition, an expression of an inherent limited pancreatic β-cell capacity in African American children has been suggested by their lack of the physiologic pubertal rise in first and second phase insulin responses compared to white adolescence, despite approximately 30% lower insulin sensitivity in adolescence compared to prepuberty.[10] These findings may reflect inherited differences in the physiologic phenotype that contributes to the increased propensity for T2DM, including both increased insulin resistance and decreased insulin secretory ability.

Family History

Many studies show a strong family history among affected youth, with 45% to 80% having at least one parent with DM and 74% to 100% having a first or second degree relative with T2DM. Therefore, genetic factors are likely to play an important role in risk for T2DM in youth in all ethnic groups. However, family history does not always imply a genetic cause, as factors such as similar environmental influences within families and the effects of obesity or DM during pregnancy on the offspring also demand consideration.

Children with T2DM are also more likely to have a family history of cardiovascular disease. The Bogalusa Heart Study found that children of individuals with T2DM were more likely to be obese and have higher blood pressures, fasting insulin, glucose, and triglycerides.

Obesity, Diet, and Physical Activity

The risk of T2DM increases with increasing weight, increased rate of weight gain, body mass index,

waist-to-hip ratio, and central fat deposition. The recent rise in T2DM incidence has paralleled the increasing prevalence of overweight in U youth and worldwide. The UK National Longitudinal Survey of Youth, found that the prevalence of overweight increased annually from 1986 to 1998 by 3.2% in non-Hispanic white youth, by 5.8% in African Americans, and by 4.3% in Hispanics. Thus by 1998, 21.5% of African Americans, 21.8% of Hispanics, and 12.3% of non-Hispanic white youth were overweight. During 1999 to 2000, 15% of 6 to 19 year olds were overweight, compared to 11% in 1994 to 1998, with the greatest increases in African American and Mexican American adolescents.[11] In 2003 to 2004, 17.1% of US children and adolescents were overweight (Figure 10-12). In addition, the heaviest children are much heavier than previously, with the greatest increases taking place in the top decile.

The findings in the United States are paralleled in other parts of the world and are of such grave concern that the World Health Organization has declared obesity to be a worldwide epidemic, declaring it the biggest unrecognized health problem in the world, affecting an estimated 22 million of the world's children. The public health importance of the obesity epidemic extends well beyond the increased risk for T2DM, because obesity is associated with increased risk for many other disabling and deadly conditions.[12]

Obesity is likely linked to recent changes in children's diets. Fast food and high fat/high sugar convenience item consumption have increased while time for family meals has decreased in many societies.[13] While diet composition may contribute to obesity, it is likely that the most important aspect in the development of obesity and insulin resistance and T2DM in youth is excess caloric intake relative to caloric expenditure. Concurrent with increases in overweight and obesity, physical activity has decreased among children and adolescents. Currently, only a small percentage of U youth report regular strenuous physical activity more than 3 times per week. One reason for the decline in physical activity is the reduction of physical education in schools, with participation rates down from 41.6% in 1991 to 24.5% in 1995. In the developed world, increasing use of computers and television also markedly decrease children's activity level.

Early Life Factors

The intrauterine environment is increasingly recognized as an important contributor to disease both in childhood and in adult life. Being either small for gestational age (SGA) or large for gestational age (LGA) is associated with the development of T2DM later in life. Both genetic and environmental factors are likely important.

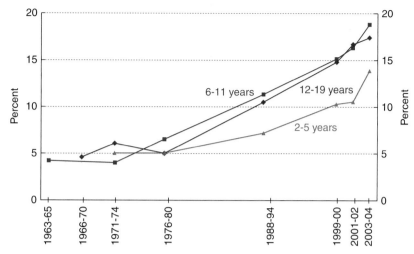

FIGURE 10-12 ■ Trends in child and adolescent overweight. Overweight is defined as BMI ≥ gender- and weight-specific 95th percentile from the 2000 growth charts issued by the Centers for Disease Control and Prevention (CDC). (*From National Health Examination Surveys II [ages 6-11] and III [ages 12-17], National Health and Nutrition Examination Surveys I, II, III, and 1999-2004, NCHS, CDC.*)

Exposure to maternal diabetes and obesity

Exposure to maternal DM *in utero* is a significant risk factor for obesity, IGT, and T2DM in youth. The offspring of women with DM during pregnancy are large at birth and more obese during childhood and adolescence than the offspring of prediabetic or nondiabetic women. Consequently, at every age before 20 years, offspring of diabetic women have more IGT and T2DM than those of prediabetic and nondiabetic women. The higher prevalence of T2DM seems to be only partially mediated by the earlier development of obesity in these offspring. There is a direct correlation between amniotic fluid insulin concentration at weeks 32 to 34 of pregnancy and obesity at ages 6 and 8 years, suggesting fetal insulin exposure as a possible mechanism of the excessive childhood weight gain.

While intrauterine exposure is often difficult so separate from genetic factors, there is evidence suggesting that the obesity and T2DM in offspring of diabetic mothers is not solely owing to genetics. To determine the role of exposure to the diabetic intrauterine environment while controlling for genetic susceptibility, the prevalence of T2DM was compared in Pima Indian siblings born before and after their mother was diagnosed with T2DM. Children born after their mother was diagnosed with DM (exposed to the diabetic intrauterine environment) had a BMI significantly higher (+2.6 kg/m^2) and had over a three-fold higher risk of developing diabetes at an early age compared to siblings born before the diagnosis of diabetes in their mother. Among Pima Indian youth, exposure to maternal diabetes and obesity in pregnancy could account for most of the dramatic increase in T2DM prevalence over the last 30 years.

Recently, the SEARCH Case-Control Study (SEARCH CC) provided evidence that intrauterine exposure to maternal diabetes and obesity are important determinants of type 2 diabetes in youth of other racial/ethnic groups (non-Hispanic white, Hispanic, and African American), together contributing to 47% of type 2 diabetes in the offspring.[14]

Breastfeeding

Breastfeeding is protective against later development of obesity and T2DM. A longer duration of exclusive breastfeeding also appears highly protective in a dose dependent manner against overweight and obesity in children of various age groups.[14] Exclusive breastfeeding for the first 2 months of life protects against the development of T2DM in adolescence and young adulthood in Pima Indians and breast feeding (of any duration) is lower among youth with T2DM than among controls in a group of youth of diverse racial/ethnic backgrounds. When BMI z-score is considered, the results suggest that the risk for type 2 diabetes is mediated through childhood weight status. Thus, these data suggest that breast feeding may be protective against development of T2DM in youth regardless of race/ethnicity, an effect that may be mediated in part by limiting weight during childhood.

CLINICAL PRESENTATION

Youth with T2DM may present with signs and symptoms ranging from acute manifestations compatible with T1DM (polyuria, polydipsia, weight loss) to mild hyperglycemia discovered incidentally. Although approximately 10% of T2DM youth presented in DKA, the majority of youth T2DM present with mild hyperglycemia and up to 50% of patients may be asymptomatic.[15] In Japan, almost one-third of T2DM youth were diagnosed by urinalysis during physical examination. Patients often display signs of insulin resistance, including hyperlipidemia, hypertension, and acanthosis nigricans (Figure 10-13a and b).

In childhood, the mean age at diagnosis is during puberty (13-15 years) and T2DM with onset at ages younger than 10 years, although possible, is extremely rare. Over 90% of adolescent type 2 patients are overweight (BMI ≥ 85th percentile for age and sex) or obese (BMI ≥ 95th percentile). Acanthosis is present in 60% to 95% and almost 90% have a family history of diabetes. There is a female to male excess risk ranging from 1.6-6 to 1. Pediatric T2DM disproportionately affects African Americans, Mexican Hispanics, Native Americans, South and East Asians, and Pacific Island Natives, but all ethnic groups may be affected.[6]

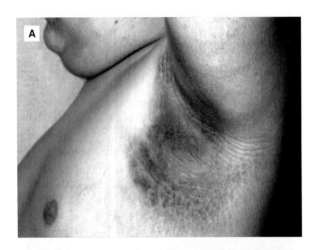

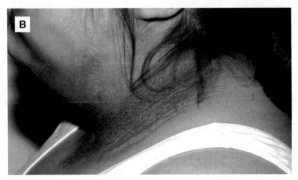

FIGURE 10-13 ■ Acanthosis Nigricans in obese teenagers. **(A)** Acanthosis nigricans in an obese teenage boy. **(B)** Acanthosis nigricans in an obese teenage girl.

DIFFERENTIAL DIAGNOSIS OF TYPE 2 AND TYPE 1 DIABETES

The differentiation of T2DM from T1DM is presented in Table 10-8, and a diagnostic algorithm is shown in Figure 10-2. As indicated in the section "Epidemiology" discussed earlier, T2DM is rare in children under 10, that is, in prepubertal children, regardless of race/ethnicity and weight, and is more common in minority youth. T2DM should be considered when an obese adolescent presents with acute onset and especially when hyperglycemia without ketosis is the initial presenting feature.[16] Additional findings of insulin resistance are also frequently present at diagnosis in T2DM and are more rare in T1DM (Table 10-8). When considering the differential diagnosis between T1DM and T2DM, it is important to remember that as obesity increases in the general population, the percent of youth presenting with T1DM who are overweight or obese will also increase. In a predominantly white population, 40% of adolescents with a BMI more than 30 kg/m² presenting with diabetes were autoantibody positive (consistent with T1DM), demonstrating that obesity may also be found in youth with new onset T1DM. In addition, data from the United Kingdom Prospective Diabetes Study (UKPDS), have shown that individuals 25 to 34 years of age with clinically diagnosed T2DM had a 33% likelihood of being GAD autoantibody positive and those with GAD positivity had a 97% risk of requiring insulin within 7 years with a mean time to insulin dependency of only 3 years.[17]

Antibodies to islet antigens should be obtained in all patients in whom classification is uncertain. This includes adolescents of minority racial/ethnic groups with new, acute onset diabetes; patients who are obese, but yet have acute onset disease; patients who are originally diagnosed with T1DM but follow a noninsulin requiring course after initial diagnosis; and, patients who are originally diagnosed as having T2DM but who require early insulin therapy to maintain adequate diabetes control and/or develop recurrent ketoacidosis in the absence of insulin therapy.[18]

The differentiation from MODY diabetes is discussed in Part A and D.

T2DM should be considered in overweight and obese youth with nonacute onset of hyperglycemia and a family history of T2DM, high-risk race/ethnicity and other signs or symptoms of the insulin resistance/metabolic syndrome. However, owing to the serious medical consequences of unrecognized T1DM, all overweight and obese young people, 10 to 34 years of age, with diabetes should be evaluated and followed carefully to determine if they have T1DM or T2DM so that insulin therapy can be promptly initiated when required.

Table 10-8.

Characteristics of Type 1 vs Type 2 Diabetes Mellitus

	Type 1	Type 2
Age onset	Throughout childhood	Pubertal
Sex distribution	F = M	F > M
Ethnic distribution	All (low frequency in Asians, Native Americans)	All (greater frequency in Hispanic, African American, Native Americans)
Obesity	Proportionate to population	>90%
Onset	Usually acute	Insidious
Acanthosis nigricans	Rare	Common
Ketosis, ketoacidosis at onset	Common	Up to 33%
Islet autoimmunity	Present >90% (if multiple antibodies tested)	Typically absent
Weight loss	Common	Common
Insulin secretion	Low	Variable
Insulin sensitivity	Normal (with BG control)	Decreased
% Probands with 1st or 2nd degree relatives affected	3%-5%	74%-100%
Inheritance	Non-Mendelian	Non-Mendelian, strongly familial

(Adapted from Rosenbloom et al, 1999 with permission)

Consideration should be given to determining diabetes autoantibodies (anti-GAD and anti-IA-2) in obese young people with diabetes to identify those at highest risk for early metabolic decompensation and insulin requirement.

TREATMENT

Goals

The goals of treatment in T2DM include

- normalization of glycemia achieving a HbA1c of less than 6.5%,
- weight loss,
- an increase in exercise capacity, and
- control of comorbidities, including dyslipidemia, hypertension, nephropathy, and hepatic steatosis.

Because of the multitude of cardiovascular risk factors associated with insulin resistance, T2DM is more likely to be associated with earlier severe complications than T1DM in childhood. In addition, reduction in the rate of complications may require more stringent blood glucose control in insulin resistant T2DM than in T1DM, and especially diligent attention to comorbidities.

As in T1DM, the physician and patient/family should set goals together to optimize understanding of the goals and maximize family adherence. Optimal goals should be adapted gradually to meet ultimate expectations in order not to make too many lifestyle changes at once, which may lead to failure. In order to maximize success, initial visits should be more frequent with the ultimate goal of visits every 3 to 6 months depending on the stability and success of metabolic control, presence of comorbidities, and family adaptation to care. The importance of education in diabetes management cannot be over emphasized. The patient and family well educated in diabetes management are generally better able to make the necessary lifestyle changes required to succeed in the goals of therapy.

Box 10-2 lists the circumstances in which a patient suspected of having type 2 diabetes should be referred to a pediatric endocrinologist.

Education

The education of the patient and family with T2DM is similar to that required for families with T1DM. Since lifestyle changes are the cornerstone of management of T2DM, the initial and on-going education for T2DM emphasizes behavioral changes (diet and activity) without which management of T2DM cannot be successful. Education in insulin therapy and hypoglycemia usually are not required immediately unless the patient has significant metabolic decompensation at presentation requiring insulin treatment.

Box 10-2. When to Refer

Diabetes Mellitus Type 2

Any of the following, isolated or in combination:

1. Clinical or chemical evidence of insulin resistance
   A. Acanthosis nigricans
   B. Elevated fasting serum insulin concentration
   C. Elevated serum triglycerides/low HDL
   D. Elevated serum transaminases (AST/ALT)
2. Abnormal carbohydrate metabolism
   A. Fasting blood glucose >100 mg/dL ≤126 mg/dL: impaired fasting glycemia (IFG)
   B. Fasting blood glucose >126 mg/dL: diabetes mellitus
   C. Random or 2-hour post oral GTT blood glucose >140 mg/dL ≤200 mg/dL: impaired glucose tolerance (IGT)
   D. Random or 2-hour post oral GTT blood glucose >200 mg/dL: diabetes mellitus
3. Clinical signs: polyuria or polydipsia

The entire family will need to "buy into" the lifestyle changes required to manage T2DM and understand the critical importance of these lifestyle changes to the successful management of T2DM. Many adolescents with T2DM have other family members with T2DM, all to frequently these individuals have been unsuccessful in managing their diabetes and are skeptical about anyone's ability to maintain diabetes control and fatalistic that any care will alter outcome. These attitudes clearly will undermine attempts at optimal care unless the diabetes education is successful in instilling hope for a good outcome and confidence that the family will be successful in helping the teen to care for diabetes.

Education should be given by team members with special expertise and knowledge of the dietary, exercise, and psychological needs of youth with T2DM. Education should be provided in a culturally sensitive manner with attention to the needs of adolescents beginning to become independent of their families. Although all socioeconomic strata are affected by T2DM, in North America, T2DM in adolescents disproportionately affects minority youth with fewer resources. Thus educational tools may need to be used which are appropriate to those with more limited financial resources and perhaps lower parental educational backgrounds. Educators will need to identify resources and provide meal suggestions that will allow families to follow the dietary recommendations optimal for T2DM, for example, how to incorporate increased fresh fruit and vegetables into meals. Likewise exercise recommendations need to be adapted to the family's circumstances and resources.

If there is uncertainty in the diagnosis of T2DM, families may be unclear if the education and advice they are given is important to them and hesitate to embrace the therapy recommended including unpleasant changes in diet and exercise. Likewise, the patient and

family may be reluctant to begin, or continue, insulin if they think the diagnosis is likely to be T2DM. This confusion can be decreased by emphasizing the importance of normalizing glucose metabolism by necessary dietary changes and if initially required, insulin, regardless of the type of diabetes. The family can be further reassured that as the metabolism improves and additional laboratory information becomes available, the optimal therapy may change depending on the individual needs of the patient.

Lifestyle Interventions

The corner stone of the management of T2DM at any age is lifestyle change with an emphasis on weight reduction and increased physical activity. The adolescent with T2DM is most frequently living in a family complicated by obesity, T2DM, and poor eating/exercise habits. For treatment to be successful all family members either directly or through providing education materials, must be included in the education and treatment planning. Teaching the health implications of obesity, high fat food intake and poor exercise habits for youth is critical for diabetes management success. Health care providers should determine key family members and target education to these members as well as the patient and parents.

An individualized plan for weight reduction is most optimal and should be provided by a nutritionist knowledgeable in culturally sensitive approaches to food management, including family resources. *Weight reduction initially may be achieved by an emphasis on eliminating sugar-containing drinks, decreasing some high fat foods, and teaching healthy portion sizes and portion management. Teaching families to eat food or beverages served on a plate or in a glass, rather than eating directly from a box, can, or bottle is the best way to teach and manage portion size.* Limiting high fat foods is important for reducing caloric intake and for decreasing cardiovascular risk by improving lipid metabolism, including a decrease hepatic fat accumulation. Dietary education should recognize that families with T2DM frequently have disordered eating behaviors including binge eating including nocturnal binge eating. A careful history to determine the frequency of disordered eating and understanding how this undermines successful diabetes management is important to diabetes management. Referral to appropriate resources to address disordered eating behaviors may be necessary before meaningful weight management can be achieved. Any improvement should be celebrated, especially family teamwork in making lifestyle changes.

Initial exercise recommendations should be limited in scope owing to the poor exercise tolerance of obese youth. In anticipation of improving exercise tolerance, a graduated exercise prescription is recommended. *Use of a pedometer and identifying a family member or friend who will participate with the adolescent in the exercise plan is important to initial success and ongoing motivation to exercise.* In addition, limiting sedentary activities including TV time and computer time is helpful in increasing activity. Maintaining a log of exercise accomplished may be motivating if points are accumulated for some type of family based reward.

Medication

Metformin and insulin are the two medications approved for treatment of T2DM in youth. Metformin is the initial treatment of choice for adolescents with T2DM (Table 10-9). Metformin has the advantages of limited risk of hypoglycemia and generally decreasing or stabilizing weight. Other medications are discussed here as they may be useful in teens more than 18 years and young adults, although the most recent recommendations of the ADA for treatment of T2DM in adults are to limit use of most of these agents since their cost effectiveness is less clear.

Lifestyle change should be continued to be emphasized in addition to pharmacologic therapy. The aim of initial pharmacologic therapy is to decrease insulin resistance.

Metformin acts on insulin receptors in liver, muscle, and fat tissue to increase insulin action. This decreases hepatic glucose production improving fasting glucose levels and improves muscle and fat glucose uptake improving waking glucose levels. A 1% to 2% decrease in HbA1c is expected with long-term, consistent use. The major side effect is intestinal complaints including abdominal pain, diarrhea, and nausea. These effects are usually transitory and can be lessened by slow dose titration over 3 to 4 weeks beginning with 250 mg daily, increasing until the desired glucose levels are achieved and/or the maximum dose of 1000 mg bid is achieved. Metformin has a low risk for lactic acidosis which may be increased in patients with renal impairment, hepatic disease, cardiac or respiratory insufficiency, or who are receiving radiographic contrast materials.

Patients at-risk for pregnancy should be counseled on the effects of diabetes and oral agents on conception and fetal development. Metformin is an FDA pregnancy category B drug and is not expected to harm the fetus, but is not approved for nursing mothers since it may be transmitted to the infant. Since metformin may normalize ovulatory abnormalities in girls with insulin resistance and polycystic ovarian syndrome (PCOS), therapy may increase pregnancy risk.

Failure of monotherapy with metformin over 3 months may indicate the need to reassess the diagnosis of type 2 diabetes and consider insulin therapy. If the

Table 10-9.

Pharmacological Treatment Algorithm in Type 2 Diabetes Mellitus

A. Initial treatment:
  1. Metabolically stable, nonacidotic, HbA1c < 8%
    ■ Start metformin at 500 mg q/d titrate as tolerated (<500 mg/wk) to maximum of 2000 mg/d
  2. Metabolically stable, nonacidotic, HbA1c >8%
    Add to metformin:
    ■ Basal insulin, glargine or detemir (15-30 units qhs)
    Once glucose control is attained, wean insulin as tolerated
  3. Metabolically unstable, acidotic
    ■ Treat as in T1DM until acidosis resolved, then
    ■ Start metformin and subcutaneous insulin as above
    Once glucose control is attained, wean insulin as tolerated
B. Intensification of therapy for failure to maintain A1c <6.5
  Reassess for compliance with metformin theray
  Add-on insulin:
    ■ Continue metformin therapy at 1000 mg bid
    ■ Add basal insulin (glargine or detemir)—start at 10–20 u/d given whenever adherence and supervision are most likely
    ■ Titrate as needed to maintain A1c <6.5
C. Failure to maintain A1c <6.5 despite 1 unit/kg long-acting insulin:
  Reassess for compliance with both metformin and insulin therapy
  Determine if there is evidence for postprandial hyperglycemia with intermittent blood glucose testing or 72 h continuous glucose monitoring, if yes:
    ■ Continue metformin and basal insulin
    ■ Add short-acting insulin or, if ≥ 18 y, meglitinide/repaglinide prior to meals with the dose determined as in type 1 diabetes (see Diabetes Part A: Type 1 Diabetes)
  Additional medication for those ≥ 18 years are listed in the text. Little data exist for any of these agents in the young adult population and they are all relatively expensive making the cost:benefit unclear

From: Diabetes Care. 2008;31:1-11. Published online October 22, 2008

diagnosis of type 2 diabetes is confirmed, failure to maintain adequate glucose regulation indicates the need to add insulin, alone or in combination with meglitinide/repaglinide. A thiazolidinedione, sulfonylurea; amylin, a GLP-1 mimetic, or a DPP-IV inhibitor may be considered in older teens and young adults. These additional oral therapies are aimed at increasing insulin secretion, further improving insulin sensitivity and/or slowing postprandial glucose absorption.[19] Only insulin and metformin are approved for use in adolescents less than 18 years of age.

Insulin may improve glucose uptake despite the presence of hyperinsulinemia and insulin resistance. Metformin should be continued to improve insulin sensitivity. Relatively small doses of a long-acting insulin analogue may provide satisfactory therapy without the addition of meal related therapy. The time of day for administration should be selected to be the time of day the adolescent can most consistently administer the insulin dose. Evening may provide the best suppression of hepatic glucose production, but this consideration should be tempered by the adolescent's schedule. If postprandial hyperglycemia occurs, rapid- or short-acting insulin may be required, however, premeal therapy may be a challenge for adolescents. If postprandial hyperglycemia persists, meglitinide/repaglinide can be substituted to determine if an oral premeal therapy is more acceptable and consistently used.

The side effects of insulin are hypoglycemia, which is not common in T2DM youth treated with insulin, and weight gain which can be a vexing problem if dietary advice is not attended to. Thiazolidinediones are not recommended in combination with insulin because of increased risk for fluid retention with the combination.

Sulfonylurea and meglitinide/repaglinide (not approved for use in those <18 years) increase endogenous insulin production. Therefore these agents are only useful when there is residual beta cell function. Sulfonylureas bind to receptors on the K^+/ATP channel complex causing K^+ channels to close, resulting in insulin secretion. Meglitinide and repaglinide bind to a separate site on the K^+/ATP channel complex and have a more rapid onset of action and a shorter duration of effect. The major adverse effects of sulfonylureas are weight gain and hypoglycemia, which can be prolonged.

Thiazolidinediones (only approved use in adults) increase insulin sensitivity in muscle, liver, and fat tissue. In contrast to metformin, the greatest effect is on muscle tissue. Treatment in adults has been shown to decrease HbA1c by 0.5% to 1.0%. Thiazolidinediones bind to ubiquitous nuclear receptors, peroxisome proliferator activator receptors (PPAR gamma). This binding activates many actions of insulin including regulation of insulin receptor activity, glucose transport into the cell, adipose cell differentiation, and muscle cell growth. Side effects include weight gain, edema, anemia, decreased bone mineral density with increased fractures, macular edema, and increased risk of heart disease, especially congestive failure, in adults. Earlier drugs in this class were associated with hepatotoxicity, including hepatic failure, but newer thiazolidinediones (rosiglitazone and pioglitazone) have not been found to have this side effect in adults. Piogliazone is not recommended because of reports of increased risk for fluid retention and potential cardiovascular side effects found in adult patients.

Glucosidase inhibitors (acarbase, miglitol) (these drugs are only approved for use in adults) reduce the absorption of carbohydrates in the upper small intestine by inhibiting breakdown of oligosaccharides, thereby delaying absorption in the lower small intestine and reducing the postprandial rise of plasma glucose. Although they have an excellent safety profile, the side effect of increased flatulence make these unacceptable to most youth.

Amylin is not approved for those under 18 years, and is only approved for use in the United States for patients with T1DM and T2DM who are taking insulin. Its action is to decrease glucagon release, slow gastric emptying, and increase satiety, thereby decreasing food intake. Amylin is produced in the pancreatic β-cells in response to food and it is decreased with β-cell failure. Amylin is administered by subcutaneous injection before meals, therefore its consistent administration may be problematic in adolescents. Adverse effects are hypoglycemia and nausea; hypoglycemia may be decreased by decreasing the insulin dose by 30% to 50% when treatment with amylin is initiated. Although weight loss is frequently a desired effect, weight loss is generally modest and the lack of more dramatic weight loss may contribute to frequent discontinuation of the medication.

Incretin mimetics (glucagon-like peptide-1 [GLP-1] receptor agonists) (exenatide) (these drugs are only approved for use in adults) have effects similar to amylin: suppressing glucagon, prolonging gastric emptying, and promoting satiety, in addition, they increase insulin secretion from the β-cell proportionate to blood glucose concentrations. In normal physiology, GLP-1 is rapidly secreted by L-cells in the small intestine into the circulation in response to food. Incretin mimetics are given as a twice-daily subcutaneous injection usually with breakfast and dinner. They are rapidly degraded by dipeptidyl peptidase-IV (DPP-IV); both native GLP-1 and the injected mimetic have a half-life of 2 minutes. Adverse effects include nausea, vomiting, diarrhea and infrequent dizziness, headache, and dyspepsia. The nausea decreases over time. A longer acting analogue is in development and may be effective when given once weekly. This analogue has not been found to promote weight loss.

DPP-IV inhibitors (not approved for use in children) inhibit the enzyme that breaks down GLP-1, resulting in higher concentrations of GLP-1 producing effects similar to those of GLP-1 mimetics. Interestingly, they do not have an effect on gastric emptying, satiety or weight loss, and are administered orally with metformin or a thiazolidinedione once daily. They are a new class of drugs and there is no experience in their use in adolescents.

Behavioral/Psychosocial Treatment

Many youth with T2DM have poor self-image, mood disorders, and disordered eating. Over 30% may be treated with mood and/or thought stabilizing medications having adverse effects on glucose metabolism (see Part D). An assessment of each patient's psychosocial functioning as well as family functioning is an important part of the evaluation and planning for many families and all patients unable to achieve appropriate metabolic stabilization. The evaluation and recommendations for treatment, if required, should be done in a culturally appropriate manner by someone skilled in caring for youth with chronic disease, ideally by some one with who also has experience evaluating families with type 2 diabetes. If English is not the primary language for one or both parents, the evaluation should be done in the primary language of the parent as well as in the language in which the child is most comfortable.

COMORBIDITIES AND COMPLICATIONS

Assessment and treatment for comorbidities, especially hypertension and lipid abnormalities are an important part of optimal management of T2DM in youth. Hypertension and dyslipidemia as well as hyperglycemia may have been present for months to years prior to diagnosis of T2DM and, with obesity, may contribute to the presence of abnormal albumin excretion at the time of diagnosis. Lifestyle changes may improve blood pressure and lipid profiles, but the addition of medication may be required for optimal management.

Insulin Resistance Syndrome

Adolescents with T2DM may have untreated insulin resistance and even mild hyperglycemia for months to years prior to presenting for medical care. Likewise, features of the insulin resistance syndrome, including low HDL cholesterol, elevated triglycerides, and hypertension, as well as PCOS in females, may be present prior to diagnosis of type 2 diabetes. This period of insulin resistance sets the stage for increased CVD risk prior to the onset of type 2 diabetes. Youth with T2DM compared to youth with T1DM have a higher prevalence of CVD risk factors with abnormalities of blood pressure, lipids, and albuminuria despite shorter duration of diabetes and lower HbA1c.[20] Compared with healthy controls, youth with T2D have higher age- and race/ethnicity-adjusted prevalence of hypertension: 27% versus 5%, obesity: 86% versus 26%, large waist circumference: 82% versus 22%, low HDLC: 25% versus 5%, and high triglycerides: 27% versus 6%, (all p <.0001).[21] Collectively 60% of T2DM youth controls have three or more CVD risk factors within 5 years of diagnosis of T2DM, many found at diagnosis. With preexisting risk factors, atherogenesis may begin years prior to diagnosis of diabetes in this population.

Smoking is a known additional risk factor for cardiovascular disease and all youth with diabetes, both T1DM and T2DM, should be evaluated for smoking and counseled to not begin to smoke, or counseled on the importance of smoking cessation.

Given the potential for preexisting comorbidities, screening for dyslipidemia, hypertension, albuminuria, smoking, and sleep apnea are recommended soon after the diagnosis of T2DM in youth.

Dyslipidemia

T2DM is associated with dyslipidemia; both are independent risk factors for cardiovascular disease in adults. Vascular lipid deposition occurs early in childhood, suggesting that lipid levels should be measured throughout childhood and intervention employed when necessary.

The Pathological Determinants of Atherosclerosis in Youth (PDAY) of 3000 young people dying of accidental causes between the ages of 15 and 34 found that the percentage of intimal surface involved with lesions in the aorta and right coronary was positively associated with VLDL and LDL cholesterol levels, with a 5% increase in surface involvement with each standard deviation increase of VLDL and the LDL cholesterol levels. Conversely, a 1 standard deviation increase in HDL was associated with a 3% decrease in intimal surface involvement. Similarly the Bogalusa Heart study found that total cholesterol, LDL cholesterol, and triglyceride levels correlated with atherosclerotic lesions.

The ADA recommendations for lipid targets in adults, LDL less than 100 mg/dL, HDL-C more than 45 mg/dL, and triglycerides less than 150 mg/dL, are modified for youth with T2DM. The most recent recommendations are to consider medication in addition to dietary and exercise changes when LDL cholesterol is more than 130 mg/dL with the therapeutic target of an LDL less than 100 mg/dL.[22] Other lipid targets are similar to those in adults. If youth with T2DM have two additional CVD risk factors (obesity, family history for early CVD, hypertension, or a positive smoking history), the latest American Heart Association and ADA recommendations for lipid assessment and care are to consider medication if LDL is more than 100 mg/dL, in accordance with recommendations for adults. Despite these recommendations, little data are available describing the results of long-term treatment of youth with lipid lowering medications.[23]

Several randomized, placebo-controlled studies in adults have demonstrated decreased risk of cardiovascular disease in subjects successfully treated with lipid-lowering agents. Any reduction in LDL-cholesterol significantly reduces the risk of cardiovascular disease by approximately 30%, even when starting LDL levels are normal (110 mg/dL). The reduction is even more pronounced in those with diabetes. Thus, although the cutoff LDL value of 100 mg/dL is currently the target standard of care, this value may be too high.

Lipid screening: Since fatty streaks and atherosclerotic plaques appear during childhood, lipid monitoring must begin early in those with the added risk of T2DM. Lipids should be measured shortly after diagnosis (when metabolic stabilization is achieved) and at 5-year intervals thereafter if lipids remain normal. Because T2DM is associated with dyslipidemia as part of the metabolic syndrome, this recommendation may not be adequate for youth with T2DM since lipid levels may increase during the teenaged years. Therefore, children who continue to gain weight, have a family history of cardiovascular risk factors, and/or have poor metabolic control should have lipid levels analyzed every 1 to 2 years.

Treatment: All youth with elevated lipid levels, LDL cholesterol level more than 130 mg/dL, or triglycerides more than 150 mg/dL should receive dietary counseling with recommendations to increase exercise and follow a Step 1 American Heart Association diet, which consists of no more than 30% of total calories from fat and of this, less than 10% should be saturated fat, up to 10% polyunsaturated fat, and less than 300 mg/day should be ingested as cholesterol. If the repeat value after 3 months has not improved, a Step 2 diet, which differs from the Step 1 diet in that less than 7% of calories are provided as saturated fat and less than 200 mg/day of cholesterol is consumed, should be prescribed. If target values cannot be achieved with the Step 2 diet and exercise, pharmacotherapy should be considered.

The pharmacologic agents recommended for children are bile acid binding resins and HMG-CoA reductase inhibitors ("statins"). The former agents are not palatable and there is a very poor compliance rate. In addition, they have only modest effects on cholesterol, with a lowering of 10% to 25%. The statins are much more effective and their use in children has been reported to be safe, with a side-effect profile similar to that noted in adults, but long-term use in children with diabetes has not been reported. Statins are currently not approved for young children and their use should be reserved for adolescents, unless marked hyperlipidemia with family history of early cardiovascular disease (in age 40s or younger) is present. Similarly, fibric acid derivatives and nicotinic acid have not been studied in the pediatric population.

Youth with LDL more than 100 mg/dL, HDL-C less than 45 mg/dL, and triglycerides more than 150 mg/dL should have lipid screening annually. Those with elevated lipids should be counseled on appropriate lifestyle interventions and, when required, pharmacologic treatment initiated, generally beginning with an HMG-CoA reductase inhibitor. The major side effects reported in adults, symptoms of myalgia, and other connective tissue complaints, need special attention as there is an increased risk of rhabdomyolysis.

Hypertension

Hypertension is a common feature of the insulin resistance syndrome and is associated with development of both microvascular and macrovascular disease. Although there have been no studies in children, clinical trials done in adults indicate that aggressive treatment of elevated blood pressure is an effective addition to glycemic control in reducing microvascular and macrovascular complications of diabetes. Guidelines for treatment in children must be extrapolated from studies performed in adults.

Hypertension is defined as blood pressure more than 95th percentile for age, height, and gender on least three occasions. The blood pressure should be taken with the child at rest, in a sitting position with a cuff size equal to two-third the length of the upper arm. Often, blood pressure measurements are obtained as the child enters the clinic, when the child is most nervous, resulting in elevated readings, the "white coat effect." Therefore, the blood pressure should be taken on at least two or three occasions before affirming that the child has hypertension. Both systolic and diastolic blood pressure elevations are important predictors of macrovascular disease. If hypertension is present, it should not be assumed that it is related to the diabetes, and laboratory evaluations to rule out primary renal disease should be performed. Blood pressure charts providing 90th and 95th percentile cut-offs based on age, gender, and height percentile are available on the web at www.//nhlbi.nih.gov/health/pof/heart/hbp/hbp_ped.pdf.

In adults with T2DM, elevated blood pressure is the strongest predictor of future development of cardiovascular disease. In a long-term follow-up study of individuals with T1DM onset before the age of 17 years, systolic blood pressure more than 130 mm Hg, and diastolic more than 85 mm Hg confers increased risk of both macrovascular and microvascular disease. Systolic blood pressures more than 110 mm Hg, 110 to 129 mm Hg, and more than 130 mm Hg confers relative risk of developing cardiovascular disease of 1.8, 2.5, and 5.6, respectively, suggesting that hypertension is also a significant risk for angiopathy in youth with diabetes.

We do not know at what age antihypertensive treatment should be initiated. We do know, however, that children can have fatty streaks in their aortas and coronary arteries at a very young age. The Bogalusa Heart Study found that 50% of children aged 2 to 15 years of age who died from accidental causes already had fatty streak lesions in the coronary arteries. The PDAY study also found that all the aortas and approximately half of the right coronary arteries in this previously healthy group 15 to 19 years at death already demonstrated lesions and 7% of the aortas and 12% of the right coronary arteries already had raised lesions or advanced lesions of atherosclerosis. The prevalence of these raised lesions involving 5% or more of the intimal surface was twice as great in both the aorta and coronary arteries if the patients had hypertension.

Therapy with an ACE inhibitor is the initial pharmacological treatment for hypertension in youth. The initial treatment should begin with the lowest dose possible and increase incrementally until hypertension is controlled or the maximum dose is reached. If hypertension is not controlled with ACE therapy alone, the addition of an ACE receptor blocker should be considered with initial reduction in the dose of the ACE inhibitor. Treatment of hypertension reduces the risk of heart disease in adults with a history of cardiovascular disease or with diabetes mellitus; the effects of the ACE inhibitors on the endothelium and on platelet function appear to be at least as important as the effect on blood pressure.

Blood pressure should be checked at every clinic visit using an appropriate sized cuff with the patient calm and resting. If the blood pressure is confirmed to be elevated it should be checked on at least two other occasions at weekly intervals and if persistently more than 95th percentile for age, sex, and height, a treatment program begun. Initial therapy should focus on weight loss, increasing exercise, moderating salt intake, and smoking cessation or avoidance. If after 3 months of attempts at lifestyle modification, blood pressure has not improved, antihypertensive drug therapy should be considered. ACE inhibitors are the initial drug class recommended. Importantly, major congenital malformations have been reported with first trimester exposure to ACE inhibitors in nondiabetic women.

Nephropathy

Microalbuminuria, defined as urinary albumin excretion rate of 20 to 200 mcg/min, and 30 to 300 mg per 24 hours in timed collections, or 30 to 300 mg/g creatinine in a "spot" collection, is predictive of both renal and cardiovascular disease. As in type 1 diabetes, proteinuria may be owing to several factors other than diabetic renal disease. Therefore, orthostatic proteinuria and exercise induced proteinuria must be ruled out before the diagnosis of macroalbuminuria secondary to diabetes is made. Furthermore, the proteinuria secondary to diabetes may initially be intermittent. High HbA1c and high baseline albumin excretion rate predict development of persistent albuminuria. Thus, intensive efforts should be made to decrease albumin excretion rates and HbA1c levels in patients with intermittent albuminuria.

It is recommended that children with T2DM have spot urine analyzed for albumin at the time of diabetes diagnosis.[24] If albumin is present, spot urine testing should be repeated on specimens obtained from voiding upon awakening in the morning and in the afternoon. If the albumin excretion rate remains elevated, two-timed urine collections on different days should be obtained. The simplest way to achieve this is to obtain a 12-hour overnight urine collection for albumin and creatinine.

ACE inhibition has been shown to decrease albumin excretion rate in patients with and without hypertension. ACE inhibition has several mechanisms of renal protective action in addition to its antihypertensive effect. In the kidney, the vasodilatory effects of the ACE inhibitors result in an increase in afferent arteriolar dilatation, with resultant decrease of elevated intra-glomerular pressure; they also have beneficial effects on the endothelium as well as on platelets and the coagulation system.

If albuminuria is persistent, the patient should be treated with an ACE inhibitor. In addition, patients should be counseled to avoid smoking, as nicotine has marked vasoconstrictive effects. The optimal ACE inhibitor dose should be determined by improvement in albumin excretion. Importantly, major congenital malformations have been reported with first trimester exposure to ACE inhibitors in nondiabetic women so female youth should be counseled on the importance of avoiding pregnancy exposure when on this therapy.

Retinopathy

Unlike type 1 diabetes, in which monitoring for complications is not recommended until the patients have had diabetes for 3 to 5 years, patients with T2DM should be monitored for presence of microvascular diseases at diabetes onset. Thus, all children with T2DM should have a dilated eye examination by an ophthalmologist at disease onset. If retinopathy is present the use of ACE inhibitors should be considered, as ACE inhibition has been shown to slow the progression of retinopathy in patients with and without hypertension.

Nonalcoholic Fatty Liver Disease

Fatty infiltration of the liver, hepatic steatosis, is associated with T2DM owing to the effect of hyperinsulinism and insulin resistance on hepatic fat metabolism. Hepatic steatosis is present in 25% to 50% of obese adolescents with T2DM, as evidenced by elevated liver enzymes, and more advanced form of nonalcoholic fatty liver disease (NAFLD), nonalcoholic steatohepatitis (NASH), is increasingly common with the increased risk for progression to cirrhosis.[25] NAFLD now represents the most common cause of cirrhosis in children and the most common reason for liver transplantation in adults in the United States. Elevated liver enzymes are present in NASH.

Initial screening for NASH should be done in all T2DM youth after diagnosis with follow-up imaging evaluation if persistent enzyme elevations are found in the absence of another explanation for the elevation. Ultrasound is a poor way to assess for NASH, with MRI the best noninvasive way to evaluate the liver for NASH. Medication, especially metformin, to reduce insulin resistance may decrease hepatic steatosis.[26] Consultation with a gastroenterologist familiar with NAFLD in youth should be considered.

Polycystic Ovary Syndrome

Included as part of the insulin resistance syndrome, adolescents with T2DM may have polycystic ovary syndrome (PCOS). This may include hirsutism and oligo-amenorrhea with anovulatory menstrual cycles. Since insulin resistance may be an important factor in the etiology of PCOS, treatment with metformin may restore ovulation. When young women with T2DM are begun on metformin, counseling on this aspect of treatment is critical to avoid unanticipated pregnancy.

PREVENTION

T2DM is a complication of obesity in susceptible children. Therefore, primary prevention of T2DM entails the prevention of obesity in children and adolescents in general, as well as in those patients who are most at risk for development of T2DM and its associated disorders. Additional targeted primary prevention efforts focus on the prevention of the development of diabetes once obesity is established. Secondary prevention includes screening for T2DM in order to modify the early clinical course of diabetes. Tertiary intervention involves efforts to prevent and control complications of T2DM in affected children.[27]

Prevention of the emergence of T2DM and comorbidities requires lifestyle changes to decrease calorie intake and increase physical activity. This is challenging in a fast food and snack culture in which there is easy availability of low-cost foods of high caloric density, and in which there has been a trend toward more eating out at fast food restaurants and larger portion sizes being served in restaurants. Physical activity has declined, with decreased time for physical education in the schools and increased time spent watching television or playing video games. Other factors include lack of safe playing environments for some children, lack of funding for after school programs, and lack of commitment to recreational facilities in many communities. Families also need to commit to increased exercise.

School-based programs have been developed to prevent obesity. Planet Health was a 2-year study of 1295 children in grades 6 to 8 who were exposed to sessions designed to encourage decreased television viewing, decreased consumption of high-fat foods, increased exercise, and increased consumption of fruits and vegetables.[28] This resulted in decreased prevalence of obesity in participating girls compared to controls. Coordinated Approach to Child Health (CATCH) is a program authorized by the Texas legislature, which was designed to train teachers and food service staff elements of a healthy diet and physically active lifestyle and convey this information to students. Following this program, school lunches had 30% of calories less in fat and physical education teachers devoting 50% of class time to vigorous physical activity. Bienestar Health Program, was designed to be a culturally relevant learning activity for 4th grade Mexican-American children involving the parent, teacher, food service workers, and after school care. This program also resulted in significantly decreased dietary fat servings and significant increases in dietary fruit and vegetables, however, there was no change in percent body fat or increase in level of physical activity.

The most successful programs have been in areas in which the population has supported exercise facilities and food modification and grass roots efforts have worked together to effect change. Attempts to modify the school food content, by addressing vending machines, school menus, and alternate school lunch lines have been ongoing in a number of localities, but the effect on children's food choices and weight are not adequately studied.[13]

The prevention of T2DM is a public health issue and must be geared toward the entire population, promoting improved dietary habits and physical activity for all children and their families. The use of pharmacologic agents to reduce weight and the use of fad diets are not appropriate for weight reduction in children. In families at risk for type 2 diabetes (diabetes onset prior to 40 years, maternal diabetes prior to pregnancy, and high-risk ethnic groups), lifestyle changes should be encouraged early in life and should include all family members.

SELECTED READINGS

1. Pinhas-Hamiel O, Dolan LM, Daniels SR, et al. Increased incidence of non-insulin dependent diabetes mellitus among adolescents. *J Pediatr.* 1996;128:608-615.
2. Dabelea D, Hanson RL, Bennett PH, et al. Increasing prevalence of type 2 diabetes in American Indian children. *Diabetologia.* 1998;41:904-910.
3. Duncan GE. Prevalence of diabetes and impaired fasting glucose levels among US adolescents: National Health and Nutrition Examination Survey, 1999-2002. *Arch Pediatr Adolesc Med.* 2006;160:523-528.
4. The SEARCH for Diabetes in Youth Study Group. The burden of diabetes among U.S. youth: prevalence estimates from the SEARCH for diabetes in youth study. *Pediatrics.* 2006 Oct;118:1510-1518.

5. Haines L, Wan KC, Lynn R, Barrett TG, Juksheild, JPH. Rising incidence of type 2 diabetes in children in the U.K. *Diabetes Care.* 2007;30:1097-1101.

6. Writing Group for the SEARCH for Diabetes in Youth Study Group, Dabelea D, Bell RA, et al. Incidence of diabetes in youth in the United States. *JAMA.* 2007; 297:2716-2724.

7. Pinhas-Hamiel O, Zeitler P. The global spread of type 2 diabetes mellitus in children and adolescents. *J Pediatr.* 2005;146:693-700.

8. Travers SH, Jeffers BW, Bloch CA, et al. Gender and Tanner stage differences in body composition and insulin sensitivity in early pubertal children. *J Clin Endocrinol Metab.* 1995;80:172-178.

9. Arslanian S. Insulin secretion and sensitivity in healthy African-American vs American-white children. *Clin Pediatr.* 1998;37:81-88.

10. Goran MI, Bergman RN, Cruz ML, et al. Insulin resistance and associated compensatory responses in African-American and Hispanic children. *Diabetes Care.* 2002;25: 2184-2190.

11. Ogden CL, Carroll MD, Curtin LR, et al. Prevalence of overweight and obesity in the United States, 1999-2004. *JAMA.* 2006 Apr 5;295:1549-1555.

12. Ebbeling CB, Pawlak DB, Ludwig DS. Childhood obesity: public-health crisis, common sense cure. *Lancet.* 2002;360:473-482.

13. Craypo L, Purcell A, Samuels SE, et al. Fast food sales on high school campuses: results from the 2000 California high school fast food survey. *J Sch Health.* 2002;72:78-82.

14. Dabelea D, Mayer-Davis EJ, Lamichhane AP, et al. Association of intrauterine exposure to maternal diabetes and obesity with type 2 diabetes in youth: the SEARCH case-control study. *Diabetes Care.* 2008;31:1422-1426.

15. Burke V, Beilin LJ, Simmer K, et al. Breastfeeding and overweight: longitudinal analysis in an Australian birth cohort. *J Pediatr.* 2005;147:56-61.

16. American Diabetes Association. Type 2 diabetes in children and adolescents: consensus conference report. *Diabetes Care.* 2000;23:381-389.

17. Turner R, Stratton I, Horton V, et al. UKPDS 25: autoantibodies to islet-cell cytoplasm and glutamic acid decarboxylase for prediction of insulin requirement in type 2 diabetes. UK Prospective Diabetes Study Group. *Lancet.* 1997;350: 1288-1293.

18. International Society for Pediatric and Adolescent Diabetes guidelines: www.ispad.org

19. Jacobson-Dickman E, Levitsky L. Oral agents in managing diabetes mellitus in children and adolescents. *Pediatr Clin North Am.* 2005;52(6):1689-1703.

20. Eppens MC, Craig ME, Cusumano J, et al. Prevalence of diabetes complications in adolescents with type 2 compared with type 1 diabetes. *Diabetes Care.* 2006;29:1300-1306.

21. Dabelea D, West N, Mayer-Davis EJ, et al. High prevalence of cardiovascular risk factors in youth with type 2 diabetes: the SEARCH for diabetes in youth case-control study. *Diabetologia.* 2008:S55.

22. American Diabetes Association: Management of dyslipidemia in children and adolescents with diabetes. *Diabetes Care.* 2003;26:2194-2197.

23. Maahs DM, Wadwa RP, Bishop F, Daniels SR, Rewers M, Klingensmith GJ. Dyslipidemia in youth with diabetes: to treat or not to treat? *J Pediatr.* 2008;153:458-465.

24. Maahs DM, Snively BM, Bell RA, et al. Higher prevalence of elevated albumin excretion in youth with type 2 than type 1 diabetes: the SEARCH for diabetes in youth study. *Diabetes Care.* 2007;30:2593-2598.

25. Nadeau KJ, Klingensmith G, Zeitler P. Type 2 diabetes in children is frequently associated with elevated alanine aminotransferase. *J Pediatr Gastroenterol Nutr.* 2005; Jul;41(1):94-98.

26. Lingvay I, Raskin P, Szczepaniak LS. Effect of insulin-metformin combination on hepatic steatosis in patients with type 2 diabetes. *J Diabetes Complications.* 2007 May-Jun;21(3):137-142.

27. Zeitler P, Pinhas-Hamiel O. Prevention and screening for type 2 diabetes in youth. In: Dabelea D, Klingensmith G, eds. *Epidemiology of Pediatric and Adolescent Diabetes.* Informa HealthCare USA, Inc, New York; 2008:201-217.

28. Gortmaker SL, Cheung LWY, Peterson KE, et al. Impact of a school-based interdisciplinary intervention on diet and physical activity among urban primary school children. *Arch Pediatr Adolesc Med.* 1999;153:975-983.

15. Rewers A, Klingensmith G, Davis C, et al. Presence of diabetic ketoacidosis at diagnosis of diabetes mellitus in youth: the Search for Diabetes in Youth Study. *Pediatrics.* 2008;121: 1258-1266.

4. Rodriguez BL, Fujimoto WY, Mayer-Davis EJ, et al. Prevalence of cardiovascular disease risk factors in U.S. children and adolescents with diabetes: the SEARCH for diabetes in youth study. *Diabetes Care.* 2006;29:1891-1896.

Part D. Other Specific Types of Diabetes Mellitus and Causes of Hyperglycemia

Lisa Gallo, Janet H. Silverstein, and William Winter

DEFINITIONS AND EPIDEMIOLOGY

A majority of cases of diabetes mellitus fall into either type 1 diabetes (T1DM), or type 2 diabetes (T2DM).

However, there are more than 50 other specific types of diabetes identified by the ADA recognizes (Table 10-1). All of these disorders collectively account for only 1% to 5% of cases of diabetes. However, ensuring a correct diagnosis is important for choosing the most appropriate therapy, managing the expected complications, anticipating associated disorders, and predicting reoccurrence in offspring and disease risk in relatives. It is important to know when to consider one of these forms of diabetes, as differentiating them from the more common type 1 and type 2 diabetes can present a significant diagnostic challenge. This chapter will help to identify some of these more unusual forms of diabetes.

Neonatal diabetes mellitus (NDM) is defined as persistent hyperglycemia occurring within the first 6 months of life, with many cases developing in the first month of life. The diagnosis of neonatal diabetes requires that hyperglycemia must persist for at least two weeks. Insulin therapy is commonly initiated.[1] NDM is comprised of two broad categories: permanent NDM and transient NDM, in which complete remission typically occurs within the first 6 months after birth, and no later than 18 months of age. Transient NDM may relapse in childhood, adolescence, or young adulthood. The incidence is 1 in 100,000 to 500,000 live births, with 50% of infants having transient NDM, and half having permanent diabetes mellitus.

Maturity onset diabetes of the young (MODY) is a heterogeneous group of disorders which result from one or more mutations in a single gene. Classically MODY is inherited as an autosomal dominant trait although spontaneous occurrence would be anticipated in some cases. Not all of the MODY genes have yet been identified, but heterozygous mutations in six genes cause the majority of the MODY cases.[2] The various MODY forms occur predominantly in Caucasians with weight distribution that mirrors that of the general population, present clinically before 25 years of age, are nonketotic, and do not initially require insulin therapy. MODY2 and MODY3 are the most frequent types, accounting for 80% of all MODY cases. It has been proposed that the term "monogenic" diabetes replace MODY because MODY is not a single disease.

Atypical diabetes mellitus (ADM), also known as "Flatbush" diabetes, is a form of diabetes in which patients initially present with ketosis or ketoacidosis, but after initial treatment with insulin, the clinical course that follows resembles that of type 2 diabetes mellitus.[3] It usually occurs in African Americans, but has been reported in other ethnic groups. ADM presents throughout childhood, and rarely has its onset after age 40. It is not associated with HLA specificities or islet autoimmunity, and the prevalence of obesity and insulin resistance in patients with ADM is no greater than that in the general population. ADM is transmitted in an autosomal dominant manner; however, there is an increased incidence in females with a male to female ratio of 1:3.

Mitochondrial diabetes has an average age of onset between 35 and 40 years. In general, patients with this form of diabetes are not obese, and do not exhibit insulin resistance. Several mutations in mitochondrial DNA (mtDNA) have been found to be associated with increased risk for developing diabetes. Most of these mutations are rare. One particular mutation, in which there is a substitution of an A for G at position 3243 in the mtDNA-encoded tRNALeu(UUR) gene, is associated with maternally inherited diabetes and deafness (MIDD) and is thought to account for 1.5% of the diabetic population in different countries and races.[4] The highest frequency of MIDD is found in Japan. The penetrance of this mutation is high, as more than 85% of the carriers will develop diabetes at some point in their lifetime.

Cystic fibrosis (CF) is the most common lethal autosomal recessive disease affecting the white population, and is less commonly found in other ethnic groups. It is caused by a defective gene on the long arm of chromosome 7, which encodes the CF transmembrane conductance regulator, a chloride channel that influences the salt content and viscosity of mucus secretions. The median life expectancy for patients with CF in North America in the year 2006 was 37 years.[5] Because of this increased survival, CF-related diabetes (CFRD) and prediabetes are emerging as common complications of the disease. The presence of CFRD predicts a poor clinical outcome and is associated with early mortality.

In 2006, the Cystic Fibrosis Foundation reported a diabetes prevalence of approximately 1% to 2% in children aged 6 to 10 years, 8% in patients 11 to 17 years, and 17.5% in patients 18 to 24 years.[5] CFRD is more common in females than males in youth less than 15 years of age, but there is no sex difference after 15 years of age.

Slowly progressive type 1 diabetes, previously known as latent autoimmune diabetes of adulthood (LADA), is clinically similar to type 2 diabetes at presentation but is considered a subtype of type 1 diabetes because of positivity for islet autoantibodies and because patients with this form of diabetes typically require insulin therapy at an earlier age than people with typical insulin-resistant type 2 diabetes.[6] These patients are usually greater than 30 years of age at diagnosis and are usually nonobese.

A variety of other uncommon forms of diabetes mellitus exist, in addition to those mentioned above, and some of these will be touched on briefly in this chapter. Although, in clinical practice, most patients who exhibit signs and symptoms typical of diabetes will subsequently be diagnosed with either type 1 or type 2 diabetes. It is important to consider one of the less common forms of diabetes described in this chapter if the patient's presentation is unusual, if the diabetes is a secondary manifestation of a primary disorder, or if there is a strong family history of diabetes suggesting an autosomal dominant mode of inheritance or maternal transmission. If one of these other specific types of diabetes mellitus is suspected, a referral to the appropriate pediatric endocrine subspecialist should be made so that further evaluation can be performed, and the proper treatment implemented (Box 10-3).

PATHOGENESIS

There are five initiating pathogenic events which result in hyperglycemia (Figure 10-1):

    a. Inadequate insulin production by the pancreas
    b. Abnormal structure or function of the insulin molecule
    c. Abnormal binding of insulin to its receptor
    d. Abnormality of the insulin receptor
    e. Insulin postreceptor defects

Inadequate Insulin Production

Neonatal diabetes mellitus

As previously stated, NDM is divided into two broad categories: transient and permanent. The genetic causes underlying all of the forms have yet to be elucidated. However, genetic abnormalities in a region of the long arm of chromosome 6 have been implicated in approximately 90% of transient forms.[7] (Table 10-10). Insulin response to glucose in these neonates, although low to absent initially, recovers within 1 to 18 months after birth, with a mean recovery at 3 months, suggesting that the etiology is a functional delay in B-cell maturation with spontaneous resolution.

Mutations in four genes cause the majority of cases of permanent neonatal diabetes (PNDM) (Table 10-11). The most frequent abnormality, accounting for 30% to 58% of cases of PNDM are activating mutations in the KCNJ11 gene on chromosome 11, which encodes the Kir 6.2 subunit of the ATP sensitive potassium channel of

Table 10-10.

Genetic Causes of Transient Neonatal Diabetes

Genetic Abnormality	Inheritance Pattern
Paternal uniparental disomy of chromosome 6	Usually a de novo, non-recurrent event
Duplication of 6q24 on the paternal allele	Autosomal dominant
6q24 methylation defect	Usually a de novo, non-recurrent event

the pancreatic B-cell.[8] A heterozygous gain-of-function mutation in the ABCC8 gene, which encodes the SUR1 subunit of the ATP-sensitive potassium channel, leads to similar abnormalities. Both of these defects result in failure of the potassium channel to close in response to increased intracellular levels of ATP, resulting in failure of β-cell depolarization and subsequent diminished insulin release (Figure 10-14). Heterozygous missense mutations in the insulin gene have recently been shown to be the underlying abnormality in 25% of cases of permanent neonatal diabetes.[9] A homozygous loss of function mutation in the gene for the enzyme glucokinase causes a loss of the "glucose-sensing" ability of the pancreatic β-cell. Mutations in the IPF-1 (insulin promoter factor-1) gene on chromosome 13 lead to pancreatic agenesis and PNDM.

MODY

Inadequate insulin production by the pancreas can result from a variety of different mechanisms, with autoimmune destruction of the B-cell in type 1 diabetes being the most well-known example. However, in the various forms of MODY, hyperglycemia results from a deficiency of insulin production as well. With the exception of MODY2, all forms of MODY are secondary to mutations in transcription factors required for B-cell differentiation and insulin gene expression. MODY2 results from a mutation in the gene coding for glucokinase, an essential enzyme in the glucose-sensing mechanism of the B-cell (Table 10-12).

In English populations, MODY3 is the most common subtype, followed by MODY2, and the two of these combined account for more than 80% or MODY cases. The remaining forms are relatively uncommon, and information available on MODY4 has stemmed from studies in single family.

Atypical diabetes

Atypical diabetes was first described in African American children who presented with acute symptoms of insulinopenia with or without diabetic ketoacidosis (DKA) and who subsequently displayed clinical and metabolic features more typical of type 2 diabetes. It has since been reported in other ethnicities. The exact etiology of ADM is not known. However, the absence of either HLA association or autoantibodies makes islet-cell autoimmunity unlikely. The strong family history in patients with ADM suggests that a genetic component may be present. First-phase insulin response to intravenous glucose injection has been shown to be lost in patients with this form of diabetes, and the fasting C-peptide-to-glucose ratio was intermediate between type 1 and type 2 diabetes patients. This group of patients appears to differ from those with typical type 2 diabetes

Table 10-11.

Most Common Genetic Causes of Permanent Neonatal Diabetes[*]

Genetic Defect	Chromosome Location	Affect
Potassium inwardly-rectifying channel, subfamily J, member 11 (KCNJ11)	11p15.1 Heterozygous gain of function mutation	Kir6.2 subunit of the ATP-sensitive potassium (KATP) channel remains open[†]
Glucokinase	7p15-p13 Homozygous loss of function mutation	Loss of the "glucose sensing" ability of the β cell
Insulin promoter factor-1 (IPF-1)	13q12.1 Homozygous loss of function mutation	Pancreatic agenesis
ATP-binding cassette, subfamily C, member 8 (ABCC8)	11p15.1 Heterozygous gain of function mutation	SUR1 subunit of the ATP-sensitive potassium (KATP) channel is activated causing the channel to remain open[†]
Insulin gene (INS)	11p15.5 Heterozygous loss of function missense mutation	Disrupts the folding of the proinsulin molecule and results in misfolded protein or retention of the protein in the endoplasmic reticulum

[*]*Permanent neonatal diabetes can also occur as part of the the following syndromes: IPEX (Immunodysregulation, polyendocrinopathy, and enteropathy, X-linked), Wolcott-Rallison, Rabson-Mendenhall, and Donahue syndrome.*
[†]*This leads to an inability of the pancreatic β cell to depolarize resulting in decreased insulin secretion.*

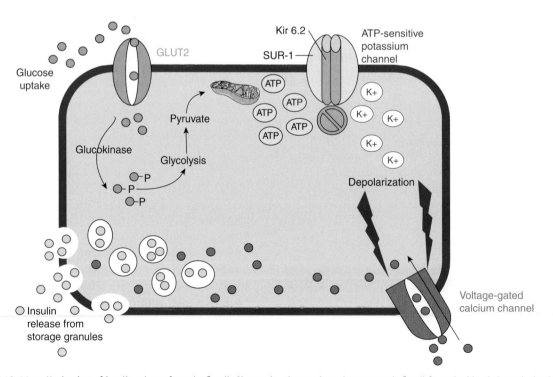

FIGURE 10-14 ■ Mechanism of insulin release from the β-cell. Glucose is taken up into the pancreatic β cell from the blood through the GLUT2 transporter. It is phosphorylated to glucose-6-phosphate by glucokinase, and then through glycolysis and the TCA cycle, ATP is produced. An increase in the intracellular ATP to ADP ratio causes closure of the ATP-sensitive potassium channel and failure of potassium to move extracellularly. The increased net positive charge within the β cell results in depolarization of the cell membrane, and opening of the voltage-gated calcium channel. Calcium then moves intracellularly and causes storage granules, containing insulin, to fuse with the cell membrane of the β cell, releasing insulin into the circulation.

Table 10-12.

Genetic Abnormalities Resulting in the Various MODY Forms

Type of MODY	Affected Gene	Defining Characteristics
1	Hepatocyte nuclear fator-4-alpha (HNF4α)	■ Progressive hyperglycemia ■ 50% reduction in serum TG ■ 25% reduction in serum concentrations of apolipoproteins AII, CIII, and lipoprotein a
2*	Glucokinase (GCK)[†]	■ Impaired fasting glucose or impaired glucose tolerance ■ Less than 50% of patients have overt diabetes (Usually obese or elderly patients) ■ 50% of women with MODY2 mutations will have gestational diabetes ■ Nonprogressive ■ May only require medication therapy during puberty or times of illness/stress
3*	Hepatocyte nuclear factor-1-alpha (HNF1α)	■ Asymptomatic glycosuria ■ Progressive hyperglycemia[‡]
4	Insulin promoter factor-1 (IPF-1)	■ Homozygous mutations result in pancreatic agenesis; heterozygous mutations cause MODY4
5	Hepatocyte nuclear factor-1-beta (HNF1β)	■ Renal cysts ■ Hypoplastic glomerulocystic kidney disease 　■ Proteinuria 　■ Nondiabetic renal failure ■ Reproductive tract anomalies 　■ Vaginal aplasia 　■ Rudimentary or bicornuate uterus ■ Elevated transaminases
6	Neurogenic differentiation 1 (NEUROD1)	■ Rare

*MODY3 and MODY2 are the two most prevalent forms, accounting for more than 80% of MODY patients.
[†]With the exception of MODY2, all forms of MODY are secondary to mutations in transcription factors required for B-cell differentiation and insulin gene expression.
[‡]In MODY 1 and MODY3, 30%-40% of patients eventually require insulin therapy, but can be managed for decades with sulfonylureas alone.
Note: All but MODY 2 may develop diabetes-related vascular complications.

in that they are not usually obese and euglycemic remission may occur without weight loss. The long-term insulin independence distinguishes ADM from type 1 diabetes, in which subjects have a high incidence of detectable islet autoimmunity. It has been hypothesized that these patients initially have inadequate insulin production to handle a glucose load following a meal, resulting in "paralysis" of the β cells caused by glucose toxicity. Recovery from the acute initial presentation of ADM results from a restoration of β-cell function following treatment of hyperglycemic β-cell toxicity.[3]

Mitochondrial diabetes

Mitochondria contain their own circular genome, which guides the synthesis of 13 of the greater than 80 subunits in the mitochondrial respiratory-chain complexes. There are more than 40 known diabetogenic mutations in the mitochondrial genome resulting in deficient insulin secretion owing to impaired mitochondrial ATP production.[10] Maternally inherited diabetes and deafness

(MIDD) is the most common phenotype, resulting from an A⇒G point mutation at position 3243 of the mitochondrial DNA, with deafness present in more than 60% of affected people.[4]

Disorders of the exocrine pancreas

Patients with disorders of the exocrine pancreas, in which abnormal glucose homeostasis is not the primary abnormality, can eventually develop diabetes once pancreatic endocrine function is compromised. For example, in patients with recurrent pancreatitis or hemochromatosis, islet cells are progressively damaged by inflammation/fibrosis and iron deposition, respectively. In patients with cystic fibrosis, the prevailing belief is that diabetes results primarily from progressive obstruction of the pancreatic ducts with thick exocrine secretions, leading to damage to both the exocrine and endocrine pancreas. Autopsy findings in CFRD patients demonstrate fibrosis and fatty infiltration of the exocrine pancreas with disruption of the islet architecture, and destruction of a majority of the islet cells.[11] However, development of CFRD is not simply a matter of the degree of islet disruption because the absolute number of β-cells does not appear to be significantly lower in CFRD patients than in those without diabetes. Deposition of amyloid within the islets appears to be the main difference between cystic fibrosis patients with and without CFRD. Recent studies in CFTR deficient mice suggest that an intrinsic defect in the islet cells of these patients may play a role as well. Insulin resistance, especially during times of acute infection, is another contributing factor underlying cystic fibrosis-related diabetes.

Slowly progressive type 1 diabetes

This form of diabetes is defined by three features: adult age at diagnosis (age >30 years), the presence of diabetes-associated autoantibodies, and a lag time of approximately 6 months or more from diagnosis to need for insulin therapy to manage hyperglycemia. There is evidence for a continuum of rate of islet cell destruction, with rapid destruction in childhood-onset type 1 diabetes to the relatively slow destruction detected in slowly progressive type 1 diabetes. Nondiabetic identical twins of patients with type 1 diabetes diagnosed at less than 25 years of age have a 38% probability of developing diabetes. Nondiabetic twins of patients diagnosed after the age of 25 years have only a 6% probability of developing diabetes. The low twin concordance for slowly progressive type 1 diabetes suggests that environmental factors play a larger role than genetic factors in the development of this disease.[6] Of the many genes that are involved in the genetic predisposition to both type 1 diabetes and slowly progressive type 1 diabetes, the most important are in the HLA region of chromosome 6.

Abnormal Structure or Function of the Insulin Molecule

The insulinopathies are caused by mutations in the insulin gene on chromosome 11 resulting in amino acid substitutions in the insulin molecule with consequent impaired ability of insulin to interact normally with its receptor.

Familial hyperproinsulinemia is a group of disorders resulting from interference in the posttranslational processing of proinsulin to insulin, resulting in increased blood levels of proinsulin.[12] Inheritance has been reported to be autosomal dominant with variable penetrance. These are very rare disorders.

Abnormality of the Insulin Receptor in Target Tissues

Mutations in the insulin receptor gene, located on chromosome 19, cause a spectrum of insulin resistance syndromes with the mildest form being type A insulin resistance, and the most severe being Donahue syndrome (Leprechaunism). Rabson-Mendenhall syndrome has an intermediate phenotype. Type A insulin resistance is not typically recognized until adolescence or young adulthood, children with Donahue syndrome usually die in infancy, and patients with Rabson-Mendenhall syndrome often survive beyond 1 year of age, but death occurs before puberty. The less severe phenotypes in patients with Rabson-Mendenhall syndrome and type A insulin resistance are believed to result from the retention of some functionality by the mutant insulin receptors. These are also very rare disorders.

Abnormal Binding of Insulin to its Receptor

Type B insulin resistance

Type B insulin resistance is a very rare disorder characterized by the presence of autoantibodies directed against specific epitopes in the insulin receptor resulting in a marked decrease of insulin-binding to its membrane receptor and severe insulin resistance. It occurs more commonly in women of African heritage, and is frequently seen in patients with a history of other autoimmune diseases, such as systemic lupus erythematosus.

Insulin Postreceptor Defects

Increased counter-regulatory hormone production

Many endogenous hormones cause hyperglycemia by increasing hepatic glucose production and decreasing insulin sensitivity. Impaired fasting glucose, impaired glucose tolerance, or frank diabetes mellitus may occur. Examples include excess secretion of growth hormone (acromegaly), cortisol (Cushing syndrome), glucagon (pancreatic glucagonoma), and epinephrine (pheochromocytoma). During times of critical illness or stress, the body's adaptive endocrine responses act to increase the release of cortisol, growth hormone, catecholamines, and glucagon, thus antagonizing insulin's effect on target tissues resulting in altered glucose metabolism, reduced hepatic and skeletal muscle glucose uptake capacity, and hyperglycemia.

Medication-induced hyperglycemia

Multiple medications have been shown to cause hyperglycemia and diabetes, with the most common offender being corticosteroids (Table 10-13).

Genetic syndromes associated with glucose intolerance

Many genetic syndromes, including Down, Turner, and Klinefelter syndromes, are associated with an increased risk of impaired glucose tolerance and diabetes. The

Table 10-13.

Medications That May Result in Hyperglycemia

- Corticosteroids
- Diazoxide
- Immunosuppressive agents
  - Tacrolimus
  - Cyclosporine
  - Daclizumab
  - Mycophenolate
- Antimicrobials
  - Pentamidine
  - Amphotericin B
  - Amphotericin B lipid formulations
  - Atovaquone
  - Gatifloxacin
  - Moxifloxacin
  - Ribavirin
  - Isoniazid
  - Nystatin
- Chemotherapeutic agents
  - Streptozocin
  - Rituximab
  - Gemtuzumab ozogamicin
  - L-asparaginase
  - Irinotecan
  - Pegaspargase
- Beta-blockers
  - Metoprolol
  - Betaxolol
  - Carteolol
  - Carvedilol
- Beta agonists
  - Albuterol
  - Levalbuterol
  - Formoterol
  - Salmeterol
  - Ritodrine
- Diuretics
  - Furosemide
  - Bumetanide
  - Chlorothiazide
  - Chlorthalidone
  - Ethacrynic acid
  - Metolazone
  - Indapamide
  - Torsemide
  - Hydrochlorothiazide
- Combination beta-blocker and thiazide diuretic
- Combination ACE-inhibitor and thiazide diuretic
- Combination angiotensin receptor blocker and thiazide diuretic

- Protease inhibitors
  - Amprenavir
  - Indinavir
  - Lopinavir
  - Ritonavir
  - Nelfinavir
  - Saquinavir
- Nucleoside analog reverse transcriptase inhibitors
  - Abacavir
  - Lamivudine,
  - Zidovudine
- Antipsychotics/antidepressants
  - Fluoxetine
  - Sodium oxybate (GHB)
  - Modafinil
  - Clozapine
  - Aripiprazole
  - Quetiapine
  - Risperidone
  - Ziprasidone
- Antiarrhythmic medications
  - Encainide
  - Sotalol
- Hormonal medications
  - Conjugated estrogens
  - Esterified estrogens
  - Levonorgestrel
  - Medroxyprogesterone
  - Norethindrone
  - Norgestrel
  - Progesterone
  - Recombinant human growth hormone
  - Corticotropin/ACTH
- Anticonvulsants
  - Phenytoin
  - Valproic acid
- Others
  - Acetazolamide
  - Baclofen
  - Caffeine
  - Isotretinoin
  - Niacin, niacinamide
  - Nitric oxide
  - Octreotide
  - Pantoprazole
  - Ursodiol
  - Megestrol

lipodystrophic diabetes syndromes have abnormal fat distribution with postbinding defects in insulin action. Discussion of the underlying mechanism for hyperglycemia in each of these disorders is beyond the scope of this chapter.

CLINICAL PRESENTATION

The symptoms of *hyperglycemia* are similar regardless of the underlying cause and include polyuria, polydipsia, polyphagia, weight loss (in cases of severe insulin deficiency), blurry vision, and fatigue. Patients may be asymptomatic if mild hyperglycemia is present. If an unusual form of diabetes is suspected it is important to obtain a thorough history and review of symptoms and to perform a full physical examination to ensure that a proper diagnosis is made. It is important to obtain a list of the patient's prescribed and OTC medications to determine if the diabetes is related to medication use (Table 10-13). In addition, a detailed family history will allow detection of similarly affected family members, which becomes especially important when trying to ascertain if type 2 diabetes, MODY (autosomal dominant), or mitochondrial diabetes (maternal transmission) are possible diagnoses.

If severe hyperglycemia is left untreated, the patient can develop nonketotic hyperosmolar syndrome or ketoacidosis; a prompt evaluation of a significant glucose abnormality is essential. In all patients, but especially in infants, close attention should be given to the presence or absence of dysmorphic features or prototypical features which can be seen in the various genetic and endocrine disorders that have diabetes as one of their manifestations. Acanthosis nigricans of the neck, axillary area, knees, or inguinal creases suggests insulin resistance.

DIFFERENTIAL DIAGNOSIS

The differential diagnosis of hyperglycemia and diabetes mellitus is listed in Table 10-1. It is important when generating a differential diagnosis to discriminate between diseases in which diabetes is the primary abnormality and those where diabetes is a secondary abnormality presenting as a symptom of another disorder or syndrome (Figure 10-3). It is also important to consider different causes of diabetes in patients who develop diabetes before versus after 6 months of age.

DIAGNOSIS

The criteria for making the diagnosis of diabetes are the same, regardless of the etiology (Table 10-2). Although type 1 and type 2 diabetes mellitus are, by far, the most common forms, atypical presentations should alert the clinician that one of the less common forms may be the actual diagnosis (Figure 10-2).

Neonatal Diabetes

Age less than 6 months at onset suggests neonatal diabetes because type 1 diabetes is very unlikely in this age group. A diagnosis of neonatal diabetes is further supported if the neonate is SGA, because insulin is a potent fetal growth factor, especially in the last trimester. In both the transient and permanent forms, in addition to hyperglycemia, these infants have low to immeasurable insulin and C-peptide levels, even in response to glucose or glucagon, and they will occasionally develop ketoacidosis. Although, one-half of patients with this form have transient diabetes, with resolution at a mean age of 3 months, and before 18 months of age. Some studies show that these patients are at an increased risk for diabetes recurrence in childhood and young adulthood, with a mean age of recurrence of 14 years and an age range of 4 to 24 years.[7] Determination of the genetic etiology of neonatal diabetes is recommended because of the need to monitor patients with transient neonatal diabetes for possible relapse in childhood and adolescence, in order to provide genetic counseling for parents and family members, and because up to 90% of patients with KCNJ11 and ABCC8 mutations can be successfully treated with oral sulfonylureas.

MODY

Patients with MODY 2 and MODY3 exhibit only mild symptoms of hyperglycemia, and therefore may only be diagnosed if glycosuria is found during school or sports physical examinations or if testing is done because of a strong family history of atypical diabetes. A diagnosis of MODY should be considered in patients who have a strong family history of diabetes, negative autoantibody testing, low or fluctuating insulin requirements, and absence of signs of the metabolic syndrome, that is, a lack of obesity, acanthosis nigricans, hirsutism in women, hypertension, and dyslipidemia. The MODY forms that are associated with a defect in genes for a transcription factor (1, 3-6) may display a progressive decline in B-cell secretion. The onset of hyperglycemia is very slow. Fasting glucose is normal in early childhood when insulin requirements are low, but progressive hyperglycemia ensues over time, generally presenting as diabetes between the ages of 5 and 25 years.

Because MODY2 and MODY3 are the most frequently encountered forms, it is important to recognize the clinical presentation of these two types. In MODY2, the abnormal glucose metabolism is a stable abnormality that is present from birth. Both fasting and postprandial hyperglycemia occur, but remain only mildly, but consistently, elevated throughout life, with fasting blood glucose levels in the 110 to 140 mg/dL range, and with postprandial values rarely above 250 mg/dL.[13] During times of critical illness, and occasionally during puberty, glycemic control may worsen necessitating more aggressive therapy. Approximately 50% of women with MODY2 mutations will have gestational diabetes. Unlike the remainder of the MODY forms, MODY2 is generally not associated with the micro- and macrovascular complications seen with typical type 1 and type 2 diabetes, reflective of the fact that HbA1c is usually just above the upper limit of the reference interval. In MODY3, the patient may remain non-insulin-dependent for a prolonged time, and often has glycosuria at blood glucose levels less than 180 mg/dL (10 mmol/L), as these patients have a low renal threshold.

Molecular genetic testing allows identification of the genetic defects linked to MODY 1-6, and can detect approximately 85% of all MODY cases in the US population. Most laboratories that offer MODY testing only test for sequence errors. Errors in gene structure (eg, deletion or inversion) would, therefore, not be detected.

Atypical Diabetes and Slowly Progressive Type 1 Diabetes

There is no specific testing to aid in the diagnosis of atypical diabetes, and the diagnosis is, therefore, based on the family history and clinical presentation described above. The initial presentation is acute, with a few days to weeks of polyuria, polydipsia, and weight loss and lack of a precipitating cause for the metabolic decompensation. At presentation, they have markedly impaired insulin secretion and decreased insulin action, but with aggressive insulin management there is significant improvement in β-cell function sufficient to allow transition from insulin therapy to sulfonylureas within a few months in many of these patients. During times of acute stress, insulin therapy may need to be temporarily reinstituted.

Slowly progressive type 1 diabetes has a much more insidious onset and is unlikely to present as DKA. It is diagnosed during adulthood and the presence of GAD autoantibodies can be helpful in differentiating it from type 2 diabetes. It should be remembered that 50% to 75% of children in the United States who present with typical type 1 diabetes do not present with ketoacidosis, but with milder symptoms of polyuris and polydipsia, or may present asymptomatically during a routine physical examination.

Mitochondrial Diabetes

Mitochondrial diabetes is very easily confused with the more common forms of diabetes, but the diagnosis should be suspected if there is a strong family history of diabetes suggestive of maternal transmission, or if the diabetes is associated with deafness. The hearing loss is sensorineural, and generally precedes the onset of diabetes by several years. Other less common comorbidities which have been reported with mitochondrial diabetes include cardiomyopathy, cardiac conduction disorders, encephalomyopathy, macular pattern dystrophy, and psychiatric disorders. The most common mutation resulting in mitochondrial diabetes is a point mutation at position 3243 in the tRNA leucine gene, leading to an A-to-G transition. An identical lesion occurs in the MELAS syndrome (mitochondrial myopathy, encephalopathy, lactic acidosis, and stroke-like syndrome); however, diabetes is not part of this syndrome, suggesting different phenotypic expressions of this genetic lesion. In a patient with suspected mitochondrial diabetes, a diagnosis can be sought by isolating mitochondrial DNA from peripheral blood lymphocytes in order to look specifically for the 3243 point mutation.

CF-related Diabetes

Because CFRD is unusual before adolescence, is usually insidious in onset, and patients are often asymptomatic in the early stages, the Cystic Fibrosis Foundation recommends annual diabetes screening beginning at age 14 years in children with cystic fibrosis.[14] In addition, any patient with signs or symptoms of diabetes should undergo immediate evaluation, regardless of age. Although patients with CF may display the classical symptoms of diabetes, such as polyuria and polydipsia, other features suggestive of poor glycemic control in CF include: delayed progression of puberty, poor weight gain, poor growth velocity, and an unexplained decline in pulmonary function. Early detection of CFRD is imperative because poor glycemic control greatly contributes to morbidity and mortality in CF. The Cystic Fibrosis Foundation reported that among the 22,000 North American patients in its registry, mortality was sixfold greater in CFRD patients than in those without diabetes.[5]

There is a spectrum of glucose abnormalities in CF including impaired glucose tolerance (IGT), CFRD with normal fasting blood glucose, and CFRD with fasting hyperglycemia. There has been controversy in recent years, as to whether fasting plasma glucose (FPG) is the best means of screening patients for CFRD because a large portion of patients (17.8% in one study) diagnosed with CFRD based on the results of an oral glucose tolerance test (OGTT) would have been missed by using FPG as the screening procedure. Some institutions are therefore using yearly OGTTs as the initial screening procedure.

Insulinopathies

Glucose abnormalities are variable in patients with an insulinopathy or hyperproinsulinemia, because although these abnormal molecules have decreased ability to interact with the insulin receptor, they often do retain some biologic activity which is sufficient to maintain normoglycemia in the absence of other diabetogenic factors.[12] These patients present with glucose intolerance or diabetes, hyperinsulinemia, and an elevated insulin:C-peptide molar ratio. Obesity is usually absent, and islet autoantibodies are negative. An adequate decline in blood glucose when exogenous insulin is administered suggests that insulin resistance is not part of the underlying cause of the glucose abnormalities in these patients. Abnormal insulin molecules or elevated proinsulin levels can be detected on biochemical testing, but such testing is not commercially available

Type B Insulin Resistance

Type B insulin resistance syndrome should be considered in patients presenting with rapid onset of insulin resistance which is unresponsive to very large doses of insulin owing to the presence of autoantibodies against the insulin receptor. For example, in two case reports of patients with this disorder, glycemic control was not reached until insulin doses reached 180 units/h and 154,075 units in a day.[15] Specific testing for insulin receptor autoantibodies can lead to a diagnosis, but such testing is not commercially available. Such patients exhibit classic findings of insulin resistance such as acanthosis nigricans.

Defective Insulin Receptor

Donahue syndrome and Rabson-Mendenhall syndrome are both characterized by growth retardation, lack of subcutaneous fat, facial dysmorphism, acanthosis nigricans, phallic enlargement, and hirsutism evident at birth or in the first months of life. Biochemical evaluation demonstrates fasting hypoglycemia, postprandial hyperglycemia, and severe hyperinsulinemia. The paradoxical fasting hypoglycemia is caused by inappropriately elevated insulin levels at the time of fasting. Because glucose release by the liver maintains blood glucose levels during times of fasting, and this function is normally suppressed by insulin, it is thought that the liver and extrahepatic tissues retain some sensitivity to the elevated insulin levels for a brief period of time after birth.[16] It has also been hypothesized that the fasting hypoglycemia is related to insulin binding to another receptor in tissues, such as the IGF-1 receptor.[16] Children with Donahue syndrome do not develop DKA, but die in infancy. Patients with Rabson-Mendenhall syndrome develop severe DKA which is minimally responsive to insulin therapy, resulting in death before 6 years of age. Type A insulin resistance is not well understood, but is thought to be related to either a defect in the insulin receptor itself or a postbinding defect in insulin

action, resulting in a phenotypic expression of mild insulin resistance. Some females with clinical features of polycystic ovarian syndrome, including insulin resistance and virilization, have been found to have a defect in the gene for the insulin receptor.

Corticosteroid-induced Diabetes

Corticosteroid therapy may result in glucose intolerance in a dose-dependent manner. Blood glucose levels should therefore be tested in patients receiving chronic steroid treatment who have glycosuria or symptoms of hyperglycemia. Fasting blood glucose levels greater than or equal to 126 mg/dL or casual blood glucose levels persistently greater than or equal to 200 mg/dL may require therapy. It can take weeks following cessation of corticosteroid therapy for the hyperglycemia to resolve.

TREATMENT

Therapy must be tailored to correct the underlying defect causing the hyperglycemia (Table 10-14).

Neonatal Diabetes

Intravenous fluid rehydration is important in the initial management of neonatal diabetes, as polyuria may be present for some time before diabetes is diagnosed and treatment is implemented. An intravenous insulin infusion is often the initial therapy in patients with both transient and permanent forms of neonatal diabetes. Once glucose control has been obtained, transition to an oral sulfonylurea agent may be attempted if genetic testing confirms one of the genetic abnormalities that have been proven to be responsive to sulfonylurea therapy, such as the KCNJ11 and ABCC8 mutations. However, a therapeutic trial of sulfonylurea therapy can also be undertaken without genetic testing. In transient neonatal diabetes, insulin therapy can eventually be weaned, but families should be counseled on the risk for diabetes recurrence in childhood or young adulthood. Infants with permanent NDM require lifelong therapy.

MODY

Patients with MODY secondary to defects in transcription factors (MODY 1, 3-6), may develop typical micro- and macrovascular complications of diabetes and thus require more aggressive management. MODY2 can usually be controlled with diet and exercise therapy alone, although some patients may require insulin therapy transiently during illness, puberty, or pregnancy. Diabetes penetrance in individuals with the genes for MODY1 and 3 approaches 80% by age 40 years.

Table 10-14.

Treatment Options

Transient neonatal diabetes	Rehydration; Transient IV or SC insulin requirement
Permanent neonatal diabetes	Up to 90% of patients with mutations involving Kir 6.2 and SUR1 respond to sulfonylureas; the remainder are usually insulin dependent
Slowly progressive type 1 diabetes	Insulin
Atypical diabetes	Insulin acutely, followed by management with sulfonylureas; usually require insulin during acute illness
MODY2	Diet and exercise; may require insulin during puberty, illness, or pregnancy
MODY1 and MODY3	Sulfonylurea initially, but may eventually need insulin therapy[*]
MODY4-6	Insulin
Mitochondrial diabetes	Insulin
Cystic fibrosis-related diabetes	Glinides with meals; small dose long-acting insulin once daily; short-acting insulin with meals
Corticosteroid-induced diabetes	Insulin
Insulinopathies	Insulin
Lipoatrophic diabetes	TZD[†], Leptin[‡]
Type B insulin resistance	HIGH doses of insulin; immunosuppressive therapy, IGF-1
Type A insulin resistance	Metformin, oral contraceptive, TZD, insulin
Rabson mendenhall syndrome	Leptin[*]; often present with severe intractable DKA despite insulin therapy
Donahue syndrome (Leprechaunism)	No known therapy

Dietary modification and lifestyle changes are important components in the therapy for most of these disorders.
[*]In MODY 1 and MODY3, 30%-40% of patients eventually require insulin therapy, but can be managed for decades with just sulfonylureas.
[†]Thiazolidinediones.
[‡]Benefits of leptin therapy in these patients is still under investigation.

Although these patients can usually be managed for decades solely with sulfonylurea therapy, many will eventually require treatment with insulin.[2] Insulin is the mainstay of therapy in MODY 4 to 6.

Atypical Diabetes

Euglycemia may be achieved rapidly in these patients using an intensive insulin regimen to eliminate glucotoxicity, resulting in a significant restoration of β-cell function and markedly improved diabetes control with near-normal glucose and HbA1c levels. Insulin requirements usually decline within a few weeks of treatment initiation as insulin production increases, and many patients are able to discontinue insulin and maintain near-normal blood glucose concentrations with sulfonylurea therapy. Insulin may be required to maintain near-normal blood glucose levels during illness.

Mitochondrial Diabetes

Treatment usually consists of diet and sulfonylureas, or insulin because the primary abnormality in these disorders is decreased glucose-stimulated insulin secretion from the pancreas. Patients with a type 2 diabetes–like phenotype can initially be treated with diet modification or sulfonylureas. Insulinopenia is often progressive, however, and as hyperglycemia worsens, most patients will require insulin therapy within a few years of diabetes onset.[10] The use of metformin is contraindicated because of the concern for lactic acidosis.

CFRD

Patients with cystic fibrosis not only have decreased energy intake, but also increased energy needs confounded by pancreatic insufficiency resulting in malabsorption. The dietary strategy in CFRD patients must provide sufficient calories for growth, frequently in excess of the amount required by healthy individuals, and to meet the increased metabolic demands that are a consequence of cystic fibrosis. The goal is to obtain a balance between food intake and insulin in order to achieve as near to normoglycemia as possible.

Insulin is the only treatment recommended currently for CFRD with fasting hyperglycemia. These patients are often treated with a small amount of basal insulin (5 to 10 units) given as twice daily NPH or detemir (Levemir), or as a once daily glargine (Lantus) injection. In addition, a rapid-acting insulin or glinide is given at mealtimes with the dose based on the amount of carbohydrate eaten. In stable CF patients, 0.5 to 1 unit of rapid-acting insulin are usually adequate to cover 15 g of carbohydrates. At times of illness or acute infection, however, a ratio of up to 1 unit per 5 g of carbohydrates may be necessary to achieve postprandial euglycemia.

Short-acting oral hypoglycemic agents, such as repaglinide and nateglinide, or rapid-acting insulin with meals can be used in the management of CFRD without fasting hyperglycemia. No specific treatment recommendations are currently available for CF patients with only impaired glucose tolerance.

Insulinopathies

Because the abnormal insulin or proinsulin molecules in these patients may retain some biologic activity, no therapy may be necessary. When treatment is indicated, it is usually with subcutaneous insulin therapy.

Type B Insulin Resistance

The initial goal when treating patients with type B insulin resistance is to manage their hyperglycemia. This generally requires large amounts of insulin. The clinical course of patients with type B insulin resistance is variable. Many patients will have a spontaneous remission but the time to remission is variable. A variety of immunosuppressive agents, including glucocorticoids, cyclophosphamide, cyclosporine, and rituximab, have been reported to induce remission, and case reports have also showed some success with recombinant IGF-1 therapy. Spontaneous regression of acanthosis nigricans in temporal association with the disappearance of circulating anti-insulin receptor autoantibodies and achievement of euglycemia in patients with type B insulin resistance has been reported.

CONCLUSION

Although these specific etiologies of diabetes represent only a small proportion of patients with diabetes mellitus, it is very important, as a primary care physician to not only know that these disorders exist, but also that they can mimic type 1 and type 2 diabetes mellitus so closely that it may be difficult to differentiate them unless close attention is paid to subtleties in the patient's history, clinical course, and family history. If one of these forms is suspected, a referral to a pediatric endocrinologist should be made so that proper evaluation and treatment can be performed and genetic counseling offered to the families.

REFERENCES

1. Von Muhlendah KE, Herkenhoff H. Long term course of neonatal diabetes. *NEJM.* 1995;333(11):704-708.

2. Timsit J, Bellanne-Chantelot C, Dubois Laforgue D, et al. Diagnosis and management of maturity-onset diabetes of the young. *Treat Endocrinol.* 2005;4(1):9-18.

3. Rasouli N, Elbein SC. Improved glycemic control in subjects with atypical diabetes results from restored insulin secretion, but not improved insulin sensitivity. *J Clin Endocrinol Metab.* 2004;89(12):6331-6335.

4. Gerbitz KD, van den Ouweland JM, Maassen JA, et al. Mitochondrial diabetes mellitus: a review. *Biochem Biophys Acta.* 1995 May 24;1271(1):253-260.

5. Cystic Fibrosis Foundation patient registry 2006 annual report. Bethesda, MD: The Foundation; 2006.

6. David R, Leslie G, Williams R, Pozzilli P. Clinical Review: type 1 diabetes and latent autoimmune diabetes in Adults: One End of the Rainbow. *J Clin Endocrinol Metab.* 2006; 91(5):1654-1659.

7. Temple IK, Gardner RJ, Mackay DJG, et al. Transient neonatal diabetes: widening the understanding of the etiopathogenesis of diabetes. *Diabetes.* 2000;49:1359-1366.

8. Gloyn AL, Cummings EA, Edghill EL, et al. Permanent neonatal diabetes due to paternal germline mosaicism for an activating mutation of the KCNJ11 gene encoding the Kir6.2 subunit of the beta-cell potassium adenosine triphosphate channel. *J Clin Endocrinol Metab.* 2004;89: 3932-3935.

9. Edghill EL, Flanagan SE, Patch AM, et al. Insulin mutation screening in 1,044 patients with diabetes: mutations in the INS gene are a common cause of neonatal diabetes but a rare cause of diabetes diagnosed in childhood or adulthood. *Diabetes.* 2008;57:1034-1042.

10. Maassen JA, 'T Hart LM, van Essen E, et al. Mitochondrial diabetes: molecular mechanism and clinical presentation. *Diabetes.* 2004;53(1):S103-S109.

11. Iannuci A, Mukai K, Johnson D, et al. Endocrine pancreas in cystic fibrosis: an immunohistochemical study. *Hum Pathol.* 1984;15:278-284.

12. Röder ME, Vissing H, Nauck MA. Hyperproinsulinemia in a three-generation Caucasian family due to mutant proinsulin (Arg65-His) not associated with impaired glucose tolerance: the contribution of mutant proinsulin to insulin bioactivity. *J Clin Endocrinol Metab.* 1996 Apr;81(4):1634-1640.

13. Fajans SS, Bell GI, Polonsky KS. Molecular mechanisms and clinical pathophysiology of maturity-onset diabetes of the young. *NEJM.* 2001;345:971-980.

14. Clinical Practice Guidelines for Cystic Fibrosis Committee. *Clinical Practice Guidelines for Cystic Fibrosis, Appendix V—Screening for Diabetes Mellitus in Patients with Cystic Fibrosis.* Bethesda, MD: Cystic Fibrosis Foundation; 1997:1-2.

15. Fareau GG, Maldonado M, Oral E, et al. Regression of acanthosis nigricans correlates with disappearance of anti-insulin receptor autoantibodies and achievement of euglycemia in type B insulin resistance syndrome. *Metabolism.* 2007 May;56(5):670-675.

16. Longo N, Wang Y, Pasquali M. Progressive decline in insulin levels in Rabson-Mendenhall syndrome. *J Clin Endocrinol Metab.* 1999;84(8):2623-2629.

CHAPTER 11

Hypoglycemia

Robert J. Ferry, Jr. and
David B. Allen

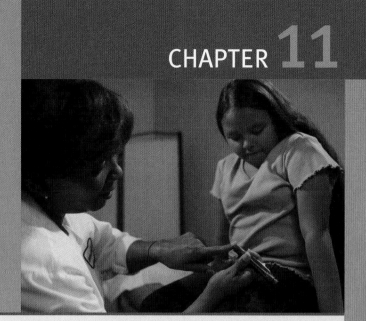

INTRODUCTION

The transition from the intrauterine to extra-uterine life requires prompt adaptations to maintain glucose homeostasis. Increased rates of glucose utilization in infants and children compared to adults heighten dependency on coordinated glycogenolysis, gluconeogenesis, and fatty acid oxidation to prevent hypoglycemia during early life. Consequently, hypoglycemic disorders often present in the neonatal period or in infancy during transitions to longer feeding intervals. Since the brain during this time is particularly susceptible to injury due to glucose deprivation, prompt recognition and treatment of hypoglycemia is paramount.

Glucose is the preferred substrate for cerebral metabolism and accounts for almost all of its energy requirements. Since the brain can neither synthesize nor efficiently store glucose, its function and health depend upon a continuous glucose supply. Metabolic demands of the developing brain raise glucose utilization rates during infancy and early childhood, when the brain is a relatively larger contributor to body mass. Thus, to avoid neurological damage, diagnosing and appropriately treating hypoglycemia is particularly critical during infancy and early childhood, when adequate glucose delivery is essential for neural growth and cognitive development. To promote the prompt diagnosis and treatment of hypoglycemia by the primary care physician and endocrinologist, this chapter integrates current molecular and clinical knowledge.

PHYSIOLOGY OF BLOOD GLUCOSE LEVEL REGULATION

Normal Pathways of Glucose Production

Regulation of blood glucose levels in the normal state relies on a delicate balance between nutrient intake and energy expenditure. Nutrition comprises the fundamental processes by which essential nutrients are absorbed by the gut and transferred through the bloodstream and across membranes for transport into cells for metabolism. All metabolic pathways which generate adenosine triphosphate (ATP) pass through glucose or key amino acids. Thus, abnormalities in the absorption, transport, storage, and metabolism of glucose provide the mechanisms for diseases resulting in low levels of glucose in blood (hypoglycemia). Clinically, low glucose levels in key body fluids (notably blood and the cerebrospinal fluid) allow initial identification of such diseases. Beyond infancy, these disorders present rarely; thus, the astute clinician recognizes that, while many patients attribute their symptoms and problems to hypoglycemia, actual hypoglycemia is seldom documented adequately and its prevalence often overestimated.[1]

Adaptation to separation from energy supplied via the placenta to self-sufficiency at birth requires rapid activation of three counter-regulatory mechanisms: glycogenolysis, gluconeogenesis, and lipolysis. These mechanisms are immature in the newborn and even more rudimentary in premature, asphyxiated, hypoxic, or small-for-gestational age (SGA) infants. The rate of glucose turnover in newborns is 6 mg/kg/min in newborns, approximately three times the adult rate. Although the demand for glucose is high, the activities of several liver enzymes involved in glucose production (eg, glucose-6-phosphatase) and ketogenesis are diminished, particularly in preterm infants. Consequently, before the first feeding, approximately 10% of normal term newborns and approximately 67% of preterm SGA infants display blood glucose levels below 30 mg/dL in the first hours of life. These data highlight the importance of administering the initial feeding, typically the fat-rich colostrum, as soon after birth as possible.

Proper storage, oxidation, and production of glucose require intact systems for glycolysis, glycogen synthesis, glycogenolysis, and gluconeogenesis coordinated through activity of the Krebs cycle and the pentose phosphate shunt. Apart from periods of active carbohydrate absorption from the gut (~30 minutes after ingestion), the majority of life is spent in the fasting state. The most immediate adaptation to fasting involves release of glucose from hepatic glycogen stores, which can typically provide substrate for up to 8 hours in older children, but for much shorter periods of time in neonates and ill patients. Thereafter, gluconeogenesis (which forms glucose from the 3-carbon precursors, lactate, pyruvate, alanine, glutamine, and glycerol) maintains homeostasis. Gluconeogenesis is relatively impaired until late childhood as a result of the decreased availability of substrates. Active recycling of intermediate metabolites occurs within the mitochondria of the hepatocyte and myocyte during glucose metabolism. The balance between glycolysis and gluconeogenesis appears to depend on the ambient flux of ATP in the hepatocyte, which is determined, under normal conditions, primarily by the extracellular glucose concentration. The maximal hepatic glucose output is approximately 8 mg/kg/min, which is close to the normal glucose requirement in infancy.

A continuous supply of glucose to the brain depends on maintaining a critical arterial plasma glucose concentration and is facilitated by glucose transport proteins (GLUT-1 and -3). Importantly, these transport proteins are up-regulated by chronic cerebral hypoglycemia, but glucoregulatory factors, including insulin, do not affect glucose uptake into the brain.

Liberation and utilization of fat as an energy source limits catabolism of lean body mass while meeting meet energy needs in a more prolonged fasting state. Free fatty acids (FFA), derived from adipose tissue, are transported via the circulation to the hepatocyte for conversion to ketones: acetone, acetoacetate (AcAc; reported by most clinical laboratories unless requested otherwise), and β-hydroxybutyrate (β-OHB). Over periods of prolonged fasting, FFA oxidation accounts for almost 80% of the body's energy sources. In contrast to gluconeogenesis, ketogenesis occurs more rapidly and to a higher level in children than in adults; after fasting for 20 hours, the ketone body turnover rate in young children is comparable to that of adults who have fasted for several days. Most body tissues (including cardiac and skeletal muscle) can use FFA for oxidative metabolism, with the notable exception of the brain, which requires β-OHB, the ketone species that predominates in human plasma (typically tenfold over AcAc) and readily crosses the blood-brain barrier. Ultimately, these adaptations to prolonged fasting decrease glucose turnover by approximately 50% and lead to a gradual decrease in plasma glucose concentrations.

Regulation of Insulin Secretion

Released from β-cells in the pancreatic islets of Langerhans, insulin is the only endocrine hormone which significantly and directly lowers the circulating glucose level. It does so by mediating glucose uptake into tissues. Pancreatic β-cells and the liver integrate the major sensors responsible for detecting high glucose and stimulating insulin release. At the β-cell level of glucose-sensing, any acute rise in the intracellular concentration of ATP or free calcium induces insulin release (Figure 11-1). Glucokinase constitutes the primary sensor for high glucose within the β-cell because its enzymatic action is the rate-limiting step for glycolysis, which results in ATP production. Oxidation of many intermediate fuels, such as glutamate, results in insulin release by raising intracellular ATP. Glutamate dehydrogenase (GDH) reversibly oxidizes glutamate to α-ketoglutarate, a direct intermediate of the Krebs cycle, for ATP production. This GDH-catalyzed reaction is enhanced by positive allosteric regulators such as *l*-leucine and inhibited by guanosine triphosphate (GTP).[2]

The primary pathway for the regulation of insulin secretion in humans is the sulfonylurea receptor (SUR1)-potassium channel complex, which accounts for more than 90% of glucose-stimulated insulin release. In humans, this complex consists of four subunit proteins of the sulfonylurea receptor (SUR1) and four inward-rectifying subunits regulating potassium (K) flux (Kir6.2 or K-ATP channel). Derived from glycolysis or other pathways, ATP binding at the intracellular nucleotide binding site of the *trans* plasma membrane SUR1 will close the associated inward-rectifying K channel. Closure to K flux depolarizes the membrane, which activates voltage-gated, L-type calcium channels. Influx of calcium raises free calcium levels intracellularly, leading to insulin release from storage granules via a pathway regulated by calmodulin-dependent kinase II.

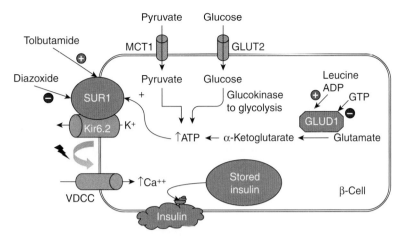

FIGURE 11-1 ■ Mechanisms of insulin secretion in pancreatic β-cells. An increase in the ATP to ADP ratio inhibits the K_{ATP} channel, resulting in its closure, depolarization of the cell membrane, influx of calcium, and release of insulin. The ATP to ADP ratio is increased (and therefore insulin secretion stimulated) by glucose oxidation via glucokinase (GK) and by leucine stimulation of glutamate oxidation via glutamate dehydrogenase (GDH also known as GLUD1). Abnormally increased pyruvate levels in the β-cell will stimulate insulin secretion. GLUT2, glucose transporter 2; MCT1: monocarboxylate transporter 1; ADP: adenosine diphosphate; ATP: adenosine triphosphate; GTP: guanine triphosphate; VDCC: voltage-dependent calcium channel; Kir6.2: inward rectifying potassium (K-ATP) channel of SUR1/Kir6.2 complex.

Counterregulation to maintain normoglycemia

Multiple counterregulatory pathways have evolved to maintain normal circulating glucose concentrations (also known as euglycemia or normoglycemia) by opposing insulin action during the stress response.

Glucagon. In response to falling plasma glucose levels, glucagon from the pancreatic α-cells enters the portal circulation to act primarily on 6-phosphofructo-2-kinase/fructose-2,6-bisphophatase in hepatocytes. The kinase and phosphatase portions of this bifunctional enzyme regulate, respectively, the key steps controlling glycolysis and gluconeogenesis. Glucagon favors the dephosphorylated state, resulting in activation of the kinase and inhibition of the phosphatase, enhancing gluconeogenesis while simultaneously inhibiting glycolysis.

Catecholamines. Catecholamines acutely rise in response to hypoglycemia. Adrenergic α_1-receptor binding enhances amino acid uptake into the liver, which increases the availability of substrates for gluconeogenesis while β-adrenergic receptor activation stimulates lipolysis by inducing phosphorylation of hormone-sensitive lipase (the enzyme that cleaves triglycerides into FFA and glycerol within adipose tissue). There, catecholamines stimulate glycogenolysis via both the α_1- and β-receptor mechanisms; in muscle, stimulation of glycogenolysis occurs solely by β_2-receptor activation and requires the presence of glucocorticoids to antagonize the effects of circulating insulin. Catecholamines also enhance FFA entry and mobilize triglycerides from skeletal muscle, but inhibit the release of amino acids from skeletal muscle, preserving this resource in muscle during stress. Effects on insulin secretion are complex and incompletely understood; β_2-adrenergic activation appears to stimulate insulin and glucagon secretion while α-receptor stimulation suppresses insulin secretion and stimulates glucagon secretion. Finally, catecholamines acutely inhibit insulin-mediated glucose uptake via β-adrenergic stimulation.

Growth hormone. Growth hormone (GH) is released in response to stress, fasting, hypoglycemia, and rapid declines in blood glucose concentrations. In the neonatal period, GH provides a primary defense against hypoglycemia via its inhibition of peripheral insulin-stimulated glucose uptake, perhaps by action of specific IGF-binding proteins to induce insulin resistance. GH also stimulates release of FFA from adipose tissue stores, thereby providing an alternate fuel to glucose during prolonged states of hypoglycemia. Hypoglycemia of significant duration (eg, hours) is a more potent stimulus than is acute hypoglycemia for GH, ACTH, or cortisol release, but this may not be the case when hypoglycemia is persistent or recurrent. For that reason, a low serum GH level found at the time of spontaneous, as opposed to acute induced, hypoglycemia does not necessarily imply GH deficiency as a cause of the hypoglycemia.

Glucocorticoids. Glucocorticoids, synthesized in the adrenal cortex upon ACTH stimulation enter the adrenal medulla and stimulate the activity of phenylethanolamine-N-methyl transferase (PNMT), which catalyzes the N-methylation of norepinephrine to epinephrine. ACTH and cortisol deficiency, therefore, result in a decrease in immediate counter-regulation by epinephrine production and secretion. Furthermore, cortisol promotes gluconeogenesis via mobilization of amino acids from muscle and activation of glucose-6-phosphatase and phosphoenolpyruvate carboxykinase.

In summary, the main insulin counterregulatory hormonal action during stress arises from adrenomedullary epinephrine, with contributions from adrenocortical cortisol, pancreatic glucagon, and pituitary GH. Although rare tumors can secrete insulin-like growth factors (IGFs) which cross-react with insulin receptors, IGFs typically exert only permissive actions on glucose transport and metabolism. Regulation of insulin-mediated glucose uptake is the primary mechanism upon which the clinician must focus. Diseases that impact this process involve the hormones of the stress response as well as inborn errors of insulin secretion, glucose transport, and ATP metabolism.

DEFINITIONS

Hypoglycemia is a common clinical problem with serious neurological sequelae when detection is delayed or treatment inadequate. Even though low blood sugar may often be transient, hypoglycemia itself is never physiological (in other words, never normal) and should not be disregarded when documented adequately. Various approaches have been applied to define an abnormally low level of circulating glucose.[3] The most pragmatic relies on glucose-level-dependent appearance and resolution of clinical signs (Box 11-1) (also see "Signs and Symptoms" later on in the chapter for specifics). Epidemiological studies of at-risk groups (infants not fed promptly and frequently after birth) may be troubled by ascertainment bias and not be representative of a truly healthy, normal population. Physiological fasting studies, which integrate sensitive and specific endocrine assessments with safe clinical outcomes, provide the most logical and compelling information.

Decades of such physiological work suggest that blood glucose at *any* age is normally more than or equal to *70 mg/dL (3.9 mM).*[4] While many complain that this therapeutic range triggers too many interventions, abundant evidence suggests that the developing brain is more susceptible to low glucose levels, which behooves clinical vigilance and use of a threshold (ie, 70 mg/dL) above which no counterregulatory response typically is triggered

to maintain glucose homeostasis. Thus, the prudent clinician feeds a newborn infant with a blood sugar less than 70 mg/dL and reassesses the blood glucose level every 15 minutes until clinical recovery is confirmed. While no specific blood glucose level will be universally accepted as the dividing line between hypo- and normoglycemia, use of *70 mg/dL as a target for normoglycemia* is reasonable. Three important caveats include: (1) this recommendation applies to the symptomatic infant with documented profound, recurrent, and/or persistent hyperinsulinemic hypoglycemia, but may not apply to newborns with a single episode of low plasma glucose; (2) for infants and children, *any documented venous plasma glucose concentration less than 60 mg/dL* should prompt a thorough evaluation; and (3) for reliable diagnostic information from the "critical blood sample" (see p. 403), a simultaneous *blood sugar less than or equal to 60 mg/dL and (preferably <50 mg/dL)* is recommended.

Casual measurement of blood glucose by fingerstick is common clinically. Blood glucose should be assessed with any new-onset seizure disorder (preferably at the time of the convulsion) at any age, or when the patient demonstrates supraphysiological glucose utilization to maintain blood glucose more than 70 mg/dL (ie, an intravenous glucose infusion rate *>5 to 8 mg/kg/min* in infants or *>3 mg/kg/min* in adolescents and adults). It is also important to assess blood glucose levels in high-risk infants, including those born SGA, premature, or large-for-gestational age (given their high incidence of known or unknown diabetic mothers).

Portable glucose meters are convenient and relatively cheap, advantages offset by their inaccuracy (up to 20% off the true laboratory glucose reading) and unreliability (simultaneous results often vary by 10%). To make a definitive diagnosis of hypoglycemia requires proper specimen collection and handling. The ideal specimen is whole blood drawn from a free-flowing intravascular catheter into a sodium fluoride (NaF)-containing, gray-top tube and processed immediately by a central laboratory (NaF inhibits glycolysis by erythrocytes which, prior to centrifugation, can decrease the glucose level by as much 20 mg/dL/h). Such results obtained by a glucose oxidase assay are both accurate and reliable within ± 1 mg/dL.

PATHOGENESIS/SPECIFIC ETIOLOGIES

Hypoglycemia results from one or more of the following:

1. Excessive glucose utilization owing to excess insulin or insulin-like action
2. Deficient energy production owing to defective glycogenolysis, gluconeogenesis, ketogenesis, or ketone utilization

---

Box 11-1. Whipple Classic Triad[3]
■ Symptoms consistent with hypoglycemia
■ Low plasma glucose level (the definition debated based on available technology and study design as discussed in the text)
■ Resolution of symptoms after raising the blood glucose level

3. Energy needs which exceed carbohydrate reserves (eg, illness with prolonged vomiting and anorexia, SGA infant)
4. Exogenous medications or toxic ingestions
5. Reactive hypoglycemia

A detailed list of etiologies of childhood hypoglycemia is presented in Table 11-1.

Excess Insulin Action or Insulin-Like Action

Transient congenital hyperinsulinism occurs most commonly secondary to *maternal* factors. Hyperglycemia as a result of uncontrolled gestational diabetes induces fetal β-cell hyperplasia and hyperinsulinism, often leading to macrosomia, risk for shoulder dystocia, and hypoglycemia

Table 11-1.

Etiologies of Hypoglycemia

1. Hyperinsulinism
   - Most often found in the setting of the infant of a diabetic mother (IDM) (usually resolves within 2-4 wk) or in infants with perinatal immaturity and/or stress
   - Inborn error of insulin regulation by the β-cell: 1 per 30,000-50,000 live births
     - Diffuse *sulfonylurea receptor* (*SUR1*) gene mutation (~50% of genetic congenital hyperinsulinism [CHI] cases): autosomal dominant or recessive
     - Focal *SUR1*: uniparental disomy with loss of heterozygosity (~40% of genetic CHI cases; one-third of the time, the focal lesion is located within the head of the pancreas)
     - Diffuse *inward rectifying potassium channel* (*Kir6.2*) gene mutation: autosomal dominant or recessive
     - Focal *inward rectifying potassium channel* (*Kir6.2*) gene mutation: postulated, but not yet reported
     - Hyperinsulinism/hyperammonemia (HI/HA) syndrome from autosomal dominant, gain-of-function mutation in the *glutamate dehydrogenase* (*GLUD1*) gene in β-cells and hepatocytes
     - *Glucokinase* (*GK*) gene mutation; other *GK* mutations result in maturity-onset diabetes of youth (MODY)
     - Congenital disorder of glycosylation (glycoprotein biosynthesis): CDG-Id[5]
   - Beckwith-Weidemann syndrome—unclear etiology; perhaps owing to SUR or Kir6.2 dysfunction (causing hyperinsulinemia) in some patients
   - Postsurgical dumping syndrome
   - Surreptitious insulin administration
   - Nonislet cell tumor hypoglycemia (NICTH) from big IGF-II[6]—can result from any of several primitive tumors including: solitary fibrous tumor, giant phyllodes tumor, gastrointestinal stromal tumor, renal cell carcinoma, hemangiopericytoma, adrenocortical carcinoma, *etc.*
2. Counterregulatory hormone deficiency
   - Isolated GH deficiency or as part of panhypopituitarism (deficient anterior pituitary hormones: GH, ACTH, TSH, FSH, and LH)[7]
     - Congenital
     - Acquired
   - Hypocortisolemia
     - Central as a result of pituitary ACTH deficiency
     - 21-hydroxylase deficiency congenital adrenal hyperplasia (CAH)
     - 11-hydroxylase deficiency CAH
     - 3-β-hydroxysteroid dehydrogenase deficiency CAH
     - Deficiency of steroid acute regulatory (STAR) protein, which transports cholesterol across the inner mitochondrial membrane for steroidogenesis
     - Congenital adrenal hypoplasia owing to a mutation of *DAX1 (NROB1)* which encodes an adrenal transcription factor
     - ACTH unresponsiveness[8]
   - Glucagon deficiency
   - Catecholamine (epinephrine/norepinephrine) deficiency
   - *l*-aromatic amino acid decarboxylase deficiency
3. Glycogen release diseases (GRD)
   - Glycogen synthase (GRD type 0)
   - Glucose-6-phosphatase deficiency (von Gierke disease)
     - GRD type 1a (enzyme defect): the most common GRD
     - GRD type 1b (transport defect) or type 1c (with neutropenia)
   - Acid maltase deficiency (Pompe disease; GRD type 2)
   - Glycogen debrancher defect (Cori or Forbes disease; GRD type 3)

(Continued)

Table 11-1. (Continued)

Etiologies of Hypoglycemia

- Glycogen branching enzyme deficiency (Andersen disease; GRD type 4)
- Muscle glycogen phosphorylase deficiency (McArdle disease; GRD type 5)
- Liver glycogen phosphorylase deficiency (Hers disease; GRD type 6)
  - X-linked variant, formerly classified as GRD type 8
  - Another variant formerly classified as type 10
- Muscle phosphofructokinase (Tarui disease; GRD type 7)
- Phosphorylase kinase (GRD type 9)
- Glucose transporter 2, *GLUT2* (Fanconi-Bickel syndrome; GRD type 11)

4. Mitochondrial fatty acid oxidation defects (first described in 1973)
- Medium chain acyl-CoA dehydrogenase (MCAD) deficiency
- Long chain acyl-CoA dehydrogenase (LCAD) deficiency
- Very long chain acyl-CoA dehydrogenase (VLCAD) deficiency
- Short chain L-3-hydroxyacyl-CoA dehydrogenase (SCHAD) deficiency
- Absent ketogenesis caused by:
  - Primary carnitine deficiency
  - Hepatic carnitine acyl transferase deficiency
    - Carnitine palmitoyltransferase 1 (CPT1A) deficiency

5. Ketone utilization defects
- Succinyl CoA transferase (SCOT) deficiency
- β-ketothiolase deficiency

6. Defective gluconeogenesis
- Severe hepatic failure
- Pyruvate decarboxylase (carboxylates pyruvate to yield oxaloacetate, reduces oxaloacetate to malate for transport out of mitochondria, and then oxidizes malate to oxaloacetate in cytosol)
- Phosphoenolpyruvate carboxykinase (decarboxylates and phosphorylates oxaloacetate to make phosphoenolpyruvate)
- Fructose-1,6-diphosphatase ([FDP1-6diPase] converts fructose-1,6-bisphosphate to fructose-6-phosphate)[9]
- Phosphoglucoisomerase (converts fructose-6-phosphate to glucose-6-phosphate)

7. Exogenous drugs
- Insulin or repaglinide misuse
- Alcohol
- Salicylates
- Sulfonylureas
- Antimalarials
- Antibiotics containing trimethoprim-sulfamethoxazole, pivalic acid, or cotrimoxazole
- Paramethoxyamphetamine
- β-blocker intoxication

8. Miscellaneous
- Ketotic (also known as fasting functional) hypoglycemia is the diagnosis of exclusion which represents normal patients who simply have a shorter fasting tolerance than expected for age; often, such a patient is small, thin, and has a straightforward, limited, intercurrent illness which taxes limited physiological reserves
- Reactive hypoglycemia[1]
- Phosphomannose isomerase deficiency (carbohydrate-deficient glycoprotein syndrome)[5]
- Islet sodium channelopathy (*Scn1b* mutation reported in mice and postulated in humans)[10]

within a few hours of birth. This usually resolves within days to 2 weeks of birth. Hyperinsulinism may also occur as a result of intravenous glucose administered during labor and delivery; secondary to tocolytic and other medications administered to the pregnant woman (terbutaline, propranolol, oral sulfonylureas, and other hypoglycemic agents used to treat gestational or type 2 diabetes); and from perinatal stress (birth asphyxia, low birth weight, preeclampsia, maternal toxemia, premature labor, or premature birth).

Congenital hyperinsulinism (CHI) is **the most common** etiology of hypoglycemia persisting beyond the immediate neonatal period (first hours of life). Several inborn errors of pancreatic β-cell function disrupt the normal coupling of insulin release to the ambient glucose concentration. These include diffuse or focal mutations of the *SUR1* or *Kir6.2* genes; mutations of the gene encoding glutamate dehydrogenase (autosomal dominant gain-of-function *GLUD1*); glucokinase deficiency (autosomal dominant *GK* gene mutation); select fatty acid oxidation gene defects (eg, *SCHAD*); and defective glycoprotein synthesis (congenital disorder of glycosylation). Genetic tests currently available can identify diagnostic mutations in 40% to 50% of patients affected by these disorders. Autosomal recessive defects caused by either homozygous mutations in the *SUR1* gene (ABDD8) or in the *Kir6.2* gene (KCNJ11) which render critical components of the K_{ATP} channel inactive (ie, constitutively open) result in diffuse β-cell dysfunction and intractable severe hypoglycemia soon after birth. Other sporadic variants may create focal adenomatous hyperplasia (40%-60% of all cases of K_{ATP}-CHI hypoglycemia) caused by loss of the maternal allele imprinted at 11p15 in a patient harboring an *SUR1* mutation on the paternal allele. It is postulated that the loss of heterozygosity either unmasks a recessively inherited *SUR1* or *Kir6.2* mutation located on the paternal allele or leads to loss of suppressor genes which normally would inhibit islet cell growth-promoting actions of *IGF-II*. The significance of identifying diffuse *versus* focal disease lies in the potential of curative, focused partial *versus* 95% pancreatectomy. Recently, PET scans with 18-fluoro-*l*-3,4-dihydroxyphenylalanine (18F-DOPA) have been shown to accurately discriminate focal CHI from diffuse CHI.[2]

Two autosomal dominant forms of hyperinsulinism tend to have milder clinical presentations and sequelae than autosomal recessive forms. Infants are frequently not large-for-gestational age and may not present symptomatically until later in infancy or even in childhood. Of these two forms, the more common activating mutation in *GLUD1*, the gene for mitochondrial glutamate dehydrogenase, causes relatively mild hyperinsulinemia accompanied by persistent mild hyperammonemia (blood ammonia levels ~100-200 µmol/L, or 3-5 times normal). These mutations in *GLUD1* cause impaired sensitivity to inhibition by GTP, resulting in gain-of-function and excessive sensitivity to activation by leucine (ie, "leucine sensitivity"). Increased conversion of glutamate to α-ketoglutarate ultimately increases the intracellular ATP to ADP ratio, stimulates insulin release, and yields excessive ammonia (which does not depend upon concurrent protein intake). A second and very rare autosomal dominant form of hyperinsulinemia is caused by a mutation in the gene encoding *glucokinase (GCK)*, resulting in increased affinity of the enzyme for glucose and an abnormally low "set point" for glucose-stimulated insulin release. Importantly, a defect in GCK can be missed if the critical sample is obtained at a blood sugar below the threshold for insulin secretion. Since the K_{ATP} channel is normal in both *GLUD1* and *GCK* mutation-mediated CHI, these disorders typically are distinguished from autosomal recessive forms of CHI first by a favorable therapeutic response to diazoxide. A description of these various causes of CHI with their genetic and clinical features appears in Table 11-2.

Hypoglycemia also occurs in 50% of infants with Beckwith-Wiedemann syndrome. This most likely results from disordered imprinting at chromosome 11p15 encompassing the *IGF2*, *SUR1*, and *Kir6.2* genes which gives rise to islet cell hyperplasia (unimprinted gene produces excess *IGF-II* action) and dysregulated insulin release from abnormalities in K_{ATP} channels of the pancreatic β-cell.

Counterregulatory hormone deficiencies clinically (although not biochemically) can resemble CHI during the first month of life, since (1) glycogen reserves may be inappropriately conserved during hypoglycemia in both the infants with CHI and those with either GH deficiency or hypopituitarism and (2) ketone production in response to hypoglycemia is limited in neonates, complicating the distinction between "ketotic" and "nonketotic" disorders at this age.

Postsurgical dumping syndrome[11] typically occurs after Nissen fundoplication or Roux-en-Y gastric bypass. Overrapid gastric emptying of elemental formulas leads to rapid transluminal absorption of glucose and rapid glucose-stimulated insulin release; the circulating insulin level climbs so high that it does not fall quickly enough to coincide with the empty gut's lack of ongoing glucose absorption, leading to postprandial hyperinsulinemic hypoglycemia. Classical dumping symptoms are loss of consciousness or mild neuroglycopenic signs within 3 hours after each meal. Nonclassical symptoms include borborygmi (loud, small bowel sounds) and adrenergic signs as the hypoglycemia resolves in response to secretion of catecholamines.

Iatrogenic hyperinsulinemic hypoglycemia may occur as a result of abruptly discontinued hypertonic dextrose infusions, including total parenteral nutrition. Excessive glucose utilization leading to hypoglycemia may also result from surreptitious insulin or sulfonylurea administration, either unintentionally from insulin overdose or, rarely, as part of either homicidal, suicidal, or Munchausen-by-proxy behavior.

Whether in isolation or as part of multiple endocrine neoplasia type 1 (MEN I), islet cell adenomas (insulinomas) are rare in children, and rarer still in infants. Hypoglycemia may result from tumors that overutilize fuel substrates or that produce IGFs. Such nonislet cell tumor hypoglycemia (NICTH) results from excessive free IGF concentrations acting via insulin and hybrid insulin-IGF receptors at the cell surface. These tumors release immature IGF molecules which nevertheless retain binding properties of the mature forms. The immature forms are often fully glycosylated, raising molecular weight and thus labeled as "big" IGFs. These variant IGF molecules may not be detected on routine commercial assays, requiring consultation with an academic center or a reference laboratory for special testing.

Table 11-2.

Classification of Genetic Forms of Congenital Hyperinsulinism

Genetic Form	Gene	Chromosome	Inheritance	Clinical Features	Treatment
K$_{ATP}$-HI	*ABCC8* *KCNJ11*	11p15	Diffuse: AR Focal: loss of hetero-zygosity with paternal mutation	Severe hypoglycemia; unresponsive to medical therapy	Pancreatectomy or "conservative" therapy with octreotide and continuous feedings
Dominant K$_{ATP}$-HI	*ABCC8* *KCNJ11*	11p15	AD	Milder hypoglycemia; responsive to diazoxide	Diazoxide
GDH-HI (HI/HA)	*GLUD-1*	10q	AD	Fasting and postprandial hypoglycemia; less severe than K$_{ATP}$-HI; protein sensitivity; asymptomatic hyperammonemia	Diazoxide
GK-HI	*GCK*	7p	AD	Variable phenotype: can range from easy to manage with medical therapy to very difficult to control	Diazoxide; pancreatectomy
SCHAD-HI	*HADH*	4q	AR	Mild to severe hypoglycemia; abnormal acylcarnitine profile	Diazoxide
MCT1 (EIHI)	*SLC16A1*	1p	AD	Exercise-induced hypoglycemia, especially anaerobic	Carbohydrate intake during exercise; limit exercise

AR, autosomal recessive; AD, autosomal dominant; HI, hyperinsulinism.

Deficient Energy Production Caused by Defective Glycogenolysis, Gluconeogenesis, Ketogenesis, or Ketone Utilization

Insufficient production of glucose during the postabsorptive state results from either: (1) intrinsic enzymatic abnormalities in glycogenolysis or gluconeogenesis; (2) deficient mobilization of glucose precursors for otherwise normal gluconeogenesis; or (3) inability to effectively produce and/or utilize fatty acids for energy.

Disorders of *glycogenolysis* are more accurately described as glycogen release diseases (GRD, listed in Table 11-1) rather than the traditional designation as glycogen storage diseases. These *GRD* patients share the clinical feature of usually minimally ketotic hypoglycemia and *markedly impaired fasting tolerance* (usually

<6 hours to onset of symptoms related to tissue ATP deficiency). Patients with GRD type 1 present most often after 6 months of age with growth retardation, cherubic facies, and hepatomegaly. Laboratory tests reveal fasting hypoglycemia, lactic acidemia, and hyperlipidemia (reflecting intact counter-regulatory hormone responses), hyperuricemia (from increased nucleic acid catabolism and decreased renal tubular secretion), and a markedly blunted glucose response to glucagon challenge. Prolonged fasting (typically over 8-12 hours) or a vigorous catecholaminergic response to hypoglycemia is usually required in patients with GRD or defective gluconeogenesis to elicit ketonuria. Neurological symptoms are usually absent in patients with GRD type 1 because the brain (and other tissues) utilize high lactate levels as an alternate fuel for ATP (an important distinction from lack of alternate substrate with hyperinsulinemic hypoglycemia). Other

forms of GRD (see Table 11-1) show similar, but milder, manifestations (GRD types 3 and 6).

Disorders of gluconeogenesis include autosomal recessive hereditary fructose intolerance (HFI; fructose-1-phosphate aldolase deficiency) and fructose-1,6-diphosphatase deficiency. HFI presents with vomiting, hypoglycemia, and seizures after initiation of fructose ingestion. Continued fructose exposure can lead to failure-to-thrive, jaundice, hepatosplenomegaly, proteinuria, aminoaciduria, and death. Fructose 1,6-diphosphatase deficiency results in fasting hypoglycemia, lactic acidosis, hepatomegaly, and ketonemia. Patients with galactosemia, an inherited autosomal recessive deficiency of galactose-1-phosphate uridyl transferase (included routinely in newborn screening programs), after exposure to lactose (hydrolyzed to glucose and galactose), develop vomiting, failure-to-thrive, cataracts, susceptibility to infection, and hepatic and renal dysfunction.

Deficient *mobilization of substrate* required for gluconeogenesis can also lead to fasting hypoglycemia. Beyond the immediate neonatal period, the second most common cause of infantile hypoglycemia arises from deficiencies of the counterregulatory (ie, energy substrate mobilizing) actions of GH and/or cortisol. This spectrum includes disorders associated with isolated GH deficiency or panhypopituitarism including congenital malformations of the hypothalamus and pituitary; disorders of the adrenal cortex; and inborn errors of cortisol synthesis. Isolated GH deficiency may have an idiopathic basis or, rarely, be owing to either autoimmune hypophysitis or a *GH* gene mutation. Congenital hypopituitarism results from malformations, such as holoprosencephaly or lissencephaly; mutations in any of the pituitary gland transcription factors (*PROP1, POU1F1, LHX3, LHX4, PITX1, PITX2, SOX2,* or *SOX3*) that can cause failure of either somatotroph (GH) and/or corticotroph (ACTH) development; and optic nerve hypoplasia/septo-optic dysplasia (associated, in some cases, with a *HESX1* mutation). Acquired GH deficiency can occur secondary to tumor, radiation, infection, and trauma. Several defects in adrenal development or steroid synthesis can cause cortisol deficiency including both congenital adrenal hyperplasia (most commonly caused by 21-hydroxylase deficiency, but also seen with many other rarer varieties) and congenital adrenal hypoplasia.

A relatively common cause of hypoglycemia in the pre-school-aged child—described simply as "ketotic hypoglycemia"—appears to result from lack of sufficient protein/alanine substrate for gluconeogenesis in an (usually, but not always) underweight child. This diagnosis of exclusion is made after careful consideration of other inborn errors of metabolism or hormonal deficiencies associated with hypoglycemia and ketonemia.

Typically, the child is light in weight for age and the clinical presentation of hypoglycemia during fasting stress occurs beyond the age of infancy, but prior to the age of 6 years. This developmental disorder of homeostasis is postulated to arise from deficient recycling of alanine or lactate in the small child.

Disorders of fatty acid oxidation/ketone production or utilization predispose the patient to **fasting** hypoglycemia owing to ongoing glucose utilization in the absence of an ability to use ketones as an energy source. Metabolic errors throughout the pathway of fatty acid uptake, activation, and β-oxidation have been described (caused by mutations in the genes encoding *MCAD, LCAD, VLCAD,* and *SCHAD;* see Table 11-1); these tend to share clinical features and to occur during prolonged fasting when normal reliance on fatty acid metabolism is maximal. Defective ketogenesis (eg, carnitine deficiency) fails to yield circulating and urinary ketones during hypoglycemia, and abnormal dicarboxylic acids are present in the urine. In addition to skeletal and cardiac muscle and liver dysfunction, a distinctive and threatening feature of some fatty acid oxidation disorders (*eg,* MCAD) is early profound neurological depression and subsequent damage that is out of proportion to the degree of hypoglycemia. This is thought to reflect direct central nervous system (CNS) toxicity of very high levels of abnormal fatty acid metabolites. Fortunately, newborn screening using mass spectrometry is increasingly allowing early detection of most of these disorders. The two known *ketone utilization defects* (β-ketothiolase deficiency and succinyl Co-A transferase deficiency) typically present with *persistent, marked ketoacidosis* in the first months of life. Defective gluconeogenesis arises from a defect in one of several enzymatic actions (in mitochondria and in the cytosol) which create glucose from noncarbohydrate carbon substrates (including lactic acid, glycerol, and amino acids [other than lysine or leucine]).

Energy Needs Which Exceed Carbohydrate Reserves—Other Causes

Hypoglycemia may occur when glucose needs exceed the patients' ability to meet them for reasons not discussed above. Occasionally, energy requirements associated with intercurrent illness can exceed carbohydrate reserves (*eg,* prolonged vomiting or anorexia). Hypoglycemia owing to a complex and multifactorial etiology is also a complication of intrauterine growth retardation. During the first several days of extrauterine life, without the placental source of nutrients, maintenance of normal glucose levels requires adequate glycogen stores; intact glycogenolytic, gluconeogenic, and lipogenic mechanisms; and appropriate counterregulatory hormone responses. The hypoglycemia in the IUGR infant is owing primarily to decreased glycogen stores with a possible contribution from diminished liver gluconeogenesis from alanine and lactate substrates. Growth-restricted infants also have limited fat stores, appear to not oxidize free fatty acids and triglycerides effectively, and may show decreased counterregulatory hormone responses to falling blood glucose levels. In addition, hyperinsulinism or excessive sensitivity to insulin appears to exacerbate hypoglycemia and, in some cases, leads to the prolonged need for high glucose infusion rates. Short-term treatment with diazoxide to reduce insulin secretion can be helpful in weaning these particular infants from dependency on intravenous glucose or continuous nasogastric feedings.[12]

Exogenous Medications or Toxic Ingestions

Most hypoglycemic agents impair hepatic gluconeogenesis, stimulate insulin release, or block ATP metabolism. Table 11-1 (subheading 7) lists the agents most commonly associated with hypoglycemia, highlighted by salicylates, antimalarials, oral hypoglycemics (sulfonylureas and acarbose), and the rodenticide, Vacor.

Reactive Hypoglycemia

Reactive hypoglycemia is a widely used term for a poorly defined and controversial condition of postprandial adrenergic symptoms in the absence of surgery or apparent pathology. Hypoglycemia cannot always be documented. Empirical therapy includes frequent small meals with limited intake of carbohydrates with high glycemic index. Acarbose may help those who fail dietary interventions.

CLINICAL PRESENTATION

Signs and Symptoms

Symptoms of hypoglycemia are nonspecific, so that a low threshold for assessing blood glucose levels is often the key to early recognition and diagnosis. Mild hypoglycemia may present as headache, hunger, anger, irritability, shakiness, absentmindedness, or overt cognitive impairment. These symptoms are age-dependent. Hypoglycemic infants typically display jitteriness, hunger, and irritability, symptoms that are usually relieved promptly by oral intake. Symptoms tend to be most severe with hyperinsulinism, in which the formation of alternate fuels such as FFA and ketones is inhibited. Alternatively, chronic and persistent hypoglycemia can lessen clinical

symptoms and hypoglycemic awareness, an adaptation thought to reflect up-regulation of CNS glucose transporters.

The full counter-regulatory response to acute hypoglycemia elicits a substantial catecholamine response, generating adrenergic symptoms that warn the patient or parents of the falling blood and CNS glucose levels. Usually seen in older children, adolescents, and adults, classic adrenergic symptoms serve as early warnings and include palpitations, sweating, and anxiety. If hypoglycemia is unrecognized and/or untreated, early neuroglycopenic symptoms, such as hunger, fatigue, anger, irritability, slowed cognitive processing, will ensue. If unrecognized, this may progress to more serious manifestations, that is, loss of consciousness and seizure activity, which are potentially dangerous at any age and certainly frighten families. Recovery from a severe or prolonged hypoglycemic episode often takes up to 6 hours, a period typically associated with nausea, vomiting, and fatigue. Diminished cognitive function may persist for several hours after a major hypoglycemic episode (eg, seizure), although physical risks from a fall or while driving are limited to the acute event.

Most concerning, recurrent or severe hypoglycemia can impose long-lasting brain damage. Recent evidence supports the possibility of impaired function of the visual cortex with ongoing, severe hypoglycemia in term neonates.[13] This is especially true in the youngest infants, whose nervous system is rapidly growing and developing. Early magnetic resonance imaging (MRI) findings appear to be more predictive of neurodevelopmental outcome of term infants than the severity or duration of hypoglycemia.[14]

History and Physical

A history of exaggerated birth length and/or large weight for gestational age, or onset of persistent hypoglycemia within the first 12 hours of life should raise suspicion for CHI. Key information to elicit is whether the mother was diabetic and whether the parents share any consanguinity. Subsequently, infants with CHI often manifest a need for more frequent and/or voracious feeding accompanied by accelerated weight gain. However, this may not occur if CNS dysfunction begins to interfere with feeding behavior. Emergence of symptoms often corresponds with changes in feeding source (eg, breast to bottle) or schedule.

GH deficiency in the newborn period typically presents as *hypoglycemia* rather than growth failure. Clinical findings associated with either isolated GH deficiency or panhypopituitarism should raise suspicion for hypoglycemia. These include mid-line facial abnormalities (either severe, *eg*, holoprosencephaly, or mild, *eg*, single central maxillary incisor), prolonged jaundice, and/or, in boys, cryptorchidism and micropenis (stretched length of the penis <2.5 cm in a term male newborn). Only later, after weaning from frequent feedings to overnight fasting (usually by corrected gestational age 4-6 months) does a decrease in linear growth velocity typically become apparent in a child with congenital GH deficiency or hypopituitarism (with or without a relative excess of weight for length or hepatomegaly).

Beyond the neonatal period, symptoms that correlate closely with introductions of specific foods suggest a metabolic intolerance syndrome (*eg*, HFI). Hypoglycemia which occurs in association with episodes of more prolonged fasting or intercurrent illness suggests disorders of impaired substrate mobilization for gluconeogenesis (*eg*, ketotic hypoglycemia) or inability to transition to effective fat utilization (*eg*, fatty acid oxidation disorders).

DIFFERENTIAL DIAGNOSIS

A variety of clinical presentations can mimic signs and symptoms of hypoglycemia and should be considered while the blood glucose is being checked.

1. Sepsis
2. Primary neurological disorder (eg, epilepsy and catalepsy)
3. Toxic ingestion (eg, illicit drug use)
4. Vasovagal syncope
5. Primary cardiac disorder (eg, "Tet" spell from tetralogy of Fallot)
6. Malnutrition
7. Cachexia
8. Panic attack

DIAGNOSIS

Definitive evaluation begins with procurement of a "critical" sample at the time of confirmed hypoglycemia (Table 11-3), and prior to administration of glucose. Although critical samples lack perfect sensitivity and specificity, they are useful for directing further diagnostic maneuvers and management. Serum and urinary levels of *ketones* and plasma *FFA*—obtained during the episode(s) of *hypoglycemia*—represent inexpensive, convenient clues to the subsequent diagnosis and management (see Figure 11-2).

Careful analysis of the critical blood sample usually allows separation of underlying etiologies into one of the following (Figure 11-2):

1. Disorders of glucose release caused by defective glycogenolysis/gluconeogenesis: increased anion gap acidosis, elevated lactate, ketonemia/

Table 11-3.

Critical Fluid Samples During Acute Hypoglycemia[15,16]

3A   Critical diagnostic serum sample
In the *absence of a clear etiology,* during empirical resuscitation and, pending further diagnostic maneuvers or subspecialty consultation, it is reasonable to collect 3-5 mL of whole blood in a plain red top tube and then separate and freeze the serum at −20°C (or preferably −70°C) within 1 h of collection.

3B   Diagnosis-directed testing
1. To evaluate **specific diagnoses**, the following collections are reliable in most hospital laboratories (key initial priority tests in italics):
   - *Glucose, lactate*, and bicarbonate (*ie, electrolytes with anion gap determination*) from 2 mL in a NaF-containing, gray top tube (1 mL minimum), collected free-flowing without a tourniquet.
   - *Insulin, GH, cortisol, alanine*, IGFBP-1, and proinsulin from 3 mL in a serum-separating, red tiger top tube (1.5 mL minimum).
   - Acylcarnitine profile from 3 mL in dark green top tube (1.5 mL minimum).
   - *FFA, β-hydroxybutyrate*, acetoacetate, and total and free carnitine from 4 mL in a dark green top tube ON ICE (1.5 mL minimum).
   - C-peptide from 2 mL in a lavender top tube (0.5 mL minimum).
   - Ammonia from 1 mL in a purple top tube ON ICE (0.5 mL minimum).
   - Pyruvate from 1 mL in a red top tube containing 0.6 M perchloric acid (1 mL minimum).
   - Send next voided *urine for quantitative determination of organic acids and ketones* (β-hydroxybutyrate and acetoacetate).
2. Additional specialized tests.
   - Saliva collection for possible future analysis of DNA (*eg*, Genotek kit).
   - For severe neuroglycopenic symptoms persisting for longer than 24 h despite normal blood glucose levels and without other apparent pathology, consider a *GLUT1* defect at the blood-brain barrier. This specific, rare diagnosis is suggested when the glucose concentration in cerebrospinal fluid (CSF) is <20% of the simultaneous circulating glucose level in the blood. The author recommends freezing (at −20°C or −70°C) any spare CSF if available after routine chemistry studies and cultures have been requested, since additional toxins or analytes may be detected in such a specimen.

Note: Prior to sample collections, discuss proper tubes and feasible sample volumes with your local pathologist or laboratory.

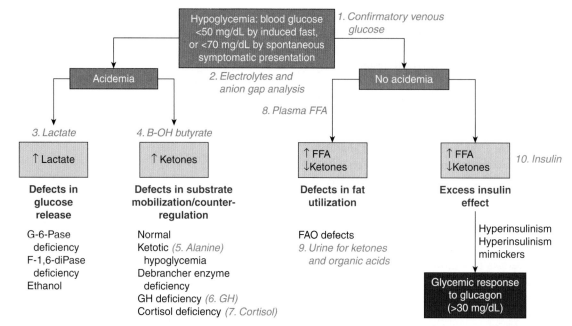

FIGURE 11-2 ■ By interpreting results from critical blood sample (numbered items, placed in proximity to their key diagnostic position) obtained at the time of hypoglycemia, the underlying cause can usually be placed into one of four categories of disease: impairment of glucose release, defects in substrate mobilization/counterregulation, defects in fatty acid oxidation (FAO) and ketogenesis, and impairment of lipolysis and ketogenesis owing to excessive insulin effect. G-6-Pase = glucose-6-phosphatase; F-1,6-diPase = fructose-1,6-diphosphatase; FAO-fatty acid oxidation; β-OHB-beta-hydroxybutyrate.

ketonuria, appropriately elevated GH and cortisol, FFA present, and insulin undetectable

2. Disorders of substrate mobilization/counterregulation: increased anion gap acidosis, normal/slightly elevated lactate, ketonemia/ketonuria (may be absent in neonates), FFA present, and insulin undetectable with: (a) low GH (GH deficiency); (b) low cortisol (ACTH or primary adrenal insufficiency); and (c) low alanine (likely ketotic hypoglycemia)

3. Defects in fatty acid oxidation: no/minimal acidosis, low lactate and ketones, elevated FFA, urine positive for dicarboxylic acids, and undetectable insulin

4. Excess insulin effect: no/minimal acidosis, low lactate and ketones, low FFA, insulin present, and glucose rise more than 30 mg/dL after glucagon

Some results can be recognized immediately as distinctive, *e.g.*, the absence of ketones in the urine within 2 hours of a hypoglycemic seizure strongly suggests the presence of hyperinsulinism. However, abnormal values have been generally been defined in the context of concurrent hypoglycemia after a formal fast, controlled in the hospital setting. As the blood glucose level falls to less than 70 mg/dL during a controlled fast in a normal child, the serum insulin level should fall and ketones should appear in both the serum and in the urine.

Although several diagnostic tests should ideally be performed on this critical specimen, such maneuvers

can be delayed during initial stabilization of the patient (from seizure, obtundation, *etc.*). At a minimum, the astute clinician should obtain 5 to 10 mL of whole blood from the acutely ill patient in a plain red-top tube (lacking anticoagulants) and *immediately* process the sample, by spinning to separate the serum and then freezing this serum at −20°C (or −70°C if available) pending an endocrinology consultation. Most patients are best served by this practical, but underutilized approach. In addition, beyond infancy, if the quantity of blood obtained is insufficient for analysis of all critical sample tests, quick dipstick assessment of urine for the presence or absence of ketones can aid in prioritizing test choices (*eg*, hyperinsulinemia is unlikely in the presence of large urine ketones).

The approach outlined in Table 11-3A is most suitable for the acute emergency setting. Plasma may be obtained in addition to serum. In contrast, the approach in Table 11-3B follows a controlled fast and requires careful, advanced planning and is most safely performed in the inpatient setting. As soon as sufficient hypoglycemia is attained (preferably <40 mg/dL but at least <50 mg/dL), the critical sample is procured. To conclude a formal fasting study (usually confined to the second approach), the clinician should perform the diagnostic glucagon challenge (Table 11-3). This test is predicated on the fact that, in the setting of hyperinsulinemia, there is continuous replenishment of hepatic glycogen so that there will be a significant rise in plasma glucose in response to the administered glucagon which will not occur with any other etiology of hypoglycemia (beyond the newborn period).

CHI is confirmed by plasma FFA concentrations less than 1.5 mM, plasma β-hydroxybutyrate levels less than 2 mM, and an excessive glycemic rise (following 1 mg of intravenous or intramuscular glucagon) of at least 30 mg/dL from a basal level less than 40 mg/dL (detailed in Table 11-4). GH deficiency can also be associated with an inappropriate glycemic rise after glucagon, especially in infancy, but not usually in older children; however, the fasting levels of ketones are usually high with GH deficiency. Lack of a glycemic rise during a glucagon challenge excludes hyperinsulinism. Although rarely requested even by experienced endocrinologists during a glucagon diagnostic challenge, a simultaneous rise in plasma lactate level by at least 2 mM confirms the diagnosis of glucose-6-phosphatase deficiency (GRD type 1), which can avoid the performance of a liver biopsy. The diagnosis of hyperinsulinism is suggested when the serum insulin level is measured to be above the lower limit of detection of the assay (usually >2 μU/mL) when the simultaneous laboratory-measured blood glucose is less than 50 mg/dL. CHI is not excluded from the differential diagnosis by the absence of absolute hyperinsulinism because the hypersecretion of insulin in CHI is erratic in both timing and amplitude with respect to the ambient glucose level.

Advanced diagnostic tests

Accurate diagnosis of the presence and cause of hyperinsulinemia may require advanced, highly specialized tests necessitating referral to pediatric endocrinologists with special expertise in this area (Figure 11-3). In addition to aforementioned laboratory testing, select imaging studies may assist the initial diagnosis. MRI of the brain (with and without gadolinium contrast) can define congenital malformations and acquired intracranial masses. Computed tomography (CT) or MRI of the pancreas rarely reveals a focal insulinoma in pediatric patients with hyperinsulinemia, although a positive result is helpful for guiding surgery. Over the past decade, minimally invasive, acute insulin response (AIR) tests have proven useful to differentiate several recognized β-cell disorders.[4,17,18] These tests take advantage of biological behaviors peculiar to the most prevalent defects in glucose-regulated insulin release. In resting, unstimulated β-cells, an open potassium channel complex (SUR1/Kir6.2) extrudes potassium from the cell, keeping the voltage-dependent calcium channels (VDCC) closed. Defective *SUR1* or *Kir6.2* function will disrupt the electrostatic homeostasis by keeping the potassium channels closed (a missing channel is equivalent to a closed channel), thus activating and opening the VDCC. Infusing calcium, therefore, to defective β-cells with open VDCCs will stimulate acute insulin release. This principle underlies the diagnostic utility of the calcium AIR tests (whether using peripheral, intravenous, or intrapancreatic arterial access). In cases where *GLUD1* mutations and the HI/hyperammonemia syndrome are strongly suspected, a similar test can be performed using leucine as a provocative agent.

Positron emission tomography (PET) is available only at specialized centers, but has demonstrated utility for identifying focal lesions.[19] Intrapancreatic, selective **A**rterial **S**timulation with calcium and portal (or hepatic) **V**enous **S**ampling (ASVS) are also limited to experienced centers and can provide additional diagnostic power.

Table 11-4.

Diagnosis of CHI

1. At the exact time of hypoglycemia, relative hyperinsulinemia with plasma insulin >2 μU/mL (varies with insulin assays), although absence of hyperinsulinemia does not exclude CHI (since insulin secretion is erratic and not necessarily related to ambient glucose level)
2. Occasionally, elevated levels of C-peptide and/or proinsulin are detected and more revealing than the insulin concentration
3. Low serum concentration of IGFBP-1 (inversely regulated by insulin)
4. Hypofattyacidemia (plasma FFA <1.5 mM)
5. Hypoketonemia (plasma β-hydroxybutyrate <2 mM)
6. Lack of urine ketonuria (outside of newborn period)
7. Inappropriate glycemic rise within 30 min following glucagon (1 mg intravenously or intramuscularly), that is, >30 mg/dL above baseline trigger level (ideally <40 mg/dL)
8. Requirement for supraphysiological dextrose infusion rate (>8 mg/kg/min in infants or children; >3 mg/kg/min in adolescents or adults) to prevent hypoglycemia

Note that criteria 4, 5, and 8 are sufficient to diagnose CHI in the absence of nonendocrine pathology (sepsis, etc.).

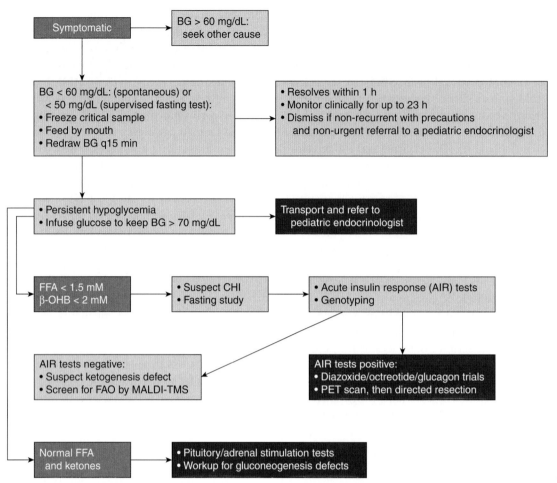

FIGURE 11-3 ■ Algorithm for detection and specific causes of hyperinsulinemia. BG: blood glucose; FFA: free fatty acids; β-OHB: β-hydroxybutyrate; CHI: congenital hyperinsulinism; AIR: acute insulin response; FAO: fatty acid oxidation defect; MALDI-TMS: matrix-assisted laser desorption/ionization–tandem mass spectrometry by reference laboratory; and PET: positron emission tomography.

TREATMENT

The primary goal of the care provider is to recognize and confirm hypoglycemia when suggested by clinical features, obtain a critical blood sample immediately if possible, and then treat with parenteral or oral glucose as indicated by the patient's mental status. It cannot be overemphasized that repeat blood glucose measurement is required every 10 to 20 minutes after any therapeutic intervention until the provider is assured that euglycemia (BG >70 mg/dL) has been restored. When a critical sample is not obtained, blood glucose levels are monitored closely during and after overnight fasting and blood obtained for analysis when the blood glucose is less than 50 mg/dL or symptoms consistent with hypoglycemia occur. Guidelines for progressive treatment of specific disorders are outlined in Table 11-5.

See Box 11-2 for elements on educating patients and families.

> **Box 11-2. Educating Families (Depending on Specific Diagnosis)**
>
> 1. Monitoring of urine ketones and appropriate responses to prevent hypoglycemia
> 2. Consultation with registered dietitian to discuss administration of uncooked cornstarch (e.g., disorders of glycogen release)
> 3. Training on emergent glucagon administration by intramuscular injection (e.g., disorders of glycogen release)
> 4. Gastrostomy placement recommendation and care
> 5. Education on pump use in case of glucagon or octreotide infusion for CHI (e.g., disorders of insulin excess)
> 6. Education regarding stress-dosing of glucocorticoids in patients with cortisol deficiency
>   - Hydrocortisone (50-100 mg intramuscularly) if vomiting or unconscious, followed by prompt medical evaluation
>   - For nonvomiting illnesses, hydrocortisone 50 mg/m² daily (divided every 8 hours if given orally at home or every 4 hours or by continuous infusion if given intravenously in emergency room)
>   - Medic-alert identification for adrenal insufficiency
> 7. Provision of "emergency letter" to all families containing information for medical personnel

Table 11-5.

Treatment and Monitoring of Specific Causes of Infantile/Childhood Hypoglycemia

Diagnosis	First-Line Therapy	Second-Line Therapy	Third-Line Therapy	Fourth-Line Therapy
Acute hypoglycemia	Cake icing, glucose gel, and glucose tablet by mouth	Dextrose infusion 0.2 gm/kg (2 mL/kg of 10% dextrose); then maintain at 8-10 mg/kg/min	Glucagon 1 mg intramuscular injection and then immediate evaluation	
CHI (unknown genotype or histology)	Diazoxide 5-15 mg/kg/d orally (divided in two doses daily)	Octreotide 5-20 µg/kg/d subcutaneously (divided in 3-4 doses daily)	Glucagon 1 mg/d as continuous subcutaneous infusion	Pancreatectomy guided by PET scan[13] or ASVS
Glycogen release disease, type 1	Frequent feedings; uncooked cornstarch 5-10 g at bedtime with protein or carbohydrate to improve palatability; titrate until euglycemic overnight[20]	Orthotopic partial or complete liver transplant		
Ketotic hypoglycemia	Avoid prolonged fasts; monitor urine ketones during periods of reduced caloric intake	Cake icing or dextrose (tablet or gel) by mouth if large urine ketones, anorexic, or vomiting *en route* to definitive care		
GH and/or cortisol deficiency	Appropriate hormone replacement therapy	Increased glucocorticoid dosing for illness or fasting stress		
Defects in fatty acid oxidation, gluconeogenesis, and ketogenesis	Avoid prolonged fasts	Immediate cake icing or dextrose if anorexic or vomiting *en route* to definitive care		
Defects in ketone utilization	Avoid prolonged fasts	Insulin daily to suppress lipolysis and ketogenesis		
Post-surgical dumping syndrome	Acarbose 12.5 mg orally or via gastrostomy immediately before meal bolus; titrate in 12.5-mg increments until post-prandial hypoglycemia resolves[11]	Surgical revision usually not required or ineffective		

GH—growth hormone
CHI—Congenital hyperinsulinism
PET—Positron emission tomography
ASVS—Arterial stimulation with calcium and portal (or hepatic) venous sampling

WHEN TO REFER

Box 11-3 lists circumstances in which a general pediatrician or internist-endocrinologist should consult a pediatric endocrinologist, rather than manage the patient independently.

REFERENCES

1. Scheen AJ, Lefèbvre PJ. Reactive hypoglycaemia, a mysterious, insidious but non-dangerous critical phenomenon. *Rev Med Liege* [French]. 2004;59(4):237-242.

2. Palladino AA, Bennett MJ, Stanley CA. Hyperinsulinism in infancy and childhood: when an insulin level is not always enough. *Clin Chem.* 2008;54(2):256-263.

3. Cornblath M, Hawdon JM, Williams AF, et al. Controversies regarding definition of neonatal hypoglycemia: suggested operational thresholds. *Pediatrics.* 2000;105(5):1141-1145.

4. De León DD, Stanley CA. Mechanisms of disease: advances in diagnosis and treatment of hyperinsulinism in neonates. *Nat Clin Pract Endocrinol Metab.* 2007;3(1):57-68.

5. Freeze HH. Congenital disorders of glycosylation: CDG-I, CDG-II, and beyond. *Curr Mol Med.* 2007;7(4):389-396.

6. Lloyd RV, Erickson LA, Nascimento AG, Klöppel G. Neoplasms causing nonhyperinsulinemic hypoglycemia. *Endocr Pathol.* 1999;10(4):291-297.

7. Mehta A, Dattani MT. Developmental disorders of the hypothalamus and pituitary gland associated with congenital hypopituitarism. *Best Pract Res Clin Endocrinol Metab.* 2008;22(1):191-206.

8. Berberoğlu M, Aycan Z, Ocal G, et al. Syndrome of congenital adrenocortical unresponsiveness to ACTH. Report of six patients. *J Pediatr Endocrinol Metab.* 2001;14(8):1113-1118.

9. Ferry RJ Jr. Fructose-1,6-diphosphatase deficiency. *eMedicine.* 2008; Available at: *http://www.eMedicine.com/ped/topic806.htm.*

10. Ernst SJ, Aguilar-Bryan L, Noebels JL. Sodium channel β1 regulatory subunit deficiency reduces pancreatic islet glucose-stimulated insulin and glucagon secretion. *Endocrinology.* 2009;150(3):1132-1139.

11. Ng DD, Ferry RJ Jr, Kelly A, Weinzimer SA, Stanley CA, Katz LE. Acarbose treatment of postprandial hypoglycemia in children after Nissen fundoplication. *J Pediatr.* 2001;139(6):877-879.

12. Rosenberg A. Intrauterine growth restriction. *Semin Perinatol.* 2008;32(3):219-224.

13. Tam EW, Widjaja E, Blaser SI, Macgregor DL, Satodia P, Moore AM. Occipital lobe injury and cortical visual outcomes after neonatal hypoglycemia. *Pediatrics.* 2008;122(3):507-512.

14. Burns CM, Rutherford MA, Boardman JP, Cowan FM. Patterns of cerebral injury and neurodevelopmental outcomes after symptomatic neonatal hypoglycemia. *Pediatrics.* 2008;122(1):65-74.

15. Kelly A, Tang R, Becker S, Stanley CA. Poor specificity of low growth hormone and cortisol levels during fasting hypoglycemia for the diagnoses of growth hormone deficiency and adrenal insufficiency. *Pediatrics.* 2008;122(3):e522-e528.

16. Antunes JD, Geffner ME, Lippe BM, Landaw EM. Childhood hypoglycemia: differentiating hyperinsulinemic from nonhyperinsulinemic causes. *J Pediatr.* 1990;116(1):105-108.

17. Kelly A, Ng D, Ferry RJ Jr, et al. Acute insulin responses to leucine in children with the hyperinsulinism/hyperammonemia syndrome. *J Clin Endocrinol Metab.* 2001;86(8):3724-3728.

18. Ferry RJ Jr, Kelly A, Grimberg A, et al. Calcium-stimulated insulin secretion in diffuse and focal forms of congenital hyperinsulinism. *J Pediatr.* 2000;137(2):239-246.

19. Hardy OT, Hernandez-Pampaloni M, Saffer JR, et al. Diagnosis and localization of focal congenital hyperinsulinism by 18F-fluorodopa PET scan. *J Pediatr.* 2007;150(2):140-145.

20. Chen Y-T, Cornblath M, Sidbury JB. Cornstarch therapy in type I glycogen-storage disease. *N Engl J Med.* 1984;310(3):1721-1725.

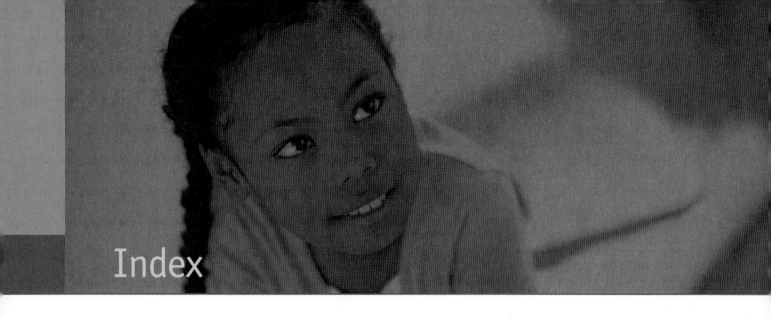

Index

Note: Page numbers followed by *b*, *f*, or *t* indicate text boxes, figures, or tables.